Psychotherapy with children and adolescents

Many difficult questions are raised when psychotherapeutic techniques are applied to young people. In this important volume, covering the principles and methods of psychotherapy in a wide range of settings, Helmut Remschmidt and an eminent team of experts examine the various problems that face practitioners who deal with disturbed young people. How, for example, to accommodate existing treatments to age and developmental status? How to adapt psychotherapeutic techniques to a broad range of specific disorders, from schizophrenia, depression, autism, anxiety and abuse to bed-wetting and stuttering? How much training and involvement should be given to parents? How best to set the treatment: group, individual, inpatient, outpatient? How to choose and assess the most effective treatment: verbal, non-verbal, behavioural? What should the criteria be for assessing treatment?

All these questions are examined, often with instructive case vignettes, alongside the most recent research findings and assessment tools available. All the major techniques of psychotherapy are covered, as are the principal disorders in which they may be of value. This will be essential reading for all mental health professionals using psychotherapy with young people.

Helmut Remschmidt is an internationally renowned psychiatrist and clinical psychologist and Professor of Child Psychiatry at Philipps-University in Marburg, Germany. His current research interests include developmental psychopathology, schizophrenia, psychiatric genetics, therapy and evaluation. He is President of the International Association for Child and Adolescent Psychiatry and Allied Professions.

Cambridge Child and Adolescent Psychiatry

Child and adolescent psychiatry is an important and growing area of clinical psychiatry. The last decade has seen a rapid expansion of scientific knowledge in this field and has provided a new understanding of the underlying pathology of mental disorders in these age groups. This series is aimed at practitioners and researchers both in child and adolescent mental health services and developmental and clinical neuroscience. Focusing on psychopathology, it highlights those topics where the growth of knowledge has had the greatest impact on clinical practice and on the treatment and understanding of mental illness. Individual volumes benefit both from the international expertise of their contributors and a coherence generated through a uniform style and structure for the series. Each volume provides firstly an historical overview and a clear descriptive account of the psychopathology of a specific disorder or group of related disorders. These features then form the basis for a thorough critical review of the aetiology, natural history, management, prevention and impact on later adult adjustment. Whilst each volume is therefore complete in its own right, volumes also relate to each other to create a flexible and collectable series that should appeal to students as well as experienced scientists and practitioners.

Already published in this series:

Specific Learning Disabilities and Difficulties in Children and Adolescents edited by Alan and Nadeen Kaufman 0 521 65840 3 PB

The Depressed Child and Adolescent SECOND EDITION edited by Ian M. Goodyer 0 521 79426 9 PB

Schizophrenia in Children and Adolescents edited by Helmut Remschmidt 0 521 79428 5 PB

Anxiety Disorders in Children and Adolescents: Research, Assessment and Intervention edited by Wendy Silverman and Philip Treffers 0 521 78966 4 PB

Conduct Disorders in Childhood and Adolescence edited by Jonathan Hill and Barbara Maughan 0 521 78639 8 PB

Autism and Pervasive Developmental Disorders edited by Fred R. Volkmar 0 521 55386 5 HB

Cognitive Behaviour Therapy for Children and Families by Philip Graham 0 521 57252 5 HB 0 521 57626 1 PB

Hyperactivity Disorders of Childhood edited by Seija Sandberg 0 521 43250 2 HB

Psychotherapy with children and adolescents

Edited by

Helmut Remschmidt

revised and translated from German by

Peter Matthias Wehmeier and Helen Crimlisk

CAMBRIDGE
UNIVERSITY PRESS

PUBLISHED BY THE PRESS SYNDICATE OF THE UNIVERSITY OF CAMBRIDGE
The Pitt Building, Trumpington Street, Cambridge, United Kingdom

CAMBRIDGE UNIVERSITY PRESS
The Edinburgh Building, Cambridge CB2 2RU, UK
40 West 20th Street, New York, NY 10011-4211, USA
10 Stamford Road, Oakleigh, VIC 3166, Australia
Ruiz do Alarcón 13, 28014 Madrid, Spain
Dock House, The Waterfront, Cape Town 8001, South Africa

http: / / www.cambridge.org

Originally published in German by Georg Thieme Verlag as *Psychotherapie im Kindes- und Jugendalter* in 1997

Revised and updated version first published in English by Cambridge University Press 2001

Printed in the United Kingdom at the University Press, Cambridge

Typeface Dante MT 11/14pt *System* Poltype ® [VN]

A catalogue record for this book is available from the British Library

Library of Congress Cataloguing in Publication data

Psychotherapie im Kindes- und Jugendalter, English
Psychotherapy with children and adolescents / edited by Helmut Remschmidt; revised and translated from German by Peter Mattheias Wehmeier and Helen Crimlisk.
p. cm. - (Cambridge child and adolescent psychiatry series)
Includes bilbiographical references and index.
ISBN 0 521 77558 2 (pb.)
1. Child psychotherapy. 2. Adolescent psychotherapy. 3. Children – Mental health.
4. Teenagers – Mental health. I. Remschmidt, Helmut. II. Title. III. Series.

RJ504.P78513 2001
618.92'8914–dc21 00–065168

ISBN 0 521 77558 2 paperback

Contents

Contributors

Eric Fombonne
Institute of Psychiatry
Denmark Hill
London SE5 8AF
UK

Richard Harrington
Department of Child and Adolescent Psychiatry
Royal Manchester Children's Hospital
Hospital Road
Manchester M27 4HA
UK

Beate Herpertz-Dahlmann
Department of Child and Adolescent Psychiatry
University of Aachen
Neuenhofer Weg 21
52074 Aachen
Germany

Ingeborg Jochmus
von-Manger-Strasse 12
48145 Münster
Germany

Matthias Martin
Department of Child and Adolescent Psychiatry
University of Marburg
Hans-Sachs-Strasse 4–8
35033 Marburg
Germany

Fritz Mattejat
Department of Child and Adolescent Psychiatry
University of Marburg
Hans-Sachs-Strasse 4–8
35033 Marburg
Germany

Uwe Müller
Kinderhospital
Iburgerstrasse 187
49082 Osnabrück
Germany

Gerhard Niebergall
Department of Child and Adolescent Psychiatry
University of Marburg
Hans-Sachs-Strasse 4–8
35033 Marburg
Germany

Kurt Quaschner
Department of Child and Adolescent Psychiatry
University of Marburg
Hans-Sachs-Strasse 4–8
35033 Marburg
Germany

Helmut Remschmidt
Department of Child and Adolescent Psychiatry
University of Marburg
Hans-Sachs-Strasse 4–8
35033 Marburg
Germany

Eberhard Schulz
Department of Child and Adolescent Psychiatry
University of Freiburg
Hauptstrasse 8
79104 Freiburg
Germany

Andreas Warnke
Department of Child and Adolescent Psychiatry
University of Würzburg
Füchsleinstrasse 15
97080 Würzburg
Germany

Doris Weber
Am Schützenplatz 2a
35039 Marburg
Germany

Preface

This introduction to psychotherapy with children and adolescents arose from our daily work with young people who suffer from psychiatric disturbances. The aim of this book is to give a comprehensive overview of the field of psychotherapy with children, adolescents and their families. It covers a broad range of topics, including diagnostic assessment, indication for psychotherapy, and choice of appropriate treatment techniques for the various types of disorder. This book reflects a concept of psychotherapy which is based on the following principles.

- Any modern approach to psychotherapy cannot be considered in an isolated manner, but should be regarded in a larger context that includes the individual patient, his/her family and other environmental factors such as peers and the school.
- It is important to perceive the developmental process to which children and adolescents are subjected.
- Psychotherapy is part of a larger treatment strategy that may include physical treatments and should allow for a combination of several psychotherapeutic techniques.
- Today, psychotherapy should be based on a pluralistic concept, which allows for an indication-informed and disorder-specific approach to treatment.
- Psychotherapy should be perceived as a skill that can be taught, in spite of the variety of methods used in practice. Thus, psychotherapy should be considered a technique like any other type of treatment. Teachers of psychotherapy with children and adolescents should have experience in treating this age group, and should share their experience with those being taught and be willing to discuss critically the cases they have treated. This approach is likely to contribute to demystification of psychotherapy and will help one to perceive psychotherapy rationally.

I sincerely hope this book will be helpful for persons treating psychiatrically disturbed young people and their families using psychotherapy. I would like to thank the authors for their valuable contributions to the original German language edition of this book, Dr Peter M. Wehmeier and Dr Helen Crimlisk for revising and translating the book, and the editorial staff at Cambridge University Press for their excellent work in preparing this volume.

Helmut Remschmidt

Marburg, March 2001

Part I

Principles of psychotherapy with children, adolescents and families

1 Definition, classification and principles of application

Helmut Remschmidt

General considerations and conceptual issues

Psychotherapy is treatment using psychological techniques, and must be distinguished from other types of treatment. Whilst it is easy to distinguish psychotherapy from techniques such as medication or physical therapy, it is more difficult to distinguish psychotherapy from approaches such as special education, occupational therapy, vocational training and encouragement and education. Placebo studies have shown that psychological factors play a significant role in all types of treatment, including those using medication. Should, therefore, any method of influencing someone by psychological means be then considered a 'psychotherapy'? The answer to this question is clearly 'no'. There are countless psychological factors which influence children and adolescents every day, and no one would suggest that all these should be considered to be psychotherapy. Nevertheless, the question in not absurd. In the course of the recent 'psychoboom', many groups and individuals have discovered that the human mind is itself a 'psychomarketplace'. Today, a profusion of different treatment methods are being offered, many of which call themselves 'psychotherapy', e.g. art therapy, music therapy, dance therapy. Such terms may in some cases be appropriate if the technique is based on a clear concept, if treatment goals are defined and if a reliable method is used to attain the goals. Ideally, these methods should be based on rational considerations and the efficacy should be measurable (Bergin and Garfield, 1994). Only those approaches to treatment psychotherapy that meet these requirements are discussed in this book.

When psychotherapeutic methods are applied, the following basic principles need to be respected (Remschmidt, 1982, 1988).

The principle of specificity

The psychotherapeutic technique used for a particular psychiatric disorder needs to be appropriate for that purpose. The wide range of psychiatric disorders in childhood and adolescence require different treatment techniques. The term specificity implies that the most appropriate and effective treatment technique for treating a given disorder needs to be chosen. Ideally, treatment will comprise a combination or package of those treatment techniques most likely to be specific and effective.

The principle of an age- and developmental-appropriate approach

When psychotherapeutic techniques are being chosen for use with children and adolescents, it is important to consider the patient's age and developmental stage. Treatment needs to be undertaken in an appropriate manner, requiring modifications by the therapist in order to achieve this.

The principle of variability and practicality

Ideally, one should be able to adapt therapeutic techniques to suit the setting in which treatment is undertaken, e.g. outpatient or inpatient treatment, individual or group setting. The treatment approach obviously needs to be practicable in order to be helpful.

The principle of evaluation and the assessment of effectiveness

The effectiveness of a therapeutic technique needs to be proven, if possible after comparison with other techniques. This principle, well established in medical treatment, is just as applicable to psychotherapy. Unfortunately, there is a paucity of empirical studies of the effectiveness of psychotherapeutic techniques in children and adolescents. This highlights the need for further studies.

Despite the fact that it is more difficult to define, undertake and evaluate psychotherapeutic techniques than medical treatment, the choice of a psychotherapeutic technique should not be arbitrary. Clear criteria derived from the results of empirical studies exist for arriving at a decision about the appropriateness of a specific technique. The American Academy of Child and Adolescent Psychiatry (AACAP) has provided practice parameters to serve as concise guidelines for the treatment of a number of specific psychiatric disorders in children and adolescents. The practice parameters have been published in the *Journal of the American Academy of Child and Adolescent Psychiatry* and are also available on the internet (http://www.aacap.org). The guidelines include information on a variety of disorders, and the series will be continued.

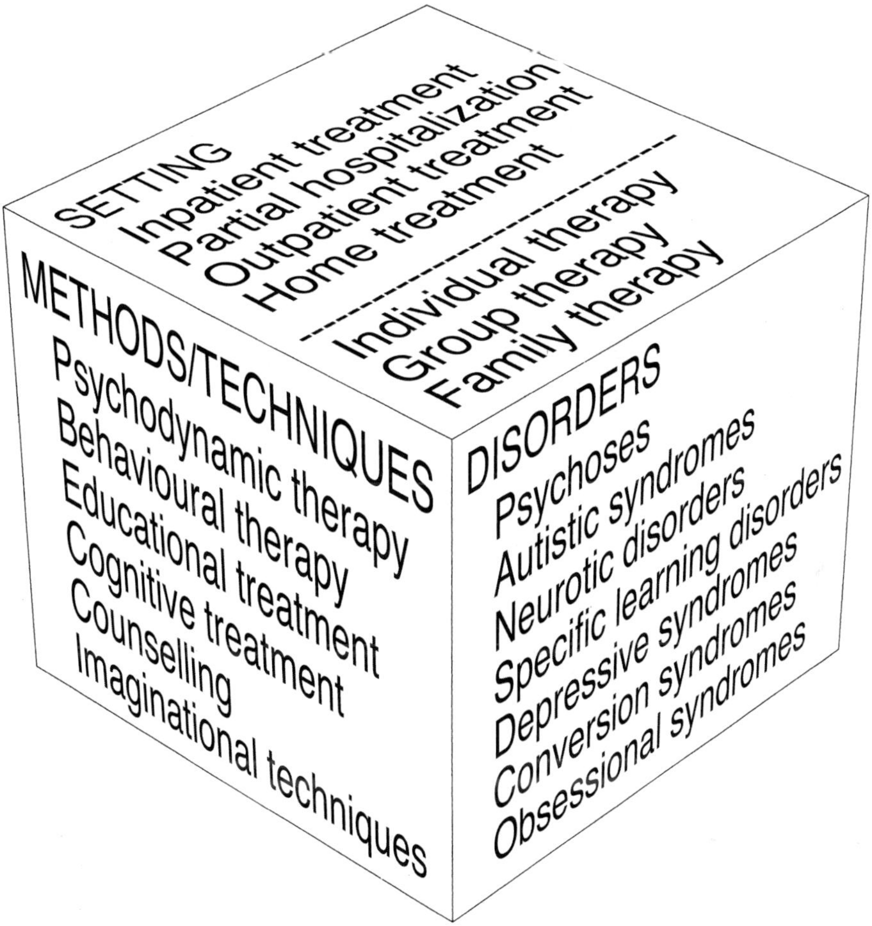

Fig. 1.1. Classification of psychotherapeutic techniques widely used in child and adolescent psychiatry.

Classification of psychotherapeutic treatment techniques

Psychotherapeutic techniques may be classified in a variety of ways, according to theoretical criteria, contents of the technique, treatment setting, or the diagnosis for which the technique is intended.

Three important criteria for classifying treatment techniques are shown in Fig. 1.1. and will be discussed here.

(i) The different approaches to treatment (methods) need to be considered. They are listed in Fig. 1.1. according to their theoretical concepts, e.g. psychodynamic therapy, behaviour therapy, counselling, etc.

(ii) The therapeutic methods may be used under various conditions (settings). Variations in setting may refer to the constellation of people present at a session (individuals, families, groups) or to the setting in which treatment is undertaken (inpatient, day hospital, outpatient).

(iii) The approach to treatment and the conditions need to be appropriate for the psychiatric disorder. Usually several options are available to the therapist. For instance, an autistic child may be treated in various settings using individual behaviour therapy: as an inpatient, on an outpatient basis or in the home. On the other hand, play therapy in an inpatient setting might also be appropriate. In both cases the child's parents would need to be offered information about the disorder. In some cases therapy may not involve the child directly at all, and intervention can remain at the level of the parents, who may be offered, e.g. couple therapy.

The issue of which method or setting to adopt for which disorder should take into account recent research findings, past clinical experience and local resources.

Selecting appropriate treatment

Several principles need to be considered for the appropriate type of psychotherapy.

Careful diagnostic appraisal to clarify indication for psychotherapy

The first step in this process is a careful diagnostic appraisal. This should include physical examination and psychological tests, and this should give some indication of the appropriate approach. In the past, psychiatric assessment has been criticized for being unhelpful in terms of therapy. However, today a child and adolescent psychiatric assessment generally includes points which help to define treatment goals, e.g. the child's developmental status, intelligence, personality traits, the situation at school and in the family. Several classification systems have tried to take these factors into account. A multiaxial classification system of psychiatric disorders in childhood and adolescence has been successfully implemented (WHO, 1996).

Adaption of psychotherapeutic techniques to specific disorders

Psychotherapy with children and adolescents requires a broad spectrum of different treatment techniques. The indication for a particular technique should be based on empirical data on the effectiveness of that technique. Unfortunately, this is not the case with many treatments. This is perhaps best illustrated by two examples. It is has been clearly established that monosymptomatic phobias and animal phobias are best treated by behaviour therapy. A good outcome has been empirically demonstrated, and the technique is widely accepted. On the other hand, it would be inappropriate to treat a disturbance of individuation during adolescence by behavioural methods. A psychodynamic approach to treatment is far more appropriate, symptoms tend to be much more varied, and treatment based on learning theory alone would be likely to encounter numerous difficulties (Remschmidt, 1979).

Adapting the treatment approach to the patient's age and developmental status

Whilst often difficult to bring about in practice, it is important that each therapist considers whether the treatment technique he considers appropriate matches the patient's age and developmental status. This point is explained in more detail (Remschmidt, 1977, 1982, 1988).

Development during early childhood (2 to 5 years) is characterized by speech development, the importance of play and fantasy, and the development of orientation. Treatment should therefore, emphasize projective techniques (totally or relatively language-free) and techniques using play. Toys, dolls, drawing and painting material, and make-believe games have been widely used and are considered very helpful as material in therapy sessions. The child's projections may be used in a therapeutic way and are usually helpful in assessing treatment results. This technique may be used during individual psychotherapy with the child (with accompanying counselling of the mother) or psychotherapy with both child and mother, in the course of which the mother is gradually integrated into therapy sessions.

Behavioural therapy techniques may also be used to treat small children. Such techniques have been used successfully in autism, phobias and anxiety disorders, tics, restlessness, enuresis and encopresis, nail-biting and thumb-sucking.

During early school age (5 to 9 years) the child's development is characterized by profound changes in perception. His perception of reality improves, his interests become more permanent and he is increasingly able to integrate in a group.

It has been suggested that regression is a very important defence mechanism at this age (Hart de Ryter, 1967, 1969). It is important to note in which situations regression occurs (is it as a fantasy, as a reaction to frustration or in the course of everyday behaviour?), and in the manner in which it occurs (on an emotional level, as a developmental delay or as impulsive and uncontrolled behaviour?). Psychotherapy needs to take these points into account.

Adolescents are easier to reach verbally than younger children; however, it may nevertheless be necessary to use non-verbal or creative techniques initially to establish rapport. Functional training may play an important role during this developmental phase.

Puberty and adolescence are characterized in terms of developmental psychopathology by the profound mental and psychosocial changes (sexual maturation, development of the self, search for identity, confrontation with authority at school, in the family and society) which occur at that age (Remschmidt, 1975). These changes bring with them new therapeutic challenges.

- Commencing and continuing psychotherapy is difficult if the patient himself has no complaints.
- The therapist's role is more difficult to define and maintain when treating adolescents.
- The problems which adolescents frequently have, e.g. a reluctance to reflect on the past, focusing on present problems, rejection of help and authority make treatment especially difficult.

These points, which make psychotherapy with adolescents difficult, have resulted in specific treatment methods being developed for this age group.

Choice of the most appropriate therapy setting

This issue refers to not only geographical setting but also to the nature of the setting, e.g. individual, family or group therapy (Fig. 1.1.). There are two aspects to this issue: the empirical data on a particular treatment technique, and secondly the practicability of establishing a working relationship with the patient and his family.

Inpatient treatment is advisable in the following circumstances:

- severe and/or chronic disorder,
- risk of self-harm or aggressive outbursts,
- necessity of separating the patient from his family, and
- the absence of appropriate nearby out-patient facilities ('relative indication').

Hospital admission rates in areas with adequate outpatient treatment facilities are usually lower than in areas lacking such facilities. However, the duration of hospitalization has been shown to be much shorter (Remschmidt and Walter, 1989).

Partial hospitalization or day-treatment can be helpful and has the following advantages:

- the duration of inpatient treatment may be curtailed
- inpatient treatment may be avoided altogether, and
- the patient may be prepared for inpatient treatment.

Whilst the first two advantages of day treatment are self evident, the third needs to be explained in more detail. This preparation is advisable when there is a clear indication for inpatient treatment (psychotherapy or medical treatment), which the patient or his family refuses. Usually these individuals are prejudiced against psychiatric hospitals and have unfounded concerns about treatment. These are addressed and reduced in the course of day treatment. Parents usually find it reassuring that their child is allowed home for the night. In many cases, admission to an inpatient unit then becomes possible. This has often proved the case in our experience with anorexia nervosa or severe separation anxiety, and hospitalization against the child's will can be avoided. Most disorders can be treated during partial hospitalization.

In some cases home treatment may be an option. The patient is here treated in his home environment. This approach may replace outpatient treatment or admission to hospital, but requires certain conditions (Eisert et al., 1985).

- At least one care-giver ('co-therapist') needs to be at home during therapy sessions.
- Sufficient space must be available for the therapist, who should not be too intrusive.
- A minimum of family structure is required.
- The distance from institution to the patient's home should not be too great (no longer than 30–40 minutes' travelling time).

The parents also need to cooperate fully with the plan, and there needs to be a working relationship between parents and child. In addition, it is necessary that the parents are willing and capable of continuing treatment during the therapist's absence.

Home treatment is helpful only when supported by a larger institution with inpatient and outpatient units, such that problems can be addressed with a modificaton of the therapeutic setting.

Many diagnoses have been successfully treated with home treatment, including neurotic disorders, anorexia nervosa, enuresis and encopresis, obesity, emotional and behavioural disturbance, and hyperkinetic disorders (Remschmidt and Schmidt, 1988).

Home treatment is contraindicated when hospitalization is deemed necessary or when treatment is manageable with partial hospizalization or on an outpatient basis. The results of home treatment have been encouraging (Reimer, 1983; Remschmidt and Schmidt, 1988); however, there is a paucity of results on the longer-term outcomes.

Integration of various therapeutic techniques in treatment

The focus of this book is psychotherapeutic treatment techniques. However, in treating child and adolescent psychiatric disorders, various other techniques may be used in addition. Such treatment techniques need to be coordinated with psychotherapeutic techniques, and this integration requires careful planning. A treatment plan is helpful in every setting, e.g. outpatient treatment, partial hospitalization, home treatment, family therapy, etc., and should include symptoms, diagnosis and additional information relevant to therapy, clearly define treatment goals, and explain treatment steps (including the role of all individuals involved). The teatment plan should also include the family and the social environment, and should suggest a timespan. Psychotherapy will usually be an essential part of such a general treatment plan, but it will usually be only one of several treatment steps. The importance of particular treatment steps is likely to vary over the course of treatment. For instance, in acute or life-threatening anorexia nervosa, medical treatment is most important. As the patient improves and gains weight, psychotherapy will become increasingly important. With younger patients, family therapy is often just as important as individual sessions, and in some cases additional antidepressant or neuroleptic medication may be required.

Limitations of psychotherapy

The term psychotherapy implies that the individuals being treated are sick. Psychotherapy is not intended to bring about general improvements. In particular, it cannot replace normal educational efforts or other supportive measures, nor does it address ideological problems or change society as a whole. Psychotherapy is not suitable for treating any mild impairment of well-being, and should therefore be restricted to treating psychiatric disorders or illnesses in childhood and adolescence. This point has been emphasized by the Deutsche Gesellschaft für Kinder- und Jugendpsychiatrie (1984), and such an endeavour would be neither feasible nor humane, potentially resulting in a diminishment of the child's or parents' ability to solve these problems.

Psychotherapy with children, adolescents and their families needs to be undertaken in a trusting atmosphere and requires the cooperation of all individuals involved. Treatment is aimed at discovering and supporting the protective factors and improving the self-healing resources of the disturbed child and his family.

REFERENCES

Bergin, A. E. and Garfield, S. L. (ed.) (1994). *Handbook of psychotherapy and behavior change*, 4th edn. New York: Wiley.

Deutsche Gesellschaft für Kinder- und Jugendpsychiatrie (1984). *Denkschrift zur Lage der Kinderpsychiatrie in der Bundesrepublik Deutschland*. Marburg.

Eisert, M., Eisert, H. G. and Schmidt, M. H. (1985). *Hinweise zur Behandlung im häuslichen Milieu ('home-treatment')*. Zeitschrift für Kinder- und Jugendpsychiatrie, **13**, 268–79.

Hart de Ruyter, T. H. (1967). *Zur Psychotherapie der Dissozialität im Jugendalter*. Jahrbuch für Jugendpsychiatrie und ihre Grenzgebiete, **6**, 79–108.

Hart de Ruyter, T. H. (1969). Psychotherapie im Latenzalter. In *Handbuch der Kinderpsychotherapie*, ed. G. Biermann, vol. I, pp. 236–40. München: Reinhardt.

Reimer, M. (1983). *Verhaltensänderung in der Familie. Home-treatment in der Kinderpsychiatrie*. Stuttgart: Enke.

Remschmidt, H. (1975). *Neuere Ergebnisse zur Psychologie und Psychiatrie der Adoleszenz*. Zeitschrift für Kinder- und Jugendpsychiatrie, **3**, 67–101.

Remschmidt, H. (1977). Therapeutische Probleme in der Kinder- und Jugendpsychiatrie. In *Diagnostische und therapeutische Methoden in der Psychiatrie*, ed. T. H. Vogel and J. Vliegen, pp. 254–65. Stuttgart: Thieme.

Remschmidt, H. (1979). Adoleszentenkrise und ihre Behandlung. In *Beratungsarbeit mit Jugendlichen*, ed. F. Specht, K. Gerlicher, and K. Schütt, pp. 44–62. Göttingen: Vandenhoeck & Ruprecht.

Remschmidt, H. (1982). Indikationen und Grenzen der Psychotherapie in der Kinder- und Jugendpsychiatrie. In: *Psychotherapie in der Psychiatrie*, ed. H. Helmchen, M. Linden and U. Rueger, pp. 280–90. Berlin: Springer.

Remschmidt, H. (1988). Gesichtspunkte zur Indikationsstellung therapeutischer Massnahmen. In *Kinder- und Jugendpsychiatrie in Klinik und Praxis*, vol. I, ed. H. Remschmidt and M. H. Schmidt, pp. 608–14. Stuttgart: Thieme.

Remschmidt, H. and Schmidt, M. H. (ed.) (1988). *Alternative Behandlungsformen in der Kinder- und Jugendpsychiatrie. Stationäre Behandlung, tagesklinische Behandlung und home-treatment im Vergleich*. Stuttgart: Enke.

Remschmidt, H. and Walter, R. (1989). *Evaluation kinder- und jugendpsychiatrischer Versorgung. Analysen und Erhebungen in drei hessischen Landkreisen*. Stuttgart: Enke.

World Health Organization (WHO) (1996). *Multiaxial classification of child psychiatric disorders. The ICD-10 classification of mental and behavioural disorders in children and adolescents*. Geneva: WHO.

2 Treatment planning

Fritz Mattejat

Diagnostic assessment and therapy as a problem-solving process

Definition

The process of assessment in medicine should determine the appropriate course of therapy. Thus, for any particular complaint, the assessment process should result in awareness of which treatments are likely to either cure the disorder (curative treatment) or reduce symptoms to a more tolerable level (symptomatic treatment).

As part of this process, the therapeutic aims need to be defined. Whilst in other areas of medicine this is often relatively straightforward, in psychotherapeutic fields, this is not the case, because the same problem can be viewed from a number of different perspectives (Schulte, 1991a).

Similar problems arise with the concept of treatment planning (Lau, 1980). The term 'planning' implies the conscious and rational weighing up of all possible therapeutic techniques, such that, in any particular clinical situation, certain aims will be set and methods will be chosen according to their appropriateness. Applied to psychotherapy, this involves the inherent assumption that psychotherapy can be viewed as a conscious and rational problem-solving process (Bartling et al., 1980; Caspar, 1987, 1989; Schmidt, 1984; Jäger, 1988; Steller, 1994; Rudolf, 1993). In contrast to this assumption, many therapists emphasize the importance of unconscious and irrational processes and come to the conclusion that many important aspects of therapy cannot be planned. Thus the concept of therapy planning remains a controversial issue (Schulte, 1991b; Schiepek, 1991).

Problem-solving model

Fig. 2.1 shows diagnostic assessment and therapy as a problem-solving process. In this schema, the assessment process and the treatment plan (with its inter-related components: problems, aims and possible interventions) are central to the model. The process begins with the collection of relevant

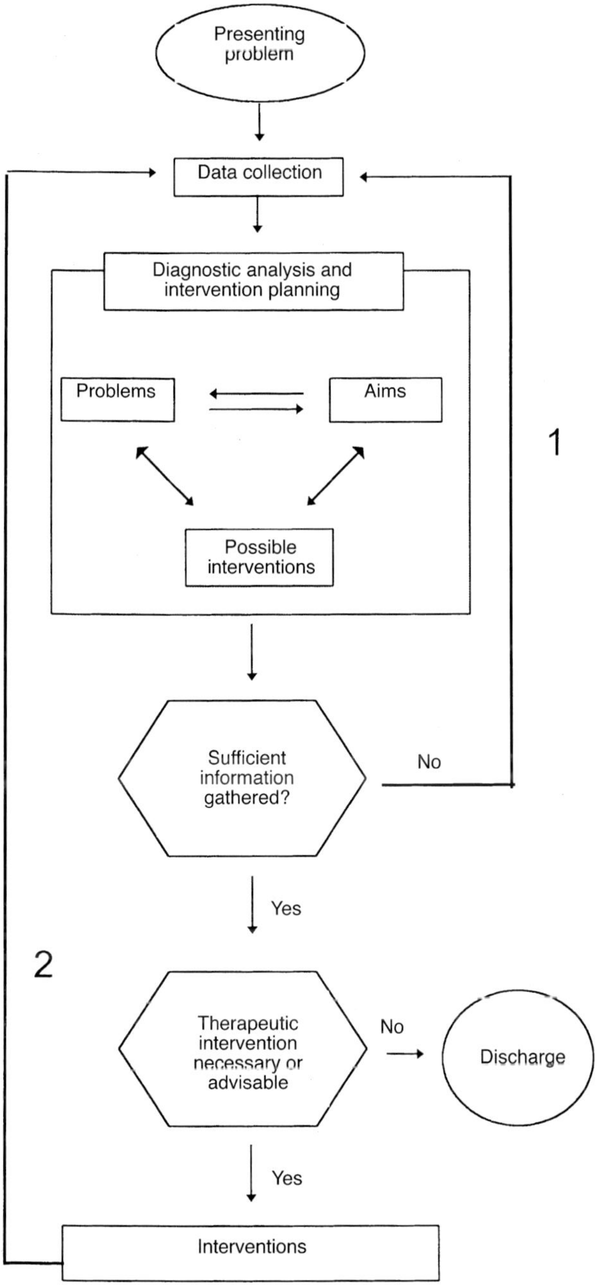

Fig. 2.1. Diagnostic assessment and treatment as a problem-solving process.

information which is then organized, in order to arrive at a diagnosis and plan the next step. Two questions are posed in this process:

(i) Is there enough information to make further plans or must additional steps be undertaken to gather more information?

(ii) Which, if any, interventions are necessary or appropriate, and in which form should they be undertaken?

If data relating to diagnoses are inadequate, a return to data gathering is necessary (path 1). If, on the other hand, therapeutic intervention is undertaken, this may itself lead to new information through a feedback process (path 2) which is then considered by working through the model again. Thus new information is constantly reviewed, altering or refining both the diagnostic and therapeutic processes.

This problem-solving model is applicable throughout various stages of assessment and treatment planning. The provisional differential diagnosis and the type of treatment planned can be modified as further information becomes available (Schulte, 1991b). Seidenstücker (1984, 1988) has subdivided this process into two steps: 'selection of interventions' and 'adaptation of interventions'. Alternatively, the process can be broken down into three different levels (Schulte, 1991b, Blaser et al., 1992). First, the selection of a therapy strategy or concept; secondly, the nature of the therapeutic technique chosen and finally, on a 'microscopic' level, which intervention will be utilized from this technique in order to best achieve the therapeutic aims. In practice, this latter process is often not preplanned, but intuitive and can only later be reflected upon.

Steps in assessment and treatment planning

Fig. 2.2 shows the typical steps undertaken in a clinical case. In the initial contact, the presenting problems are investigated (data gathering) with the aim of reaching a diagnosis and/or concept regarding the nature of the problem. In association with this, the clinician must begin to consider whether any treatment is indicated. At this point it is also necessary to make a decision on the aims of therapy and on the range of treatments open to the patient. The objective of this process is to formulate a treatment plan, which can be proposed to the patient and his family. The next step involves negotiation and modification of the proposal if necessary. In some cases, it may be advisable to draw up a written treatment contract, which can include both psychotherapeutic or more practical measures to be undertaken.

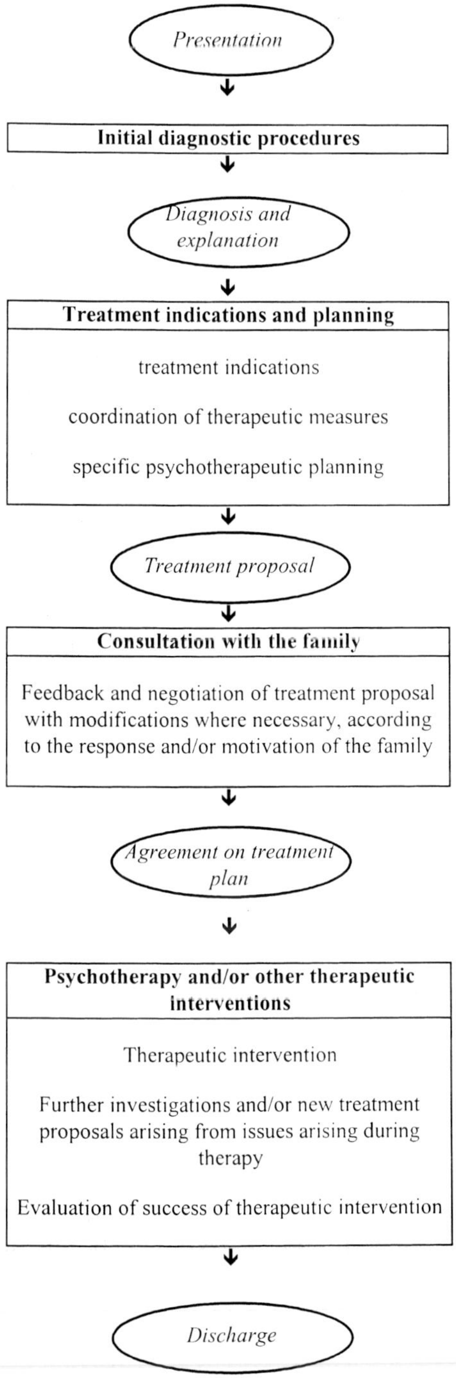

Fig. 2.2. Typical steps in a clinical process.

Clarification of the basic issues: is therapy really necessary and what are the options?

The basic requirement of an assessment is to carry out appropriate diagnostic measures aimed at reaching a diagnosis, and to form a concept of the important aetiological factors and specific issues relevant to the individual patient (WHO, 1996). The next essential step is to decide whether treatment for the problem is desirable and if so what type of therapy would be most appropriate in this particular case.

In order to answer these two questions, it is necessary to consider the natural history of the problem, i.e. its likely course without therapeutic help and whether spontaneous remission is possible and the predicted response to any intervention, i.e. to what degree treatment is likely to help the problematic symptoms. The issues of assessment shown in Fig. 2.3 are influenced to a great degree not only by the child but also by his family and wider social circle.

General planning measures: focus, setting and coordination of interventions

The planning of intervention should not be limited to disciplines within the psychotherapeutic field. It is important to draw upon the resources available from a wide range of disciplines, e.g. psychotherapeutic, psychosocial, educational and medical measures, and often several techniques can be utilized simultaneously. Psychotherapeutic planning should be clearly distinguished from other professional help, which may or may not be advisable (see Fig. 2.4). Three issues need to be addressed at this stage:

(i) Which discipline should act as the main source of help and who from that discipline is most appropriate to undertake the key role?

(ii) Under what conditions can the expectations of therapy best be realized (abode, home conditions, therapeutic setting, etc.)?

(iii) In what way can the different therapeutic components be optimally combined?

Focus of treatment

Psychotherapy often comprises only a secondary or subordinate component of the treatment plan. Fig. 2.5 gives an overview of the most important measures which may be considered in the treatment of children or adolescents with psychiatric disorders. These measures can be classified according to where their predominant effect is intended, here shown in relation to the six axes of the Multiaxial Classification Scheme (WHO, 1996).

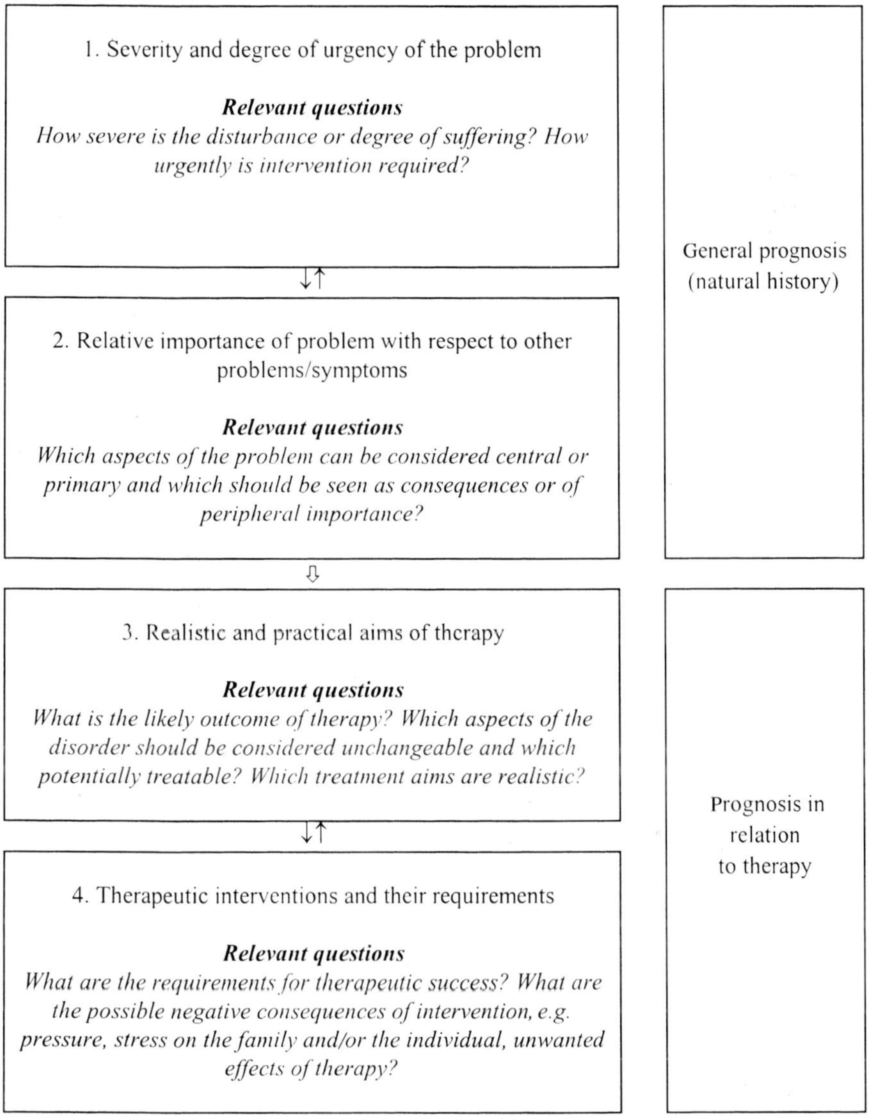

Fig. 2.3. Basic issues of indication for therapy.

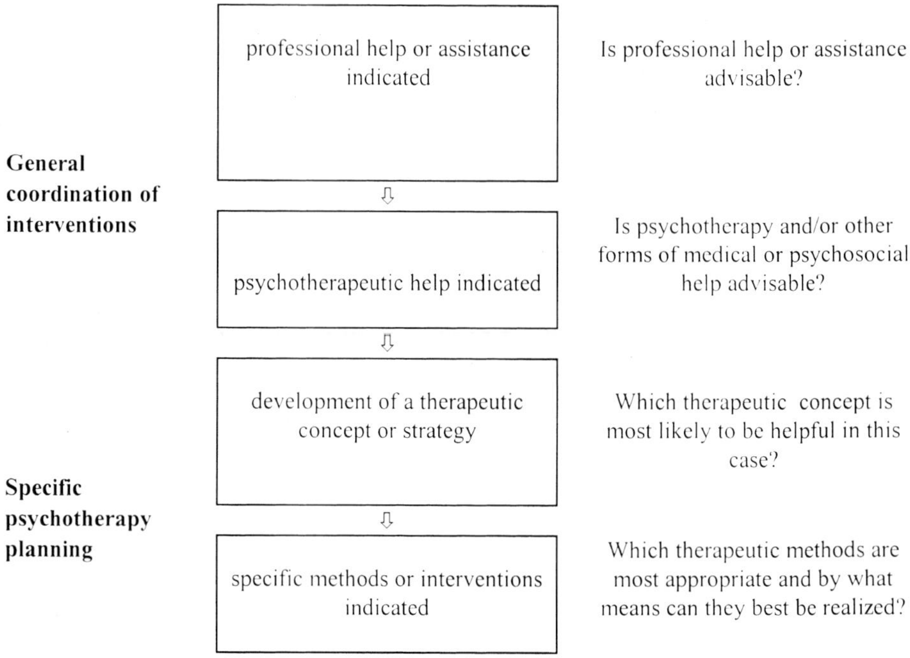

Fig. 2.4. Decision-making steps in assessment and treatment planning.

Treatment modality and setting

Options for therapy include:

- inpatient treatment,
- partial inpatient treatment (e.g. in a day hospital),
- treatment in the naturalistic setting (e.g. home treatment),
- outpatient treatment.

These specific treatment modalities are described in more detail in subsequent chapters of this book.

Coordination of therapeutic measures

All measures brought into play should have the same ultimate therapeutic aims. The more clearly therapeutic aims are prioritized, the easier it will be to coordinate therapeutic interventions. When several professionals or institutions are involved, it is especially important to ensure that the communication between them is optimized. Many treatment plans fail because of communication difficulties or misunderstandings between different professionals. This

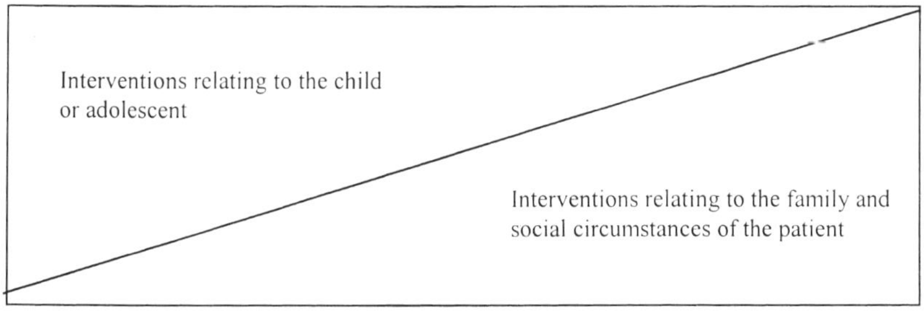

Inter-ventions:	Treatment with medication or other medical measures	Practically orientated training exercises and educational interventions	Psychotherapy		Social service inter-ventions	Outside agencies or other interventions related to the social circum-stances
			Relating to the presented patient	Related to the family and social milieu		
Multiaxial classification* of areas of disturbance	IV	II and III	I	V	V	V

Fig. 2.5. Overview of the most important interventions. *Multiaxial classification of child and adolescent psychiatric disorders (WHO, 1996). The Roman numerals represent the different axes of the multiaxial classification scheme.

cooperation should occur from the planning stage on, and should be implemented throughout treatment. What this should not mean, however, is that the 'responsibility' for the case is delegated elsewhere. Each member of the therapeutic team should bear a shared responsibility for the patient.

Planning therapeutic options: the development of a specific therapeutic proposal

The following issues need to be considered in the consideration of the most appropriate type of therapy (see Remschmidt and Mattejat, 1994):

Content: on which area or aspect should the psychotherapeutic input focus?

Method: which methods are most appropriate?

Setting and intensity: what are the most appropriate settings and the optimal frequency of sessions?

Compatibility of therapeutic components: how can the chosen settings and methods best be coordinated?

Psychotherapeutic options

According to Grawe (1992, 1997) and Grawe et al. (1994), psychotherapeutic methodology can be subdivided into five groups (see also Wetzel and Linster, 1992):

Humanistic therapies: these comprise person-centred therapies, e.g. client centred psychotherapy and play therapy, Gestalt therapy and psychodrama.

Psychodynamic therapies: these comprise classical long-term psychoanalysis, short psychodynamic therapies and other analytically orientated therapies.

Cognitive and behavioural therapies: this group includes classical behaviour therapies such as operant conditioning, systematic desensitization, exposure therapy, biofeedback, social skills training, cognitive behavioural therapy, problem-solving therapies and cognitive therapies such as the rational emotive therapy.

Interpersonal and systemic therapies: included in this group are interpersonal psychotherapies, couple or family therapies from different theoretical backgrounds and systemic individual therapy.

Additional special therapy forms: the last, heterogeneous group includes techniques which are otherwise difficult to classify, e.g. relaxation training, meditation and imaginative techniques such as ink blot drawings, hypnosis, music, dance and art therapy and other movement or bodily techniques.

The psychotherapeutic assessment is often thought of as involving the choice of a particular therapeutic school (see Seidenstücker, 1984, 1988). In fact, this is, and only ever has been, a partial truth. Over recent years, many therapeutic schools have broadened the range of patients for which their form of therapy is claimed to be appropriate. Thus, a patient previously said to have specific indications and/or contraindications for a certain therapeutic school, is often no longer seen in such narrow terms and many different therapeutic approaches can be justified. Furthermore, there is a growing tendency to integrate methods from different psychotherapeutic schools into a more general frame. This tendency is exemplified by the 'generic psychotherapy' (Orlinsky and Howard, 1988). A further tendency is the establishment of 'disorder-specific' therapies, which do not have a common theoretical background, but rather make up a 'package' which is thought to be appropriate for a particular disorder (see relevant chapters in this book). Current practice is often an eclectic, pragmatic procedure, which is to some degree a consequence of many younger therapists being trained in a variety of psychotherapeutic techniques and of their desire to offer their patients a personalized, integrated therapy.

Mechanisms of change in psychotherapy

A therapeutic plan that encompasses approaches from a variety of schools, must nevertheless formulate a clear concept as to the nature of the disorder, and in addition, develop a problem-related strategy with specific therapeutic aims. Following this, appropriate therapeutic techniques and individual interventions can be selected. Research findings, which aim to review the empirical evidence for certain therapeutic techniques, have been compiled to help therapists with this task, notably, the work of Orlinsky and Howard (1988), and Grawe et al. (1994), who have been especially influential in German-speaking countries. Grawe identified the following 'mechanisms of change', which are the main components of successful therapies.

Mastery/coping: problem-solving and other behaviour-oriented therapy components

Grawe et al. (1994) consider active and concrete support of the patient with the aim of improving his capacity for problem-solving or coping the 'most powerful therapeutic factor of successful psychotherapy'. This type of assistance forms a constituent part of most behaviour or cognitive therapies. Although this aspect is less important in more 'insight'-orientated therapies, supportive measures such as encouragement and help with motivation, may nevertheless also be experienced as 'problem-solving' help. The problem-solving component can be characterized by two specific factors.

(a) The therapist only picks up on problems that the patient brings to therapy. These are difficulties experienced by the patient which he would like to overcome, but does not feel in a position to tackle. The therapist does not search for hidden motives nor does he try to interpret the presented symptoms (see Pohlen and Bautz-Holzherr, 1995).

(b) The therapist actively helps the patient to overcome these problems by introducing the patient to a problem-solving technique. How this is undertaken is naturally dependent to some degree on the nature of the problem, the characteristics of the patient's disorder and the patient's competence to carry out the problem-solving exercise.

The aim of a problem-solving oriented therapy is the acquisition of new skills and competencies, either which the patient has never previously had, or which he has lost.

Clarification of meaning: interpretation and other insight-orientated therapy components

According to Grawe et al. (1994), the second 'equally or almost equally important components of successful therapy' are techniques which are directed at a 'clarification of meaning'. By this is meant that 'the therapist helps the patient to better understand his own experiences'. Through the help of the therapy the patient should be able to 'better comprehend his strengths and weaknesses, and consciously learn to understand the effects of his behaviour on other people'. The therapist should encourage self-exploration through interventions such as interpretation, confrontation and focusing methods. These principles can be subdivided into a process of 'working through emotional issues' and 'improving insight' (see Blaser et al., 1992; Ambühl, 1993). Under this component, emotional and motivational aspects rather than skill acquisition are the focus of attention.

The relationship component

Grawe's third area is the 'relationship component' (Grawe et al., 1994). It was shown empirically that the therapeutic relationship has a quite strong association with therapeutic outcome: the better the quality of the relationship, the better will be the therapeutic result. Another reason for highlighting this factor is that psychological disturbance often manifests itself through difficulties in relationships. Analysis of the therapeutic relationship provides some of the best material for bringing about positive change. Without attention to the nature of the patient–therapist relationship, interpretational and behavioural techniques will be less successful. On the other side a healthy therapeutic relationship automatically leads to an improvement in the patient's feelings of self-worth, increases his readiness to disclose problems to the therapist and expands the patient's capacity to take on the challenges of additional therapeutic interventions.

As a result of his research, Grawe (1997) proposed that a 'research-informed' or 'generic' psychotherapy ('Allgemeine Psychotherapie') is the natural successor of the traditional psychotherapeutic schools. In practice, their proposal is that every psychotherapist should be in the position to offer:

(a) active behaviour-orientated help and guidance to support the patient in developing better problem-solving skills and coping behaviours,

(b) insight-orientated interventions, and

(c) a therapeutic relationship which the patient experiences as positive and encouraging, with the therapist being seen as an ally.

This type of eclectic programme is now quite widely established, and from the onset was empirically research based. Another way of overcoming the boundaries of traditional psychotherapy schools is the development of therapies which address specific problems or questions, that is of 'disorder specific therapies'. Such developments can ease the task of creating an individualized,

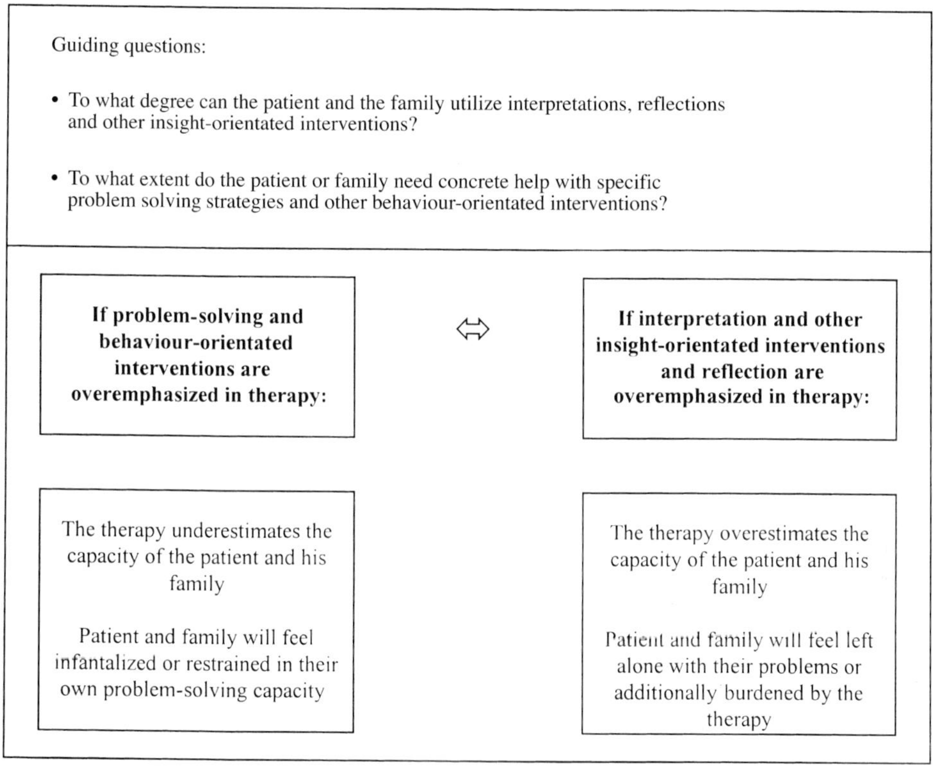

Fig. 2.6. Choosing the optimal therapeutic balance for work with a patient or family.

therapeutic plan, but do not replace the necessary planning procedure. In practice, the optimal therapeutic plan is only revealed following a problem-orientated planning procedure.

Therapeutic options with regard to the main mechanisms of change

When deciding upon particular psychotherapeutic interventions, it is initially important to consider whether insight-orientated methods or behaviour-orientated interventions should be emphasized. The correct balance of these components should be aimed for. Overemphasis of interpretational components in a family with urgent or pressing problems, may cause a further sense of overburdening, whereas, on the other hand, too much emphasis on psychoeducation and problem-solving techniques involves the risk of infantalizing families, and limits the degree to which they can access their own problem-solving strategies (see Fig. 2.6).

The decision should not be made purely on the basis of fundamental

Therapy components

Criteria	**Insight-orientated methods ('clarification of meaning', interpretations, reflections)** ⇔	**Behaviour-orientated methods ('mastery/coping', problem-solving)**
Formal aspects of the symptoms	Diffuse, non-specific symptoms or those difficult to define	Specific or well-defined symptoms
Principal content of symptoms	Internalized symptoms, symptoms predominantly expressed in terms of cognitive or emotional aspects	Externalized symptoms, symptoms predominantly expressed in terms of behaviour
Association with developmental disorder or bodily symptoms	No developmental disorder or bodily symptoms	Development disorder or bodily symptoms
Severity	Mild to moderate	Moderate to severe
Acute threat to patient	Low immediate threat to patient or requirement for immediate intervention	High risk patient, immediate intervention deemed necessary
Psychological capacity for dealing with stress and conflict	High capacity for dealing with conflict or stress, low risk of decompensation	Low tolerance of conflict, significant risk of decompensation

Fig. 2.7(*a*). Criteria for psychotherapeutic methods: psychopathological aspects.

principles; however, it should be weighed up according to the current needs of the individual patient and his family and the likely productiveness of a particular intervention at that time. The patient and the family themselves should play an important role in this decision-making process. Thus, the therapist should continuously monitor the wishes or expectations of the patient and/or the family and modify the intervention strategy accordingly. Successful therapy depends on this ability to be flexible and to allow plasticity within the therapeutic plan. Figs 2.7(*a*) and (*b*) summarize the most important criteria for the

	Therapy components		
	Insight-orientated methods ('clarification of meaning', interpretations, reflections)	⇔	**Behaviour-orientated methods ('mastery/coping', problem-solving)**
Criteria			
Individual aspects:			
Age and developmental status	Older age groups (school children and adolescents)		Younger age groups (school and preschool children)
General social functioning	Good functioning		Poor functioning
Intelligence and capacity for introspection	High intelligence and capacity for introspection		Low intelligence and capacity for introspection
Dominant coping style	Intrapsychic or abstract coping styles		Concrete or behavioural coping styles
Therapeutic expectations	Preference for less structured and non-directive treatment		Preference for structured or directive treatment
Family and social aspects:			
Degree of family problems	Socially well-integrated family with few other problems		Family with multiple problems or sociocultural conflicts
Degree of cohesion and structure within the family	Family with high cohesion and capacity to deal with stresses		Family with low cohesion and little capacity for dealing with stress
Family relationship structure	Rigid or enmeshed family structures		Chaotic or disintegrated family structures

Fig. 2.7(*b*). Criteria for psychotherapeutic methods: individual, familial and social aspects.

different therapeutic components (see Seiderstücker 1984, 1988). This overview is, of course, an oversimplification of the actual situation, as most patients and/or families will not conform to one category. For this reason, it is important to develop an individually constructed therapeutic plan in each case.

Therapeutic options regarding the main focus of therapy

The most important criteria for the decision, regarding the main focus of therapy are:

- the manifestation of symptoms,
- the possible aetiological factors,
- the possibilities for change, and
- how the family looks at the problem.

The manifestation of symptoms

Many psychiatric disorders occur relatively independently of the context, whereas others have a high degree of situation specificity, with a manifestation predominantly causing family interactional disturbances, e.g. conflicts or aggression within the family or family relationship disturbances, e.g. autonomy conflicts with adolescents. The therapist should first consider the domain of the reported abnormalities. If these are predominantly non-situation specific, distinct behavioural characteristics, an individual approach to therapy may be most appropriate. Whereas situation specific problems or those which commonly involve particular family members, invite a family orientated approach.

The possible aetiological factors

The manifestation of the disturbance cannot, however, be the only criterion; disturbances that predominantly take place outside the family can nevertheless have their origins within the family and its constituent relationships. Thus in children with symptoms of conduct disorder, e.g. truancy or stealing, there is often concern over the degree of parental supervision or responsibility.

The therapist must therefore also consider the likely aetiological contributory factors. In many cases, it is relatively easy to arrive at a conclusion about this, based on knowledge of the specific disorder and its explanatory models, e.g. aetiological and risk factors, exacerbating and maintaining factors, natural course and prognosis. For example, disorders relating to neglect or abuse should not be limited exclusively to individual-orientated therapy, at least not while the child or adolescent remains within the family environment. On the other hand, disorders such as psychosis or psychiatric disorders, related to specific developmental disorders such as dyslexia, lend themselves better to individually orientated therapy. Exclusive reliance on family or relationship-orientated therapy in these conditions would be inappropriate. In most cases, however, both individual and interactional components are present and, again, it is the job of the therapist to weigh up the most appropriate balance of therapy and to estimate the relative importance of individual factors (organic, developmental, psychological) and interactional or social factors (relationships, environmental) in the aetiology and maintenance of the disorder. Of particular importance is the consideration of factors which are most likely to be related to the risk of the disorder becoming chronic.

The possibilities for change

Exclusive reliance on an aetiological model does not, however, make sense – as in the vast majority of cases, the 'causes' of a disorder cannot be established with certainty. Much more likely is the production of a list of likely contributing relevant factors. Indeed, the very concept of a 'cause' or a 'responsible agent' often makes little sense in psychiatry and leads to a fruitless discussion unlikely to be of assistance to the patient. Symptoms cause interactional problems which, in turn, cause further symptoms. This pattern is conceptualized in systems theory as 'circular causality' and 'co-evolution': The problems to be dealt with in therapy comprise biological, psychological, interactional and social aspects, whereby the components of the system develop together, reciprocally perpetuating each other. The alteration of one component has an effect on other components (and with it the whole system), such that a constellation with altered components is constituted, which again fits together. Individual, relationship and family problems are so tightly bound up with one another that change in one area invariably affects all the others.

Thinking along these lines, it becomes possible to see the focus of therapeutic intervention from a different perspective. Instead of trying to consider the primary or original state (which in any case is no longer accessible), the system is analysed for components which are potentially modifiable: At which point and on which level (individual, interactional, social) is change most likely to occur? This question steers the view away from the problem, to the possible solutions. Attention is shifted away from pathological aspects to the positive resources of the patient and the family. Finally, the issue returns to the nature of the therapeutic relationship: which kind of therapy can the patient utilize?

Thus, the third criterion for the main focus of therapy states that the decision should take into account where change is possible, and resources should be focused on areas in which a positive way forward has been identified.

As with the other criteria, this can also only be considered a partial principle, as therapy cannot be limited to those areas in which it is clear that change is possible, but should also consider where change is desirable or necessary. The criteria are not mutually exclusive, but rather complement one another.

How the family looks at the problem

The criteria mentioned up to this point should not be considered exclusively from the perspective of the therapist, but also from the perspective of the family. The final decision as to the kind of therapy is arrived at only after negotiation between therapist and family. It is therefore important that the therapist is aware of the following issues:

- the family's view as to which problems are most important,
- how these problems are accounted for (explanation of the patients and their parents), and
- where they see the possibilities of change.

The fourth criterion for the constellation of therapy is how the family views the problem. The decision as to the focus of therapy should be based to a large degree on their wishes. Even this criterion, however, is not absolute. The therapist can only go along with the family's wishes in so far as it complies with his own sense of professional responsibility and ethical views.

Choice of setting and intensity of therapy

The most important psychotherapeutic settings in work with children, adolescents and their families are:

- individual therapy with the child or adolescent,
- working with parents (couselling, advice and psychoeducative interventions),
- family sessions,
- group therapeutic sessions.

Individual therapy may take the form of a number of different therapeutic models, e.g. counselling, play therapy, behaviour therapy, etc., but is defined by involving a single patient with a therapist. The parental sessions can likewise be very varied in nature including counselling, psychoeducation and parent training, and may occur with either one or both parents. Family sessions are defined by including participants from more than one generation. This may, at the most minimal, simply mean the patient and one parent, but more commonly both parents and others, e.g. siblings take part. The group therapy sessions include not only 'patient'groups, but also parent and relative groups. Family and group sessions are more commonly co-therapied by two therapists, which offers the advantage of having an additional person who can observe the dynamics and content of sessions, as when many people are present, it can be difficult for a single therapist to achieve an overview of the session.

The issue of therapy intensity refers both to the frequency and the duration of therapy. Outpatient individual therapy invariably occurs weekly and lasts the classical 50 minutes. There is no reason, however, why this intensity cannot be varied according to the particular needs and wishes of the patient. Inpatient psychotic patients, for example, may benefit from having shorter sessions of 5–20 minutes at shorter intervals, whereas group therapy sessions can often be somewhat longer (1.5 hours). Likewise, the frequency of family sessions is often arranged such that several weeks pass between sessions, whereas it is not uncommon to undertake inpatient individual therapy several times a week.

The most appropriate intensity is also influenced by the content and focus of work to be undertaken (see above).

(i) The setting should allow the reported symptoms of the disorder to be seen or manifested, in order that they can be directly addressed in the session. There should therefore be some degree of affinity between the therapeutic session and that in which the problems occur, e.g. problems with social interaction might be best addressed in a group setting with peers.

(ii) All those necessary for addressing and resolving the patient's problems should be present in the therapeutic setting. (The most commonly observed problem with regard to this point is absence of the father.)

(iii) The chosen setting should provide the opportunity for productive change. Therefore, settings in which the problems manifest, but are for some reason inaccessible to therapeutic action should be avoided. (The most common example of this problem is the family in which conflict further escalates, with the therapist feeling unable to intervene.)

(iv) The chosen setting must be agreed upon by all relevant parties.

Fig. 2.8 shows an example of the options for different constellations of focus and setting.

Coordination of components into a therapeutic plan

Fig. 2.9 shows the most important therapeutic methods used with children, adolescents and families. There are two aspects shown here which need to be considered in the coordination of a therapeutic plan:

- the combination of behavioural and insight-orientated interventions,
- the combination of patient-orientated and family-orientated interventions.

Both these aspects remain a topic of controversy. Many authors continue to

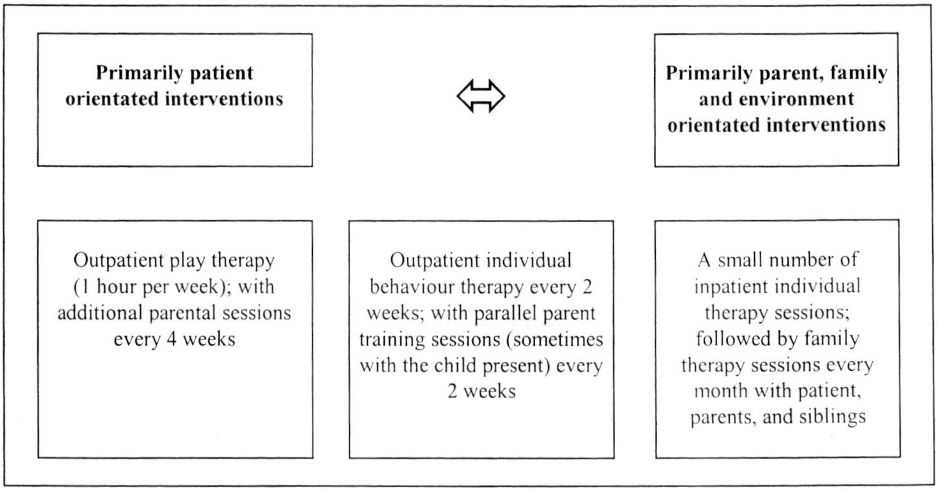

Fig. 2.8. Examples for different therapy constellations.

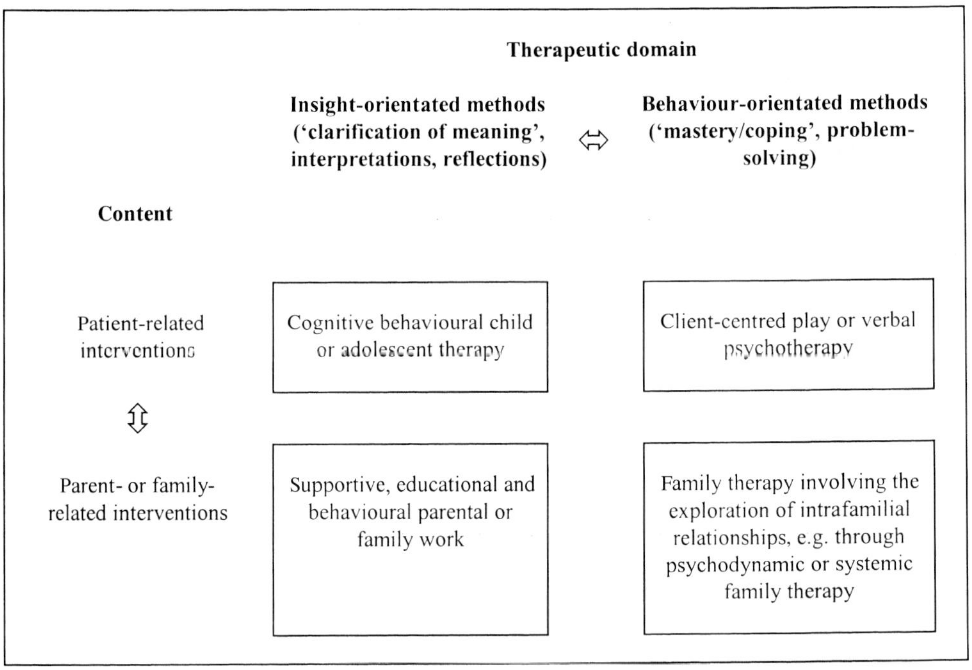

Fig. 2.9. The most important methods of therapy involving children, adolescents and families.

insist that, for example, client centred and behaviour therapy work antagonistically, or that patient and family-orientated therapies should not be undertaken in parallel, as the therapeutic models are incompatible. These types of discussion come down to the issue of how closely one should adhere to the particular schools of therapy. The more closely a therapist associates himself with a particular therapeutic school, the more likely he is to perceive these incompatibilities. Such a therapist is likely to view the involvement of other therapy models in the therapeutic plan as unnecessary and irksome. But such rigid fixation can today no longer be justified. Rather than stick to the dogma of any particular therapeutic school, it is important to take into consideration the results of empirical research. Furthermore, the question should not be whether two different established therapeutic approaches are compatible, but rather how therapeutic techniques can be combined in order to attain the best possible results for the patients.

In practice, this means that, for example, play therapy can be combined with behaviour therapy techniques, when this combination appears to be in the best interests of the patient (as advocated by Schmidtchen, 1989). Thus the application of a therapeutic concept such as 'unconditional acceptance' need not be absolute, but can be calibrated according to the patient's needs (Döpfner, 1993) (see Fig. 2.10). In this way, therapy can be altered across a number of therapeutic dimensions:

- the degree of structuring through the preselection of play material and content,
- the degree of structuring through the application of certain boundaries and rules within therapy,
- the level of supportive assistance offered, for example, links are made between cognitions and emotional responses or actions,
- the extent to which advice, suggestions or encouragement are utilized,
- the degree to which the therapist reacts in the face of undesired behaviour (see Döpfner, 1993 for a more detailed explanation of this dimension).

In choosing a combination of patient, and family or parent-related interventions, it is important to bear in mind that even when the focus of therapy is child orientated (such as individual therapy), this cannot be undertaken in complete isolation, and some level of contact with the parents is always necessary. This may lead to some difficulties.

- Parents may expect that the therapist will report back to them the contents of therapy. The therapist must recognize this need and ensure that he provides the parents with feedback concerning his professional opinion. On the other hand, the parents need to know that the content of therapy is a private matter

Problem area for the child	Therapist behaviour dimension: *Structuring* — Of play material or situation	*Structuring* — Through boundary setting	*Support*	*Advice*
Children with emotional disturbances, e.g. anxiety	+	+	++	+
Children with developmental delay	++	+	+++	++
Children with hyperactivity or attention deficits	+++	+++	++	+++
Children with aggressive (acting out) behaviour	+	+++	++	++

Fig. 2.10. Therapeutic modifications in play therapy format, according to the nature of the child's problem.

between therapist and child, which cannot be shared without breaking confidences. Naturally, this needs to be achieved without offending the parents or giving any impression of there being a conspiracy against them.

- A similar situation can occur when the therapist is told important information 'in confidence' with the instruction that it should not be revealed to other family members. The therapeutic relationship demands that (as far as is professionally responsible) this is respected. It is usually advisable, however, to work towards supporting the person (who gave the information), such that he is prepared to bring this information out into the open.
- A further common problem can arise when family therapy is begun, following a period of intensive individual child therapy. Having seen the problem until this point predominantly through the eyes of the child, the therapist may experience difficulty in identifying or sympathizing with the family members (so-called 'identification with the patient' or 'difficulties with loyalty or neutrality'). A family therapy perspective can only be productive if the therapist is able to treat each member impartially. In addition to addressing this issue in supervision, it can also be useful to introduce a co-therapist at this juncture.

Assessment as a cooperative process: negotiation and compromise

The assessment and treatment-planning processes are only the first steps towards coming to an agreement on the most appropriate way forward. The most expert planning is useless if it is not endorsed by the patient or family. The purpose of a post-assessment consultation with the parents is to arrive at a therapy agreement that involves those members of the family most relevant for a good outcome.

- The best chances of a successful therapeutic outcome and the lowest drop-out rate occur when the therapeutic plan is accepted and valued by both the parents and the child or adolescent.
- The more that the child and parents can be motivated to work with and for one another, the better are the chances of a good outcome. The therapeutic plan will be more binding if the therapist can build up a good relationship with the family members and also encourage closeness between the patient and his family.
- The more closely that therapy reflects the views of the family members and takes their views, suggestions and initiatives into account, the greater are the chances of success.
- The family will benefit from clearly stated and transparent therapeutic aims.

The feedback and consultation process should involve everyone relevant in the attempt to help the child or adolescent. This normally involves, at a minimum, the presented child and his parents. It is particularly important to involve both parents where possible, particularly if there are problems in the parental relationship. There is otherwise a significant risk that therapy will be undermined or even boycotted, for example, by an absent father who may feel rejected or resentful if not involved at this stage.

Before proposing any particular therapeutic intervention, the therapist should have discussed the following aspects with the family.

(i) The nature of the problem: how do the family members define and view the main current problems?; physical, psychological, interactional, social problems; perceived cause of the problem; 'problem carrier'; views as to what therapy is necessary.

(ii) Family relationships: how do family members relate to one another? (emotional bonds, degree of autonomy or independence possible).

(iii) Treatment expectations: what are the wishes, hopes and fears associated with therapy in the minds of the family?

(iv) Therapeutic relationships: what are family's preconceptions about 'therapy', e.g. cautious and guarded, interested but worried, hopeful and trusting? It is also useful at this point to gather information about contacts with other agencies, both those already underway and those which the family is holding 'in reserve'. It is not uncommon for families to seek help from a number of different agencies, although they may feel reluctant to discuss this. It is important, however, that this is brought out into the open as soon as possible to avoid an uncoordinated approach. The therapist should be prepared to accept the decision of the family, if they reject his offer of help and opt for that from another agency.

After having discussed these topics, the therapist should explain the results of the investigations performed and propose a therapeutic plan. This should include a discussion as to the severity of the condition and the reasons for treatment, the possible causes and the likely course of the symptoms, the therapeutic options and the likely prognosis with, and without, treatment. The discussion should also cover the realistic likelihood of being able to relieve symptoms and any possible unwanted effects or disadvantages of therapy. The therapist should bear two things in mind during this.

- The information should be presented in a way that is understandable for all family members, using the models which the family have offered and adopting their terminology as far as possible. This process is described in psychotherapeutic terms as 'joining' with the family.
- Whilst it is important to respect the position of the parents within the family, all relevant information, including that which may be painful for the family to hear repeated, must be addressed. It should be clearly stated whether the child suffers from a psychiatric disorder and whether or not treatment is considered desirable or necessary. This issue is just as important to address when the therapist finds no 'disorder' in the child or adolescent, even though this may be difficult for the parents to accept. It is the role of the therapist to be clear and matter of fact at this point.

In the following discussion as to the way forward, the therapist must clarify where the responsibility of the parents lie and what his professional duties are. The therapist him/herself needs to be clear about this issue, as ambiguous feelings can lead to him/her becoming embroiled in a confused and contradictory family system.

If the disorder is not too severe, the therapist should emphasize that his suggestions should be seen as advice only, and that the parents themselves should come to a decision about the future course of action. If the parents or the patient are of the opinion that they can deal with the problem without recourse to professional help, this view should be respected and the therapist should not try to limit their autonomy or competence. It should always be

		Need for therapy in the patient's and/or family's view	
		High	*Low*
Need for therapy in the therapist's view	*High*	1. **Consensus** Therapy is considered necessary and desirable by all	2. **Dissent** Patient and family are not interested in therapy, although the professional recommendation is that it would be beneficial
	Low	3. **Dissent** Therapy is requested, however, professional opinion is that therapy is not necessary	4. **Consensus** Therapy is not undertaken by mutual agreement

Fig. 2.11. Possible situations in cooperative treatment planning.

borne in mind that spontaneous remission is not a rare event in psychiatry, and there are considerable advantages to a solution emanating from within the family, rather than being imposed from outside. Finally, the therapist should acknowledge that treatment is an irrevocable step, which may have long-term negative consequences for the patient. Objections raised by the family to therapy should be respected and their autonomy and decision-making capacity should be restricted as little as possible. More serious symptoms or a greater perceived risk must, however, be reflected in the feedback given to the family. If the family fails to respond appropriately in the event of a serious threat to the child or adolescent's well-being, the therapist may be required to consider his professional duty and take the necessary legal recourse to ensure that the patient receives the help or protection he requires.

The aim of the consultation is to arrive at an agreement as to how to proceed which is accepted by all participants. There are four theoretical situations which can be envisaged (see Fig. 2.11).

(i) Therapist and family have no major disagreements as to the appropriate intervention and can reach a therapeutic agreement.

(ii) The therapy suggested is refused, despite there being, in the therapist's view, a clear need for intervention. This can be a difficult situation to handle; however, the therapist should consider it part of his responsibility to try to improve the motivation and/or insight of the family. This process requires care and experience and is unlikely to be achieved at one setting. The aim should be to offer concessions to the family, without giving ground on what the therapist sees as essential components of the treatment plan. He should be careful not to offer false hopes or promises that are not in his power to keep. It may be more appropriate to try to reach short-term agreements. It is not uncommon, for example, for patients with school phobia or anorexia nervosa, to insist that they can deal with their problems without help, or with outpatient help alone. This puts the parents in a difficult situation and they may be reluctant to insist on an inpatient stay against the will of their child. In these situations, the offer of a strictly time-limited period outpatient appointment can be offered, in order to clarify to all concerned the aims and goals for this period, e.g. school attendance, weight gain, etc. The further course of action can be made conditional on these goals being achieved. Under these circumstances it is particularly important to be absolutely clear about the conditions, if necessary using a written contract. If the family turns down this suggestion, the therapist should not allow his disappointment or frustration to show, and not take this outcome personally but rather to ensure that there is always a 'door left open'.

(iii) A situation, which is often easier for the therapist to deal with, is the family who express the desire for therapy, when in the view of the therapist, no treatment is necessary. In these cases, a clear explanation should be offered to the family and they should be reassured. It is important under these circumstances to inquire a little more as to how the referral came about, in order to clarify how a well child came to be referred. Common reasons include: over-concerned parents (as a result of insecurity, depression or other formal mental illness in the family), or the presentation of a child as a 'ticket of entry' for dealing with other issues (such as marital or family conflicts). The purpose of such a discussion is to clarify how such a situation arose and to direct the family to more appropriate help. If the underlying problem is not identified, it may be advisable to offer the family the opportunity to attend a follow-up appointment in a couple of months.

(iv) Another more straightforward situation is where family and therapist are in agreement that no intervention is necessary. This may arise following the reassurance given as a result of a normal diagnostic test. In these cases also, however, the family should be advised that a re-referral is always possible should they change their minds.

These four constellations are an oversimplification of the situation with which the therapist is usually faced. It is relatively common, for example, to find that the family members have very divergent opinions as to the nature of the problem and what should be done. In this situation, it can be a very challenging, although invariably also an interesting task, to try to arrive at a consensus which everyone can accept. This task is of central importance in the subspecialty of child and adolescent psychiatry, but often also very time consuming. It has a significant influence on the outcome of any ensuing therapy. During this process, the therapist must also take care to reflect upon his own reactions to the family. Very quickly, the therapist can find him or herself entangled in the family system, and once this has occurred it can be difficult to reassume neutrality in the sessions.

Continuous assessment during therapy

The issues of assessment discussed above should not be considered relevant only to the initial assessment procedure, but rather as part of an ongoing process, which continues throughout therapy. Appraisal and review of the therapy process is particularly important in work with children, adolescents and families, as it is usually only possible to plan ahead for a few months at the most. Long-term aims can only be made in vague terms and it is therefore important that both family and therapist keep in mind an overview of the onset and the ending of different therapeutic phases. This can be achieved by the use of periodic 'review' sessions every 2 to 3 months where progress can be appraised and the next goals defined. Involvement of the family at this point is vital, binding them to therapeutic process and avoiding any sense of loss of control or helplessness. Depending on the progress made up to this point, plans for further interventions can be developed in these review sessions and a variety of shifts of emphasis, alterations and additions to the original plan can be conceived. At the beginning of therapy, it is impossible to predict the developments which may occur both in the patient's perceived problems and also in the nature of the goals which they set. This should by no means be regarded as representing an error or a faulty initial assessment. It is rather the nature of successful therapy that 'preparedness for change' is maintained.

In practice, a number of specific developments in therapy are common. Therapeutic interventions often initially concentrate on relationships and behaviour, whilst as time progresses, an exploratory or cognitive process often becomes more appropriate. Therapy also tends to become wider in its perspective – initially concentrating on the current problems of the individual, and subsequently broadening the field of interest to the individual's past experiences and family background.

Alongside these content-related developments, the arrangements for therapy will also change over time. Thus, for example, the interval between sessions will typically increase as therapy progresses, from perhaps 1–2 sessions a week at the beginning to sessions every few months during the later phases of treatment. Therapy started as an inpatient treatment will usually initially be very intensive, with a number of parallel strands of therapy being undertaken at once. Usually, as time progresses, both the intensity and the number of therapeutic techniques used will be reduced. This 'winding down' of therapy can be used as a signal that the therapist is relinquishing more responsibility to both patient and family. Other chapters of this book cover examples of this in practice in specific disorders.

REFERENCES

Ambühl, H. (1993). Was ist therapeutisch an Psychotherapie? Eine empirische Überprüfung der Annahmen im 'Generic Model of Psychotherapy'. *Zeitschrift für Kinder- und Jugendpsychiatrie*, **41**, 285–303.

Bartling, G., Echelmeyer, L., Engberding, M. and Krause, R. (1980). *Problemanalyse im therapeutischen Prozess*. Stuttgart: Kohlhammer.

Blaser, A., Heim, E., Ringer, C. and Thommen, M. (1992). *Problemorientierte Psychotherapie*. Ein integratives Konzept. Bern: Huber.

Caspar, F. (1987). Was ist aus der guten alten Verhaltensanalyse geworden? In *Problemanalyse in der Psychotherapie. Bestandsaufnahme und Perspektiven*, ed. F. Caspar, pp. 1–19. Tübingen: Deutsche Gesellschaft für Verhaltenstherapie (DGVT).

Caspar, F. (1989). *Beziehungen und Probleme verstehen. Eine Einführung in die psychotherapeutische Plananalyse*. Bern: Huber.

Döpfner, M. (1993) Grundlegende Interventionsmethoden und ihre Integration. In *Kinderpsychiatrie im Vorschulalter*, ed. M. Döpfner and M. H. Schmidt, pp. 65–94. München: Quintessenz.

Grawe, K. (1992). Psychotherapieforschung zu Beginn der neunziger Jahre. *Psychologische Rundschau*, **43**, 132–162.

Grawe, K. (1997). Research-informed psychotherapy. *Psychotherapy Research*, **7**, 1–19.

Grawe, K., Donati, R. and Bernauer, F. (1994). *Psychotherapie im Wandel. Von der Konfession zur Profession*, 3rd edn. Göttingen: Hogrefe.

Jäger, R. S. (1988). Der diagnostische Prozess. In *Psychologische Diagnostik*, ed. R. Jäger, pp. 382–6. München: Psychologie Verlags Union.

Lau, C. (1980). Planungstheorie. In *Handbuch wissenschaftstheoretischer Begriffe*, vol. 2 (G–Q), ed. J. Speck, pp. 481–5. Göttingen: Vandenhoeck & Ruprecht.

Mattejat, F. (1993). *Subjektive Familienstrukturen*. Göttingen: Hogrefe.

Orlinsky, D. E. and Howard, J. U. (1988). Ein allgemeines Psychotherapiemodell. *Integrative Therapie*, **4**, 281–308.

Pohlen, M. and Bautz-Holzherr, M. (1995). *Psychoanalyse. Das Ende einer Deutungsmacht*. Reinbek: Rowohlt.

Remschmidt, H. and Mattejat, F. (1994). Psychotherapeutische Ansätze in der Behandlung von Kindern und Jugendlichen. *Monatsschrift für Kinderheilkunde*, **142**, 250–7.

Rudolf, G. (ed.) (1993). *Psychotherapeutische Medizin. Ein einführendes Lehrbuch auf psychodynamischer Grundlage*. Stuttgart: Enke.

Schiepek, G. (1991). *Systemtheorie der Klinischen Psychologie*. Wissenschaftstheorie, vol. 33. Braunschweig: Vieweg.

Schmidt, L. R. (1984). Überblick zur Psychodiagnostik. In *Lehrbuch der Klinischen Psychologie*, 2nd edn, ed. L. R. Schmidt, pp. 131–8. Stuttgart, Enke.

Schmidtchen, S. (1989). *Kinderpsychotherapie*. Stuttgart: Kohlhammer.

Schulte, D. (ed.) (1991a). *Therapeutische Entscheidungen*. Göttingen: Hogrefe.

Schulte, D. (1991b). Therapie aus der Perspektive des Therapeuten. In *Therapeutische Entscheidungen*, ed. D. Schulte, pp. 7–14. Göttingen, Hogrefe.

Seidenstücker, G. (1984). Indikation in der Psychotherapie: Entscheidungsprozesse – Forschung – Konzepte und Ergebnisse. In *Lehrbuch der Klinischen Psychologie*, 2nd edn, ed. L. R. Schmidt, pp. 443–511. Stuttgart, Enke.

Seidenstücker, G. (1988). Indikation und Entscheidung. In *Psychologische Diagnostik*, ed. R. S. Jäger, pp. 407–420. München: Psychologie Verlags Union.

Steller, M. (1994). Diagnostischer Prozess. In *Psychodiagnostik psychischer Störungen*, ed. R-D. Stieglitz and U. Baumann, pp. 37–46. Stuttgart: Enke.

Wetzel, H. and Linster, H. W. (1992). Psychotherapie. In *Handwörterbuch Psychologie*, 4th edn, ed. R. Asanger and G. Wenninger, pp. 627–39. Weinheim: Psychologie Verlags Union.

World Health Organization (WHO) (1996). *Multiaxial classification of child psychiatric disorders. The ICD-10 classification of mental and behavioural disorders in children and adolescents*. Geneva: WHO.

3

Psychotherapy research

Helmut Remschmidt and Fritz Mattejat

Psychotherapeutic treatment methods must, as with all treatment in children and adolescents, take into consideration the following issues.

- Developmental aspects: in all psychiatric disorders affecting children and adolescents, the developmental stage and their implications should be borne in mind. They are relevant not only in terms of the symptom profile but also in the choice of an appropriate therapy.
- Family relationships: the family or group of people comprising the household in which a child lives make up the closest contacts a child or adolescent has. Children are much more dependent on their immediate social surroundings than adults, and any psychiatric disorder needs to be viewed in this context.
- Educational or vocational aspects: beyond the family, educational or training institutions such as nurseries, schools or colleges are very important with respect to a child's development. This must be considered when treating the psychiatric disorder of a child or adolescent.
- Risk factors for developmental variability and psychiatric disorders: a number of known risk factors are modifiable, especially those in social areas; attempts should therefore be made to identify them at the earliest possible stage and to minimize their potentially harmful effects as part of a treatment plan.
- Protective factors and prevention: childhood and adolescence are the optimal times for bringing protective or preventative measures into play. Intervention during this critical period can prevent, for example, psychotic episodes becoming chronic.
- Coping mechanisms: most ill children or adolescents develop their own coping mechanisms. The therapist has the responsibility of identifying these both in the patient and his family in order to encourage their utilization in therapy.

All the above-mentioned aspects are of particular importance in psychotherapy research. They should be taken into account during assessment, as well as over the course of therapy. They will have an influence on the course and the outcome of therapy, and they must also be considered when evaluating the effects of therapy.

Epidemiology

The purpose of epidemiology is not primarily to examine specific treatment methods, but rather to attempt to answer a number of comprehensive questions, which are of importance with regard to the application of therapeutic interventions, in particular, those in the field of psychotherapy. Examples of these are as follows.

(i) How common are psychiatric symptoms and disorders in children and adolescents?
(ii) How many of those seek help or treatment?
(iii) Whose help do they seek, i.e. child psychiatrist, family practitioner, psychologist?
(iv) What influences the help-seeking behaviour of parents and children?
(v) What is the role of social factors such as community or cultural influences, social class, and educational level of the parents?
(vi) What factors will influence the length of treatment?
(vii) How is the need for therapy defined?
(viii) How many children remain untreated, despite a therapeutic need having been established?

A research programme, supported by government grant, enabled us to investigate some of these questions in an almost complete population of children and adolescents who utilized the available psychiatric and psychotherapeutic facilities in a defined area (three counties) over a year. The study included 37 different institutions, including baby and toddler clinics, child guidance centres, child and adolescent psychiatric practitioners, outpatient clinics, hospitals, etc. By also investigating nearby institutions outside the region to whom presentations might have occurred, we were able to ensure the inclusion of all referrals from the region, and thus an analysis of an entire presenting population was possible. The results of this analysis demonstrated to us the influence of external factors in presenting patterns. For example, increasing distance between home and inpatient services had the effect of reducing the likelihood of admission, but increasing the length of stay. Patients who were not admitted to a local hospital were also on average a year older, had more complex or severe psychiatric diagnoses and were treated for twice as long as those from local communities, where there was an option of local outpatient therapy.

Table 3.1. Treatment measures for outpatients (1983–1990)

	Patients		Sessions	
Treatment measure	*N*	%	Total	Mean
Patient-orientated psychotherapy	1124	36.84	11 998	10.67
Parent and family related interventions	2352	77.08	10 096	4.29
Skills-based therapy, e.g. for dyslexia	308	10.09	10 508	34.29
Other interventions	917	30.05	2136	2.32
Total[a]	3051	100		

[a]Patients who received psychotherapy. The figures are not mutually exclusive, due to the common occurrence of more than one therapeutic intervention being carried out at a time.

Outpatient and inpatient psychotherapy

Before beginning to look at the more complex issues of therapeutic research, such as effectiveness or therapeutic evaluation, it seems sensible to first consider the more straightforward, but centrally important, issue of the extent to which psychotherapeutic treatment is being undertaken, both in inpatient and in outpatient settings and which techniques are principally being used. In the literature there is relatively little pertaining to this issue, most of which looks at single therapeutic techniques (see Wuchner and Eckert, 1995; Podeswik et al., 1995; Heekerens, 1989a). We have audited the activity within the Hospital for Child and Adolescent Psychiatry, University of Marburg (Germany) and its associated institutions (wards, day hospital, outpatient clinics, outreach services, and child guidance centres) over an 8-year period (Remschmidt and Mattejat, 1994; Mattejat et al., 1994). The next section of this chapter outlines the results of this audit.

Psychotherapy in outpatient settings

Over the 8-year period of observation, 7969 patients were assessed. In 1992 no further contact took place. In 2991 patients, one further session (e.g. couselling, crisis intervention) was provided. In 3051 further sessions (e.g. ongoing psychotherapy or other treatments) were undertaken.

Table 3.1 shows an overview of these 3051 outpatients. It can be seen that, in 36.8% of cases, an individual therapy was undertaken with the patient, in 10% a skills-based therapy was instituted and in 77% therapeutic interventions consis-

Table 3.2. Form of psychotherapy in outpatients (1983–1990)

	Patients		Sessions	
Treatment measure	*N*	%	Total	Mean
Verbally based psychotherapy[a]	592	52.66	4124	6.96
Play therapy	402	35.76	5546	13.79
Psychodynamic psychotherapy	58	5.16	957	16.50
Behaviour therapy	179	15.92	1131	6.31
Other methods	48	4.27	240	5.00
Total[b]	1124	100		

[a]See Chapter 10.
[b]Patients who received psychotherapy. The figures are not mutually exclusive, due to more than one form of therapy being carried out consecutively.

Table 3.3. Medication in outpatients (1983–1990)

	Prescription			
	No		Yes	
Drug	*N*	%	*N*	%
Anticonvulsants	2941	96.42	109	3.57
Neuroleptics	2978	97.63	72	2.36
Antidepressants	3019	98.98	31	1.01
Tranquillizers	3025	99.18	25	0.81
Stimulants	3015	98.85	35	1.14
Total[a]	2783	91.24	267	8.75

[a]Outpatients who received medication. The figures are not mutually exclusive, due to more than one medication sometimes being prescribed.

ted of parent counselling or training. In 30% other methods were used.

Table 3.2 shows a breakdown by type of therapy (individual and group therapy are grouped together) for the 1124 patients who received psychotherapy. In over half of the cases, individual verbally based therapy was undertaken, the next most common forms were play therapy, especially with younger children, behavioural therapy, psychoanalytic therapy, etc.

Table 3.3 shows the use of medication in the outpatient clinic population. By far the most common drugs, used in 3.6% of the patients, were anticonvulsants. These were prescribed almost exclusively in conjunction with the presence of

Table 3.4. Treatment measures in inpatients (1983–1990)

	Patients		Sessions	
Treatment measure	*N*	%	Total	Mean
Patient-orientated psychotherapy	1342	88.40	39 010	29.06
Parent- and family-related interventions	1286	84.71	8402	6.53
Functional training therapy, e.g. for dyslexia	976	64.29	54 686	56.03
Other interventions	662	43.61	2491	3.76
Total[a]	1518	100.00		

[a]Inpatients who received psychotherapy. The figures are not mutually exclusive, due to more than one form of therapy being carried out consecutively.

seizures. 2.4% of the cases were treated with neuroleptics and approximately 1% received antidepressants and stimulants, respectively. The use of tranquillizers at less than 1% was minimal. It can be seen that over 90% of this population received no medication at all, dispelling the myth that child and adolescent psychiatric institutions invariably resort to drug treatment. In outpatient settings, drugs are rarely used, and only in the presence of a clear indication.

In summary, looking at outpatient treatment:

- in around half of cases, crisis intervention or advice was followed by psychotherapy;
- the most common form of psychotherapeutic intervention was patient orientated in either a group or individual setting;
- in 77% of cases, parent counselling sessions or parental training were undertaken;
- verbally based therapy was the most common form of therapy, followed by play and behavioural therapy;
- medication played only a minor role.

Psychotherapy in the inpatient population

Over the study period (1983–1990) 1608 patients were treated as inpatients in our hospital for child and adolescent psychiatry. Sixty-one of these were admitted only briefly for diagnostic purposes, leaving 1547 who received treatment or crisis intervention. Of these, 1518 underwent psychotherapy or ongoing counselling sessions, and only 29 did not.

Table 3.4 gives an overview of the therapeutic interventions undertaken in

Table 3.5. Form of psychotherapy undertaken in inpatients (1983–1990)

	Patients		Sessions	
Form of therapy	*N*	%	Total	Mean
Verbally based psychotherapy	975	72.65	23 236	23.83
Play therapy	251	18.70	4626	18.43
Psychodynamic psychotherapy	83	6.18	2028	24.43
Behaviour therapy	345	25.70	5891	17.07
Other methods	190	14.15	3229	16.99
Total[a]	1342	100		

[a]Patients who received psychotherapy. The figures are not mutually exclusive, due to more than one form of therapy being carried out consecutively.

Table 3.6. Drug therapy in inpatients (1983–1990)

	Prescription			
	No		Yes	
Drug	*N*	%	*N*	%
Anticonvulsants	1415	93.21	103	6.78
Neuroleptics	1119	73.71	399	26.28
Antidepressants	1370	90.25	148	9.74
Tranquillizers	1466	96.57	52	3.42
Stimulants	1426	93.93	92	6.06
Total[a]	820	54.01	698	45.98

[a]Patients who received medication. The figures are not mutually exclusive, due to more than one medication sometimes being prescribed.

these 1518 inpatients. Even more pronounced than in the outpatients, psychotherapy, whether group or individual, can be seen to be focused more intensely on the patients themselves. Treatments using functional exercises play a greater role than in the outpatient setting (64.3%) and parent-related training or sessions are also more common (84.7%) and intensive.

Here also (Table 3.5), verbally based (72.5%) is the most common form of therapy administered, followed by behaviour therapy (25.7%) and play therapy. Psychoanalytic psychotherapy is carried out in only around 6% of cases.

Table 3.6 shows the use of medication in the inpatient sample. Medication was used in less than half of those patients receiving a psychotherapeutic intervention (1518). In comparison to the outpatient sample, the use of medication is higher.

In summary, looking at inpatient treatment:

- psychotherapeutic treatment is undertaken in nearly 90% of all inpatients, normally in individual sessions (occasionally in groups);
- in around 85% of cases, parents were also included in the treatment;
- functional training therapies play a more important role in the inpatient setting;
- verbally based psychotherapy is the most commonly utilized psychotherapeutic intervention (72%), followed by behaviour therapy and play therapy;
- in the inpatient group, the proportion of patients treated with medication is higher than in the outpatient group.

The most important conclusions which can be drawn from the audit of the work of our Department of Child and Adolescent Psychiatry and its associated institutions can be summarized as follows.

(i) Therapeutic work with parents plays an essential role. This work consists mainly of sessions offering information and advice, as well as supportive sessions for parents. Formal family therapy was carried out less often and least common were therapeutic interventions for parents themselves. The extent of this type of work was relatively similar for all institutions covered by the audit, and work with parents was influenced little by the individual's diagnosis.

(ii) The most commonly undertaken treatments for children and adolescents were verbally based and play therapy. Pragmatic or problem-related approaches were used more than therapies based on a single therapeutic school or theoretical concept. Behavioural techniques play a much greater role than psychodynamic techniques.

(iii) The degree of medication used varies enormously across the different institutions. These differences relate predominantly to the nature of the disorders represented and to their severity, as well as to the nature of the institutions involved in the audit. Treatment involving medication was limited to specific disorders in which there are clear indications such as epilepsy, psychosis, affective disorders and attention deficit syndromes.

The results underline a pragmatic and problem-related mode of working, where complex problems can be addressed on a number of different levels. These comprise a variety of treatment components integrated into an appropriate overall plan. The exclusive adoption of the theoretical concepts of a

particular school would be unable to do justice to the complex nature of the problems presented. A better model is that of a combination treatment plan with various components, worked out individually for each patient. In practice, the treatment of such patients does not follow 'textbook' descriptions, but is a more complicated and multilayered approach.

We consider these principles to be representative of a general trend in child and adolescent psychiatry, and would expect similar results to be obtained in many other clinics and hospitals throughout Europe.

The evaluation of psychotherapeutic treatments

Evaluation remains one of the most difficult tasks in the field of child and adolescent psychiatry. Evaluation differs from the audit process described above in that it looks at the efficacy of therapy (Grawe, 1997). In brief, psychotherapy research consists of examination of efficacy, comparisons of efficacy of different therapies and therapy process research (see Fig. 3.1). There are a number of further research methodologies that can be used to evaluate and improve upon the therapeutic options offered (see Fig. 3.2).

Proof of efficacy

The most fundamental issue is whether a certain psychotherapeutic treatment method can be shown to be efficacious. For this purpose, efficacious appropriate methods to measure relevant changes must be chosen. The aim of psychotherapy is usually an improvement in symptomatology. Above and beyond this, therapeutic measures often aim to alter the personality structure or behavioural aspects relevant to the disorder. The general social functioning of the child or adolescent must also be taken into account. Social competence can be examined in a number of different areas: social and family environment, school or workplace and out-of-school activities. The assessment of the efficacy of a particular psychotherapeutic measure must also look at changes which occur in the child or adolescent's environment, for example, the attitude and behaviour of parents towards their child, as well as changes in the extended family (altered family relationships, particular stresses, present and social support utilized). Thus not only must the child's symptoms be assessed, but also the general development of the child, behaviour at school, integration within the family and in the wider social field. Fig. 3.3 shows the relationships of these different areas of the child's social functioning. The variety of data which can be collected is shown in Fig. 3.4.

Investigation	Question to be answered	Research design
Efficacy (general evaluation of the success of treatment)	Does psychotherapy (or any other specific technique) produce the desired therapeutic improvements?	A treatment group, compared to a non-treated or placebo control group
Comparative efficacy and specific indications (specific evaluation of the relative efficacy of treatments in different settings)	Does the efficacy of treatments differ and which treatment is the most appropriate for a certain problem (diagnosis), patient (age, co-morbidity, etc.) or setting (Inpatient/outpatient, etc.)?	Two or more treatment groups with different treatments being compared in the same clinical problem, e.g. diagnosis
Components of effectivity (process examination)	Which processes occur over the course of therapy and which of these have an influence on the therapeutic result?	One or more treatment groups in which the interaction between patient and therapist is examined or a correlation study looking at the relationship between certain processes and outcome markers

Fig. 3.1. The 'classical' categorization in psychotherapeutic research (see also Kazdin, 1991 and Grawe et al., 1994).

Comparative effectiveness

When comparing different psychotherapeutic treatments, the aim is to establish whether one or more therapies is better in the treatment of a particular disorder.

Research into this area requires therapies to be classified under relevant headings. The research group headed by Grawe et al. (1994) has developed such a classification. (Although designed with adults in mind, it is also relevant in child and adolescent therapy). The following therapeutic forms are listed:

- behaviour therapy,
- humanistic therapies,
- psychodynamic therapy,
- biological or medically orientated therapy,
- relaxation and hypnosis,

Research strategy	Question to be answered	Research design
Investigation of the general efficacy of a therapeutic programme	Does the therapy programme produce the desired therapeutic improvements?	A treatment group in comparison to a non-treated or placebo control group
Comparative effectivity of therapeutic programmes	Which therapeutic programme is most effective for a certain problem (diagnosis), patient (age, co-morbidity, etc.)?	Two or more treatment groups with the same clinical problem in different treatment programmes
Identification of meaningful therapeutic components	Which components of a treatment are necessary, sufficient and conducive to therapeutic improvement?	Two or more treatment groups which differ with regard to treatment components
Combination of meaningful therapeutic components	Which components or other treatments could be added in order to raise the efficacy of treatment?	Two or more treatment groups, with differing therapeutic components, or a correlation study looking at the relationship between therapeutic components and outcome
Optimization of therapeutic parameters	How can a specific treatment be altered to improve its efficacy?	Two or more treatment groups, which differ in one or more therapeutic dimensions; or a correlation study which compares therapeutic parameters and outcome
Identification of meaningful individual or context parameters	How is the effectivity of therapy affected by patients, families or therapeutic parameters?	The comparison of a number of treatment groups, which differ according to these factors; or a correlation study looking at the relationship between these factors and outcome

Fig. 3.2. Different research strategies used in psychotherapy to develop effective treatments (after Kazdin, 1991).

Patient		Social environment
Symptoms	General behaviour and personality	1. Relation of the parents and other important carers towards the patient
	Social functioning: - social contacts - out-of-school activities - school or workplace	2. Extended family or wider social field

Fig. 3.3. Areas to be considered when researching the efficacy and effectiveness of therapy in children or adolescents (Mattejat and Remschmidt, 1988).

		Type of data	
		Subjective ⟷	***Objective***
		(implicit data and criteria individual and/or subjective assessments)	(explicitly defined data with good inter-rater reliability and assessment)
	From within	Assessment of outcome by patients and family	Behaviour observation by patients and family
Perspective of assessment	↕	Assessment of outcome by involved professionals	Behaviour observation by involved professionals
	From without	Assessment of outcome by external evaluators	Behaviour observation by external evaluators

Fig. 3.4. Types of data which can be used to evaluate therapy.

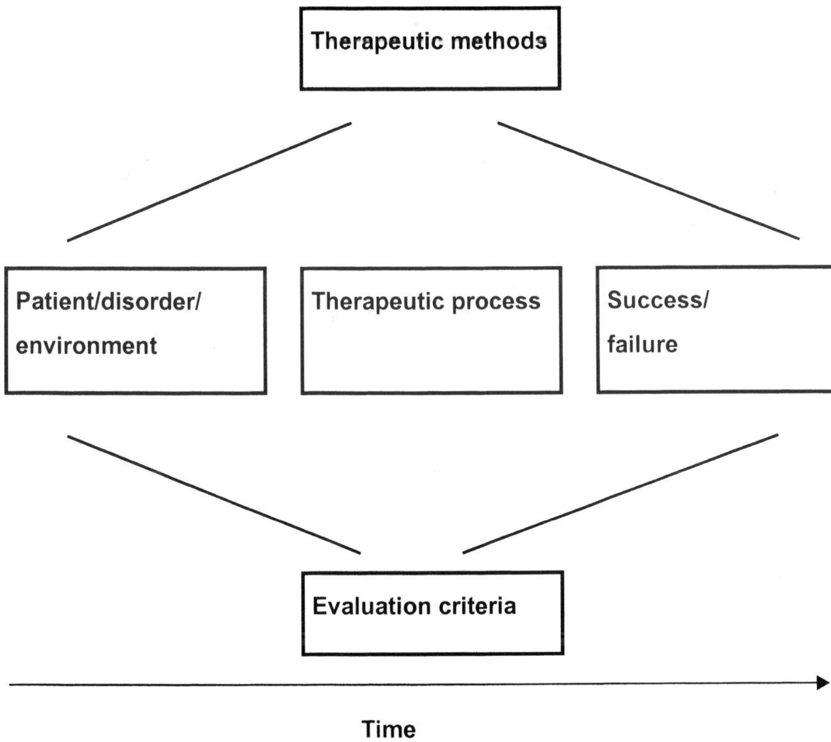

Fig. 3.5. The central role of the therapeutic processes within psychotherapy.

- communication therapy and systemic therapies,
- eclectic therapy,
- milieu therapy,
- psychotherapy or counselling, not otherwise specified.

In the field of child and adolescent psychiatry, there are as yet few systematic studies comparing the outcome using different therapeutic approaches. The most important results from the studies available are described in a later section.

Therapy process research

Traditionally, in psychodynamic approaches, the phenomena of transference and counter transference were considered to be essential variables of therapy. These and other interactional aspects of psychotherapy are considered to influence therapy outcome and are studied in therapy process research. Fig. 3.5 shows a simplified schema of the central role of the therapeutic process in the evaluation of a psychotherapeutic treatment. Five different domains are differentiated, which are characterized by a number of variables.

First, the therapeutic method being used, e.g. behaviour therapy, analytic therapy, then the particular characteristics of the patient and the problem, e.g. personality, nature of disorder, family constellation and cooperation and other relevant environmental factors. The therapy process deals, in individual therapy, with the nature of the relationship between patient and therapist, covering not only verbal aspects of the relationship, but also non-verbal exchanges. The domain of success/failure concerns the intrinsic assessment of effectiveness by patient and therapist.

At present, in the therapy of children and adolescents we are still only starting to understand the nature of therapeutic process and what influence it has on outcome. In the field of adult psychotherapy, this has been studied in much more detail. Studies have shown that the structure of the patient–therapist relationship is an important intrinsic prognostic factor for therapy success (Mintz and Luborsky, 1979). The early establishment of a supportive and empathic relationship between patient and therapist has a positive influence on outcome. Earlier studies, e.g. Luborsky et al., 1971 hinted at the fact that patient and therapist variables alone were unable to explain the differences in outcome by a therapeutic intervention, but that it was rather the interaction between these factors that needed to be taken into consideration. These findings suggest that it would also be well worth looking in more detail at these interactions in child and adolescent psychotherapy.

Evaluation of therapeutic programmes

The phrase 'therapeutic programme' is used here to denote the combination of two or more treatment elements, e.g. medication + behaviour therapy + parental education sessions that are integrated in a treatment plan. The treatment plan should comprise defined treatment aims, the interventions to be used to achieve these aims and a time-scale indicating when and for how long the interventions will be applied. Such a treatment plan need not, and should not, however, be adhered to rigidly. Modifications should be made and documented in accordance with information gathered over the course of therapy (see Eisert, 1986).

In contrast to studies on 'process' described earlier, a number of studies have been performed to evaluate a range of treatment programmes in the field of child and adolescent psychiatry, many with encouraging results. This type of research will be illustrated with three examples.

Therapeutic programmes for attention deficit syndromes

Many studies have now demonstrated the benefits of a multimodal treatment programme over single measures such as play therapy, medication or behaviour therapy alone. These programmes usually consist of a combination of the following interventions: structured help for day-to-day management (the promotion of practical daily living skills and social skills training), direct patient-related interventions (medication with stimulants, a behavioural contingency programme, occupational therapy and interventions to improve motor skills) and interventions acting on the environment (parent training, involvement of the school and other relevant institutions). Stimulants have a dose-dependent effect on hyperactivity, cognitive parameters, and social adaptive behaviour. Improvement can be demonstrated not only on measures of perception, e.g. vigilance and reaction times but also on measures of the mother–child interaction (Mash and Johnston, 1982; Barkley, 1988). These results have been replicated many times. As a consequence of an overall improvement in the disturbed behaviour of the child, parents are able to summon renewed strength and it is often possible to reconstruct a healthier parent–child relationship.

Therapeutic programmes in schizophrenic adolescents

In this group of patients, too, combined therapeutic programmes, comprising neuroleptic treatment, supportive psychotherapy, occupational therapy and family work, have been shown to be effective. In adolescents and in young adults with schizophrenia, all studies with adequately prescribed medication and structured, supported family programmes have been proved worthwhile (King and Goldstein, 1979; Martin, 1991; Remschmidt and Martin, 1992). The combination of these two measures has two important effects: the structured family interventions result in a reduction of exaggerated or hostile emotions within the family, whilst the medication ensures that a protective mechanism is in place to enable the patient to deal better with emotional difficulties without decompensating into psychosis. These programmes have been shown to be more effective than individual measures.

Comparison of therapeutic programmes under various conditions

Clinical experience shows that the conditions under which therapy is undertaken can have a significant influence on outcome. A study by Remschmidt and Schmidt (1988) looked at 109 patients with ten different psychiatric disorders, from two hospitals. According to well-defined inclusion and exclusion criteria, these patients were allocated randomly to either home treatment, inpatient or day hospital treatment regimens. In each case, similar treatments were used, but naturally the conditions varied according to the treatment modality.

The therapeutic methods chosen were principally dependent on the diagnosis: with relatively straightforward or circumscribed disorders, behavioural techniques were the most commonly used, whereas in more complex disorders, psychoanalytic or family therapy was seen as the treatment of choice. The course of action was chosen to reflect the multifactorial nature of child and adolescent psychiatric disorders and was usually multidisciplinary. The results were as follows.

- No significant differences were found in therapeutic outcome among the three different treatment groups, although the outcome differed, as would be expected, according to the disorder being treated. Thus neurotic and emotional disorders had the best outcome, whereas conduct disorder had a generally worse outcome.
- No significant differences were found in the length of treatment between the three groups.

The results of this study therefore support the notion that, for a defined proportion of well-selected patients, treatment in a day hospital or home treatment can be considered an acceptable alternative to inpatient treatment. In practice, the percentage of patients suitable for such treatment is likely to be around 10–15% and if this became policy, a considerable reduction in health expenditure could be achieved, with the proviso that this selection should be made carefully and prudently (see also Remschmidt et al., 1988).

The relevance of the family for therapeutic success

The most important factor responsible for therapeutic outcome is the nature of the disorder itself. For example, it is well established that externalizing disorders such as conduct disorder have a poorer untreated course and a worse outcome with therapy than internalizing disorders such as emotional disorders Similarly, prognostic factors are also apparent within disorders. For example, it is generally accepted that some subgroups of schizophrenia have a better prognosis that others. Knowledge about the likely course and outcome in a particular patient is important when deciding on a treatment plan for a particular patient, which should aim to achieve an optimal but realistic outcome (see Chapter 2).

However, these factors are often not the most important factor in predicting outcome or in planning therapy. Clinical experience has shown repeatedly that familial situation and intrafamilial relationships are of enormous importance with respect to both the feasibility and success of any therapy offered. It is, at present, difficult to assess which particular familial factors are of the most importance, as little empirical work has been undertaken in this field. We have undertaken some studies to address these issues.

An initial study (Mattejat and Remschmidt, 1989) looked at 50 patients and their families before the onset of treatment using an inventory called 'Profile of Psychosocial Adversities'. Therapeutic success (with regard to patient symptomatology) was recorded at the end of the treatment period in order to assess the prognostic relevance of a range of family characteristics as measured at the onset of therapy. The results of this analysis revealed that most psychosocial factors could not be shown to have a specific effect on outcome. Two factors did, however, seem to be of particular relevance.

- The presence of rejecting or hostile behaviour in a parent towards the child had a negative prognostic effect. The prognosis was particularly poor in those children who were the only ones on the receiving end of this hostile or rejecting behaviour, in other words where the child had the role of scapegoat in the family.
- The ability of the parents to offer guidance and control to their child was also found to be an important positive prognostic factor. This factor related to their ability to demonstrate a sense of responsibility and confidence with regard to discipline. Children from families with parents lacking these qualities (who felt weak, helpless and had little ability to structure or to be consistent when disciplining their child) had a particularly poor prognosis.

These two prognostically relevant factors predicted therapy outcome (measured in terms of symptom improvement) correctly in approximately three-quarters of cases in this study. A further study (Mattejat and Remschmidt, 1991) looked into this in more detail. A sample of 131 inpatients and their parents were studied on the day of admission and upon discharge (interview was limited to this family triad to assist comparison of data). The diagnostic instrument used was the 'Marburg Family Scales'. This semi-structured interview and observational rating scale assesses the dynamics of family relationships allowing subscores to be obtained for 'proximity-seeking behaviour' and 'distance-seeking behaviour'. The results of the study are described below and shown in Fig. 3.6.

First, the 'proximity-seeking' subscores had little influence on the success or otherwise of the therapy undertaken, whereas the 'distance-seeking' subscore revealed a clear relationship with outcome. Of particular significance were the father and the mother's behaviour towards the patient and the patient's behaviour towards his/her father. All detected differences are in the direction expected, thus unsuccessful therapy groups had higher 'distance-seeking' sub-

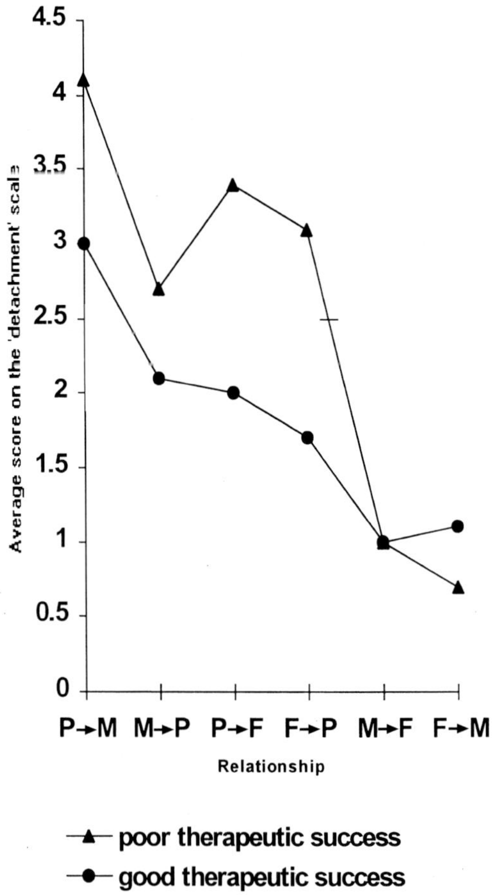

Fig. 3.6. The relationship between family characteristics and therapeutic success.

scores prior to therapy. In the relationship between mother and father, no differences were found between the successful and unsuccessful groups.

Furthermore, patients had the best outcome if they were from families where neither parent showed distance-seeking behaviour towards the patient. Where just one parent showed this behaviour, the chances of successful outcome were already significantly reduced, and where both parents showed this behaviour outcome was severely jeopardized. In families where neither parent showed distance-seeking behaviour, the chances of a successful therapy outcome were over 80%, whereas in those with two parents with this behaviour, the outcome was poor in almost 80% of cases.

We have further extended our work to look not only externally at the nature of the relationships, but also using a self reporting instrument called the 'Subjective Family Image' (Mattejat and Scholz, 1994). Using this instrument, mother, father and child/adolescent rate how they view themselves and their relationships. Again, two aspects were looked at: the positive emotional binding of each family member to one another and the individual autonomy of each family member in interaction with one another.

A high degree of positive emotional binding in a relationship was reflected by interest, warmth and understanding for the other, whilst relationships characterized by low emotional binding were described as cold and intolerant, showing little interest in the other person. A high score on the individual autonomy scale was obtained when family members felt independent, self-assured and capable of making decisions for themselves. Those relationships with a low score on the individual autonomy scale, on the other hand, were characterized by feelings of anxiety, dependence and indecisiveness in interaction with the other family members.

The results obtained at assessment prior to therapy from the 'Subjective Family Image' instrument were able to predict therapeutic outcome in approximately 80% of cases (Mattejat, 1993). The main results were as follows.

- There was a poor prognosis when parents felt rejected by their child or adolescent.
- Likewise there was a poor prognosis when the child or adolescent viewed parents as being indecisive, anxious or incapable of independent action.

The results of the study looking at the family's subjective feelings about one another thus confirm those of our previous observational study. We interpret this to imply that parents whose behaviour appears to us to be hostile and rejecting, themselves feel rejected by their child. They feel exhausted and demoralized, and desire a sense of recognition or positive endorsement from their children, which is not forthcoming. The parents have reversed roles and moved into the 'child position', a shift which the child experiences as disturbing. They experience the parents as no longer autonomous or in control and yearn for an expression of a greater sense of decisiveness or safety. Because of this shift in roles, these families on assessment at interview come across as lacking structure. Fitting the results of the two studies together suggests the following conclusions.

(i) Subjective self-reports and objective observations both emphasize the relevance and validity of the family or system-orientated perspective. It is clear that the family has an enormous influence on the outcome of therapy.

(ii) These results also serve to demonstrate the limits of therapy. Successful therapy depends to a large degree on what the patient and the family bring with them into therapy. This does not mean that one should become fatalistic about the effectiveness of therapeutic intervention. However, it does mean that we should be more attentive in trying to address family-related factors which have a significant influence on outcome. How can we encourage and develop a process in which the parent is seen by the child as becoming more decisive, self-assured and competent whilst the parents feel less of a sense of rejection from their children?

Meta-analyses

Methodology and general results

The aim of meta-analyses in psychotherapeutic research is to summarize the results of a number of studies in a systematic manner. Through the statistical accumulation and integration of relevant data, an overview of the current state of knowledge can be achieved. Smith et al. (1980) have used the term 'effect size' as a quantitative measure of the efficacy of a therapeutic intervention. The effect size, e.g. Cohen's *d* is calculated by dividing the difference of the mean values of the therapy group and the untreated control group at the end of the treatment period, by the standard deviation of the control group. With this standardized measure, different studies can be compared directly with one another. The measure is constructed such that positive values reflect a positive therapeutic effect. Thus, an effect size of 1 indicates that the average results of the therapy group are one standard deviation better than those of the untreated control group.

The meta-analyses performed by Smith et al. (1980), which looked predominantly at psychotherapy in adults, independent of the psychotherapeutic approach, found an average effect size of 0.85. Thus the average values obtained in the psychotherapeutically treated patients were 0.85 standard deviations higher (better) than those of the control group. Expressed in percentages, this means that the results of the average psychotherapeutically treated patient were better than 80% of the untreated patients. Smith et al. also looked at the efficacy of a number of different therapy approaches in comparison with one another. The behavioural methods, e.g. behaviour and cognitive behavioural therapy had the best effect sizes (average effect sizes 0.68–1.13), with non-behavioural therapies, e.g. client centred, insight orientated, psychodynamic scoring somewhat lower (average effect sizes 0.62–0.89). These results have since been replicated (see Grawe et al., 1994). There remains, however, controversy as to how to interpret these meta-analyses and what conclusions can be drawn from them.

The calculation of effect size (as defined above) depends on the comparison of a treated group and an untreated control group. When this comparison is not possible, because of the lack of an untreated control group (which is often the case), it is nevertheless possible to calculate an analogous measure, which is valid, but not identical to that described above. In this calculation, for each treatment group, the measure used is the difference between pre- and post-treatment. This is then divided by the pooled standard deviations of the pre-test values of the treated groups (see Grawe et al., 1994). This 'pre–post-effect size', in contrast to Smith's 'control group effect size', includes not only the effects caused by therapeutic interventions, but also non-specific treatment effects and changes relating to spontaneous remission. The 'pre–post effect size' for psychotherapeutic treatments therefore tends to result in somewhat higher, i.e. more favourable values than those of the classical 'control group effect size'.

Using these measures, Grawe et al. (1994) have compiled a comprehensive overview and meta-analysis of the results of a number of studies using the most important psychotherapeutic techniques of psychotherapy in adults. They drew the following conclusions. The improvement in the therapy groups showed an average total pre–post-effect size of 1.21, the improvement in the placebo groups had an average pre–post-effect size of 0.36 (this reflects non-specific placebo effects and spontaneous remission). Subtracting the effect size of the placebo group from the treatment groups, one is left with an average effect size of 0.85, which is astonishingly close to the control group effect size arrived at by Smith et al. (1980) in their meta-analysis.

Effect sizes can also be converted to correlation coefficients (the correlation between the variables 'treatment' and 'improvement'). An effect size of 0.85 is equivalent to a correlation coefficient of 0.39 and an explained variance of 0.15 (see Rosenthal, 1991). The explained variance of only 15% appears rather unimpressive; however, the meaning of this in practical terms can be demonstrated by calculating the binomial effect size display (BESD) (see Rosenthal, 1991). In the BESD, the success or improvement scale is dichotomized (improved/not improved) and the groups are standardized to comprise 100 people. Table 3.7 shows the (rounded off) BESD for an effect size of 0.85.

Results in child and adolescent psychotherapy

In comparison to the work in adults, where a large number of controlled therapy studies have been performed (Grawe et al., 1994 looked at 897 studies), the number of studies in children and adolescents leave a lot to be desired. The most important meta-analyses looking at effectiveness of psychotherapy in children and adolescents are those by Casdey and Berman (1985), Weisz et al.

Table 3.7. Binomial effect size display (BESD) for an effect size of 0.85

	No significant improvement	Significant improvement	Total
Psychotherapy treatment group	30	70	100
Control group without psychotherapy	70	30	100
Total	100	100	

Adapted from Rosenthal (1991).

(1987) and Kazdin et al. (1990). A good review article has been put together by Heekerens (1989b).

Casdey and Berman (1985) analysed 64 studies with untreated control groups published between 1952 and 1983 looking at the effectiveness of psychotherapy (both behavioural and non-behavioural) in children under 13. They found an average effect size of 0.71. This means that treated children showed a better outcome than 76% of the untreated control children. For the behavioural methods, the effect size was calculated as 1.0 and for the non-behavioural methods, 0.4. A problem with this calculation was that the measurements used to assess the behavioural treatments were often similar to the procedures used in therapy. Thus, children were trained to achieve certain skills, which were then measured in the post-test assessments. The exclusion of such studies reduced the difference in effect size between behavioural and non-behavioural methods (0.55 vs. 0.34). The authors also demonstrated that the effect sizes were dependent on the measures used, the sources of information (teachers, parents, therapists, etc.) and the nature of symptoms. For example, better scores were achieved when the outcome of anxiety or phobias was looked at. A weakness of this meta-analysis was that the majority of the studies included patients who were especially recruited and only a relatively small percentage of studies (24%) used clinical patients. This raises questions about the representativeness of the study.

Weisz et al. (1987) analysed 163 therapeutic studies in their meta-analysis of the therapy of children between 4 and 18 years of age. They found a mean effect size of 0.79. The treated children thus lay, on average, on the 79th percentile of the control group. The behavioural therapeutic methods used consisting of 126 studies, had a better effect size (0.88) than the 27 studies using non-behavioural methods (0.44). Here also, this difference was reduced considerably when studies using measures similar to the treatment procedures were excluded. Only three studies used psychodynamic therapies and here the mean effect size was negligible (0.01). A further important result was that children under the age of 12 had a considerably better effect size than adolescents.

Kazdin et al. (1990) undertook a meta-analysis of 108 studies of children between the ages of 4 and 18. The majority of interventions were behavioural or cognitive behavioural, although Kazdin et al. did not compare the therapeutic methods with one another. They found an overall mean effect size of 0.88 (comparing treatment groups with true non-treatment control groups). Comparison with placebo-controlled groups revealed a mean effect size of 0.77.

Hazelrigg et al. (1987) and Markus et al. (1990) have undertaken meta-analyses in the discipline of family therapy. Both analyses looked at approximately 20 studies (10 were included in both analyses). Hazelrigg et al. found an effect size of 0.46 (looking at family interaction measures) and 0.5 (for child behavioural measures). Markus et al. found a somewhat more impressive mean effect size of 0.7.

In summary, the following conclusions can be drawn.

- The number of studies available for inclusion in a meta-analysis of psychotherapy in children is considerably smaller than that in adults. Less than 10% of controlled psychotherapy studies have been performed in children or adolescents. It cannot be taken for granted that studies in adults are relevant to children and adolescents and for this reason it is important that further work in this is carried out.
- The available studies make it clear, however, that psychotherapy in children and adolescents is effective. Significant differences are apparent not only in comparison with untreated control groups, but also with placebo-controlled groups, where a number of other non specific factors may come into play. The effect sizes of therapies with children and adolescents are comparable to those found in adult psychotherapy.
- Children under the age of 12 appear to have a considerably better treatment effect compared with adolescents. The likelihood of a successful outcome is further influenced by a number of other factors, e.g. the nature of the disorder.
- There are also consistent differences apparent between different treatment methods. Behavioural techniques appear to be more effective than non-behavioural techniques, whilst techniques such as client-centred and family therapies are more effective than psychodynamically orientated therapies.
- The differences found should be interpreted with care as there remain a number of methodological problems running through all the studies. The majority of controlled studies have used recruited subjects and can therefore

not be considered representative of the general clinical population. In addition, a number of other factors have been shown to influence the results; not only the measurements made, e.g. content, source of information and assessor but also the theoretical orientation of the researcher has been shown to have a clear influence on the results obtained (Shirk and Russell, 1992).

Summary and further open questions

Although there are considerable deficits in the research on psychotherapy in children and adolescents, considerable steps forward have been taken in recent years that have added to our knowledge in this area (see Reinecke, 1993).

(i) Many studies are in concordance with the view that traditional long-term psychotherapy is less effective than short-term focused psychotherapeutic interventions (Rutter, 1983). As in adults, behavioural and cognitive behavioural techniques appear to be most effective. Also of value, although probably less effective, are client-centred and family therapy. Psychodynamic approaches show less promising results; however, one should be cautious when drawing conclusions, because considerable methodological difficulties, e.g. small number of methodologically well-founded studies have to be taken into account.

(ii) An active role of the therapist, as has been shown in adults, is more effective than a reserved or detached relationship.

(iii) The perceptions and beliefs of the patient and family are of considerable importance and should be borne in mind during therapy. Weisz (1986) found that the chances of success were considerably improved when patients became convinced that their problems were solvable and when they had confidence that the therapist would be able to help them.

(iv) The development of a trusting relationship with the therapist appears to be of central importance for the course and success of therapy, just as in adults.

There remain a number of unanswered issues regarding psychotherapy in children, which urgently need addressing.

- The development of effective therapeutic methods for conduct disorders and antisocial behaviour. There have been far fewer studies performed in this area in comparison to internalizing disorders.
- Further research into the therapeutic process. This area relates not only to the interaction between therapist and patient but also to the complex interactions between child and parents, which needs to be looked at in more detail.
- The comparison of effectiveness of different therapeutic methods and therapeutic programmes. The evaluation of psychotherapeutic techniques and treatment programmes still needs to be developed more in the future.

- Assessment of combination of psychotherapeutic treatments with other treatment modalities, e.g. medication. Again here, relatively little work has been done in this area, which is likely to be of increasing importance in the years to come.

REFERENCES

Barkley, R. A. (1988). The effects of methylphenidate on the interaction of preschool ADHD with their mothers. *Journal of the American Academy of Child and Adolescent Psychiatry*, 27, 336–41.

Casdey, R. J. and Berman, J. S. (1985). The outcome of psychotherapy with children. *Psychological Bulletin*, **98**, 388–400.

Eisert, H-G. (1986). Programmevaluation. Definitorische, konzeptuelle und praktische Probleme. In *Therapieevaluation in der Kinder- und Jugendpsychiatrie*, ed. H. Remschmidt and M. H. Schmidt, pp. 1–23. Stuttgart, Enke.

Grawe, K. (1997). Research-informed psychotherapy. *Psychotherapy Research*, **7**, 1–19.

Grawe, K., Donati, R. and Bernauer, F. (1994). *Psychotherapie im Wandel. Von der Konfession zur Profession*, 3rd edn. Göttingen: Hogrefe.

Hazelrigg, M. D., Cooper, H. M. and Borduin, C. M. (1987). Evaluating the effectiveness of family therapies. An integrative review and analysis. *Psychological Bulletin*, **101**, 428–42.

Heekerens, H-P. (1989a). *Familientherapie und Erziehungsberatung*. Heidelberg: Asanger.

Heekerens, H-P. (1989b). Effektivität von Kinder- und Jugendlichenpsychotherapie im Spiegel von Meta-Analysen. *Zeitschrift für Kinder- und Jugendpsychiatrie*, **17**, 150–7.

Kazdin, A. E. (1991). Treatment research. The investigation and evaluation of psychotherapy. In *The clinical psychology handbook*, 2nd edn, ed. M. Hersen, A. E. Kazdin and A. S. Bellack, pp. 293–312. New York: Pergamon Press.

Kazdin, A. E., Bass, D., Ayers, W. A. and Rodgers, A. (1990). Empirical and clinical focus of child and adolescent psychotherapy research. *Journal of Consulting and Clinical Psychology*, **58**, 729–40.

King, C. E. and Goldstein M. J. (1979). Therapist ratings of achievement of objectives in psychotherapy with acute schizophrenics. *Schizophrenia Bulletin*, **5**, 118–29.

Luborsky, L., Chandler, M., Auerbach, A., Cohjen, J. and Bachrach, H. (1971). Factors influencing the outcome of psychotherapy. A review of quantitative research. *Psychological Bulletin*, **75**, 145–85.

Markus, E., Lange, A. and Pettigrew, T. F. (1990). Effectiveness of family therapy. A meta-analysis. *Journal of Family Therapy*, **12**, 205–21.

Martin, M. (1991). *Der Verlauf der Schizophrenie im Jugendalter unter Rehabilitationsbedingungen*. Stuttgart: Enke.

Mash, E. J. and Johnston, C. (1982). A comparison of the mother–child interactions of younger and older hyperactive and normal children. *Child Development*, **53**, 1371–81.

Mattejat, F. (1993). *Subjektive Familienstrukturen*. Göttingen: Hogrefe.

Mattejat, F. and Remschmidt, H. (1988). Explorative Untersuchung methodischer Fragen und Probleme. In *Alternative Behandlungsformen in der Kinder- und Jugendpsychiatrie. Stationäre Behandlung, tagesklinische Behandlung und Home-Treatment im Vergleich*, ed. H. Remschmdt and M. H. Schmidt, pp. 81–101. Stuttgart: Enke.

Mattejat, F. and Remschmidt, H. (1989). Family variables as predictors of differential effectiveness in child therapy. In: *Children at risk. Assessment, longitudinal research and intervention*, ed. M. Brambring, F. Lösel and F. Skowrinek, pp. 440–56. Berlin: de Gruyter.

Mattejat, F. and Remschmidt, H. (1991). Die Bedeutung der familialen Beziehungsdynamik für den Erfolg stationärer Behandlungen in der Kinder- und Jugendpsychiatrie. *Zeitschrift für Kinder und Jugendpsychiatric*, **19**, 139 50.

Mattejat, F., Gutenbrunner, C. and Remschmidt, H. (1994). Therapeutische Leistungen einer kinder- und jugendpsychiatrischen Universitätsklinik mit regionalem Versorgungsauftrag und ihrer assoziierten Einrichtungen. *Zeitschrift für Kinder- und Jugendpsychiatrie*, **22**, 154–68.

Mattejat, F. and Scholz, M. (1994). *Das subjektive Familienbild*. Göttingen: Hogrefe.

Mintz, J. and Luborsky, L. (1979). Measuring the outcomes of psychotherapy: findings of the PENN Psychotherapy Project. *Journal of Consulting and Clinical Psychology*, **47**, 319–34.

Podeswik, A., Ehlert, U., Altherr, P. and Hellhammer, D. (1995). Verhaltenstherapie bei Kindern und Jugendlichen. Eine versorgungsepidemiologische Untersuchung. *Zeitschrift für Kinder- und Jugendpsychiatrie*, **21**, 149–60.

Reinecke, M. A. (1993). Outpatient treatment of mild psychopathology. In *Handbook of clinical research and practice with adolescents*, ed. P. H. Tolan and B. J. Cohler, pp. 387–410. New York: Wiley.

Remschmidt, H. and Martin, M. (1992). Die Therapie der Schizophrenie im Jugendalter. *Deutsches Ärzteblatt*, **89**, 387–96.

Remschmidt, H. and Mattejat, F. (1994). Psychotherapeutische Ansätze in der Behandlung von Kindern und Jugendlichen. *Monatsschrift für Kinderheilkunde*, **142**, 250–7.

Remschmidt, H. and Schmidt, M. H. (1988). Alternative Behandlungsformen in der Kinder- und Jugendpsychiatrie. Stuttgart: Enke.

Remschmidt, H., Schmidt, M. H., Mattejat, F., Eisert, H-G. and Eisert, M. (1988). Therapieevaluation in der Kinder- und Jugendpsychiatrie. Stationäre Behandlung, tagesklinische Behandlung und home treatment im Vergleich. *Zeitschrift für Kinder- und Jugendpsychiatrie*, **16**, 124–34.

Rosenthal, R. (1991). *Meta-analytic procedures for social research*. London: Sage.

Rutter, M. (1983). Psychological therapies. Issues and prospects. In *Childhood psychopathology and development*, ed. S. B. Guze, F. J. Earls and J. E. Barrett. New York: Raven Press.

Shirk, S. R. and Russell, R. L. (1992). A reevaluation of estimates of child therapy effectiveness. *Journal of the American Academy of Child and Adolescent Psychiatry*, **31**, 703–9.

Smith, M. L., Glass, G. V. and Miller, T. I. (1980). *The benefits of psychotherapy*. Baltimore: Johns Hopkins University Press.

Weisz, J. R. (1986). Contingency and control beliefs as predictors of psychotherapy outcomes among children and adolescents. *Journal of Consulting and Clinical Psychology*, **54**, 789–95.

Weisz, J. R., Weiss, B., Alicke, M. D. and Klotz, M. L. (1987). Effectiveness of clinic-based psychotherapy with children and adolescents. *Journal of Consulting and Clinical Psychology*, **55**, 542–9.

Wuchner, M. and Eckert, J. (1995). Frequenz – Dauer – Setting in der Gesprächspsychotherapie heute. Teil 2: Klientenzentrierte Einzelpsychotherapie bei Kindern und Jugendlichen. *GwG Zeitschrift*, **26**, 17–20.

4 Quality assurance

Fritz Mattejat

Introduction

The concepts of quality assurance and quality management (here used synonymously), which were originally developed by the business community, are now seen as being of increasing importance in the health services of today (see Schramm, 1994; Riordan and Mockler, 1997). Quality assurance is intended to be of benefit not only to the interests of the patients, but also to the contractors in health services. For the insurance companies for example, financial considerations are of primary concern: they only want to reimburse that diagnostic or therapeutic work which has been recognized by the profession as justifiable and appropriate. For the professionals (providers), here in particular those from the discipline of Child and Adolescent Psychotherapy, the most important issues are to have the diagnostic and therapeutic procedures which they see as being necessary recognized, and to work towards an improvement in the standards of their practice which will further benefit patients. Quality assurance should protect the patient from inappropriate management and treatment by unqualified personnel. Each patient should be provided with the best treatment available, within the known limitations of the system. As a result of the different interests of the providers and the contractors, conflicts are not uncommon. When planning and trying to implement quality assurance measures, it is necessary to bear these potential conflicts of interest in mind and to attempt to balance them in an appropriate manner.

Definitions and setting standards

The terms quality, quality assessment and quality assurance have been defined by Eichhorn (1993) as follows:

Quality is the sum of characteristics, which it is deemed must be fulfilled by a product or service according to predetermined standards which have been set. It follows that quality assessment should assess whether and to what degree the characteristics of the actual product or service deviate from those prerequisites. A quality assurance system can be set up to implement a systematic analysis of any deviations detected and institute corrective measures to ensure that future quality deficits are minimised or avoided.

From these definitions it is clear that 'quality' is not an absolute characteristic, but can be defined only in terms of predetermined aims or standards. This results in considerable variation in the interpretation of the term by different professional groups. As well as economic (business) and objectively determined quality characteristics, e.g. the objective efficacy of therapeutic interventions, a number of more subjective aspects can also be considered, e.g. patient acceptability of aspects of treatment, general levels of satisfaction, etc. The Deutsche Institut für Normung [German Institute for Standards] has produced a document: 'Quality Management and Elements of Quality Assurance Systems' (DIN, 1992) relating to health care institutions and services which emphasises 'customer satisfaction': 'The establishment and maintenance of a satisfactory level of quality is dependent on the systematic application of a quality management system, whose task is to ensure that the requirements of customers are understood and fulfilled.' Several German insurance agencies also express this view but with a different emphasis, namely, that the aim of the quality assurance system in health settings should be the achievement of transparency, efficacy and efficiency (VDR, 1992).

Quality management in health care systems can be therefore seen as operating on three different levels.

(i) On a subjective measure of quality assessment through patients, relatives and personnel (doctors, psychologists, nursing staff and paramedical staff), whereby the satisfaction of patients is usually given predominant weight.

(ii) On objective quality indicators (e.g. benefit and efficacy of interventions, unwanted side effects, etc.).

(iii) And finally, on the efficiency (cost–benefit analysis) of the work undertaken whereby cost does not only imply financial considerations but also other costs, e.g. time, anxiety or stress caused by treatments, etc. The economic efficiency should only be considered as one part of this equation, even though it is often given overriding importance.

Dimensions of quality assurance: scope, tasks

Aspects

Donabedian (1966) defined three aspects of quality assurance. This subdivision has subsequently been integrated into the legal framework: The structural quality of care comprises the demographic, financial and material aspects of the care institution, including for example, available personnel resources and the qualification of medical and paramedical professionals. The process quality of health care relates to the quality of the treatments offered and the manner in which these are organised. Finally, the outcome quality relates to the effectiveness and the efficiency with which diagnostic and therapeutic procedures are performed and the outcomes of such interventions.

Scope

The concept of quality assurance can be applied across a number of different areas of health care:

- diagnostic procedures,
- therapeutic interventions,
- nursing and educational tasks,
- organizational or administrative aspects such as finance, bed capacity and provision of food.

In addition to these areas, which are concentrated on patient care, the principles of quality assurance can also be applied to other areas such as the basic and specialist training of clinical and non clinical personnel.

Tasks

The implementation of quality assurance in the above-mentioned areas requires a number of prerequisites to be fulfilled:

(i) The definition of quality standards and criteria (the intended standards)
(ii) The assessment and documentation of the current situation (the actual standard being achieved)
(iii) A comparison of the intended and actual standards (a comparative analysis)
(iv) The planning and implementation of measures to correct any shortcomings detected with the aim of improving the quality of patient care (see also Wilkinson et al., 1994; Firth-Cozens, 1993).

These tasks can be further specified, together they are often referred to as 'quality management system' (DIN, 1992). For further information see the document produced by the British Working Party on Audit in Child Psychiatry (1991), and 'Focus on Clinical Audit', College Research Unit, Royal College of Psychiatrists (Hardmann and Joughin, 1998).

Two levels of activity can be distinguished: first, the development of quality assurance systems and secondly, the concrete realization of such systems in clinical practice, in hospitals, clinics and other psychotherapeutic institutions. The first of these levels is determined to some degree by legal requirements and comprises the development of general principles of psychotherapeutic quality management. Quality standards need to be defined for different institutions or departments, which then act as guidelines to be reviewed and revised as necessary. In addition, means of collecting, storing and analysing data must be developed in order to enable the implementation of the desired measures. It may also be necessary to design pilot studies to assess the quality of the measures put in place. Institutions should also participate in local, regional and supra-regional working parties or committees to ensure the development of consensual guidelines across geographical boundaries. The second level, the concrete implementation of these systems in clinical practice, can be facilitated through local quality assurance committees or working parties whose task it is to assess how the general guidelines can be interpreted in a way meaningful and relevant to the local setting, and to set in motion mechanisms by which they can be implemented locally. This often demands extensive discussion within the working party, the consideration of representations from a number of interested parties, the assessment and analysis of existing local data and the promotion of skills required for audit, through the provision of training for staff.

Development of quality standards

When developing standards for quality assurance, the following questions should be addressed:

- Which diagnostic and therapeutic procedures should be available for which patients?
- What are the indication criteria which need to be met in order for these procedures to be realizable?
- How can these procedures be realized in practice?
- What are the prerequisites (e.g. institutional characteristics, qualification of personnel, etc.) which need to be fulfilled?
- How can the quality features of these procedures be measured, documented, controlled and improved?

The development of quality standards for patient care should be based on analyses of need and the results of scientific research. In the discipline of Child and Adolescent Psychiatry and Psychotherapy there is still considerable controversy as to how these standards should be set and developed (Mattejat and Remschmidt, 1995; Schmidt and Nübling, 1994).

The 'Working Group on Quality Issues' of the American Academy of Child and Adolescent Psychiatry (AACAP) has set quality standards ('practice parameters') for diagnostic procedures, therapeutic interventions, and outcome in various disorders (AACAP, 1997). These documents set down:

(i) which diagnostic procedures should be carried out in the presence of certain symptoms (for example, following information obtained through the personal history of the child, the family history, the mental state examination etc.);

(ii) what features are necessary for a diagnosis to be applied and which investigations should be carried out to exclude potential differential diagnoses;

(iii) what the essential components of a treatment programme should be, which components of treatment are of proven value and which aspects should be observed or assessed over the course of therapy.

Most of the proposals made are deliberately general and non-specific, particularly those concerning therapeutic aspects. Possible therapeutic measures are listed, but there is rarely any reference to more specific details of indications or therapeutic implementation. Summaries of these practice parameters are available on the internet (http://www.aacap.org).

These attempts at the development of quality standards in Child and Adolescent Psychiatry serve to demonstrate the difficulties involved in determining quality criteria and should act as a reminder of the limitations of this activity. A fundamental problem is how generalized or specific criteria should be: quality criteria cannot simply replicate the diagnostic scheme of the ICD or DSM classificatory systems, neither can they constitute a therapeutic manual. The most they can hope to achieve is to emphasize the most important and relevant aspects on which to concentrate during assessment or treatment. Likewise, much more than knowledge of these quality standards is required in order to carry out the relevant diagnostic procedures or treatment. What the quality standards can, however, offer is a simplified and therefore more transparent and comparable understanding of the important issues of the disorder, and despite their inadequacies, the current standards can be seen as a useful adjuvant which needs further work to improve their precision and usefulness. A further consideration is whether disorder specific standards are the most appropriate means of setting and applying standards. An alternative is to set general standards with respect, for example, what should be achieved at an outpatient assessment with a psychiatrically disordered child or adolescent, and to give the diagnostic standards secondary consideration. Working within this model, it would then be possible to develop standards for other working modalities such as crisis intervention, etc.

Analysis and documentation

The acquisition, synthesis and documentation of data in the clinical setting can present serious problems and in this respect much can be gained by looking at the similar activities carried out in research projects, which make similar demands (see Esser et al., 1990; Remschmidt and Walter, 1989, 1990; Grawe et al., 1994; Grawe, 1997; Remschmidt and Schmidt, 1988 for further details relating to data collection in epidemiological, health care and therapeutic evaluation research, respectively). In many clinics data collection systems will already be in place which can then be utilized, with modifications where necessary, for quality assurance or audit (see Remschmidt, 1988; Wienand, 1993). The data collection needs to be as accurate and as complete as possible, and consideration should be given to developing economic, practicable and efficient means of data collection so as not to unnecessarily place an additional burden on staff.

The basic data which need to be collected are listed in Table 4.1 along with suggestions as to what should be encompassed. The last question is likely to present the most difficulties, but reflects the most important aspect, relating to assessment of the quality of the intervention. A particular problem relates to the issue that there are still no universally accepted methods relating to process and outcome quality. This issue raises fundamental questions which have not yet been adequately assessed (see Callias, 1992; Parry, 1992). For example, therapeutic evaluation is primarily understood to mean assessment of therapeutic outcome. Process variables, i.e. the means by which success is achieved are often neglected. If success is measured simply by the responsible therapist with a rating scale, i.e. in terms of symptom improvement, a number of problems will be encountered (subjectivity, therapist bias, etc.). On the other hand, the use of objective measures of therapeutic success is often considered too time-consuming and expensive for routine use in the clinical setting.

This issue has been looked at in more detail by Mattejat and Remschmidt (1993), who have developed an instrument which is appropriate to the clinical setting. The Therapy Evaluation Questionnaire (TEQ) (see Table 4.2) provides the opportunity to assess and document the quality of treatment from a number of different perspectives. The instrument is applicable regardless of the nature of the therapeutic intervention carried out and can be used in both inpatient and outpatient settings. It is relatively quick and easy to complete and is therefore appropriate for use in a wide range of clinical settings in the field of Child and Adolescent Psychotherapy and Psychiatry. It exists in three versions: for therapist, patient and parents. The scales, which are calculated in each

Table 4.1. Collection and documentation of data relevant to quality assurance

Question	Data collection/ documentation	Area	Example
Who undertakes which tasks under which conditions?	Documentation of individual and structural characteristics	Characteristics of the quality within the structure (institutional and personal characteristics)	Type of worker; their assignments and qualifications; diagnostic and therapeutic capability and their means of recompense
For whom and for what indications?	Demographic documentation	Patient and environmental characteristics	Age, sex, social characteristics; diagnostic and symptom profile
What is undertaken?	Documentation of the nature of the intervention	Type, extent and expense of intervention	Main diagnostic or therapeutic procedures, their duration and frequency of application
What level of quality is achieved?	Objective quality measures	Benefit and effectivity of the utilized intervention	Effectivity of therapies through pre- and post-assessment with standardized instruments
	Subjective quality measures	Subjective quality of care provided and treatment satisfaction	Assessment of treatment satisfaction by patients, relatives and clinical personnel

version were defined on the basis of factor analyses. In all three versions, there are two main components to the assessment: the 'success' and the 'acceptability' of the treatment (the therapy satisfaction). The 'success' component relates to the effectiveness and efficiency of the treatment, whilst the 'acceptability'

Table 4.2. Overview of the Treatment Evaluation Questionnaire (TEQ)

TEQ-Questionnaire	Abbreviation of subscale	Name of subscale	Aspect of quality measured
Therapist version TEQ-T	Scale 1: patient success	Therapeutic success with regard to the patient	Outcome
	Scale 2: family success	Therapeutic success with regard to the family	
	Scale 3: patient cooperation	Cooperation with the patient	Process
	Scale 4: mother cooperation	Cooperation with the mother	
	Scale 5: father cooperation	Cooperation with the father	
Adolescent version TEQ-A	Scale 1: success	Success of treatment	Outcome
(Patient version)	Scale 2: relationship	Relationship to the therapist	Process
	Scale 3: nuisance	Degree of nuisance associated with therapy	
Parent version TEQ-P	Scale 1: success	Success of treatment	Outcome
	Scale 2: relationship	Relationship to the therapist, attitude towards the hospital or clinic, general satisfaction	Process

component attempts to measure the quality of the co-operation, the nature of the therapeutic relationship achieved, the negative stresses caused by treatment and general satisfaction. Thus the questionnaire aims to give equal weight to aspects of results and process (see Crombie and Davies, 1998).

Use to date has shown the questionnaire to be a reliable instrument in the subjective assessment of quality of treatment. Agreement between the three groups has been shown to be limited, showing that the treatment is often differently appraised by the various participants, which emphasises the importance of this multiple-perspective approach to assessment.

Future tasks and problems

Having developed standards and obtained information on the nature of the current manner in which health services are being offered, the next step is the comparison of these data and their utilization to improve the delivery of health care. The data obtained inevitably refer to a number of different areas and the integration of this data into a meaningful result can be difficult. (How to weigh up and compare the importance of economic factors and patient satisfaction together?) Ways have been proposed in the field of evaluation research as to how this can be meaningfully undertaken (see Wottawa and Thierau, 1990). Finally, methods need to be developed to feed this data back and implement changes to improve health care delivery. Here, it is useful to borrow from the work which has been undertaken in the business world (controlling) and from methods developed in occupational psychology which can be further developed for use in the field of psychotherapy (see Doppler and Lauterburg, 1994; Schuler, 1993). The process of quality assurance in the field of Child and Adolescent Psychotherapy still includes a wealth of unresolved issues; however, we are beginning to be able to recognize possible solutions to some of these problems.

The future development of this area will, nevertheless, require a degree of restructuring in the way that we are used to thinking about these issues.

- The development of generally accepted quality criteria requires the acceptance that, in psychotherapy, as in all other areas of health care, objectifiable and refutable criteria must be utilized. Objectivation means that standards and criteria will have to be developed which are relevant to all psychotherapeutic schools. This implies changes in the therapeutic ideology: the importance of psychotherapeutic schools decreases.
- An essential feature of quality assurance is the aspect of 'control'. That is the preparedness to permit therapeutic and organizational activities to be open to external and internal review. One of the aims of quality assurance is to achieve maximal transparency in health care services. Psychotherapy must move from its previous position of cryptic, opaque closed shop to a more open, accessible discipline welcoming or at least tolerant of being observed and criticized. This change is required not only of the discipline, but also of the professionals working within it. It is well known from the experience of supervision groups

that the open presentation of individual work can be a precarious business even when only in front of colleagues.

- The transparency gained as a result of new working methods will inevitably lead also to a change in the patient–therapist relationship. Quality assurance means the exchange of information and involvement of the patient in treatment planning. Decisions should be made, wherever possible not only for, but with, the patient. Authoritative or paternalistic behaviour will become obsolete. Therapy will need to be seen not longer as a one-sided intervention, but rather as a problem-specific and time-limited collaborative cooperation between therapist, patient and relatives.

Quality assurance thus represents a modern developmental trend, which offers enormous possibilities for positive change. The potential dangers must, however, also be recognized. If undertaken without due care to accuracy, competence and ethical considerations, the measures could lead to worsening health care delivery. In this respect, the following issues are particularly important.

- Quality standards should not be allowed to handicap or hinder innovative developments. If quality standards are defined in too restrictive or narrow a manner, or become immovable or 'written in stone' over a long period of time, it will be difficult or impossible for new methods, or developments, to become incorporated in health care. Standards only make sense if they are continually reviewed and revised where necessary.
- Quality assurance should not lead to excess bureaucracy. If measures used to obtain data in quality assurance exercises are perceived as being too time-consuming, irrelevant, adding to work loads without bringing positive benefit, or taking away valuable time from face-to-face patient work, not only will morale suffer, but the quality of the data obtained will also deteriorate. The implementation of quality assurance systems must therefore always be accompanied by measures to protect both therapist and patient from unnecessary bureaucracy.

REFERENCES

American Academy of Child and Adolescent Psychiatry (AACAP) (1997). Practice parameters. *Journal of the American Academy of Child and Adolescent Psychiatry*, **36**(10), pp. 1S–202S (Supplement).

British Working Party on Audit in Child Psychiatry (1991). *Audit in child psychiatry*. Document.

Callias, M. (1992). Evaluation of interventions with children and adolescents. In *Child and adolescent therapy. A handbook*, ed. D. A. Lane and A. Miller, pp. 39–64. Buckingham: Open

University Press.

Crombie, I. and Davies H. (1998). Beyond health outcomes. The advantages of measuring process. *Journal of Evaluation in Clinical Practice*, **4**, 31–8.

Deutsches Institut für Normung (DIN) (ed.) (1992). *DIN ISO 9004, Teil 2. Qualitätsmanagement und Elemente eines Qualitätssicherungssystems. Leitfaden für Dienstleistungen*. Berlin: DIN.

Donabedian, A. (1966). Evaluating the quality of medical care. *Milbank Memorial Fund Quarterly*, **44**, 166–203.

Doppler, K. and Lauterburg, C. (1994). *Change management. Den Unternehmenswandel gestalten*. Frankfurt: Campus.

Eichhorn, S. (1993). Qualitätssicherung im Krankenhaus als ärztliche Aufgabe. In *Förderung der medizinischen Qualitätssicherung durch den Bundesminister für Gesundheit*, ed. Projektträgerschaft 'Forschung im Dienste der Gesundheit' in der Deutschen Forschungsanstalt für Luft- und Raumfahrt, pp. 35–54. Bonn.

Esser, G., Schmidt, M. H. and Woerner, W. (1990). Epidemiology and course of psychiatric disorders in school-age children. Results of a longitudinal study. *Journal of Child Psychology and Psychiatry*, **31**, 243–63.

Firth-Cozens, J. (1993). *Audit in mental health services*. Hove: Earlbaum.

Grawe, K. (1997). Research-informed psychotherapy. *Psychotherapy Research*, **7**, 1–19.

Grawe, K., Donati, R. and Bernauer, F. (1994). *Psychotherapie im Wandel. Von der Konfession zur Profession*, 3rd edn. Göttingen: Hogrefe.

Hardmann, E. and Joughin, C. (1998). *Focus on clinical audit in child and adolescent mental health services*. Gaskell.

Mattejat, F. and Remschmidt, H. (1993). Evaluation von Therapien mit psychisch kranken Kindern und Jugendlichen. Entwicklung und Überprüfung eines Fragebogens zur Beurteilung der Behandlung (FBB). *Zeitschrift für Klinische Psychologie*, **22**, 192–233.

Mattejat, F. and Remschmidt, H. (1995). Aufgaben und Probleme der Qualitätssicherung in der Psychiatrie und Psychotherapie des Kindes- und Jugendalters. *Zeitschrift für Kinder- und Jugendpsychiatrie*, **23**, 71–83.

Parry, G. (1992). Improving psychotherapy services. Applications of research, audit and evaluation. *British Journal of Clinical Psychology*, **31**, 3–19.

Remschmidt, H. (ed.) (1988). *Siebenjahresbericht 1981–1987. Klinik und Poliklinik für Kinder- und Jugendpsychiatrie der Philipps-Universität*. Marburg.

Remschmidt, H. and Schmidt, M. H. (1988). *Alternative Behandlungsformen in der Kinder- und Jugendpsychiatrie. Stationäre Behandlung, tagesklinische Behandlung und Home-Treatment im Vergleich*. Stuttgart: Enke.

Remschmidt, H. and Walter, R. (1989). *Evaluation kinder- und jugendpsychiatrischer Versorgung. Analysen und Erhebungen in drei hessischen Landkreisen*. Stuttgart: Enke.

Remschmidt, H. and Walter, R. (1990). *Psychische Auffälligkeiten bei Schulkindern. Mit deutschen Normen für die Child Behavior Checklist*. Göttingen: Hogrefe.

Riordan, J. and Mockler, D. (1997). *Clinical audit in mental health. Towards a multidisciplinary approach*. Chichester: Wiley.

Schmidt, J. and Nübling, R. (1994). Qualitätssicherung in der Psychotherapie. Teil 1: Grundlagen,

Hintergründe und Probleme. *GwG-Zeitschrift*, **96**, 15–25.

Schramm, D. (1994). Qualitatskontrolle in 'Sozialen Einrichtungen'/Nonprofit-Organisationen. *Sozialmagazin*, **19**, 22–8.

Schuler, H. (ed.) (1993). *Lehrbuch Organisationspsychologie*. Bern: Huber.

Verband Deutscher Rentenversicherungsträger (VDR) (ed.) (1992). *Bericht der Reha-Kommission des Verbandes Deutscher Rentenversicherungsträger. Empfehlungen zur Weiterentwicklung der medizinischen Rehabilitation in der gesetzlichen Rentenversicherung*. Frankfurt: VDR.

Wienand, F. (1993). Qualitätssicherung/Therapieevaluation in der Praxis. *Forum der Kinder- und Jugendpsychiatrie und Psychotherapie, Mitgliederrundbrief 2*, pp. 63–4.

Wilkinson, I., McDonald, J. and Searson, S. (1994). Setting and evaluating standards for family services. *Association for Child Psychology and Psychiatry Review and Newsletter*, **16**, 70–6.

Wottawa, H. and Thierau, H. (1990). *Lehrbuch Evaluation*. Bern: Huber.

Part II

Psychotherapeutic methods and settings

5 Psychodynamic therapy

Helmut Remschmidt and Kurt Quaschner

Principles of psychodynamic therapy

The term 'depth psychology' was introduced in 1910 by the Swiss psychiatrist Eugen Bleuler in his publication *Die Psychoanalyse Freuds*. Sigmund Freud first used the term in his publication *Das Interesse an der Psychoanalyse* in 1913, intending to distinguish his ideas from the psychology of conciousness which was dominant at that time (Pongratz, 1983).

Today, the term 'depth psychology' encompasses several different schools of psychotherapy, which are based on similar assumptions. The terms 'psychoanalytically orientated psychotherapy' or 'psychodynamic therapy' are generally considered synonyms. Psychoanalytically orientated therapy is based on the following assumptions:

- the significance of the unconcious for mental functioning and individual behaviour;
- the importance of drives for the determination of human behaviour;
- the importance of developmental phases during which libidinous energy, i.e. drives are variably expressed;
- the belief that symptoms are caused by conflicts determined by specific developmental phases; these symptoms in turn influence the manner in which an individual adapts to his environment;
- the concept of transference, by which the patient projects past emotions and experiences on the therapist, who then interprets the material.

Further common ground between the psychoanalytically orientated schools is discussed in more detail by Pongratz (1983), Greenson (1966) and Brenner (1955). This chapter uses the structural model suggested by Rapaport (1973), in which he distinguishes between several different theoretical aspects of psychoanalytic theory (Table 5.1) (Remschmidt, 1992; Remschmidt and Heinscher, 1988).

Table 5.1. A structural model of psychodynamic psychotherapy

The topical aspect	Almost all psychoanalytically orientated schools have a topical idea of psychic functioning. The most well known is Freud's idea of agencies ('Instanzen'), according to which the human psyche comprises three such agencies: id, ego, and superego. The id is the unconscious source of drives which acts according to the pleasure principle. The ego represents conscious thoughts and actions (reality principle), whilst the superego contains internalized moral values and acts as one's conscience. All three agencies interact vigorously.
(ii) The dynamic aspect	The dynamic aspect is also an important part of psychoanalytically orientated psychology. The term dynamic is used to describe those factors which propel human behaviour: needs, instincts, drives, emotions. Psychoanalytically orientated theory proposes a few distinct drives to explain all behaviour. Initially, Freud assumed only one drive which he designated 'libido'.
(iii) The genetic aspect	The genetic aspect of psychoanalytically orientated psychology reflects human development. The first few years of life are of particular interest, as they fundamentally influence the development of psychiatric disturbance. The most widely acknowledged theory was developed by Freud, and other theories are often just modifications of Freud's ideas. Freud classified child development in five phases: oral, anal, genital or oedipal, latency and a second genital phase. These phases are discussed below. The oral phase extends from birth to the age of about 18 months. During this phase, libido is restricted to the oral region, which has the characteristics of an 'erotogenic area'. The anal phase extends from the age of about 18 months to 3 years old. During this phase the anal region becomes the primary erotogenic area. The phallic phase is also termed first genital or oedipal phase, and extends from about 3–5 years old. During this phase the genital region becomes the primary erotogenic area with which the libido is associated. During this time an 'Oedipus complex' develops, which, briefly, can be summarized as affection of a son towards his mother or a daughter towards her father. The sequelae of this Oedipus complex significantly affect future sexual and social development.

Table 5.1. (*cont.*)

	The subsequent latency period continues from about 6–11 years old. During this period, sexual impulses no longer play any significant role. Such impulses recur in a reinforced way in the course of puberty. Earlier conflicts are reactivated during this second genital phase. In contrast to child development, adolescence has not been of great interest to psychoanalytically orientated theory. Only decades after Freud have theoretical concepts been developed which are as complex and detailed as any theories about early childhood, e.g. Blos (1967).
(iv) The social and cultural aspect	This aspect reflects the influence of environmental factors. Human development is influenced to a great degree by the behavioural rules of one's environment. The degree of social adaptation largely depends upon the individual's identification with those rules. Social and cultural influences also determine the development of ethical and moral standards and one's conscience. Further developments of psychoanalytically orientated theory, such as those elaborated by Anna Freud (1936), cannot be addressed here. In later years, new branches of psychoanlytic theory developed, some based on the work of Hartmann (1964). These newer theories were eventually designated 'ego psychology'.

Modified after Rapaport (1973).

The relationship between psychotherapy in adults, children and adolescents

Prior to discussing psychoanalytically orientated psychotherapy in children and adolescents, the use of this approach in adults needs to be addressed, as this preceded the treatment of children both historically and theoretically. Although the approaches are essentially comparable, the techniques used with children have been modified. However, as the treatment of adults has widely been considered as a reference to which other psychoanalytically orientated treatments are usually compared, this technique will be briefly discussed here, although the practical importance of the approach has decreased considerably.

The classical psychoanalytic technique

The aim of classical psychoanalytic treatment is to lift the constraints of repression by making the unconcious accessible to conciousness. This process is undertaken in a specific situation or 'setting'. The setting is determined by formal factors such as the time, place and frequency of sessions, and specific rules to guide the interaction between patient and therapist. The fundamental rule is that the patient reports all his spontaneous thoughts in a process of free association, i.e. without exerting any control over his/her own thoughts. The rule of abstinence requires that the therapist adopts a passive role in his interaction with the patient. Regression is encouraged as the patient is usually required to lie on a couch without eye contact with the therapist, and regression facilitates keeping the rule of abstinence. Despite regression, the patient is expected to maintain therapeutic rapport with the therapist in order to encourage introspection and ensure the continuation of treatment.

The most important treatment technique is the therapist's interpretation of the patient's revelations during free association. The aim of interpretation is to make the patient concious of previously unconcious pathogenic mechanisms. The material suitable for interpretation includes spontaneous thoughts, dreams, transference and resistance. The term transference designates uncompensated emotional attitudes which persist from early stages of childhood, which the patient shows towards the therapist, i.e. transfers on to him. The term resistance designates the opposition against the psychoanalytic process, i.e. resistance against the therapist's influence and change.

Differences between psychotherapy in adults, children and adolescents

The psychoanalytic approach used with adults cannot be applied to children and adolescents without modifications accommodating the patients' developmental stage. The most important modifications apply to free association, the establishment of therapeutic rapport and transference.

Whilst adolescents maybe have a restricted capability for free association, children almost entirely lack this ability. Rather, free association is replaced in therapy by actions such as activities, games, or outings in adolescents, and by play in children.

Establishing and maintaining therapeutic rapport is usually much more difficult with children and adolescents than with adults. Scharfman (1973) has suggested several explanations:

- children and adolescents usually have no desire to change, which makes it difficult to motivate them for treatment;
- children have a different time perspective, which makes it difficult for them to

anticipate the improvements which may result from treatment;
- children tend to regard problems as being caused by external factors rather than being the result of intrapsychical disorder;
- the ego of children and adolescents tends to be so intensely preoccupied with defence that therapeutic rapport can be difficult to establish or maintain;
- the capacity for introspection (which requires therapeutic splitting of the ego) is reduced or absent;
- particular developmental phases such as the end of the oedipal phase or adolescence are characterized by turning away from the past, which makes therapeutic access difficult.

It has been widely acknowledged that the transference of children and adolescents is unlike that of adults, but the nature of children's and adolescents' transference has remained controversial. For example, it is unclear whether children and adolescents can develop the transference neurosis (or tranference reaction) described in adults.

Modifications of technique

The modifications necessary due to differences between children and adults have resulted in play becoming as an essential part of psychoanalytically orientated child psychotherapy. Therapy with adolescents has resulted in significant modifications of the treatment setting, e.g. dispensing with the couch.

Comprehensive modifications of long-term individual psychotherapy have also been undertaken. Some of the more recent approaches derived from psychoanalytically orientated psychotherapy include crisis intervention, group and family therapy (Seiffge-Krenke, 1986; Müller-Küppers, 1988).

Seiffge-Krenke (1986) has suggested several guidelines for the treatment of children and adolescents:
- psychoanalytically orientated psychotherapy with children and adolescents should be directive;
- the therapist needs to be more flexible and active with his techniques than when treating adults; he needs to consent to any practical suggestions the patient may have;
- adolescents should not be exposed to the same degree of frustration as adults might be; this, for example, applies to extended periods of silence, boredom, or elaborate interventions;
- regression must be dealt with very carefully; the therapist needs to give adolescents much more assistance during reality testing than adults, and encourage ego function.

Treatment with children

Treatment with children should always take into account the child's developmental stage. This determines the required modifications of technique.

It is possible to divide treatment according to whether it occurs before or during latency, approximately equivalent to the treatment of preschoolers and schoolchildren, respectively. Some authors further restrict the period before latency to the phallic-oedipal phase, as the developmental prerequisites for psychoanalytically orientated therapy are supposed to be absent until this age (Scharfman, 1973). Two arguments have been used to support this view. First, internalized conflicts do not occur prior to this phase, and second, a stable representation of objects has developed by this time, so that transference is possible. This does not mean that psychoanalytic theory cannot be applied to younger children; however, it is doubtful whether therapy at this age can truly be considered psychoanalytically orientated (Scharfman, 1973).

Indications

In contrast to treatment with adults, the indications for psychoanalytically orientated psychotherapy with children have always been rather indistinct (Müller-Küppers, 1988). Thus, different authors propose a wide range of indications for this treatment, and many indications are contradictory. The abilities to internalize conflicts and bring about transference have been mentioned as prerequisites for psychoanalytically orientated treatment.

Childhood neurosis with regression of libido, putting further development at risk, is a clear indication for treatement. Symptoms would include many that develop in the phallic–oedipal phase, such as phobias, conversion reaction, psychosomatic problems, sleep disturbance and obsessive-compulsive symptoms (Scharfman, 1973).

Following Anna Freud, Scharfman (1973) suggests that impairment of ego development through the excessive influence of specific defence mechanisms should be considered a criterion for treatment. For example, defence mechanisms such as reaction formation and isolation may make a child with obsessions appear overadapted and emotionally inhibited, with a tendency to intellectualization.

Any problems in connection with gender roles, e.g. problems with gender identity or perversion may also be regarded as an indication for treatment.

Undertaking treatment

Although psychoanalytically orientated psychotherapy with children has been the focus of more attention than that with adolescents, and several different approaches to treating children have been proposed, no single technique comparable to the treatment of adults has been developed. This is unlikely to occur in the future, because the practical importance of the approach has decreased considerably. A wide range of different schools exist, however, and they do have several common characteristics (Dührssen, 1980).

- As a result of the different role of the therapist treating children, in contrast to adults, the therapeutic relationship may become very close and intimate.
- The high level of parental dependence of a child has a significant influence on the nature of therapy.
- The therapeutic technique must generally be modified according to the child's age and developmental status.
- The use of play, in addition to verbal interactions, means that actions are also permitted in therapy.

In contrast to these common charateristics of psychoanalytically orientated therapy with children, a number of issues continue to be a source of controversy:

- the degree to which parents should be involved in therapy and how they should support treatment;
- the relationship between child therapy and upbringing education;
- the relevance of transference for therapy; and
- the importance of interpretation.

These issues have been extensively discussed in the debate between the schools of Anna Freud and Melanie Klein.

The establishment of therapeutic rapport with children is more difficult and time-consuming than in adults. Anna Freud (1980) attributed this to the fact that children lack the desire to change, and also fail to anticipate treatment success, and generally have not chosen to attend therapy. It has been suggested that children need to be 'trained' to accept psychoanalysis. Others, e.g. Scharfman (1973) emphasize the fact that children need time to develop a trusting relationship to appreciate the potential benefits of treamemt. The therapist's most important 'tools' in this context are patience, willingness to listen and the ability to understand.

Another difficulty is that the therapist needs to establish 'double therapeutic rapport' (Müller-Küppers, 1988), with both the child and his/her parents.

From the start, cooperation with parents is an essential part of therapy. Dührssen (1988) has emphasized the psychodynamic aspect of the formalities such as discussing and organizing therapeutic steps with parents. This issue relates to the frequency and number of sessions, distance between the child's home and place where therapy is undertaken, the child's timetable and other factors such as activities in the child's free time. In some cases it may be necessary to assess whether the parents would also benefit from psychotherapy.

The essential role of play in therapy is universally accepted. Children's inability to engage in free association makes play the most important means of accessing the unconscious, although dreams, daydreams and conscious recollections may also be helpful.

Opinions differ widely with respect to assessing and interpreting play. Whilst Melanie Klein regarded play as a type of symbolic language and attempted to interpret it from an early age, Anna Freud was of the opinion that play is more than just a type of symbolic language and was much more cautious in making interpretations. In his interpretation-free child analysis Zullinger (1988) even dispensed with verbal interpretation entirely.

Dührssen (1988) suggested distinguishing between symbolic play and joint or common play. Symbolic play has always played an important role in psychoanalytically orientated therapy. Often unstructured, amorphous material is recommended (Scharfman, 1973) to encourage the child's creativity and expression. However, children with neurosis may find it difficult to express themselves using amorphous material, and it may then be more appropriate to use prepared material, e.g. manufactured toys. All types of role play, including the use of dolls, enable children to express their internal emotional world.

The term joint or common play is used to describe games that are based on rules which all participants must keep, such as hide-and-seek, dexterity games and games with explicit rules. From a psychological point of view, it is interesting to observe how the child copes with the rules, deals with rivalry and reacts to winning or losing.

Joint or common play requires that the therapist joins in and participates (Dührssen, 1988), for example, by helping the child to construct something, complete a puzzle, look for material, etc. The most important aspect of this interaction is to establish a trusting relationship rather than to discuss conflicts.

The issue of the therapeutic relationship reflects the phenomenon of transference. The issue of transference in therapy with children has been very controversial. Again, the contradictory views of Anna Freud and Melanie Klein are the source of this dissent. Whilst Klein (1932) asserted that children were capable of developing transference neurosis, Freud (1980) contested this and suggested that a child's psychological make-up did not permit transference, the therapist being perceived by the child as an individual independent of tranference, who nevertheless exerted a considerable amount of influence on the child. Therapists still disagree about this, their view relating to their own theoretical background. Dührssen (1980) has taken an intermediary stance by pointing out that interpretation of transference and the unconscious makes up only a fraction of what constitues therapy.

Both the term transference and countertransference have previously played an insignificant role in child therapy. They are, however, central to the issue of 'double therapeutic rapport' mentioned earlier, which demands that the therapist encourages not only the patient, but also his/her parents. When assessing a child's transference towards the therapist, it is important to bear in mind the child's libidinous bonds with his parents, such that any therapeutic intervention will automatically affect the entire family system (Müller-Küppers, 1988). The therapist also needs to keep in mind feelings about his/her own parents when assessing countertransference. A common theme is the therapist who inadvertently takes on the role of a 'better father' or 'better mother', which parents can find very difficult.

The issue of when to terminate therapy is closely associated with the aims of treatment. Despite different opinions in matters of technique, most therapists agree that the aims of therapy are similar in most cases (Dührssen, 1988). These include dissolution of anxiety, improved coping with impulses and drives, clarification of the patient's position with relation to his parents, improved reality testing, a higher degree of emotional stability, etc. Scharfman (1973) explicitly states four criteria for the termination of therapy both during prelatency and latency: (i) the disappearance of neurotic symptoms, (ii) the maturation of the libido and the ego such that age-appropriate relationships and behaviour are possible, (iii) the dissolution of fixation and repression, (iv) and the presence of a stable relationship between the child and his parents.

The practical relevance of psychoanalytically orientated approaches in child and adolescent psychotherapy has decreased considerably. Although many therapist still consider their work 'psychoanalytic', they tend to use various more or less psychoanalytically orientated techniques rather than psychoanalytic psychotherapy in the strict sense (Merydith, 1999).

Treatment with adolescents

Psychoanalytic concept of adolescence

Adolescence has been called the 'step-child of psychoanalysis' (Lampl de Groot, 1965) or a 'white spot on the map of psychoanalysis' (Müller Pozzi, 1980). Interest in this transitional phase between childhood and adulthood has, to a great degree, been of theoretical nature. Aspects associated with treatment have been considered unimportant, a fact which is reflected by the paucity of publications on this topic.

In his publication *Three essays on the theory of sexuality* (1905) Freud characterized puberty by two major changes: first, the subjugation of all other sources of sexual excitement to the genital area, and second, the process of object choice. Freud's idea that the Oedipus complex is reactivated during adolescence and ultimately disolves was very influential, and was considered a point of theoretical reference for many years. From a practical point of view, the work of Bernfeld (1923) and Aichhorn (1971) have contributed greatly to the understanding of adolescence.

Anna Freud (1936) also addressed this issue, and considered puberty the end of a period of calm development. She found, that the increased drives as a result of physical change causes anxiety in adolescents as a result of a power conflict between the ego and id. In addition to its earlier defence mechanisms, the ego develops new puberty-specific mechanisms of defence. Such mechanisms typical for adolescence include asceticism, which helps to suppress drives and prevent gratification, and intellectualization, which helps to repress drives through abstract thoughts and rational ideas. As drives from all pregenital phases are repressed during adolescence, psychopathology fluctuates and tends to be unpredictable, resulting in a potentially wide range of symptoms.

Erikson (1968) elaborated on Freud's theory of psychosexual development and emphasized the social dimension of development. Erikson distinguishes eight developmental phases in adolescence. He associates the fifth phase with the conflict between consolidation and the diffusion of identity. Ego development is said to comprise the gradual integration of all identifications, and the synthesis of accumulated ego values such as trust, autonomy, initiative and diligence. This integration is said to be a delicate process, which can easily be disturbed and may fail altogether, resulting in a diffusion of identity rather than a consolidation, putting further development at risk.

A very detailed model of adolescence has been proposed by Blos (1967), who distinguishes five distinct phases in development from childhood to adulthood. The five phases are summarized in Table 5.2. Blos's theory has been controversial and criticized as ignoring environmental factors such as interactional aspects of transition (Seiffge-Krenke, 1986).

Indications

The issue of psychoanalytically orientated treatment of adolescents has been extremely controversial, and opinions have ranged from approval to total rejection. The approach is considered futile by many, due to the difficulties that

Table 5.2. Five phases of adolescence

Pre-adolescence (about 9–11 years old)	During this phase, an increase in instinctual impulses causes arbitrary cathexis of all libidinous and aggressive types satisfaction, which have served the child well during previous years.
Early adolescence (about 12–13 years old)	During this subsequent phase, both boys and girls impetuously direct their attention towards libidinous objects outside the family. Thus, the process of true separation of early object–relationships begins.
Intermediate adolescence (about 14–16 years old)	During this phase of adolescence proper, the search for new object cathexis takes on a new quality. By giving up narcissistic and bisexual dispositions, heterosexual object relationships become possible.
Late adolescence (about 17–19 years old)	This is a phase of consolidation. Ego-functions and sexual disposition stabilize, resulting in relatively constant object cathexis and self-image.
Post-adolescence (about 20–24 years old)	This phase designates transition from adolescence to adulthood. The young adult continues to address the problem of bringing about more harmony in his personality. This integration is associated with activation of social roles, including courtship, marriage and parenthood.

Modified after Blos (1967).

some therapists have had with resistance and transference during treatment, caused by the emotional fluctuations which are normal at this stage of development. On the other hand, there have always been proponents for the technique, which reflects the importance of psychoanalysts' theoretical background concerning this issue.

Hysterical or obsessional neuroses have been considered the ideal indication for psychoanalytically orientated treatment in adolescents (Scharfman, 1973). The spectrum of suitable disorders was expanded by Anna Freud (1958), who considered psychoanalytic therapy urgently indicated in cases of retraction of libido to the self. She illustrated this with a case of narcisstic withdrawal, ideas of grandeur and hypochondriac anxieties. She also considered the treatment of 'ascetic' adolescents indicated.

Pearson (1968) attempted to determine the indications for therapy according to the subphases of adolescence. Regardless of developmental level, he considered anxious hysteria, conversion reaction, and obsessional neurosis indications for treatment. Friend (in Wolman, 1972) proposed assessing the following functions prior to treatment:

- the capacity for stable object-relationships,
- the ability to tolerate anxiety without decompensation,
- adequate verbal expression,
- the ability for introspection
- the gradual approach to the stage of genital primacy.

Treatment may commence if these criteria are fulfilled. After a probation time, the patient and therapist make a decision as to whether to continue analysis.

Many psychoanalysts, however, are reluctant to treat children or young adolescents. Significant modifications of technique are usually considered necessary. Agreement is greater concerning the treatment of older adolescents with neurosis or neurotic character. Psychoanalytically orientated psychotherapy may also be appropriate in severely disturbed adolescents with borderline personality disorder, especially when other attempts at treatment have failed or cannot be undertaken. However, again in such cases significant modifications of technique are usually necessary (Scharfman, 1973).

Undertaking treatment

In contrast to the treatment of children, treatment of adolescents is much closer to that of adults, although several important differences still exist.

Low treatment motivation in adolescents is a problem, the cause of which may be developmental factors, personality traits, and the patient's environment. Initiation of treatment is influenced to a great extent by parents, who usually choose the therapist, expect their child to attend sessions, and furnish the child's history. This puts the adolescent's sense of autonomy under pressure.

However, psychological factors play a much more important role, e.g. concern about dependence, fearfulness about emotional injury, and, in contrast to this, the wish for autonomy.

All of these factors require a much longer assessment phase than with adults, and some authors, e.g. Scharfman (1973) propose an extended period of prepartion prior to therapy proper, designated 'probational treament'.

Many authors propose that the therapist should take on a more active role in treatment with adolescents than he would with adults (Dührssen, 1986; Scharfman, 1973; Seiffke-Krenke, 1986). Intervention should initially aim to demonstrate to the patient the therapist's willingness to understand his problems, inform him fully, resolve any misunderstandings, and improve introspection

(Scharfman, 1973). When undertaking verbal interventions, the therapist should take into account the patient's way of expressing himself and his language milieu. Sessions should initially revolve around everyday topics which are less anxiety provoking. Dührssen (1988) considers it a severe mistake to induce loyalty conflicts in the patient, e.g. by asking the patient directly about conflicts with his mother or father.

The establishment and maintenance of therapeutic rapport may be rendered difficult by the 'psychoanalytic stiuation', i.e. the setting which promotes regression and anxiety. Thus, it may be necessary to modify the setting, such as dispensing with the couch.

The course of therapy depends to a considerable degree on the extent to which a transference relationship can be established, and on the question as to whether the strucure of such a relationship is equivalent to that in adults remains controversial (Seiffge-Krenke, 1986). Therapy initiates a process in the course of which the patient gradually detaches from primary objects that previously have been close to him, and assumes new non-incestuous object relationships. The patient may, however, not find any suitable objects in his environment, with cathexis of the self with libido being a potential result. This mechanism is considered relevant for the aetiology of narcissistic traits typical in adolescents, and may prevent regressive cathexis of the therapist or previous objects with libido.

Additional problems may occur as a result of the therapist having to adopt a variety of roles. The therapist is not entirely neutral and distant, but a real object who represents the expectations and functions of the patient's parents. These multiple roles disrupt the development of transference and cause the transference relationship to vacillate. Considering these problems, it may not be surprising that transference resistance is significantly more common than acceptance. This tends to result in a worsening of symptoms, which frequently causes patients to discontinue treatment. Thus, with adolescents transference interpretation should be undertaken with great caution (Seiffge-Krenke, 1986).

In addition to dealing with transference, resistance analysis is an essential part of psychoanalytic technique. Several types of resistance and defence typical for adolescence are explained below.

The defence mechanisms of asceticism and intellectualization, both characteristic of adolescents, have already been mentioned. Secondary narcissism has also been mentioned as a defence mechanism which may occur as a result of oedipal incestuous objects being reactivated. In this case, libido is diverted to the self.

'Defensive passivity' is a type of regression. Fundamentally, this is a defence mechanism against mourning over infantile wishes, dreams and fantasies which have remained unfulfilled during development from childhood to adulthood. The defence against infantile relationships results in renewed cathexis of early objects (Seiffge-Krenke, 1986).

Some authors consider the systematic analysis of resistance and defence mechanisms in the context of developmental phases a central aspect of treating adolescents with this technique (Settlage, in Harley, 1974).

Although the tendency to act out is age-appropriate in adolescence, such behaviour may disrupt therapy to a considerable degree. Acting out also makes it difficult to keep to the rule of abstinence and remain neutral. Adolescents tend to involve the therapist in conflicts through actions, and will request an opinion on various topics to a much greater degree than adults will. As the secure setting of classic psychoanalysis is not usually used with adolescents and treatment is much closer to reality through the use of activities, games and conversations, patients have more opportunity for acting out conflicts. This greater proximity to reality must be taken into account when undertaking therapy with adolescents.

Problems which may occur in connection with transference have been mentioned above. However, countertransference is influenced significantly by the function which the 'new object', i.e. the therapist, fulfils. The therapist is at risk of identifying excessively with the adolescent as a result of countertransference, e.g. when the therapist feels pity for the patient. Countertransference may also occur in connection with parents. The therapist may feel obliged to fulfil parents' expectations, but he will also need to consider their contribution to the adolescent's disorder. This may result in covert bias either towards or against parents.

Cooperation with parents during treatment of adolescents is a difficult technical task. Initally, the therapist needs to select an approach to cooperation. The adolescent's actual dependence on his parents usually makes some degree of cooperation necessary, even when treatment aims ultimately to assist in the separation of the patient from his parents. It is also important to avoid regarding children exclusively as 'designated patients', and suggesting family therapy in every case (Dührssen, 1988).

Cooperation always requires clear agreements with parents, despite which parents may still attempt to intervene in the course of treatment, especially when symptoms worsen or change, or when a crisis occurs. Scharfman (1973) has proposed training and educating parents to develop some degree of understanding for the therapeutic process their child is going through and to tolerate temporary problems.

The approach to terminating treatment differs to a significant degree between adolescents and adults. Some authors have proposed designating this step 'interruption' rather than 'termination' (Friend, in Wolman, 1972). This view seems to be determined by the fact that developmental ('external') factors connected with detachment from the family often have a significant influence on treatment.

As in adults, the dissolution of transference neurosis is a criterion in favour of the termination of therapy with adolescents. However, the ongoing controversy about transference in adolescence has shown that adolescents tend to be capable of elaborating considerably fewer aspects of transference than one would consider ideal. Thus, the therapist will often need to restrict the goals of therapy. Potential goals may include clarifying the genetic aspects of individual development, expanding the ego-ideal and consciousness in multiple areas, improving understanding of anxiety and reactions to anxiety, as well as encouraging the capacity for establishing and maintaining close and trusting relationships (Friend, in Wolman, 1972).

Many therapists who do consider their work 'psychoanalytic' actually use a variety of different techniques, which may be more or less psychoanalytic (Merydith, 1999). However, as the practical relevance of psychoanalytically orientated approaches in child and adolescent psychotherapy is decreasing, psychoanalytic psychotherapy in a narrower sense is no longer used very often.

Evaluation

The empirical basis of psychoanalytically orientated psychotherapy with children and adolescents is flimsy. There is an almost total lack of systematic and controlled studies of the efficacy of this treatment method, as empirical research has widely been considered incompatible with the approach to therapy (Marans, 1989). In a review of available studies, Heekerens (1989) suggests that the efficacy of psychodynamic therapy of children and adolescents has still not been empirically proven. Thus, no conclusive data on the efficacy of the technique can be presented here.

This inadequate state of affairs has resulted in increased efforts to obtain empirical data, which have led to identification of several trends (Marans, 1989). First, research has gradually evolved from the study of effectiveness to the study of the course and process of disorders, such that the focus of interest is shifted away from global parameters to determine outcome towards assessing those parameters which influence the course of the disorder. Secondly, research has gone beyond the evaluation of individual cases. For this purpose, index scales have been developed in order to amalgamate cases for research purposes, e.g. 'Hampstead Index', 'Diagnostic Profile'.

Heinecke and Ramsey-Klee (1986) have undertaken controlled group studies to study associations between psychoanalytic parameters and other factors, whilst Moran and Fonagy (1987) have attempted to correlate the contents of psychoanalytically orientated therapy with biological factors.

Whether such research strategies will result in any significant contribution to the empirical data base is unclear. Because of the enormous methodical difficulties of this type of research the issue of empirical proof is likely to remain the 'Achilles' heel' of psychoanalytically orientated therapy for some time to come.

REFERENCES

Aichhorn, A. (1971). *Verwahrloste Jugend*, 7th edn. Bern: Huber.

Bernfeld, S. (1923). Über eine typische Form der männlichen Pubertät. *Imago*, **9**, 169–88.

Blos, P. (1967). *On adolescence*. New York: Free Press.

Brenner, C. (1955). *An elementary textbook of psychoanalysis*. New York: International Universities Press.

Dührssen, A. (1980). *Psychotherapie bei Kindern und Jugendlichen*, 6th edn. Göttingen: Vandenhoek & Ruprecht.

Dührssen, A. (1988). Analytische Psychotherapie bei Kindern und Jugendlichen. In *Kinder- und Jugendpsychiatrie in Klinik und Praxis*, vol. I, ed. H. Remschmidt and M. H. Schmidt, pp. 672–85. Stuttgart: Thieme.

Erikson, E. H. (1968). *Identiy: Youth and crisis*. New York: Norton.

Freud, A. (1936). *The ego and mechanisms of defence*. New York: International Universities Press.

Freud, A. (1958). Adolescence. I. Adolescence in the psychoanalytic theory. In *The psychoanalytic study of the child*, vol. XIII, ed. A. Freud. New York: International Universities Press.

Freud, A. (1980). *Einführung in die Technik der Kinderanalyse*, 3rd edn. München: Kindler.

Freud, S. (1905). Three essays on the theory of sexuality. In *Standard edition of the works of Sigmund Freud*, vol. 7, ed. J. Strachey, pp. 125–243. London: Hogarth Press.

Greenson, R. R. (1966). *The technique and practice of psychoanalysis*. Madison, C.T.: International Universities Press.

Harley, M. (1974). *The analyst and the adolescent at work*. New York: Quadrangle.

Hartmann, H. (1964). *Essays on ego psychology*. London: Hogarth Press.

Heekerens, H. P. (1989). Effektivität von Kinder- und Jugendlichenpsychotherapie im Spiegel von Meta-Analysen. *Zeitschrift für Kinder- und Jugendpsychiatrie*, **17**, 150–7.

Heinecke, C., and Ramsey-Klee (1986). Outcome of child psychotherapy as a function of frequency of session. *Journal of the American Academy of Child and Adolescent Psychiatry*, **25**, 247–53.

Klein, M. (1932). *The psychoanalysis of children*. London: Hogarth Press.

Lampl de Groot, J. (1965). Zur Adoleszenz. *Psyche*, **19**, 477–85.

Marans, S. M. (1989). Psychoanalytic psychotherapy with children: current research trends and challenges. *Journal of the American Academy of Child and Adolescent Psychiatry*, **28**, 669–74.

Merydith, S. P. (1999). Psychodynamic approaches. In *Counselling and psychotherapy with children and adolescents. Theory and practice for school and clinical settings*, 3rd edn, ed. H. T. Prout and D. T. Brown, pp. 74–107. New York: Wiley.

Moran, G. and Fonagy, P. (1987). Psychoanalysis and diabetic control. *British Journal of Medical Psychology*, **60**, 357–72.

Müller-Küppers, M. (1988). Kinderpsychotherapie. In *Psychiatrie der Gegenwart*, 3rd edn, vol. 7, ed. K. P. Kisker, H. Lauter, J-E. Meyer, C. Müller and E. Strömgren, pp. 429–54. Berlin: Springer.

Müller-Pozzi, H. (1980). Zur Handhabung der Übertragung in der Analyse von Jugendlichen. *Psyche*, **34**, 339–64.

Pearson, G. H. J. (1968). *Handbuch der Kinder-Psychoanalyse*. Frankfurt: Fischer.

Pongratz, L. J. (1983). *Hauptströmungen der Tiefenpsychologie*. Stuttgart: Kröner.

Rapaport, D. (1973). *Die Struktur der psychoanalytischen Theorie. Versuch einer Systematik*. Stuttgart: Klett.

Remschmidt, H. (1992). *Psychiatrie der Adoleszenz*. Stuttgart: Thieme.

Remschmidt, H. and Heinscher, H. G. (1988). Psychodynamische Ansätze. In *Kinder- und Jugendpsychiatrie in Klinik und Praxis*, vol. I, ed. H. Remschmidt and M. H. Schmidt, pp. 233–49. Stuttgart: Thieme.

Scharfman, M. A. (1973). Psychoanalytic treatment. In *Handbook of treatment of mental disorders in childhood and adolescence*, ed. B. B. Wolman, J. Egan and O. R. Ross, pp. 47–69. Englewood Cliffs: Prentice Hall.

Seiffge-Krenke, I. (1986). *Psychoanalytische Therapie Jugendlicher*. Stuttgart: Kohlhammer.

Wolman, B. (1972). *Handbook of child psychoanalysis*. New York: Van Nostrand-Reinhold.

Zulliger, H. (1988). Die deutungsfreie psychoanalytische Kinderpsychotherapie. In *Handbuch der Kinderpsychotherapie*, ed. G. Biermann, pp. 110–18. Frankfurt: Fischer.

6 Behaviour therapy

Uwe Müller and Kurt Quaschner

Introduction

Behaviour therapy is the attempt to modify human behaviour and emotions, positively based on the rules of learning theory (Eysenck, 1964). The term 'behaviour therapy' obviously refers to behaviour, however, Eysenck extended the definition to include those internal processes we call 'emotions'. Since cognitive behaviour therapy was introduced in the 1960s, verbal, cognitive and motivational factors have increasingly been taken into account. Earlier views, which held that all internal mental factors should be ignored for methodical reasons, are no longer tenable.

The theoretical basis of behaviour therapy has been expanded considerably since its introduction. Until the 1950s, behaviour therapy had been based to a considerable extent on learning theory, especially Pavlov's concept of classical conditioning, Thorndike's learning theory of the association between stimulus and response, Hull's formal learning theory, and Skinner's paradigm of operant conditioning. Subsequently, the theoretical basis of behaviour therapy extended beyond this to include findings and theories from general and social psychology, as well as from neuropsychology. Related fields such as physiology and neurophysiology have also contributed to the development and application of behavioural methods, which today form an essential part of the relatively new discipline of behavioural medicine.

In contrast to the changing theoretical foundations, some basic methodological problems retaing to behaviour therapy have persisted. Behaviour therapy should, however, be informed by empirical and experimental findings (Graham, 1998).

The concept of the human being in behaviour therapy has gradually changed. In contrast to previous views, where human beings were regarded as organisms who react passively to environmental stimuli, today human beings are considered active subjects with a self-conscience, who plan and undertake actions in an organized way. This change in perspective is reflected in the newer concepts of behaviour therapy, such as self-control, self-expression, attribution styles, plans, coping strategies and competency to act (Watson and Gresham, 1998).

The continuous expansion of behaviour therapy has made it increasingly difficult to define the field concisely. Thus, in contrast to Eysenck's definition of behaviour therapy, newer definitions merely seem to be detailed lists of criteria, e.g. Ammerman and Hersen (1995), Margraf and Lieb (1995), Rimm and Masters (1979).

Treatment with children and adolescents

In the past few years, behavioural treatment of children and adolescents has increasingly incorporated age-specific considerations. Several trends have consistently been noted in the literature, e.g. Kendall (1991), Mash (1989).

It is important to view diagnostic appraisal and treatment from a systemic perspective. This takes into account the fact that behaviour of children and adolescents depends to a high degree on their environment. The family environment is of utmost importance; however, other factors such as school, peer groups, and other social relationships also influence behaviour considerably. With the growing influence of the systemic perspective, behavioural family therapy has become increasingly popular.

Emphasis of the developmental perspective is an additional trend in behaviour therapy. Developmental considerations are relevant in various ways. In addition to conceptualizing psychiatric disorders, i.e. aetiology and pathogenesis, developmental considerations are helpful for specifying diagnostic procedures and therapeutic interventions. Although behavioural techniques have been used to treat children and adolescents for a long time, e.g. operant conditioning, critics have pointed out that children and adolescents have been treated with 'diluted' and inadequately adapted techniques which were originally developed for adults (Kendall, 1991).

In addition to the two major trends mentioned above, other approaches have been developed (Mash, 1989), most of which comprise revisions of theoretical models and practical interventions.

Learning theory: the basis for behaviour therapy

In the following section several important principles of learning theory are explained, as they constitute the basis for behaviour therapy.

Classical conditioning

In classical conditioning, organisms learn to associate certain stimuli with specific consequences. The principle of classical conditioning was discovered by the Russian physiologist Pavlov, who studied the physiology of the gut in dogs at the turn of the century.

Pavlov found that presenting a piece of meat resulted in salivation. When the presentation of food was associated with some other stimulus normally irrelevant to dogs (e.g. a sound or light), the presentation of the stimulus alone eventually also resulted in salivation.

The paradigm of classical conditioning is based on the following general principle: when a stimulus causing an inadvertent reaction in an organism is closely associated with a neutral stimulus, the presentation of the neutral stimulus eventually also results in that inadvertent reaction.

This principle which was derived from experiments with animals has been applied to human beings. Classical conditioning seems to play an important role in the aetiology of several mental and psychophysiological disorders, e.g. anxiety disorder.

Instrumental or operant conditioning

With instrumental or operant conditioning, organisms learn to associate specific behaviours with resulting consequences. This paradigm is based on the theory introduced by the American learning theorist Thorndike in 1911, who designated the phenomenon the 'law of effect'. The American psychologist Skinner developed this theory in the 1940s, and it later became known as 'operant conditioning'.

The term instrumental or operant conditioning is used to describe a process by which specific consequences result in a significant increase in the probability of a particular behaviour occurring when a stimulus is presented. The specific consequences are known as 'reinforcers'.

The paradigm of operant conditioning was first applied on a large scale in the 1960s. The attempt was made to modify the behaviour of severely disturbed adolescents in institutions using 'operant conditioning schedules', and schools used operant conditioning techniques to develop 'programmed learning'.

Modelling

Human learning processes are so complex that they cannot be explained by the prinicples of classical and instrumental conditioning alone. Behaviour can be acquired through 'modelling', without the individual having to actually act out the behaviour, i.e. by closely observing the behaviour of other individuals. The idea of learning by modelling was developed by the American psychologist Bandura (1977). This technique was also widely applied in the 1960s.

This therapeutic technique has been successfully used in social skills training and in the treatment of phobias. Modelling is also appropriate when patients are unable to comprehend verbal instructions, for example, children with learning difficulties and/or autism.

Cognitive learning theories

Most supporters of conditioning theories, including Skinner, considered the organism a 'black box', influenced by environmental stimuli, resulting in visible reactions to the stimuli. The objective description of the processes occuring within the 'black box' was considered neither possible nor neccessary.

Cognitive learning theories, which have nearly as long a tradition, took up an opposing stance. Tolman (1959), known as an early supporter of cognitive learning theories, studied learning processes in rats using labyrinths in the 1930s to 1950s. He eventually developed concepts such as 'insight', 'purpose' and 'cognitive maps' to explain behaviour (Hilgard and Bower, 1975).

According to cognitive learning theory, learning is a result of information processing. This process is said to be influenced by cognitive factors such as expectations and assumptions about oneself and the environment, as well as by selected perceptions and memories.

In the 1960s and 1970s, cognitive learning theories increasingly influenced behaviour therapy, which had previously been determined by the theory of classical conditioning. Based on cognitive theories, several treatment techniques have been developed, which aim to modify cognition, such as cognitive restructuring in depressed patients or self-control techniques to treat dependency or eating disorders. Improvements on a cognitive level are expected to influence behaviour on both an emotional and physiological level.

The process of assessment and diagnostic appraisal in behaviour therapy

An important feature of behaviour therapy is the close association between diagnostic appraisal and treatment. This distinguishes behaviour therapy from other types of treatment. Theoretical considerations emphasize the logical and operational unity of diagnostic appraisal and therapy, and the two aspects interact closely (Braun, 1978). Diagnostic appraisal does not end when treatment begins, but continues throughout the course of therapy, and feeds back into treatment success.

The behavioural approach to the process of diagnostic appraisal and therapy can be divided into several steps (Braun, 1978; Schulte, 1976a, b):

(i) use a functional model to record the present state;
(ii) illustrate the association of conditions with symptomatic behaviour;
(iii) define treatment aims (target behaviour) in terms of:
  - the functional model and
  - an analysis of environmental conditions;
(iv) draw up a detailed treatment plan;
(v) undertake treatment;
(vi) assess treatment success;
(vii) compare outcome with the initial hypotheses and target behaviour.

This series of successive steps can be regarded as a feedback system, which is repeatedly applied over the course of treatment. The output of the system serves as input for the next cycle.

Although classical behavioural analysis has evolved to a more comprehensive 'problem analysis' (Hautzinger, 1993), the approaches to behavioural analysis proposed by Kanfer and Saslow (1969) and Schulte (1976b) are still relevant today. The analysis of symptomatic behaviour using the functional model may be an oversimplification; however, the model can be very helpful in structuring data to develop the working hypothesis to be tested, along which specific treatment steps can then be defined.

The original working model of behavioural assessment used five steps to describe behaviour and determine the functional relationship of various parts:

S: stimulus, preceding situational conditions
O: biological features of the organism
R: reaction, behaviour
K: reinforcement schedules
C: consequences

The practical approach to this model requires the following steps.

Defining target behaviour (R)

Behavioural analysis is based on a precise qualitative and quantitative assessment of a symptom (frequency, duration, intensity, extent). Behaviour is described not only in terms of motor behaviour but also as its emotional, cognitive and physiologic components. It is important that the description is accurate and detailed, omitting any general or imprecise statements.

Analysis of preceding situational conditions (S)

The features of any situation preceding the behaviour need to be described in detail. For example, it is important to note whether discriminatory stimuli (as in operant conditioning), or precipitating stimuli (as in classical conditioning) are relevant.

More recent developments in behavioural analysis have considered cognitive factors such as attitudes, perceptions and expectations as behaviour-relevant stimuli (Hautzinger, 1993).

Analysis of organism variables (O)

Originally, these were used to describe the strictly biological and physiological conditions of behaviour. However, today the term is used to designate those 'individual differential variables' (Braun, 1978), which determine individual disposition.

Analysis of consequences (C) and reinforcement schedules (K)

In order to assess the consequences following target behaviour, the quality and frequency of the consequences, i.e. the 'pattern' or 'reinforcement rate' must be known. It is also important to know whether the consequences occur shortly or at a latent interval after the behaviour, and whether they are external or internal.

Methods and approaches to diagnostic appraisal in behaviour therapy

Although the scope of diagnostic appraisal in behaviour therapy differs considerably from the usual trait-orientated assessment, it uses a similar approach, because behavioural assessment lacks its own spectrum of elaborate instruments. Thus, the list of frequently used diagnostic approaches includes both specifically behavioural methods as well as other techniques. Reinecker (1987) and Braun (1978) have suggested using the following 'strategies for obtaining information':

Systematic verbal interview about behaviour (Braun, 1978), especially when undertaken as part of a functional behavioural analysis, is the most important technique for obtaining information. However, as behavioural assessment may be difficult with children and adolescents due to their age, developmental level, and/or symptoms, behaviour observation is also recommended in this age group.

Self-observation training may also be helpful with children as well as systematic behaviour observation. Interviews with parents or other care-givers such as teachers are also very important in this regard.

Diagnostic role play or 'situational behavioural tests' may also contribute to obtaining pertinent information. Questionnaires, behaviour inventories, and assessment scales are often used in assessment, and standardized psychological tests may also be necessary.

Today, behaviour therapy is understood as a complex problem-solving process which is not merely restricted to eliminating symptoms or establishing target behaviours.

During the past few years, the concept of disorder, patient motivation, and the therapeutic relationship have gained importance in behaviour therapy.

Fig. 6.1. shows a summary of the strategies considered important by Hand (1986) in his 'five-phase-model' of behaviour therapy.

Behavioural interventions

The following section gives a summary of several methods commonly used in behaviour therapy, including both traditional and modern techniques (Braun and Tittelbach, 1978).

Operant techniques

These traditional techniques are used to encourage or discourage behaviour. The method is based on the principles of operant learning theory, as developed by Skinner.

Operant techniques are used to achieve desired behaviour modifications by means of systematic exposure to the positive or negative consequences of behaviour. The use of reinforcements is an essential part of operant techniques. Reinforcements are awarded or withheld to modify the probability with which a behaviour is likely to occur.

Operant methods include several specific interventions, some of which will be discussed here.

When the technique of shaping is used, the patient gradually approaches complex target behaviour, encouraged by positive reinforcement of distinct behavioural steps, e.g. speech in children with autism.

Reinforcement schedules are based on contracts between the therapist and patient, defining target behaviour and the reinforcements used when the behaviour is achieved. Such reinforcement schedules are often used to treat disorders in childhood, eating disorders, dependency and delinquency.

Token economy uses non-specific reinforcements, e.g. plastic tokens, which can be exchanged for primary reinforcements later, e.g. activities, watching television, sweets. Token economy programmes generally tend to be useful only for treating patients in institutions such as hospitals or residential homes, e.g. to motivate long-stay patients or treat children with chronic behaviour disorders.

One general feature of all operant conditioning techniques is the relatively

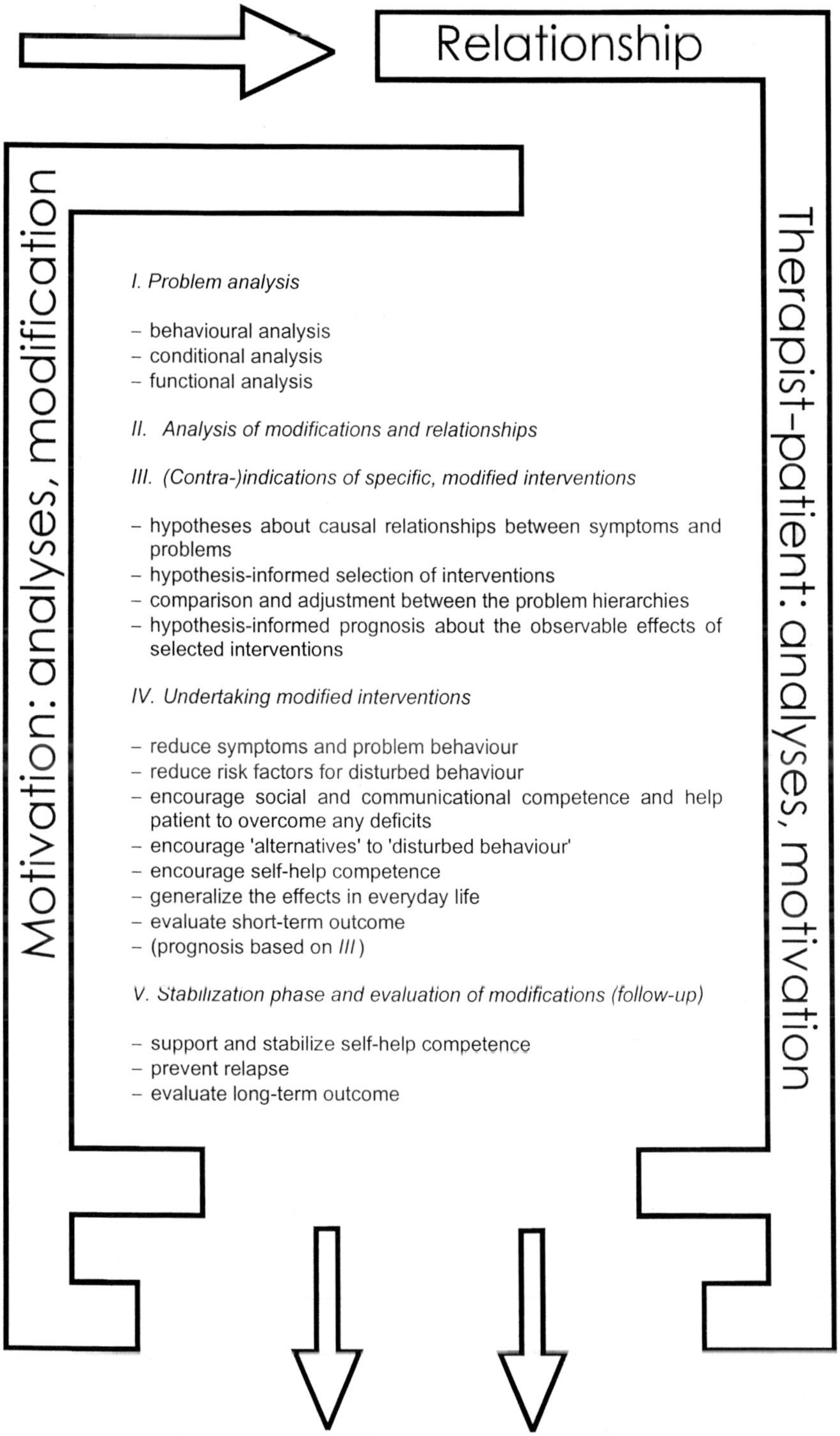

Fig. 6.1. A strategy for behaviour therapy in five phases (Hand, 1986).

high degree of external control which is required. The awarding or withdrawal of reinforcements is controlled by the therapist, teacher or other care-giver rather than the patient. This largely determines the indications for operant techniques: the approach is helpful when the patient has insufficient capacity for self-control as a result of his age, developmental level, intellectual capacity, and/or psychiatric symptoms. Such restrictions must be taken into account when operant techniques requiring external control are used with adults. However, operant techniques remain very useful in children.

In contrast, more recent behavioural approaches such as self-control techniques are characterized by a much lower degree of external control. Thus, where possible, operant methods should be gradually replaced by techniques over the course of therapy in order to encourage the development of a sense of responsibility. This gradual switchover of behavioural techniques is common, for example, in patients with anorexia nervosa.

Systematic desensitization

This method was developed by Wolpe and Lazarus (1966) in the 1950s. For a long time this was the most important and well-known behavioural therapy technique. However, in recent years it has been increasingly replaced by exposure techniques such as flooding.

The classical indication for systematic desensitization is in phobic disorders, although the technique may also be used to treat other disorders associated with anxiety, such as sexual dysfunction, obsessions, depression or stuttering. The technique is inappropriate, however, for the treatment of disorders characterized by 'free-floating' anxiety.

Systematic desensitization is the method of choice for treating children and adolescents with phobias. Prior to commencing treatment, the therapist needs to assess whether the patient has the capability to imagine the anxious situation. In some cases it may be appropriate to expose the patient to the anxious stimulus using illustrations or models rather than simply a mental representation.

Systematic desensitization is undertaken in several steps: initially, the patient learns a relaxation technique, usually progressive relaxation training. In the next step, the patient is assisted in draws up an individual anxiety hierarchy (see case report in Chapter 15).

During the desensitization phase proper, the patient is asked to imagine exposure to the anxious situation, beginning with the least anxious, gradually progressing to increasingly anxious situations as treatment progresses. Should the patient experience anxiety during sessions, he is asked to undertake relaxation training exercises.

Only when the patient is able to imagine an anxious situation without experiencing any anxiousness is he asked to continue and imagine the next most anxious situation. The aim is to achieve generalization of desensitization through exposure to less anxious situations outside treatment sessions.

Exposure techniques

These are characterized by exposing the patient to situations which cause anxiety, whilst simultaneously preventing any avoidant behaviour. Exposure is especially appropriate in treating phobias, and has been shown to be effective both in the short and long term. It is now used more often than systematic desensitization.

Indications

Exposure techniques can be used in the treatement of phobias, obsessional ideas and compulsions. The technique can also be used to treat severe and persistent grief-reactions after traumatic experience or loss. This approach, in which patients are confronted with the loss retrospectively, was developed by Ramsay in the 1970s.

During in vivo exposure, the patient is exposed to an anxiety-provoking situation (e.g. going shopping in a supermarket or using public transport for a patient with agoraphobia), accompanied by the therapist. It is important that the patient remains in the situation for as long as it takes for the anxiety to substantially decrease. During exposure, any avoidant behaviour such as retreating from the situation must be prevented. In most cases, anxiety decreases considerably within several minutes, in some cases it can take up to half an hour. Most patients experience less anxiety than they had expected. As treatment progresses, patients are gradually expected to bear more responsibility, and may eventually undertake exposure without the therapist's assistance.

Prior to beginning exposure treatment, the individual steps and the principles on which the treatment is based must be carefully explained. The patient should understand that he has to remain in the anxious situation until he feels almost no anxiety, and is expected to refrain from any avoidant behaviour. It is especially important for the therapist to motivate the patient during this preparatory phase, in which the dropout rate is highest.

Exposure treatment is usually an extremely stressful experience for the patient. The use of the technique with children is therefore controversial. If, however, exposure techniques are used with children, it is important that a trusting relationship between child and therapist has first been built up, and that the child has been well prepared for treatment. The successful treatment of school anxiety in children with exposure techniques has been reported in the literature.

Case report

The following case report summarizes the inpatient treatment of an adolescent with anxiety disorder and extreme physical symptoms of anxiety.

S., a 14-year-old boy who had been attending secondary school was unable to continue going to school because of nausea and vomiting in the morning. At presentation, he had been absent from school for 1 year because of the symptoms.

Problem analysis during the first phase of treatment revealed that the nausea and vomiting were symptoms of marked school anxiety. During the phase of cognitive preparation, the disorder was explained to him in terms of an appropriate model, emphasizing the importance of his avoidant behaviour (being so long absent from school) in maintaining the disorder. In addition, S. was also taught about the nature of in vivo exposure treatment. After obtaining consent from S. and his parents, exposure training commenced at school the following day.

S. was accompanied to school by the therapist, who noticed increasing signs of anxiety in the patient as he approached the school (anxiety, trembling, sweating, nausea and vomiting shortly before entering the building). The patient's anxiety decreased a short while after entering the building, and after about 1 hour he felt no anxiety at all.

The next day, exposure was undertaken in an identical way. On the fourth day, he no longer vomited, and this recurred only occasionally, ceasing permanently after the 27th day of treatment. The nausea and anxiety also improved, and after several weeks, the patient was able to resume school attendance without any symptoms.

The final phase of inpatient treatment included social skills training, because the patient's absence from school had resulted in insecure interaction with peers. Follow-up 15 months after discharge revealed that the improvements made had been retained.

Cognitive restructuring

Cognitive phenomena such as perceptions, expectations, attitudes, interpretations, attributions, etc. are involved in many psychiatric disorders. Irrational and distorted thoughts tend to encourage the genesis, maintenance and aggravation of psychiatric disturbance. The modification of such cognitions as part of therapy is likely to have a positive influence on other areas as well, e.g. motor behaviour and emotions.

The main aim of cognitive restructuring is to modify maladjustive cognitions. This technique has been the most commonly used in depression, but anxiety, dependency and obsessional disorders have also been treated successfully.

In the 1960s, Beck developed a cognitive approach for treating depression which has received considerable recognition. According to this theory, a depressed individual has a negative and hopeless attitude towards himself, his environment and the future. Such negative thoughts occur almost 'automatically' to the depressed individual. During cognitive therapy, negative thoughts and associated attitudes are identified, following which the logical validity, actuality, and consequences of the thoughts are critically appraised. Finally, alternative ways of assessing and interpreting cognitions are developed and practised using real situations.

In the treatment of depression, cognitive restructuring is usually combined with techniques which directly address behaviour, such as physical activity or social skills training.

The standard technique of cognitive restructuring was initially developed to treat adults with depression. Today, it is a common approach, whose success has been demonstrated. The treatment of children and adolescents, however, requires several modifications, such as an emphasis on the importance of actions. Cognitive techniques alone, which require a considerable amount of introspection and verbal skills, are likely to exceed the capability of most children.

Assertiveness training

Assertiveness involves many aspects: the ability to express one's own thoughts and emotions, and perceive those of others; being able to say 'no'; initiating, continuing, and terminating conversations; behaving appropriately; tolerating public attention, etc.

Indications for assertiveness training include social anxiety and interactional difficulties, but the technique is also appropriate in the treatment of aggressive behaviour, hyperactivity, mental retardation and in the rehabilitation of long-stay psychiatric patients.

Assertiveness training has two main aims: reducing social anxiety and encouraging social skills. A wide range of different techniques can be used to achieve these aims, such as role play and behavioural training exercises, daily life training sessions, modelling, operant techniques, video feedback, group therapy, self-control techniques, etc. Thus, assertiveness training is usually undertaken as an integrated training programme with a defined schedule.

Assertiveness training programmes have been developed to treat children with social anxieties and interactional difficulties using individual and group training sessions, as well as parent education (Petermann and Petermann, 1989; Rimm and Masters, 1979).

Self-control techniques

Self-control techniques, initially developed by Kanfer and Karoly (1972), have gained considerable importance since the 1970s. Self-control techniques require the patient to bear a considerable amount of therapeutic responsibility. This reduces therapist dependency and emphasizes the patient's own responsibility for his behaviour.

Patients are helped to anticipate problem behaviour, and direct their attention towards achieving specific aims using techniques acquired during therapy. The therapist's role is to instruct the patient in behavioural techniques, motivate him in the initial phase, and assisst him in acquiring the necessary skills.

Self-control techniques have a wide range of potential applications, e.g. learning disorders, motivational difficulties, eating disorders, anxieties, phobias. These techniques are appropriate for children and adolescents, and may be used to treat impulsive and aggressive behaviour. In some situations it may be helpful to use material such as games or comic books to encourage the patient.

Self-control programmes usually include various techniques with different theoretical backgrounds. The following techniques are often used: self-observation, e.g. keeping a behavioural diary, external stimulus control, e.g. the removal of all high-calorie foods from the environment in a patient with bulimia, self-reinforcement, e.g. the self-reward by a patient following the achievement of a goal, self-induced relaxation, self-instruction, e.g. the use of internal verbalization to control behaviour, and thought-stopping, e.g. the interruption of obsessional thoughts. Patients may also be instructed to undertake in vivo exposure or cognitive restructuring without direct assistance from the therapist.

Evaluation

Behavioural approaches range among the most effective psychotherapeutic techniques (Petermann and Warschburger, 1993). Behavioural approaches have been evaluated in great detail and invariably been found to be effective (Kazdin et al., 1990). However, despite great acclaim, evaluation studies should be reviewed carefully, as they may contain inconsistencies. For example, some samples may include patients with inadequate clinical criteria, results may be derived from adult samples or interpretations based on flawed methods. Thus, it is advisable to refer to established texts (Mash and Barkley, 1989; Kendall, 1991) when discussing the outcome of behaviour therapy techniques.

REFERENCES

Ammerman, R. T. and Hersen, M. (ed.) (1995). *Handbook of child behavior therapy in the psychiatric setting*. New York: Wiley.

Bandura, A. (1977). Self-efficacy. Toward a unifying theory of behavioral change. *Psychological Review*, **84**, 191–215.

Braun, P. (1978). Verhaltenstherapeutische Diagnostik. In *Handbuch der Psychologie. Klinische Psychologie*, ed. L. J. Pongratz, pp. 1648–725. Göttingen: Hogrefe.

Braun, P. and Tittelbach, E. (1978). Verhaltenstherapie. In *Handbuch der Psychologie. Klinische Psychologie*, ed. L. J. Pongratz, pp. 1955–2081. Göttingen: Hogrefe.

Eysenck, H. J. (1964). The nature of behavior therapy. In *Experiments in behavior therapy*, ed. H. J. Eysenck. Oxford: Pergamon Press.

Graham, P. J. (ed.) (1998). *Cognitive-behaviour therapy for children and families*. New York: Cambridge University Press.

Hand, I. (1986). Verhaltenstherapie und Kognitive Therapie in der Psychiatrie. In *Psychiatrie der Gegenwart*, 3rd edn, vol. 1, ed. K. P. Kisker, H. Lauter, J-E. Meyer, C. Müller, and E. Strömgren, pp. 277–306. Berlin: Springer.

Hautzinger, M. (1993).Verhaltens- und Problemanalyse. In *Verhaltenstherapie*, 2nd edn, ed. M. Linden and M. Hautzinger, pp. 27–32. Berlin: Springer.

Hilgard, E. R. and Bower, G. H. (ed.) (1975). *Theories of learning*, 4th edn, Englewood Cliffs, NJ: Prentice-Hall.

Kanfer, F. H. and Karoly, P. (1972). Self-control. A behavioristic excursion into the lion's den. *Behavior Therapy*, **3**, 398–416.

Kanfer, F. H. and Saslow, G. (1969). Behavioural diagnosis. In *Behaviour therapy. Appraisal and status*, ed. C. M. Franks, pp. 417–44. New York: McGraw-Hill.

Kazdin, A. E., Bass, D., Ayers, W. A. and Rodgers, A. (1990). Empirical and clinical focus of child and adolescent psychotherapy research. *Journal of Consulting and Clinical Psychology*, **58**, 729–40.

Kendall, P. C. (1991). *Child and adolescent therapy. Cognitive-behavioral procedures*. New York: Guilford Press.

Margraf, J. and Lieb, R. (1995). Was ist Verhaltenstherapie? Versuch einer zukunftsoffenen Neucharakterisierung. *Zeitschrift für klinische Psychologie*, **24**, 1–7.

Mash, E. J. (1989). Treatment of child and family disturbance. A behavioral-systems perspective. In *Treatment of childhood disorders*, ed. E. J. Mash and R. A. Barkley, pp. 3–36. New York: Guilford Press.

Mash, E. J. and Barkley, R. A. (ed.) (1989). *Treatment of childhood disorders*. New York: Guilford Press.

Petermann, U. and Petermann, F. (1989). *Training mit sozial unsicheren Kindern*, 3rd edn, München: Psychologie Verlags-Union.

Petermann, F. and Warschburger, P. (1993). Neue Trends und Ergebnisse in der Kinderverhaltenstherapie. Ursachenforschung und Interventionen. In *Verhaltenstherapie mit Kindern*, ed. F. Petermann, pp. 6–84. München: Röttger.

Reinecker, H. (1987). *Grundlagen der Verhaltenstherapie*. München: Psychologie Verlags-Union.

Rimm, D. C. and Masters, J. C. (1979). *Behavior therapy*, 2nd edn. New York: Academic Press.

Schulte, D. (1976a). Der diagnostisch-therapeutische Prozess in der Verhaltenstherapie. In *Diagnostik in der Verhaltenstherapie*, 2nd edn, ed. D. Schulte, pp. 60–73. München: Urban & Schwarzenberg.

Schulte, D. (1976b). Ein Schema für Diagnose und Therapieplanung in der Verhaltenstherapie. In *Diagnostik in der Verhaltenstherapie*, 2nd edn, ed. D. Schulte, pp. 75–104. München: Urban & Schwarzenberg.

Tolman, E. C. (1959). Principles of purposeful behavior. In *Psychology. A study of a science*, vol. 2, ed. S. Koch, pp. 92–157. New York: McGraw-Hill.

Watson, T. S. and Gresham, F. M. (ed.) (1998). *Handbook of child behavior therapy*. New York: Plenum Press.

Wolpe, J. and Lazarus, A. A. (1966). *Behaviour therapy techniques*. Oxford: Pergamon Press.

7 Cognitive behaviour therapy

Richard Harrington

The cognitive behaviour therapies have been used in many different psychiatric disorders of children and adolescents. The management of many of these disorders is discussed in other parts of this book. The present chapter provides an overview of cognitive behavioural techniques that are used with young people, the kinds of disorders that they are most often used for, and the evidence for their effectiveness. Before reviewing these issues, however, it is necessary to consider briefly how cognitive behaviour therapy is defined.

Definition of cognitive behaviour therapy

Cognitive models of psychopathology view children and adolescents as actively involved in constructing their reality. Cognitive behaviour therapy (CBT) is therefore based on the assumption that psychopathology in young people is due, at least in part, to cognitive processing deficiences or deficits. A very wide variety of procedures has been included under the broad umbrella of the term 'cognitive behaviour therapy'. At the core of most techniques is an emphasis on certain cognitive interventions, which are designed to produce changes in thinking. For most cognitive therapists these changes in thinking are hypothesized to lead to changes in behaviour, mood, or actions. Nevertheless, while recognizing the importance of cognitions and development of mental disorder among children and adolescents, cognitive behavioural formulations also emphasize the learning process, and the ways in which the child's family or environment can change both cognition and behaviour. Cognitive behaviour therapy for young people therefore usually has a significant emphasis on behavioural performance-based procedures. Indeed, in younger children, behavioural techniques form the core of the therapy, and there may be relatively little application of so-called cognitive techniques (see later). In addition, there is at all ages a major emphasis on the involvement of the family. Some forms of cognitive-behaviour therapy also involve the school.

Cognitive behavioural techniques

A variety of different techniques are used when working with children and adolescents. The choice of technique will depend on many factors, particularly the child's motivation, the child's developmental level, the type of problem being treated, and the clinician's formulation of the causes of the child's disorders. Most of the cognitive-behaviour therapies have, however, the following features in common.

The therapist

The mental posture of the cognitive behaviour therapist working with young people has been described as consultant or educator (Kendall, 1991). The therapist should be active and involved. However, he or she should not be too didactic, or give the impression of having all the answers. Rather, there is an emphasis on the development of a collaboration between the therapist and the young person. The therapist stimulates and educates the child to think for him or herself. In many cognitive behavioural programmes, children are encouraged to learn through experience. This can be gained through tasks that the child carries out during the session or through homework assignments.

Assessment and goal setting

The initial assessment aims to provide a detailed cognitive behavioural formulation. This is a written explanation of the problem that highlights the key cognitive and behavioural factors that are hypothesized by the therapist to contribute to both the onset and maintenance of the child's difficulties. It is very important that the formulation should also reflect the role of external factors, such as family difficulties, as well as internal factors such as the young person's views of him or herself.

The initial interview should also provide a detailed analysis of the presenting problem, in order to generate a short list of difficulties that are most distressing to the child and which are most amenable to treatment. Cognitive behaviour therapists often use standardized measures of the child's behaviour both to define problems and as a method for measuring change. In collaboration with the child, the therapist then endeavours to identify behaviours or cognitions that seem to be maintaining the problem. It is essential that a thorough assessment of the child's social context is made, and that strengths or weaknesses within this context are identified.

Engaging the family

The cognitive behaviour therapies are usually individual or group-based treatments. However, there is a growing trend towards encouraging other members of the family, especially the parents to have a role. Parents are often very helpful in implementing certain aspects of therapeutic programmes, particularly behavioural techniques. Thus, for example, parents will often be involved in the reinforcement of homework assignments. It is also very important to involve parents because parental behaviours and attitudes may be important predisposing or maintaining factors.

Cognitive techniques

Most of the cognitive therapies have, at their core, a set of techniques for monitoring and correcting distorted beliefs about the world. All techniques therefore, have an emphasis on self-monitoring. That is, on recording the relationship between thoughts and other phenomena, such as experiences or mood. In younger children, it is often necessary to use special techniques to elicit and monitor cognitions. In older adolescents, cognitions can usually be elicited using the same techniques as in adults.

Once negative cognitions have been elicited, an important next step in many CBT programmes is some form of cognitive restructuring. Once a thought has been identified, the thought itself is written down. Arguments and evidence for and against the thought are then considered. The idea is that the young person should reach a reasoned conclusion based on the available evidence both for and against their thinking.

Negative cognitions are often underpinned by prevailing attitudes and assumptions about the world or about the self. A typical example would be a child with conduct disorder who believes that fighting is a legitimate way of dealing with problems with his peers. These kinds of assumptions are seldom fully articulated in the young person's mind, and usually have to be inferred from the person's behaviour. With older, psychologically minded adolescents, it may be possible for the young person to look for stable reactions to situations that betray these underlying assumptions. However, this is seldom possible in younger children, in whom much more emphasis is made on behavioural techniques.

Behavioural techniques

Exposure techniques are often used when the patient avoids a feared situation, such as school. Most cognitive behavioural programmes, particularly those that are used with younger children, include a system of behavioural contingencies. This involves setting up a system of rewards that are appropriate for the young person in order to reinforce desirable behaviours. Parental involvement in reward systems is crucial, but in some instances there may be an emphasis on self-reinforcement that does not involve tangible external reward. For instance, the child might be told to think 'congratulate yourself . . . you did really well in that situation!'.

Inactivity is a common correlate of many child psychiatric disorders, particularly emotional disorders such as depression. Activity scheduling involves the establishment of goal-directed, enjoyable activities throughout the child's day. The therapist, child, and parents collaborate to plan the young person's activities hour by hour.

Cognitive-behaviour therapists also make much use of specific behavioural techniques for specific kinds of symptoms. Relaxation training, for example, can be very useful for somatic anxiety symptoms. Sleep hygiene measures are commonly used to help with sleep disturbance, which is associated with many child psychiatric disorders.

Social problem-solving

Whilst many emotional and behavioural disorders in children and adolescents are associated with abnormal cognition or behaviours, it is very commonly the case that these are provoked by an external problem of one kind or another. Many of these problems involve interpersonal difficulties, usually with family or peers. An important component of many cognitive behavioural therapies, then, is to help children to solve interpersonal difficulties more effectively. Social problem-solving involves a sequence of steps. First, the child is encouraged to identify a problem capable of being solved. Next, he or she is encouraged by the therapist to generate several possible solutions. The young person then chooses one solution, and works with the therapist to identify steps to carry it out. Finally, the child tries out the solution, and evaluates the results.

Indications for cognitive-behaviour therapy

The cognitive behaviour therapies have been applied to almost all child psychiatric disorders. However, the conceptual basis and evidence base is strongest for four problems: depression, anxiety, aggression, and attentional problems.

Depression

Depressive symptoms and depressive disorders are less common in children than in adolescents (Angold et al., 1998). Can children experience the same cognitive symptoms that are found in adult depressive disorder? The evidence suggests that, by the preschool years, children start to differentiate the basic emotions and to understand their meaning (Kovacs, 1986). With the onset of concrete operational thinking (age range 7 through 11 years) the child begins to discover what is consistent in the course of any change or transformation. The child starts to develop self-consciousness and to evaluate his own competence by comparison with others. During early adolescence the self is also perceived more in psychological than physical terms, and concepts such as guilt and shame therefore become more prominent.

It seems, then, that enduring relatively stable negative attributions about the self become possible by early adolescence. At the same time, the young person's emotional vocabulary expands and the child starts to make fine-grain distinctions between emotions such as sadness and anger. So, by early adolescence, most young people can both experience and report the negative cognitions that are found in adult depression.

Research findings show that depressed young people have a set of cognitive distortions that are similar to those found in depressed adults. They often have low self-esteem and frequently show cognitive distortions, such as selectively attending to the negative features of an event (Kendall et al., 1990).

Several different cognitive behavioural programmes have been developed to treat these cognitive distortions (Harrington et al., 1998b,c). Most programmes have the following features in common. First, the therapy begins with sessions on emotional recognition that aim to help the young person to distinguish between different emotional states (for instance, between anger and sadness). Secondly, the child or adolescent is taught to self-monitor thoughts, and to start linking external events, thoughts, and feelings. Thirdly, behavioural tasks are often used to reinforce desired behaviours and thence to help the young person to gain control over symptoms. Self-reinforcement is often combined with activity scheduling. At this stage, it is quite common to introduce other behavioural techniques to deal with the behavioural or vegetative symptoms of depression. Fourthly, cognitive techniques are used to reduce depressive cognitions. For instance, adolescents and older children may be helped to identify cognitive distortions and to challenge them using techniques such as pro–con evaluation.

Anxiety disorders

Anxious children often show cognitive distortions, particularly a tendency to be overcritical and overconcerned about self-evaluation, and a bias towards picking up a threat in an ambiguous situation (Kendall & Chansky, 1991). They expect bad things to happen. Like anxious adults, anxious children tend to catastrophize physiological symptoms of anxiety, constructing symptoms such as panic attacks as heralding imminent death (Ollendick et al., 1993). As anxiety worsens, the young person typically begins to engage in avoidance behaviour and may eventually refuse to go to school.

One of the most widely used programmes for dealing with anxiety disorders is the four-step coping, or FEAR, plan (Kendall et al., 1992). The acronym FEAR stands for: Feeling frightened? (awareness of anxiety symptoms such as somatic symptoms); Expecting bad things to happen? (negative self-talk); Attitudes and actions that can help (problem-solving strategies); Results and rewards (rewards for success, learning to deal with failure). A typical programme starts with sessions to help the child identify anxious feelings and link these to somatic symptoms and to anxiety-provoking situations. Relaxation training is then introduced. The next few sessions help the child to identify anxious, self-talk (e.g. 'everyone is looking at me'), and to correct these thoughts using positive coping strategies. Finally, the child is helped to practise the skills learned in the first part of the programme in realistic situations. These may involve trips out of the clinic to real-life settings that invoke anxiety, such as school.

Aggression and behavioural problems

According to social learning theory, aggression is not just triggered by environmental events, but rather by the ways that these events are perceived. Research on aggressive children has shown a number of cognitive biases (Kazdin, 1985). They are more likely than non-aggressive children to read hostility into ambiguous social situations. They tend to view the world as hostile. This view has some basis in reality. Aggressive children are, in fact, more likely to be treated aggressively by their peers. This treatment by other children tends to perpetuate the reciprocal hostility of the aggressive child. Children with aggression and behavioural problems also have difficulties in sorting out testing social situations.

Cognitive behavioural programmes for young people who are aggressive usually have a strong focus on both changing social cognitions and on interpersonal problem-solving. Several programmes have been developed and most have the following features in common. Self-monitoring of behaviour helps young people to monitor and label thoughts, emotions and the situations in which they occur. Social perspective taking helps them to become aware of the intentions of others in social situations. Problem-solving skill training attempts to remedy the deficits in cognitive, problem-solving processing abilities that are often found in aggressive young people. One of the best-known programmes is the Hahnemann programme (Spivack et al., 1976). This programme has an emphasis on the development of simple word concepts that are necessary for problem-solving. These words emphasise that there are alternative ways of solving a problem ('I can hit him or tell him that I am cross. Hitting is different from talking'). The Hahnemann programme also fosters skills in information gathering and understanding motives.

Attention deficit disorder

Current models suggest that children with attention deficit disorder have deficits in certain 'executive' functions, particularly of self-regulation and inhibition. The key problem is thought to be the way that children inhibit or delay behavioural responses to external cues. They are unable or unwilling to inhibit actions and to wait for delayed consequences. Cognitive behavioural programmes for children with attention deficit usually include three elements: increasing the structure of the child's environment; behavioural therapy programmes with parents; and cognitive behavioural interventions with the child. Environmental changes emphasize the importance of constructing a structured environment that reduces the likelihood that the child will be overactive or impulsive. Behavioural interventions include techniques such as reward systems. Parents and other carers are taught that children with attention deficit/hyperactivity need more instructions and reinforcement than other children. Some of them require extra help in class or at times when the environment is less structured, such as during the morning break. Cognitive procedures generally aim to enhance self-control. At the core of most programmes are 'stop–think–do' approaches. The child is first taught to stop and then to think out aloud while performing various tasks. The idea is that the child learns techniques to recognize problems and to apply strategies to deal with them. These techniques are commonly taught to children using cartoons as in the Think Aloud Programme (Camp and Bash, 1985).

Contraindications

Although the cognitive behaviour therapies (CBT) have been applied across a range of child psychiatric problems, there are some relative contraindications to their use. The first is developmental stage. Many of the more 'advanced' cognitive techniques require that the child has some knowledge about cognition, and is able to use executive processes, or both. For example, many cognitive programmes require the child to complete homework assignments that may involve some degree of planning, such as phoning a friend to see if the friend is still cross. Younger children are likely to find this difficult as they are less likely to plan activities before carrying them out. Similarly, a key task in many cognitive programmes is to evaluate the evidence for and against a particular belief. However, the ability to hold mental representations of 'theory' vs. the 'evidence' emerges only gradually during adolescence. Developmental stage is therefore an important determinant of the best technique for the child. As a general rule, older children and adolescents respond better to cognitive treatments than younger children. Different techniques need therefore to be applied to children of different ages.

Another relative contraindication to CBT, at least on current evidence, is severity of disorder. It has to be said that much of the research that has been conducted with the CBT up to now has been based on samples recruited through advertisements or through schools. Furthermore, most of the literature on the treatment of childhood emotional disorders such as depression and anxiety appears to be based on relatively mild cases. It cannot be guaranteed that CBT will be effective in the most severe forms of depression or conduct disorder.

A final contraindication is environmental adversity. Child psychiatric disorders are deeply embedded in a social context. No treatment is going to succeed if basic needs such as adequate educational opportunities or security of family placement are not met. For example, children whose home life is repeatedly disrupted by parental arguments and violence are unlikely to be helped by CBT, or indeed by any other form of individual psychological intervention.

Evidence base for cognitive-behaviour therapy

There have been many randomized trials of the efficacy of the CBT for child and adolescent disorders. Thus, for instance, there have been at least six randomized controlled trials of CBT in samples of children with depressive symptoms recruited through schools (Harrington et al., 1998a,b,c). In four of these trials cognitive therapy was significantly superior to no treatment. Encouraging results have also been obtained with clinically diagnosed cases of depressive disorder, in whom a meta analysis found a significant improvement in the CBT group over comparison interventions (Harrington et al., 1998a,b,c). Similarly, positive findings have been reported for the use of the CBT in childhood anxiety disorders. Thus, two randomized trials from the same research group suggest that CBT is an effective treatment for anxiety symptoms (Kendall et al., 1997).

The cognitive behaviour therapies have also been applied to aggressive or conduct disordered children. For instance, Kazdin and colleagues (Kazdin et al., 1987) used a 20-session problem-solving skills programme with psychiatric inpatient children. Compared with two control conditions, the intervention led to significant reductions in parents' and teachers' ratings of aggressive behaviour after treatment and at 1-year follow-up. Other groups, too, have found that CBT has significant beneficial effects on antisocial behaviours that persist at 1-year follow-up. These results are very encouraging, though a significant minority of children with aggression do not respond.

Behavioural interventions improve certain targeted behaviours and social skills in children with attention deficit. However, these improvements tend not to persist over time or to generalize to new situations. Moreover, behaviour modification alone appears to be less effective than medication alone (American Academy of Child and Adolescent Psychiatry, 1997). Certain cognitive techniques, such as self-instruction, have also been used to help children with attention deficit. However, the evidence thus far suggests that cognitive techniques are not a particularly effective treatment for attention deficit, and add little to the effects of medication (American Academy of Child and Adolescent Psychiatry, 1997).

In summary, there is evidence from randomized trials that supports the efficacy of the CBT in depression, anxiety, and aggression. However, CBTs are not a 'cure-all'. Some conditions do not appear to benefit significantly, and it has not yet been established that the CBT are effective in very severe forms of emotional or behavioural disorder. Another key, yet relatively unexplored issue, is how they are best combined with other treatments, such as medication.

Conclusions

Increasing numbers of mental health professionals are adopting cognitive-behavioural approaches to the treatment of emotional or behavioural disorders in children and adolescents. Great progress has been made in understanding the negative cognitions that accompany many child psychiatric disorders. The cognitive-behaviour therapies appear to be an effective treatment for some, but by no means all, of these conditions. Future research on these CBTs in this age group needs to establish whether or not they are effective in the most severe forms of emotional and behavioural disorder.

REFERENCES

American Academy of Child and Adolescent Psychiatry (1997). Practice parameters for the assessment and treatment of children, adolescents, and adults with attention-deficit/hyperactivity disorder. *Journal of the American Academy of Child and Adolescent Psychiatry*, **36** (10 Supplement), 85S–121S.

Angold, A., Costello, E. J. and Worthman, C. M. (1998). Puberty and depression. The roles of age, pubertal status and pubertal timing. *Psychological Medicine*, **28**, 51–61.

Camp, B. W. and Bash, M. A. S. (1985). *Think aloud. Increasing social and cognitive skills. A problem-solving approach for children*. Champaign, IL: Research Press.

Harrington, R. C., Whittaker, J. and Shoebridge, P. (1998a). Psychological treatment of depression in children and adolescents. A review of treatment research. *British Journal of Psychiatry*, **173**, 291–8.

Harrington, R. C., Whittaker, J., Shoebridge, P. and Campbell, F. (1998b). Systematic review of efficacy of cognitive behaviour therapies in child and adolescent depressive disorder. *British Medical Journal*, **316**, 1559–63.

Harrington, R. C., Wood, A. and Verduyn, C. (1998c). Clinically depressed adolescents. In *Cognitive behaviour therapy for children and families*, ed. P. Graham, pp. 156–93. Cambridge: Cambridge University Press.

Kazdin, A. E. (1985). *Treatment of antisocial behaviour in children and adolescents*. Homewood, IL: Dorsey Press.

Kazdin, A. E., Esveldt-Dawson, K., French, N. H. and Unis, A. S. (1987). Effects of parent management training and problem-solving skills training combined in the treatment of antisocial child behavior. *Journal of the American Academy of Child and Adolescent Psychiatry*, **26**, 416–24.

Kendall, P. C. (1991). *Child and adolescent therapy. Cognitive-behavioural procedures*. New York: Guilford.

Kendall, P. C. and Chansky, T. E. (1991). Considering cognition in anxiety disordered youth. *Journal of Anxiety Disorders*, **5**, 167–85.

Kendall, P. C., Stark, K. D. and Adam, T. (1990). Cognitive deficit or cognitive distortion in childhood depression. *Journal of Abnormal Child Psychology*, **18**, 255–70.

Kendall, P. C., Chansky, T. E., Kane, M. T. et al. (1992). *Anxiety disorder in youth. Cognitive behavioral interventions*. Needham Heights, MA: Allyn and Bacon.

Kendall, P. C., Flannery-Schroeder, E., Panichellie-Mindel, S. M., Southam-Gerown, M., Henin, A. and Warman, M. (1997). Therapy for youths with anxiety disorders. A second randomized clinical trial. *Journal of Consulting and Clinical Psychology*, **65**, 366–80.

Kovacs, M. (1986). A developmental perspective on methods and measures in the assessment of depressive disorders. The clinical interview. In *Depression in young people: developmental and clinical perspective*, ed. M. Rutter, C. E. Izard and R. B. Read, pp. 435–65. New York: Guilford.

Ollendick, T. H., Mattis, S. G. and King, N. J. (1993). Panic in children and adolescents. A review. *Journal of Child Psychology and Psychiatry*, **35**, 113–34.

Spivack, G., Platt, J. J. and Shure, M. B. (1976). *The problem-solving approach to adjustment.* San Francisco, CA: Jossey-Bass.

8 Interpersonal psychotherapy for adolescents

Eric Fombonne

Interpersonal psychotherapy (IPT) was first developed in the mid-1960s as a brief, time-limited psychotherapy for depressed adults (Klerman et al., 1984; Weissman and Markowitz, 1994). Since then, modifications of IPT have been provided to treat specific psychiatric disorders such as eating disorders (Fairburn et al., 1991; Fairburn et al., 1993), drug addiction (Carroll et al., 1991), late depression (Reynolds et al., 1999), antepartum depression (Spinetti, 1997), or to address specific situations such as marital problems, counselling patients with HIV or bipolar disorders (Klerman and Weissman, 1993; Weissman and Markowitz, 1994). A downward extension for adolescents with major depression has also been developed by the Columbia Group (Moreau et al., 1991; Mufson et al., 1993). The goal of this chapter is to outline the main features of interpersonal psychotherapy with depressed adolescents and to review efficacy studies on IPT as a treatment of depression.

Interpersonal psychotherapy for adolescents (IPT-A) is a time-limited treatment for adolescents with major depression, which is suitable for 12- to 18-year-olds with the exclusion of those with high suicidal risk, psychotic depression or bipolar disorder. IPT-A is structured around 12 weekly sessions, and therefore lasts for about 3 months. Unlike most supportive, expressive forms of psychotherapy which are often used to treat depressed adolescents and which are not standardized, IPT-A has a treatment manual available (Mufson et al., 1993) and specific training is required for the therapist. The specific goals of IPT-A are: (i) to alleviate depressive symptoms; and (ii) to improve interpersonal functioning of the depressed adolescent. Thus, IPT-A is a symptom-orientated, highly focused intervention.

Conceptual background of IPT-A

The development of IPT was inspired by the work of influential theoreticians such as Meyer, Sullivan and Bowlby who emphasized the role of relationship disturbances and of a patient's environment in the onset of psychiatric disorder, as well as the importance of attachment and bonding as a primary biological need. Empirical studies establishing an association between stress, life events, loss of social attachments and the onset, course and outcome of adult depression, have supported this earlier theoretical work (Mufson et al., 1993). Clinical studies of depressed adults have also consistently shown the importance of social impairment in both acutely depressed and recovered patients, whilst intimacy and social support have been shown to be protective and to increase resilience in the face of adversity (Klerman et al., 1984).

IPT is not tied to a particular aetiological model of depression and recognizes that depression can occur through different pathways where biological, psychological, genetic and social factors act in various combinations. IPT, however, emphasizes that depression, irrespective of its particular cause, occurs in a social and interpersonal context which influences the onset, course and outcome of depression. More specifically, three processes are considered to contribute to depression: (i) a set of biopsychosocial mechanisms which lead to symptom formation; (ii) social functioning which reflects the combination of early childhood experiences and current social interactions; and (iii) personality, representing enduring traits and behaviours unique to the person which might predispose to symptom development. IPT aims to have an impact on the two first levels of processes, i.e. symptom formation and social functioning but, because IPT is a therapeutic intervention of low intensity with a focus on current depressive episodes, no attempt is made to impact on character pathology or underlying personality.

The role of the therapist in IPT-A

In IPT-A, the therapist is the patient's advocate and does not remain neutral. The therapist must speak for the patient, explain his problems and find practical solutions to them. The therapist must be active and not passive, engaging in various activities of liaison with the family and the school when the need arises. Similarly, the therapist may involve the parents at the end of some sessions, with the agreement of the patient, in order to facilitate communication between the therapist, the patient and his family. The therapeutic relationship is not interpreted in IPT as transference, although it might help the therapist to recognize such transference if it facilitates the understanding of the patient's current problems. The focus, however, remains on the here and now of the patient's network of relationships. Finally, the therapeutic relationship is not a friendship and clear boundaries need to be maintained.

Many of the features of the therapist's role are not specific to IPT-A. Thus, the therapeutic stance and most of the therapeutic techniques used in IPT-A do not differ from other forms of psychotherapies. IPT-A differs from other interventions in the strategies used to apply the therapeutic stance and techniques for specific tasks.

Techniques used in IPT-A

A wide array of techniques is used in IPT-A tailored to the particular patient's problems. Education is an important initial component of IPT-A and consists in providing information about depression, its symptoms, its nature, and its outcome to both patients and to significant others, and this educative component is seen as an important initial step in the therapy. Exploratory techniques of a non-directive kind are used by the therapist to acknowledge the patient's difficulties in a supportive way, and to convey to the patient a sense of being accepted and understood. More directive techniques are also used in IPT where the therapist actively elicits some material from the patient, as in each session's symptom review and in doing the interpersonal inventory in the initial phase of the treatment. Clarification is used to help the patient recognize, understand and communicate his feelings and emotions. This might take the form of making links between behaviours, feelings and thoughts, as they occurred in a relational context meaningful to the patient. Clarification of expectations within specific relationships is also used, particularly for adolescents whose roles are changing under various developmental pressures, and which require that the adolescent and his relatives adapt their own expectations in a reciprocal and flexible manner. Problem-solving can be used to help the patient address specific problem areas and conflicts, for instance, by helping the patient to generate alternative solutions. Encouragement of affect is a commonly used technique which aims at facilitating the expression, understanding and management of affects by adolescents. It may consist, for instance, of facilitating the acceptance of painful affects or encourage the development of new ones. Enhancement of communication skills is obtained using various techniques including role play within therapeutic sessions or social skills training for adolescents with deficient interpersonal skills. Communication analysis is used in sessions where the script of problematic relationships is reviewed with the patient in order to detect incorrect assumptions in the relationship, or ambiguous or paradoxical non-verbal communication features. Finally, straightforward behavioural change techniques can also be used in role play sequences, or in helping the patient generate solutions to actual problems (decision analysis).

Table 8.1. Goals of the initial phase of IPT-A

Sessions 1 to 4

(a) Deal with depression
  - (i) Review of depressive symptoms
  - (ii) Give the syndrome a name
  - (iii) Educate about depression (child + parent)
  - (iv) Give the patient a limited sick role
  - (v) Evaluate other aspects

(b) Relate depression to the interpersonal context
  - (i) Inventory of relationships
  - (ii) Identify expectations, (un)satisfying aspects, changes that patient wants to make, etc.

(c) Identify problem areas
  - (i) Determine problem area related to current depression
  - (ii) Treatment goals, i.e. which aspects of which relationships are related to depression and might be changed

(d) Assess suitability of patient for IPT-A

(e) Set a treatment contract
  - (i) Outline your understanding of the problem(s)
  - (ii) Agree on treatment goals
  - (iii) Discuss practical issues

To a large extent, the implementation of behavioural measures remains non-directive.

Outline of IPT-A

IPT-A is conveniently divided into an initial phase (sessions 1 to 4), a middle phase (sessions 5 to 8) and a termination phase (sessions 9 to 12), although some flexibility is permitted regarding these time divisions.

Initial phase

The goals of the initial phase are numerous and for convenience are summarized in Table 8.1. The first major target is to educate the adolescent as to what depression is, how it affects the patient's life, and how it impinges on his relationships with significant others. It is useful to start treatment by reviewing the depressive symptomatology reported by the patient and to assess the severity of each symptom. Diagnosing depression as a disorder, or giving it the name that the patient may have spontaneously used for his/her bad mood, allows the patient and his family to establish some distance from the disorder and helps communication about its effects. It is also useful to give the patient a

Table 8.2. Problem areas in the middle phase of IPT-A

(i)	Grief
(ii)	Role disputes
(iii)	Role transitions
(iv)	Interpersonal deficits
(v)	Single-parent family

limited sick role in order to avoid the criticism which depressed adolescents often experience when they withdraw from relationships or fail to fulfil social expectations as a result of their depression. For instance, this might consist of reducing the amount of homework that the patient has to do for the school in order to reduce the pressure on the adolescent, or else to limit the home chores that are expected by the relatives at home. Other issues relating to adolescent depression need to be carefully assessed in the first two sessions, such as the occurrence of co-morbid psychiatric disorders and, in particular, alcohol and substance abuse. The therapist will need to evaluate the possibility of using antidepressant medication in selected cases, and to address issues regarding school attendance or underachievement. The second goal of the initial phase is to establish the links between depressive symptoms and the interpersonal context in which they occur. An inventory of relationships is drawn up which provides a panoramic view of the network of relationships which are significant for the patient, to identify those relationships which are dysfunctional and those which are protective and supportive, to pinpoint communication problems, and clarify expectations within and from relationships, and to gauge which changes the patient wants to make in his specific relationships. When completing the interpersonal inventory, the therapist constantly makes links between interpersonal events and fluctuations in depressive symptomatology which help both the therapist and the patient to understand the depression as influenced by the interpersonal context. This inventory of relationships also helps the therapist to identify one or two key problem areas which will form the focus of the rest of the treatment, depending upon the particular predicament of the patient. The determination of problem areas should be discussed with the patient and should lead to agreement on a set of tenable treatment goals which the patient wants to achieve.

One goal of the initial phase is to assess the suitability of the patient for IPT-A which requires from the patient a willingness to work in a one-to-one relationship and some degree of psychological mindedness. Agreement must also be reached between the therapist and the patient on what are the key problem areas and the therapist must ensure that reasonable family support is available to the patient when embarking on psychotherapy. If the family is too dysfunctional, it might well be that other forms of intervention would take precedence over individual treatment, i.e. inpatient admission or Social Services involvement. When the initial phase is completed, a treatment contract must be set between the therapist and the patient which makes explicit the understanding of the current problems and the specific treatment goals to both the subject and his/her parents. A discussion of the practical issues regarding the time and frequency of sessions, what to do about missed sessions, issues of confidentiality, and ways in which the therapist may handle suicidal risk, must then be held openly.

Middle phase

One or two problem areas are selected from those listed in Table 8.2 as the focus of the middle phase of IPT-A. The congruence between these problem areas and the normal challenges occurring during adolescent development is striking. The first area, grief, is selected when the depression relates to a form of distorted, delayed or chronic grief following the loss of a loved figure. It will aim at helping the adolescent to acknowledge the loss and the feelings of abandonment which accompany it, to re-evaluate the pros and cons of the lost relationship, and to more realistically appraise the remaining relationships and social networks available to him/her. Role disputes is an area selected for conflictual relationships, typically between the adolescent and his parents, when a link between these conflicts and depressive symptomatology is found. The aims are to open new negotiations between the involved parties, to acknowledge role changes and modify expectations within the relationships, and to modify communication patterns. The third problem area, role transitions, will be selected when the depressive symptoms relate to difficulties in changing roles within the developmental process, either because the parents do not accept new roles in the adolescent or because the adolescent has his/her own difficulties in coping with new demands and expectations. This typically occurs with the passage from group to dyadic relationships, with the emergence of intimate sexual relationships, and with key normative transitions such as leaving home or planning a career, or with unforeseen circumstances such as adolescent pregnancy. The fourth problem area, interpersonal deficits, is addressed when a link has been established between the onset and maintenance of depressive symptoms in the adolescent and a chronic lack of interpersonal skills and social isolation which can be improved using communication analysis and direct teaching of relevant social skills. The fifth problem area, single parent family, has been added specifically for the adolescent version of IPT, recognizing the fact that, nowadays, many, if not the majority, of adolescents live within single-parent families or have had to deal with the departure of one of their parents from the home. This area will help to address feelings of loss and rejection, to clarify expectations from the relationship with the parent who left, to negotiate harmonious and working relationships with custodial parents, and to accept the permanence of the separation between the parents.

Termination phase

The last four sessions will be devoted to reviewing progress and changes which have been accomplished in therapy and to assess residual symptoms of depression. The review of progress and remaining difficulties should involve both the child and the parents. An explicit discussion of the termination before the last session ought to be initiated by the therapist and an acknowledgement of the difficulties of terminating the therapeutic relationship should be facilitated. This may be used to promote the recognition of independent competence in the adolescent by the therapist. The issue of full or partial relapse should also be addressed and the adolescent should by then have a clear knowledge of which symptoms to monitor and how to recognize the initial phases of a relapse. Appropriate assistance should be available in case of relapse.

Involving parents and the school

As previously mentioned, the parents will be involved especially at the beginning of the treatment to ensure their participation in the diagnostic assessment and to improve their own understanding and knowledge of depression, presentation, outcome and treatment. It is also important to involve parents in the initial phase when a specific treatment contract is to be set up between the therapist and the patient. Parents should be informed of the practical goals of the treatment, what will be left untouched by the therapist, and issues of both confidentiality and communication between the therapist and themselves if the circumstances indicate this, i.e. suicide risk. The parents will often also be involved in the middle phase during work with the adolescent on specific targets. This may take the form of the therapist spending some time with the adolescent and his/her parents at the end of sessions to discuss issues relevant to family life which are considered to impinge on treatment progress.

Liaison with the school is also a key component of intervention and the therapist, or a professional colleague from the same team, may need to explain to the school the nature of the depression and why it has resulted in failure to attend or to achieve at school (educational aspect). It may also be necessary to negotiate the practical steps which can be taken to facilitate reattendance, and to create conditions which will improve achievement as recovery occurs (interventional aspect). The reader is referred to the treatment manual (Mufson et al., 1993) for practical examples of IPT-A treatments.

Efficacy of IPT and IPT-A

Several well-designed randomized controlled trials have been conducted with IPT in both the treatment of acute depression in adults and in maintenance studies (Weissman and Markowitz, 1994). Acute treatment studies showed in the early 1970s that IPT and tricyclic antidepressant intervention had roughly equal efficacy against control conditions in the treatment of acute depression, with an improved effect for the combination of drug and psychotherapy (Klerman et al., 1974). Although antidepressant medication had a slightly quicker effect in alleviating symptoms, IPT appeared to be associated with a better psychosocial functioning at one year follow-up, an effect which was delayed. The recent NIMH study of the Treatment of Depression Collaborative Research Programme (16-week treatment of 250 depressed adults) confirmed that cognitive behavioural therapy (CBT), IPT and imipramine had similar benefits over control conditions, with a trend towards superiority of IPT over CBT in the most severe cases (Elkin et al., 1989). In a recent study, combined pharmacotherapy and psychotherapy has been found to produce better results when the major depression is severe (Thase et al., 1997a). Similarly, the response to IPT was less good amongst adult depressives with abnormal sleep profiles indicating more neurobiological disturbance (Thase et al., 1997b). The limited research evidence on the cost-effectiveness of psychotherapy and pharmacotherapy suggests slight superiority of pharmacotherapy (Lave et al., 1998) but data are so far too scarce to draw even preliminary conclusions on this issue.

The first maintenance treatment studies showed that IPT was shown to improve social functioning after six months of treatment, and the combination of IPT with drug treatment appeared to result in the best effect (Klerman et al., 1974; Weissman et al., 1979). Broadly similar results were found in a 3-year maintenance trial comparing high-dose imipramine with a low frequency form of IPT (one session per month) which was superior to placebo and more efficacious in combination with drug treatment (Frank et al., 1991). The same pattern of better maintenance with combined nortriptyline and IPT over single modality treatments has been shown for older depressives (Reynolds et al., 1999).

As IPT for adolescents has been developed recently, there are fewer systematic studies investigating its efficacy. In one open trial, the Columbia University group described the pre- and post-treatment differences in a group of 14 adolescents (12 girls and 2 boys) with a mean age of 15.5 years during a 12-week course of IPT-A (Mufson et al., 1994). Post-treatment, 90% of this small sample had recovered from their major depression, and exhibited a significant decrease over time in depressive rating scales including the Beck Depression Inventory and the Hamilton Rating Scale for Depression. Improvement was also noted in several areas of social functioning. While this study was useful in showing the acceptability of IPT-A for adolescents, caution is needed in interpreting its results since no comparison group was available, the treatment was administered by one single therapist, ratings were not blind, and the particular pilot sample was rather unrepresentative. The same group published 1-year follow-up data on ten subjects of this initial sample (Mufson and Fairbanks, 1996) and only one subject fulfilled criteria for major depression at follow-up, a rate of recurrence which is consistent with other studies. There had been no hospital admissions in the treated group, no unplanned pregnancies, no suicidal attempts, and all subjects were attending school regularly. In addition, they expressed a positive attitude towards the treatment which they had received. The Columbia group has now completed a randomized clinical trial assessing the efficacy of IPT-A in a controlled experiment, whose results show efficacy over a control psychological intervention (Mutson et al., 1999). Furthermore, a randomized comparison of IPT-A against CBT and a waiting-list control modality has confirmed the benefits of IPT-A in reducing depressive symptoms and improving social functioning, with a trend towards superiority of IPT-A over CBT (Rossello and Bernal, 1999). The current evidence therefore suggests that IPT-A is a useful treatment for adolescent depression. Alongside other therapeutic interventions, IPT-A is one of the suggested treatments for adolescent depressive disorders in the practice parameters published by the American Academy of Child and Adolescent Psychiatry (AACAP, 1998).

Differences between IPT-A and other psychotherapies

Table 8.3 provides a list contrasting the features of IPT, cognitive behavioural therapy (CBT) and psychodynamic therapy. Therapists used to psychodynamic approaches will probably find it easier to adopt an IPT model of brief focused psychotherapy rather than that embodied by cognitive vulnerability models. The focus on the adolescent's self and on the subject's meaningful relationships and the emphasis on emotional learning in IPT provides natural bridges between IPT and psychodynamic therapy. However, IPT and CBT also share many characteristics. The main difference between these two focused, time-limited therapies lies in the adoption of a highly specified theoretical model in CBT which determines the focus of action for the therapy. By contrast, IPT is not tied to a particular theoretical model and generally focuses on higher order

Table 8.3. IPT-A, CBT and psychodynamic therapy

	IPT	CBT	Psychodynamic
Depression	Primary, multifactorial	Due to dysfunctional beliefs and distorted cognitive style	Derives from guilt, anger hostility
Focus	Here and now	Here and now	Past experiences
	On actual relationships	On cognitions and belief systems	On intrapsychic processes
Goals	Symptom relief	Symptom relief	Personality change
Time frame	Time-limited	Time-limited	Longer term
Therapist	Active, supportive	Active, supportive	Neutral, not intervening
Technique	No interpretation of therapeutic relation	No interpretation of therapeutic relation	Transference is interpreted
	No homework, within session practice	Task assignment	No active techniques

levels of organization. Whether or not the processes of change in each of these two therapies are different is, however, uncertain. It has, for instance, been shown that improvement in depressive symptomatology with CBT was not obviously linked to corresponding changes in the negative cognitions of the patient (Lewinsohn et al., 1990; Harrington et al., 1998). Conversely, the significant improvements described with IPT in psychosocial functioning and in relationships are bound to be mediated, at least partially, in changes in the subject's beliefs and cognitions. Thus, the main obvious difference lies in the strategies used in each therapy to promote change rather than in specific processes. With very few exceptions (Ablon and Jones, 1999), studies of processes of change with these therapies are non-existent and much could be gained from a more fine-tuned understanding of how change occurs with these respective psychotherapeutic strategies.

Issues for future research

ITP-A has, as yet, not been as intensely assessed as CBT (Wood et al., 1996; Harrington et al., 1998; Reinecke et al., 1998; Brent et al., 1997). Assuming that

IPT-A will continue to show superiority over control conditions in treating the depressed adolescent, the practitioner will have to select between two forms of time-limited psychotherapy (CBT and IPT-A) and active psychopharmacological agents of the SSRI group (Emslie et al., 1997). With the exception of the study by Rossello and Bernal (1999), no studies so far have performed a direct comparison of each of these active treatments in adolescent samples, and undoubtedly this will be a major task for the forthcoming years (Fombonne, 1998). It is noteworthy that psychopharmacological studies conducted on samples of depressed adolescents were, on average, more severely impaired than those included in psychotherapy studies. In addition, as for adult studies, the issue will arise as to whether combination treatment (psychotherapy and medication) is associated with more rapid improvement and better overall efficacy in the treatment of acute major depression. A further question to be answered is whether certain features such as abnormal sleep profile, neuroendocrine abnormalities and symptom severity predict a better clinical response to certain treatment modalities. When comparing each modality, it will be necessary to undertake longer follow-ups than are usually performed in short-term clinical trials. Studies in adults indicate that IPT has a delayed effect, with superiority detected only at 6-month or 1-year follow-up. If so, it will be important to document the long term effects of each treatment, particularly looking at outcome criteria such as relapse rate which is typically high in adolescent samples. Finally, the use of either of the psychotherapies or medication as a maintenance treatment in recurrent depression will have to be assessed.

Clinical vignette

Sophie is a 15-year-old girl, a single child, living with two old-fashioned parents who raised her according to strict moral principles. During her summer holiday in Spain, Sophie had a brief romantic relationship with a 16-year-old boy from a local family. It was her first romance and, following the end of her summer vacation, she became increasingly sad as she did not receive a reply to the letters which she sent to her ex-boyfriend. She developed sleep difficulties, lost her appetite, had increasing concentration difficulties at school and her school performance had dropped considerably by the end of the first term. At referral a few weeks later, she was very tired, lacking in energy, and bored with most of her usual activities. Her parents had reacted to her initial difficulties by being dismissive of the importance of this brief summer relationship. As a result, Sophie became very angry, had several severe arguments with them, and withdrew more and more from her relationship with her parents, spending most of her time in her bedroom, isolated, usually lying in bed. When her parents tried to engage her, it was only to emphasize her need to improve her school performance.

In the initial phase of IPT, the therapist identified and discussed the depression with Sophie and her parents. The abnormal quality of Sophie's symptoms was explained to both Sophie and her parents whose views on Sophie's behaviour progressively shifted from a superficial adolescence crisis towards a recognition of the depression and an acknowledgement of its detrimental effect on Sophie's functioning. The assignment of a sick role to Sophie allowed the parents to be less critical, less demanding regarding her school work, and more supportive of her. An inventory of Sophie's relationships showed that she had always been very close to her mother and that she had been very disappointed by her lack of support over recent months; the ongoing arguments with her mother were actively maintaining her depressive symptomatology. In the initial sessions, the therapist connected the depressive symptoms, both in terms of onset and later exacerbation, with the relationship difficulties with the mother; the problem area which was defined in agreement with Sophie was an interpersonal role dispute.

The middle phase sessions allowed Sophie more effectively to express her feelings to her mother, to request more directly her support, to clarify the mutual expectations on their relationship, and to resume more flexible and effective communication patterns. The conflicts with her mother decreased in both frequency and intensity and both mother and Sophie were able to resume an open and supportive relationship. The depressive symptomatology rapidly decreased in parallel.

Sophie's case illustrates how well IPT suits depressed adolescents' needs. Sophie was stuck in her relationship with her parents, but during the therapy sessions she could express her feelings of disappointment and anger at them, and, with the help of the therapist, connect these feelings with the depressive symptoms and the relational context. This was achieved without relying on homework assignments which might have proved too difficult for Sophie (considering her extreme tiredness and apathy, and her concentration difficulties) and for her parents (in view of their lack of psychological-mindedness and inappropriate grasp of the problem initially). The focus by the therapist on the emotional meaning of the depressive experience brought the therapy sessions into close line with her daily experiences. Sophie wanted to share her feelings and talk about her actual relationships, her feelings of anger and disappointment; a narrow cognitive focus would have been less naturalistic and less motivating for Sophie. Generally, the focus on the interpersonal context in IPT is congruent with most adolescents' ways of talking about their daily psychological experiences. Therapists coming from a psychodynamic perspective will probably find it easy to grasp the IPT techniques and strategies which share with psychodynamic approaches a focus on emotions and on their meaning in an interpersonal context.

REFERENCES

Ablon, J. S. and Jones, E. E. (1999). Psychotherapy process in the National Institute of Mental Health Treatment of Depression Collaborative Research Program. *Journal of Consulting and Clinical Psychology*, **67**(1), 64–75.

American Academy of Child and Adolescent Psychiatry (AACAP) (1998). Practice parameters for the assessment and treatment of children and adolescent with depressive disorders. *Journal of the American Academy of Child and Adolescent Psychiatry*, **37** (10 Suppl.), 63S–83S.

Brent, D. A., Holder, A., Kolko, D. et al. (1997). A clinical psychotherapy trial for adolescent depression comparing cognitive family, and supportive therapy. *Archives of General Psychiatry*, **54**, 877–85.

Carroll, K. M., Rounsaville, B. J. and Gawin, F. H. (1991). A comparative trial of psychotherapies for ambulatory cocaine abusers: relapse prevention and interpersonal psychotherapy. *American Journal of Drug and Alcohol Abuse*, **17**, 229–47.

Elkin, I., Shea., M. T., Watkins, J. T. et al. (1989). National Institute of Mental Health Treatment of Depression Collaborative Research Program: general effectiveness of treatments. *Archives of General Psychiatry*, **46**, 971–82.

Emslie, G. J., Rush, A. J., Weinberg, W. A. et al. (1997). A double-blind, randomized, placebo-controlled trial of fluoxetine in children and adolescents with depression. *Archives of General Psychiatry*, **54**(11), 1031–7.

Fairburn, C., Jones, R., Peveler, R. et al. (1991). Three psychological treatments for bulimia nervosa: a comparative trial. *Archives of General Psychiatry*, **48**, 463–9.

Fairburn, C., Jones, R., Peveler, R., Hope, R. and O'Connor, M. (1993). Psychotherapy and bulimia nervosa: longer-term effects of interpersonal psychotherapy, behavior therapy, and cognitive behavior therapy. *Archives of General Psychiatry*, **50**, 419–28.

Fombonne, E. (1998). The management of depression in children and adolescents. In *Handbook on the management of depression*, pp. 345–63, ed. S. Checkley. Oxford: Blackwell.

Frank, E., Kupfer, D. J., Wagner, E. F., McEachran, A. B. and Cornes, C. (1991). Efficacy of interpersonal psychotherapy as a maintenance treatment of recurrent depression: Contributing factors. *Archives of General Psychiatry*, **48**, 1053–9.

Harrington, R. C., Wood, A. and Verduyn, C. (1998). Cognitive behavioural treatment of clinically depressed adolescents. Principles and practice. In *Cognitive-Behavioural Therapy in Children and Adolescents*, ed. P. Graham. Cambridge: Cambridge University Press.

Klerman, G.L., Weissman, M. M., Rounsaville, B.J. and Chevron, E. S. (eds.) (1984). *Interpersonal psychotherapy for depression*. New York: Basic Books.

Klerman, G. L., DiMascio, A., Weissman, M. M., Prusoff, B. A. and Paykel, E. S. (1974). Treatment of depression by drugs and psychotherapy. *American Journal of Psychiatry*, **131**, 186–91.

Klerman, G. L. and Weissman, M. M. (ed.) (1993). *New applications of interpersonal psychotherapy*. Washington, DC: American Psychiatric Press.

Lave, J., Frank, R., Schulberg, H. C. and Kamlet, M. S. (1998). Cost-effectiveness of treatments for major depression in primary care practice. *Archives of General Psychiatry*, **55**, 645–51.

Lewinsohn, P. M., Clarke, G. N., Hops, H. and Andrews, J. (1990). Cognitive-behavioural treatment for depressed adolescents. *Behaviour Therapy*, **21**, 385–401.

Moreau, D., Mufson, L., Weissman, M. M. and Klerman, G. L. (1991). Interpersonal psychotherapy for adolescent depression: description of modification and preliminary application. *Journal of the American Academy of Child and Adolescent Psychiatry*, **30**(4), 642–51.

Mufson, L. and Fairbanks, J. (1996) Interpersonal psychotherapy for depressed adolescents: a one-year naturalistic follow-up study. *Journal of the American Academy of Child and Adolescent Psychiatry*, **35**(9), 1145–55.

Mufson, L., Moreau, D., Weissman, M. M., Wickramaratne and Samoilov, A. (1994). Modification of interpersonal psychotherapy with depressed adolescents (IPT-A). Phase I and II studies. *Journal of the American Academy of Child and Adolescent Psychiatry*, 33(5), 695–705.

Mufson, L., Moreau, D., Weissman, W. and Klerman, G. (1993). *Interpersonal psychotherapy for depressed adolescents*. New York: Guilford Press.

Mufson, L., Weissman, M., Moreau, D. and Garfinkel, R. (1999). Efficacy of interpersonal psychotherapy for depressed adolescents. *Archives of General Psychiatry*, **56**, 573–9.

Reinecke, M. A., Ryan, N. E. and DuBois, D. L. (1998). Cognitive-behavioral therapy of depression and depressive symptoms during adolescence. A review and meta-analysis. *Journal of the American Academy of Child and Adolescent Psychiatry*, **37**(1), 26–34.

Reynolds, C., Frank, E., Perel, J. et al. (1999). Nortriptyline and interpersonal psychotherapy as maintenance therapies for recurrent major depression. *Journal of the American Medical Association*, **281**(1), 39–45.

Rossello, J. and Bernal, G. (1999). The efficacy of cognitive-behavioural and interpersonal treatments for depresssion in Puerto-Rican adolescents. *Journal of Consulting and Clinical Psychology*, **67**, 734–45.

Spinetti, M. (1997). Interpersonal psychotherapy for depressed antepartum women: a pilot study. *American Journal of Psychiatry*, **154**(7), 1028–30.

Thase, M., Buysse, D., Frank, E. et al. (1997a). Which depressed patients will respond to interpersonal psychotherapy? The role of abnormal EEG sleep profiles. *American Journal of Psychiatry*, **154**(4), 502–9.

Thase, M., Greenhouse, J., Frank, E. et al. (1997b). Treatment of major depression with psychotherapy or psychotherapy–pharmacotherapy combinations. *Archives of General Psychiatry*, **54**, 1009–15.

Weissman, M. M. and Markowitz, J. C. (1994). Interpersonal psychotherapy. *Archives of General Psychiatry*, **51**(8), 599–606.

Weissman, M. M., Prusoff, B. A., DiMascio, A., Neu, C., Goklaney, M. and Klerman, G. L. (1979). The efficacy of drugs and psychotherapy in the treatment of acute depressive episodes. *American Journal of Psychiatry*, **136**, 555–8.

Wood, A., Harrington, R. and Moore, A. (1996). Controlled trial of a brief cognitive-behavioural intervention in adolescent patients with depressive disorders. *Journal of Child Psychology and Psychiatry and Allied Disciplines*, **37**(6), 737–46.

9 Play therapy with children

Gerhard Niebergall

Introduction

Concepts about the mechanisms of change in play therapy are closely associated with theories of play. Almost all theories of play assume that play is biologically useful, because it facilitates development of the human organism and gives young children the opportunity to experiment with the coping mechansims they develop as they grow up. Most theories of play agree that play performs an important educational function and helps in the socialization process of the child. They emphasize certain aspects of play as being important, such as the joy of effectance, e.g. exercising motor functions or fine motor skills, the increase in the degree of spontaneous activity, the opportunity to practise the rules of social interaction and the possibility of confronting oneself with the idea of being in dangerous situations.

Children, with or without a psychiatric disorder, learn to cope with the problems and conflicts of everyday life spontaneously through play. The child has the opportunity to act out emotions (in the sense of 'catharsis'). Through spontaneous play, the child has the opportunity to experience a feeling of creativity and effectiveness, thus improving his/her self-esteem. In this way, the child's sense of self-esteem is built up. At play, the child is involved in a 'dialogue' between himself and his environment. Through watching a child at play, adults can gain insight into his/her internal world and extend their understanding of the child. Children frequently incorporate experiences from real life into their play, making these experiences accessible.

Beyond its spontaneous therapeutic effect, play is important in clinical practice because of its diagnostic function, e.g. in children who have been physically or sexually abused. Such children often relate their experiences, either overtly or covertly, when provided with appropriate toys or play material. All these observation have resulted in the development of the concept of 'play therapy' with children. Play therapy is a technique which relies to a great extent on play with the child as therapeutic medium (Moore et al., 1999).

The most widely used approaches to play therapy have been psychodynamic and client centred. However, client-centred play therapy often includes a number of concepts from behaviour therapy models (Landreth, 1991).

Approaches to play therapy

Play therapy is associated with the names of a number of prominent child and adolescent psychotherapists. The basic concepts of the psychoanalytically orientated child and play therapies as developed by Anna Freud, Melanie Klein, Hans Zulliger, Donald Winnicott and Annemarie Dührssen are shown in Table 9.1. Virginia Axline, who worked with Carl Rogers, played a major role in developing the technique of non-directive play therapy. This is based on the following assumptions (Axline, 1947; Moore et al., 1999).

- The therapist should develop a warm, friendly relationship with the child, in which a good rapport is established as soon as possible.
- The therapist should establish a feeling of permissiveness in the relationship such that the child feels free to express his feelings openly.
- The therapist should accept the child exactly as he or she is.
- The therapist should be alert to the feelings the child is expressing and reflect those feelings back to him or her in a manner such that the child will gain insight into his or her behaviour.
- The therapist should maintain a deep respect for the child's ability to solve his (or her) own problems when given an opportunity to do so. The responsibility to make choices and to institute change must remain with the child.
- The therapist should not attempt to direct the child's actions or conversation in any manner. The child leads the way, the therapist follows.
- The therapist should not try to hurry the pace of therapy. It is a gradual process and it should be recognized as such by the therapist.
- The therapist should place only such limitations as are necessary to anchor the therapy to the world of reality and to make the child aware of his (or her) responsibility within the relationship.

As play therapy continues to evolve, client-centred play therapy with children and adolescents continues to be widely used, although approaches to play therapy based on learning theory are becoming increasingly important (see also Chapter 11).

Play therapy in clinical practice

Play therapy is usually undertaken in an individual setting. The room in which sessions are undertaken should be suitable for the purpose. An adequate but

Table 9.1. Psychoanalytically orientated play therapy: basic approaches and specific techniques

Author	Basic approach	Therapeutic techniques
A. Freud	The approach is psychoanalytical, with therapeutic and educational elements. Emphasis is placed on both the therapist's and the patient's needs and expectations.	No interpretation. Conflicts are expressed symbolically through play. Conflicts can be solved through catharsis and adaptation.
M. Klein	Modification of classical psychoanalysis. This presupposes early partial object relations, which generally involve strong emotions. The individual deals with such emotions through defence mechanisms such as introjection or projection.	Drive impulses, anxieties and fantasies are interpreted verbally during play, with the aim of bringing those impulses and emotions into consciousness and thus subsequently reducing anxiety.
H. Zulliger	Psychoanalytical approach, with emphasis on educational and other directive elements.	No verbal interpretation. The aim of therapeutic interventions is to uncover conflicts at a symbolic level during play (acting-out together with the child).
D. Winnicott	Modification of the psychoanalytical approach. Combination of interpretation, encouragement and support. The experience of a positive relationship is considered more important than gaining insight into particular conflicts.	Acting-out together with the child and interpreting early childhood conflicts in terms of bonding and detatchment. Combination of supportive and demanding elements in therapy.
A. Dührssen	Neo-analytical concept. Emphasis is placed on practical educational interventions rather than the interpretation of unconscious conflicts.	The aim of therapy is to offer an 'expansive space' to encourage the child to express his inhibited impulses. The therapist's function is to clarify, compensate and direct the child's behaviour.

Modified from Kampmann-Elsas, 1997.

not overwhelming quantity and range of toys and other material should be provided. Toys should be attractive to a wide range of children of different ages, interests and capabilities. Such play material may include toys which help children to express their anxieties and behavioural difficulties, e.g. weapons to express aggressive impulses, a sandbox to allow imaginative play, toys demanding dexterous skills, competitive games and board games for the expression of issues arising from the observance of rules.

Commonly, sessions are undertaken once a week, one session lasting 45 minutes. An average of about 30 sessions is often enough to bring about improvement over the course of therapy. However, the number of sessions necessary may vary considerably.

The content of play therapy sessions obviously depends on the specific technique used and the therapist's theoretical background, i.e. his understanding of the disorder's aetiology. Most therapists agree that the principal aim of play therapy is to facilitate normal psychological development. The therapeutic setting should be an environment suitable for addressing the child's basic needs in terms of secure relationships, empathy, positive regard, recognition and encouragement. Play is the most important mode of communication between the child and the therapist. Thus, play therapy should focus on encouraging the child to express himself and deal with emotions at a non-verbal level. However, verbal expression should also be encouraged, because it is an important additional mode of communication in play therapy. Verbal communication is essential for achieving an appropriate balance between cognitive and emotional processes, and improving congruence of the child's emotional experience and behaviour.

Play during therapy will reflect the child's internal world. The therapist should give the child the opportunity to use the available toys and material to play. The degree of active participation by the therapist will largely depend on his theoretical background. However, this should not be the only determining factor. The child's symptoms and behavioural difficulties should also influence considerably the extent of structuring, steering and direct assisstance that is given by the therapist (see also Chapter 2, Fig. 2.10).

During play therapy, the therapist should demonstrate those qualities which are considered important in client-centred psychotherapy, i.e. genuinness, unconditional positive regard and empathic understanding towards the patient (Rogers, 1951). In a play therapy setting this implies a warm and friendly attitude in a pleasant and relaxed atmosphere, which will enable the child to express those impulses which seem most important to him through play. In this way, the child will be able to approach previously suppressed, avoided, or partially unconcious topics and emotions. As in verbally based psychotherapy with adolescents, the therapist's permissive attitude during play therapy encourages the child's tendency towards self-realization. On the other hand, certain boundaries must exist in terms of the child's behaviour during play therapy sessions, including basic rules such as not assaulting the therapist, tidying up after sessions, and not being destructive with the toys and other play material. In contrast to children with extraverted behaviour disorders, for whom keeping these rules is particularly important, children with introverted disorders often require encouragement and support in experiencing their impulses and transforming them into actions.

Mechanisms of change, indications and contraindications

Indications and contraindications for play therapy also depend on the therapist's view on the mechanisms of change, i.e. the way in which this type of treatment is considered to bring about change. The same mechanisms of change which apply to other types of psychotherapy also apply to play therapy (Grawe, 1997): the problem-solving component ('mastery' or 'coping'), the explanatory component ('clarification of meaning'), and the relationship component ('problem actuation').

From a psychoanalytical perspective, psychopathological symptoms are considered to be the result of unconscious conflicts. Play therapy is intended to encourage the symbolic expression of such latent conflicts, and make them accessible to conscious contemplation by means of verbal interpretation. In this context, the aim of play therapy is to identify the latent conflicts expressed symbolically through play and treat the conflicts in therapy by means of verbal interpretation during play with the child.

Client-centred approaches to psychotherapy emphasize the beneficial effect of treatment in terms of the capacity for spontaneous self-realization ('self-cure'), particularly in children who have been impaired in their normal development as a result of external circumstances and who have suffered consequently an emotional disturbance or adjustment disorder. However, behaviour in play therapy can also be understood in terms of learning theory. Thus, behavioural approaches are often useful in this setting, including systematic desensitization for anxious children, exposure, operant conditioning techniques for externalizing behaviour etc.

Based on these considerations, play therapy can be considered particularly suitable for the treatment of anxious and inhibited syndromes and other emotional disturbances, but is also widely applied in the treatment of adjustment disorders, conduct disorders, interactional difficulties at school and family conflicts. It is important to include the child's parents (or the whole family) in treatment, especially when the child's behavioural or emotional problems are associated with issues arising from or within his/her family.

In contrast, play therapy is usually contraindicated in children with intellectual impairment, extremely aggressive behaviour and severe acting-out. In general, however, play therapy has a broad spectrum of indications, especially if the approach to play therapy is wide and includes educational measures ('broad spectrum technique'). Whilst play therapy is especially appropriate for children between 3 and 12 years old, some techniques have been used successfully to treat adults (especially in a group therapy setting). Thus, there are no strict age limits for play therapy (see also Chapter 11).

Evaluation

Unfortunately, there is a paucity of empirical evaluation studies of child and adolescent psychotherapy, play therapy in particular. Many of the available studies are narrow in scope and have methodological faults. In many cases, the authors report subjective evidence for treatment success and consider this a sufficient basis for evaluation. In contrast, several empirical studies have shown the efficacy of a non-directive, client-centred approach, e.g. Schmidtchen (1996), Goetze and Jaide (1974). Psychoanalytically orientated approaches to play therapy have also been reported to be effective (Fisher and Greenberg, 1977), although the approach has remained controversial (Luborsky et al., 1975; Smith et al., 1980; Enke and Czogalik, 1993).

REFERENCES

Axline, V. (1947). *Play therapy*. Boston, MA: Houghton Mifflin.

Enke, H. and Czogalik, D. (1993). *Allgemeine und spezifische Wirkfaktoren in der Psychotherapie*. Stuttgart: Dietmar Fischer.

Fisher, S. and Greenberg, R. P. (1977). *The scientific credibility of Freud's theories and therapies*. New York: Seymour Harvester.

Goetze, H. and Jaide, W. (1974). *Die nicht-direktive Spieltherapie*. München: Kindler.

Grawe, K. (1997). Research-informed psychotherapy. *Psychotherapy Research*, 7, 1–19.

Kampmann-Elsas, C. (1997). Spieltherapie. In *Psychotherapie im Kindes- und Jugendalter*, ed. H. Remschmidt, pp. 114–19. Stuttgart: Thieme.

Landreth, G. L. (1991). *Play therapy. The art of the relationship*. Bristol, PA: Accelerated Development.

Luborsky, D. H., Singer, B. and Luborsky, L. (1975). Comparative studies of psychotherapy. *Archives of General Psychiatry*, **32**, 995–1008.

Moore, H. B., Presbury, J. H., Smith, L. W. and McKee, J. E. (1999). Person-centered approaches. In *Counselling and psychotherapy with children and adolescents. Theory and practice for school and clinical settings*, ed. H. T. Prout and D. T. Brown, pp. 155–202. New York: Wiley.

Rogers, C. (1951). *Client-centered therapy*. Boston: Mifflin.

Schmidtchen, S. (1996). Neue Forschungsergebnisse zu Prozessen und Effekten der Kinderspieltherapie. In *Personenzentrierte Psychotherapie mit Kindern und Jugendlichen*, ed. C. Boeck-Singelmann, B. Ehlers, T. Haensel, and C. Monden-Engelhardt, pp. 99–140. Göttingen: Hogrefe.

Smith, M. L., Glass, G. V. and Miller, R. I. (1980). *The benefits of psychotherapy*. Baltimore: Johns Hopkins University Press.

10 Individual psychotherapy with adolescents

Gerhard Niebergall

Introduction

Various psychotherapeutic techniques have evolved out of the 'client-centred' methods developed by Rogers (1951). In these, the therapist plays a non-directive role, restricting his interventions to comments on the emotional significance of the patient's statements. Although there are many approaches, the basis of this type of therapy is invariably verbal interaction between the patient and the therapist. The verbal interaction is intended to bring about the following changes (Wolberg, 1969; Kind, 1982): (i) remove, reduce or modify symptoms, (ii) minimize disordered behaviour, (iii) encourage normal development and personality maturation.

Verbal therapeutic methods vary according to the degree to which attempts are made to influence the patient (Fig. 10.1). Thus, while client-centred therapy is considered an essentially 'non-directive' technique, rational emotive therapy involves a more directive approach, and psychoanalytically orientated psychotherapy lies somewhere between the two.

In clinical practice, especially with adolescents (Lehmkuhl et al., 1992), therapists do not usually adhere strictly to a single technique. A combination of several different techniques may be better suited to meet the specific needs of patients. An excessively rigid approach should be avoided, and sessions should be flexible, responding to the reactions of the patient to avoid feelings of being misunderstood or not being taken seriously.

It is important to bear in mind the developmental stage of a child or adolescent when undertaking psychotherapy (see also Chapter 1 and 2).

Rogers considered the relationship between patient ('client') and therapist to be of paramount importance in psychotherapy. This view, of course, is not unique to client-centred therapy, and the importance of an appropriate therapeutic relationship is widely accepted. In this method, however, the relationship includes a number of specific features (Rogers, 1951):

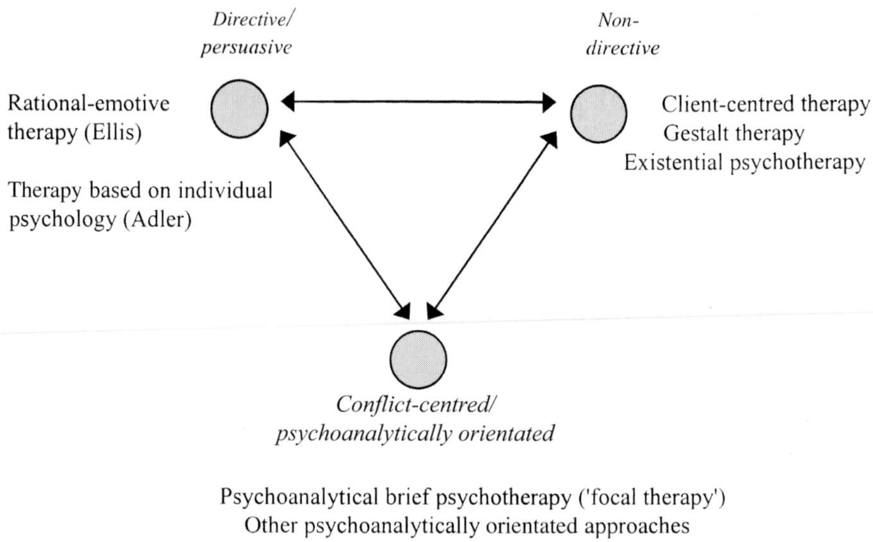

Fig. 10.1. Degree to which the patient is directly influenced with verbal approaches to psychotherapy (Kind, 1982).

(i) unconditional positive regard and emotional warmth towards the client;
(ii) empathic understanding and an attempt to convey back to the patient what the therapist has understood;
(iii) genuiness in the therapist's behaviour towards the client.

The therapist's empathy, support, uncomplicated language and particularly the 'reflection of feelings' intend to convey to the patient the feeling of being understood. Eventually this should enable the patient to integrate those aspects of his personality that he has previously been unable to accept. This is an important prerequisite for the development of a 'fully functioning person', congruent with his own personality. The aim is for the patient to be able to adapt appropriately to a constantly changing environment. This does not imply that opportunistic behaviour should be encouraged; however, the patient should be supported as he/she reorganizes the subjective world, enabling the patient to become a more spontaneous, autonomous and confident individual. The process of cathartic abreaction may facilitate this process and help to release emotions which have been hidden or denied and are thus inaccessible to the patient. The verbal outpouring of emotions should help the patient to improve introspective abilities and support self-help capacity.

Although the principles of client-entered therapy described here were developed in adults, they apply equally in the treatment of adolescents. Indeed, Rogers (1951) emphasized the developmental nature of client-centred therapy as a constantly developing human relationship, facilitating growth and change. The approach is based on the assumption that every human being has the potential for change which can be released with the help of a supportive relationship. A further essential component is that this individual is experiencing feelings of positive regard, sensitive, empathic understanding, and that these feelings can be conveyed to the client. In its emphasis on the interpersonal relationship rather than symptoms and techniques, this approach is unique.

Obviously, the therapist's attitude is of paramount importance in this type of treatment. With adolescents, the therapist should adopt the role of a friendly companion, who can understand the patient's difficulties and problems, reflect back emotions, and subsequently help the patient to find his way out of difficult situations. The therapist should not offer advice to the patient directly, but should encourage him to find solutions of his own. If the therapist's attitude is genuine and congruent, he may choose to reveal some of his own experiences. By helping the patient to realize that the therapist is not perfect, the therapist's credibility can be enhanced (Remschmidt, 1992).

In a way, both therapist and client experience a similar process, in which the client is helped to direct his attention towards his emotional state and fully experience the emotional and physical sensations associated with a specific person, object or situation in his life (Kind, 1982). Rogers designated this process 'experiencing'.

In contrast to psychoanalytically orientated psychotherapy, client-centred therapy focuses on current problems and feelings. The past is discussed only if the patient explicitly raises an issue. Thus, counselling with adolescents tends to focus on everyday anxieties, problems associated with relationships, difficulties at school or work, conflicts with parents and siblings, etc.

Indications and contraindications

Client-centred psychotherapy was used by Rogers in parents, adolescents and students. The technique is especially useful in these clients, particularly when dealing with identity crises, difficulties with achievement at school or work, acute reactions to conflicts, and antisocial behaviour. There are several preconditions for successful psychotherapy with adolescents. These include an adequate introspective capability, the capacity to verbalize emotions, and to transfer any progress from therapy sessions to everyday life

Client-centred therapy is not indicated in the treatment of severe psychiatric disturbances whether they may be 'neurotic' or psychotic disorders such as schizophrenia. It is also inappropriate to treat 'psychosomatic' disorders. The technique was developed as a brief psychotherapy, and is usually limited to a total of 20–25 sessions (Remschmidt, 1992). When used in a manner resembling 'counselling', it is an appropriate adjuvant technique to support children and adolescents requiring long-term psychiatric treatment.

In clinical practice an eclectic approach to treatment is often adopted, integrating several different therapeutic techniques. Depending on their background, therapists are likely to emphasize specific techniques. However, when treating adolescents with verbal methods, it is important to bear in mind the special characteristics of this age group.

The practice of verbally based psychotherapies

As adolescents progress, a significant change occurs in the patterns of communication of adolescents. In particular, there is a shift in their preparedness to disclose intimate information (Seiffge-Krenke, 1986). As they grow older, adolescents tend to seek less support from their parents and other adults, whilst the role of peers become increasingly important.There is also a difference between males and females regarding the acceptance of psychotherapy, females being more likely to accept psychotherapeutic help. It is important to bear in mind that the developmental phases of adolescence are associated with specific characteristics, which play a significant role during psychotherapy.

Blos (1962) has summarized the developmental phases of adolescence in a five-phase model (see Chapter 5). Each phase is associated with specific problems and conflicts, during which the adolescent learns to deal with issues such as social rules (often represented by the adolescent's parents) and detatchment from the family. The adolescent is also likely to feel that the therapist represents social values and rules. Thus, conflicts with social rules are likely to be transferred to the therapist, resulting in suspicion and defensiveness. These and any other difficulties need to be addressed during therapy.

It is helpful to distinguish five phases of psychotherapy (Lipitt, 1961). These are discussed in detail below:

(i) motivating the desire for change,
(ii) establishing a relationship,
(iii) working towards change,
(iv) stabilizing improvements,
(v) terminating the relationship.

Motivating the patient for change

Prior to commencing psychotherapy, a framework should be defined, concerning details such as the number, frequency, duration and content of sessions. The therapist should assess factors such as the patient's and his parents' desire to change, willingness and ability to cooperate, verbal skills, and the need for any adjuvant therapeutic measures. Whilst it is often difficult to predict exactly the number of sessions that will be required, clinical experience has shown that a small number of sessions, i.e. 15–20 is sufficient in many cases ('focal therapy'). In the presence of a chronic psychiatric disorder, such as anorexia nervosa, longer-term adjuvant counselling may be required.

The initiative for therapeutic help is usually taken by the parents. They often feel at least partly responsible for their child's problems and any guilty feelings need to be addressed. If the parents can be reassured, the prognosis of treatment can be improved.

The adolescent's desire for change depends largely on his/her degree of suffering. It is often the case, however, that other individuals in the environment, e.g. family members, teachers suffer more than the adolescents themselves. This can result in considerable problems, with the family being more motivated than the adolescent himself. Psychotherapy will be difficult if the adolescent sees no point in treatment and refuses to cooperate.

To facilitate a degree of cooperation, it is important to gain the patient's trust at an early stage. An atmosphere free of anxiety, with assertions about the confidentiality of treatment sessions will help in this, as will explaining clearly the triangular relationship which exists between the therapist, patient and parents.

The therapist should refuse the role of 'surrogate parent', whilst avoiding forming a coalition with the adolescent against his parents. In order to develop an appropriate relationship, the therapist should define the therapeutic goals together with the patient and discuss any benefits that may realistically be expected of psychotherapy. Therapeutic goals depend to a considerable degree on the nature of the symptoms, and will also determine the techniques which are appropriate. The therapist should aim to keep therapeutic options open when choosing treatment methods, and avoid being put under pressure or being limited by the patient, his parents or other care-givers.

The patient's trust in psychotherapy will be strengthened by the demonstration of professionalism and competence. This may be demonstrated, for example, by offering information about the likely course and prognosis of the problem, although it is also important to explain that symptoms may fluctuate over the course of treatment to avoid disappointment. Experience shows that problems often improve following the initial phases of psychotherapy, but that improvements may be difficult to maintain over time. Crises are often associated with an increase in symptoms, and should be expected to occur over the course of psychotherapy. They can be used as an opportunity to discuss with the patient the possible causes of the crisis and develop appropriate coping strategies. Any alterations of therapeutic technique should be explained in detail to the patient to help him feel involved in the process, and to maintain confidence in the therapist.

The personalities of patient and therapist have a significant influence on the nature of the therapeutic relationship. Riemann (1961) identified four types of personality structure which differ in terms of the way individuals deal with anxieties. He designated these types of personality 'schizoid', 'depressed', 'hysterical', and 'obsessional'. When two such personalities encounter one another during psychotherapy, predictable patterns of interaction ensue. The four personality types can be arranged in opposing positions.

'Schizoid' or 'depressesd' personalities are placed at opposite ends along an axis representing 'relationship', whilst 'hysterical' and 'obsessional' mark the ends of an 'order' continuum. The theory developed by Riemann (1974) predicts that certain combinations of personality traits will result in characteristic conflicts. For example, a 'schizoid' therapist is likely to maintain a certain distance between himself and his 'depressed' patient. The patient is likely to react by feeling rejected and misunderstood, as he is (consciously or unconsciously) in need of closeness and security.

An 'obsessional' therapist may find it difficult to accept a 'hysterical' patient's breaking of social rules. In contrast, a 'hysterical' therapist may induce anxiety in an 'obsessional' patient as he attempts to modify the patient's preoccupation with order, rituals and regulations, without appreciating the role which such mechanisms play in reassuring the patient and reducing his anxiety. Whilst this model offers some help in predicting the nature of the likely therapeutic conflicts, reality is obviously much more complex.

The content of psychotherapeutic sessions is also an important factor in building up motivation for change in the adolescent. Whilst adolescents usually enjoy conversation, they may find it difficult if the topics for discussion seem irrelevant, or if they are required to initiate rather than respond to issues. Particularly in the initial phase of therapy, the topics for discussion should either be based on the adolescents symptomatology, or determined by the therapist using dynamic interactional methods (Cohn, 1997). Some adolescents are able to demonstrate a good understanding of the nature and relevance of their symptoms, whilst others either lack insight into their problems or develop their own elaborate theory about their symptoms.

In contrast to the 'rule of abstinence' so important in psychoanalytically orientated therapy, in client-centered psychotherapy it has been considered beneficial that the therapist points out to the patient the connection between symptoms, potential causes (conflicts), and theories which may explain the disorder. By attempting to understand the patient's symptoms, the therapist helps the adolescent to develop the feeling of being accepted. A bond of trust is thus established between therapist and patient. Whilst it is important to avoid unnecessary criticism, excessive praise and encouragement are also inappropriate, and may result in the patient overestimating his capacity to deal with the inevitable future difficult situations.

Establishing a therapeutic relationship

When attempting to establish a therapeutic relationship, it is helpful to adapt to the adolescent's developmental phases and be flexible in treatment technique as therapy progresses. Psychotherapy should not only consist of verbal sessions, but include activities such as games and walks together with the patient. Verbal sessions should focus on the patient's specific interests and needs. This approach not only encourages a trusting relationship, but also enables the therapist to identify the patient's resources and encourage his self-help capacity. Thus, the patient can improve his autonomy and develop coping strategies to deal with problems.

During this unstable phase the therapist should remember that the patient is likely to see the therapist as an authority figure and react accordingly. In some cases this can result in premature discontinuation of treatment. However, if a trusting relationship develops, the patient's cooperation can usually be maintained for a number of months.

Other factors may put therapy in jeopardy for a number of reasons, e.g. dissatisfaction of the parents either with the nature or results of treatment. Müller-Küppers (1988) has used the term 'double therapeutic rapport' to describe the need to establish rapport with both the patient and his parents.

During this phase of therapy, the way in which the therapist behaves towards the patient is especially important. It is usually necessary to adopt a more proactive manner with adolescents. The focus should be on current problems, and it should be borne in mind that treatment may bring about a limited improvement. The therapist should not entertain unrealistic expectations or make excessive demands of the patient. If an adolescent feels overwhelmed during psychotherapy, e.g. by inappropriate communication, elaborate speech, use of theoretical terms, long pauses, etc., he is likely to discontinue treatment.

Bringing about behavioural change

The issue of which symptoms require treatment needs to be addressed at an early stage. The aims of treatment will influence the choice of technique.

The positive effect of most psychotherapy is thought to result from a learning process, e.g. development of insight, modification of attitudes, cognitive restructuring, etc. However, how these learning processes occur with different approaches remains unclear. Above, we have outlined the theoretical basis for this learning process according to Roger's 'client centred therapy', however, other theoretical explanations have also been put forward. The psychoanalytically orientated therapist, Hilde Bruch (1977) considered several questions to be useful as guidelines in therapy sessions: 'What?', 'How?', 'When?' (for the first time), 'With whom?', 'Why?', and 'With what results?' These questions are considered and analysed by the patient and therapist together to initiate a cognitive process which encourages the patient to perceive his current emotions in parallel. This may help to clarify how earlier experiences relate to the patient's current condition. If the patient can understand this association, he is then more likely to be able to modify his behaviour. From a therapeutic perspective, a further technique may be helpful, which is to bring about cathartic experiences. The therapist encourages the patient to acknowledge and permit the experience of strong emotions such as sadness, hopelessness, anger and rage. As patients tend to suppress such emotions, this may be difficult, especially if they relate to individuals close to the patient such as family members. Cathartic experiences usually result in temporary emotional relief, and one method of facilitating them is through the use of a technique designated by Rogers (1951) as 'reflection of feelings'. During these phases of intense emotional experience, adolescents may suddenly understand how previous occurences are connected with their present situation. This type of experience should be followed by a detailed re-assessment of factors which previously and currently still play a role. These may include specific individuals or emotions, e.g. anger, sorrow, disappointment, anxiety, affection, love which may have been acted out without being conciously experienced. The aim of this approach is to modify the patient's emotional state through involving him emotionally in therapy, and to demonstrate how his feelings can cause specific behaviours. Over time, the patient learns to recognize the advantages of change and can modify his behaviour.

The therapist should use plain and simple language, avoiding stereotyped or impersonal communication styles, especially when reflecting the patient's feelings. Excessively long pauses during sessions can make the patient feel insecure. An appropriate therapeutic attitude will allow the therapist to comfort, praise and advise the patient in therapy (Dührssen, 1986).

Although the phase of 'bringing about change' is not generally based on psychoanalytically orientated theories, such considerations may be useful in some situations. For example, an adolescent refusing to cooperate at school may be regarded as an authority conflict involving transference. The cause of the problem can be considered an unresolved conflict with his parents, or persisting from childhood, which now influences current relationships with others. Seen from this perspective, the aim of treatment is to make the adolescent conscious of these connections and to help him to modify his attitude towards persons in authority. For example, this therapeutic approach might be initiated by saying: 'Can you remember having experienced anything like this before?'

Some symptoms may be helped by a careful analysis of psychological 'defence mechansims'. Obsessional symptoms frequently protect the patient against instinctual impulses, i.e. sexual or aggressive drives. This type of defence mechanism is called 'reaction formation'. From a therapeutic perspective, it is important not only to uncover the unconscious connection, but also to encourage the adolescent to test changes of attitude and behaviour in reality. Without such reality testing, the therapist may have the impression that progress is being made, whilst the patient is actually incapable of coping with the demands of everyday life. Thus, when working with adolescents, it is important to give the patient the opportunity to actually try out behavioural modifications and subsequently discuss the experience in feedback sessions.

In contrast to the 'rule of abstinence' in psychoanalytically orientated therapy, when counselling adolescents, therapists may choose to reveal something of themselves. The therapist may speak about his own experiences and emotions to demonstrate his introspective capacity. In this way, the therapist acts a 'model' for the patient. Other topics which can be touched upon are experiences with one's own children, other patients and one's own adolescence. This may help the patient to perceive the motives by which other individuals act, and learn to accept their behaviour.

As psychological changes usually require a considerable amount of time, sessions may go on over an extensive period.

Stabilizing behavioural change

Improvements brought about by therapy can be put in jeopardy as a result of a number of factors. Parents may have different expectations of therapy, and whilst it is important to remember that the adolescent is the patient, parents' expectations cannot be ignored. Parents need to be informed about the aims of therapy and progress being made. At times, it may also be appropriate to include parents in treatment, to help them understand and accept behavioural changes occuring in the family context. New conflicts are likely to arise, putting any gains at risk. It is not uncommon for familial conflicts to persist, and in this case, individual sesssions may be more appropriate to help the adolescent cope with the situation. The aim is to strengthen the adolescent such that over time he develops sufficient independence.

Derogatory comments from peers can make adolescents feel insecure, and thoughtless comments from teachers may put treatment success at risk. In such cases it may be appropriate to discuss this with the relevant authority, having first gained permission from the adolescent and parents to do so.

The therapist can work on factors which are likely to stabilize the changes achieved. The experience of 'success' through successful reality testing will improve the adolescent's self-esteem and self-concept. He will learn to cope better with everyday stresses, and also to avoid situations which are likely to precipitate crises or impair his sense of well-being. Therapy should always have a sense of direction, encouraging and facilitating the development of new coping strategies, but the therapist should be careful not to make treatment aims inappropriately high, which will tend to be discouraging for the adolescent.

Terminating the therapeutic relationship

At an appropriate point, both therapy and the therapeutic relationship must be brought to an end. In contrast to educational relationships, the duration of the therapeutic relationship must be limited. The appropriate time to end the relationship depends on a number of factors. The adolescent's symptoms are the most obvious indicator of success, and they can usually be assessed without difficulty. However, with emotional and interactional disorders, additional information from parents or teachers are often also neccessary. Standardized psychological tests (e.g. personality questionnaires, specific behaviour scales) may be useful to evaluate the course objectively. Therapy should be brought to an end in a graded manner, and the intervals between sessions are usually increased progressively, enabling the therapist to intervene quickly if an acute crisis occurs. Many adolescents value knowing that their therapist is available for support and advice after therapy has been terminated.

Abrupt discontinuation of therapy does not neccessarily imply that treatment has failed and prognosis is poor. Many adolescents and their families lose their motivation to change over the course of therapy and discontinue treatment when symptoms have improved somewhat. In some cases spontaneous improvement may occur, resulting in premature discontinuation of therapy.

Evaluation

There is a paucity of systematic studies on the effectivity of non-directive psychotherapies with adolescents. Schmidtchen (1989) found that verbally based techniques, psychoanalytically orientated therapy and behaviour therapy are more effective than no treatment. Remschmidt and Schmidt (1988) found that psychotherapy with children and adolescents with psychiatric disorders had positive effects, and that improvement was better in cases of 'internalizing' than 'externalizing' disorders. Heekerens (1989) has reviewed several meta-analyses of the outcome of psychotherapy with children and adolescents. He found that 'non-directive, client-centred' techniques are generally effective and had a better outcome than 'psychoanalytically orientated' approaches. 'Behavioural methods' have been shown to be slightly more effective.

In a comprehensive study, Grawe et al. (1994) showed that the effects of pschotherapy can be reduced to the following 'mechanisms of change', independently of the psychotherapeutic technique used (Grawe, 1997):

(i) the problem-solving component, which involves helping the patient to actively deal with his problems,

(ii) the explanatory component, which involves discussing the patient's motives, value system and aims,

(iii) the relationship component, which is based on the assumption that psychiatric disorders are associated with a disturbance of interpersonal relationships. Psychotherapy always implies personal interaction, and the quality of interaction affects the outcome of psychotherapy.

Grawe et al. (1994) suggest that significant changes can be brought about using client-centred psychotherapy. The therapeutic effect of the sessions largely depend on the way in which the sessions are held. These results were obtained in adult patients, however, with some modification, they may also be considered true for children and adolescents (also see Chapter 2).

Case vignette

A 17-year-old female patient presented to the outpatient clinic for assessment of her eating disorder. She reported an average of three bulimic attacks per day, and a previous phase of anorexia. Symptoms had persisted for 2 years, with fluctuating severity. The patient was 176 cm tall, her maximum weight had been 76 kg

Table 10.1. Case vignette: treatment of a 17-year-old female patient with anorexia and bulimia nervosa

Phase of therapy	Principal interventions	Topics, problems, conflicts
Motivation of the desire for change (duration: 5 sessions/4 weeks)	Diagnostic appraisal Feedback and education (father, stepmother, patient)	Explain the results of physical examination and psychiatric and psychological assessment Educate the patient and parents about symptoms and the course of anorexia nervosa with bulimic symptoms The patient and her parents are motivated for change
	Explain indications for therapy (inpatient, outpatient)	The patient is motivated for outpatient psychotherapy; her capacity for introspection and verbal skills are good
Establish a relationship (duration: 6 sessions/3 weeks)	Commence counselling sessions Improve the therapeutic relationship	The patient's interest include: horse riding, cooking, going out with her boyfriend. Achievement at school, preparations for final exams, vocational plans.
	'Non-directive' sessions: 'reflection of feelings'	The role of her mother's death Reactions of the patient's peers and family to her anorexic and bulimic symptoms
	Additional sessions with the father and stepmother	Current family situation (rivalry between siblings, style of upbringing, the stepmother's jealousy of the patient)
Bring about behavioural change (duration: 50 sessions/2 years)	Direct confrontation: hospitalization if symptoms deteriorate	Marked increase in bulimic attacks Diet: scheduled meals at home Observation by her stepmother, resulting in conflicts Patronized by family members (grandparents)

Table 10.1. *(cont.)*

Phase of therapy	Principal interventions	Topics, problems, conflicts
	Increase the frequency of sessions ('non-directive')	Crisis in the relationship with her boyfriend: deterioration of anorexic symptoms
	Psychoanalytically orientated sessions	Sexual experiences, social role of women
		Clarification of the patient's relationship to her stepmother
	Family therapy	The stepmother's personal problem (self-esteem)
		Contrary opinion of the parents concerning child-raising
	Individual psychoanalytically orientated sessions	Stepmother/patient/the issue of self-esteem/anorexic and bulimic symptoms
		The father's role in the patient's life
		The patient's role as 'surrogate mother' for her two younger sisters
	Bring about cathartic experiences	Hospitalization of the patient's mother for several months when the patient was 13 years old; death due to stomach cancer
		Extreme grief reaction (resulting in emotional relief), gradual clarification of relationships in the family
	Educate about ways to modify eating behaviour (based on behaviour therapy)	Improvement of symptoms
	Positive feedback about the course of treatment (hospitalization not required)	Stable body weight
	Psychoanalytically orientated sessions	Recurrence of conflicts in the family, reproachful stepmother
		Connection of self-esteem with anorexic symptoms (patient often compares herself with her mother and friends)

Table 10.1. (*cont.*)

Phase of therapy	Principal interventions	Topics, problems, conflicts
		Developing relationship with her boyfriend; the psychosexual role of women
	Give advice about eating behaviour	Class trip: recurrence of bulimic symptoms
	'Non-directive', psychoanalytically orientated sessions	Anxieties, conflicts, wishes: sexuality, identification with her role as a woman
		Increasing detachment from the family: final exams at school, plans for university, new conflicts with her stepmother
	Give direct advice	Occupational choice
	Develop behavioural strategies	Preparation of final exams at school
		Fear of exams
Stabilize behavioural changes (duration: 12 sessions/10 weeks)	Encourage the patient to modify eating behaviour	Improvement of bulimic episodes
	'Non-directive' therapy sessions focusing on the relationship with a new boyfriend	Stabilization of the relationship with her boyfriend; conflicts
	Give a direct advice	Eating behaviour in company, e.g. visiting a restaurant
		Occasional insecurity about the size of servings
		Successful final exams; occupational considerations
	Advise the patient together with her parents	Initiation of detachment from the therapist
		Reflection of the treatment course, changes in the family, anxieties about the future, etc.
	Plan the future, anticipate problems	Preparation for leaving home to begin vocational training as a graphic designer

Table 10.1. (*cont.*)

Phase of therapy	Principal interventions	Topics, problems, conflicts
Terminate the relationship (duration: 2 sessions / 3 weeks)	Review the course of therapy	Difficult phases during therapy: risk of recurrence of anorexic and bulimic symptoms
	Offer additional interventions if necessary	Telephone call about 9 months after the end of therapy: personality and eating behaviour are fairly stable Telephone call after 4 years: personality development had been good, but bulimic episodes still occur occasionally

(BMI = 24.5), and her minimum 56 kg (BMI = 18.0). Based on the history and diagnostic appraisal, the patient was diagnosed as having 'bulimia nervosa'. She reported that low self-esteem had precipitated the anorexic phase ('other girls in my class were very thin, and I felt clumsy compared to them'). The family then went through a difficult phase over the period when her mother died. Her father remarried 2 years later, and the relationship between the patient and her stepmother and step-siblings was difficult. She attended secondary school, where she was well integrated, achieved good results, and had friends, including a boyfriend. The patient was treated using verbally based psychotherapy. The course is summarized in Table 10.1.

REFERENCES

Blos, P. (1962). *On adolescence*. New York: Free Press of Glencoe.

Bruch, H. (1977). *Grundzüge der Psychotherapie*. Frankfurt: Fischer.

Cohn, R. (1997). *Von der Psychoanalyse zur thermenzentrierten interaktion*, 13th edn. Stuttgart: Klett-Cotta.

Dührssen, A. (1986). *Psychotherapie bei Kindern und Jugendlichen*. Göttingen: Vandenhoeck & Ruprecht.

Grawe, K. (1997). Research-informed psychotherapy. *Psychotherapy Research*, 7, 1–19.

Grawe, K., Donati, R. and Bernauer, F. (1994). *Psychotherapie im Wandel. Von der Konfession zur Profession*, 3rd edn. Göttingen: Hogrefe.

Heekerens, H-P. (1989). Effektivität von Kinder- und Jugendlichen-Psychotherapie im Spiegel von Meta-Analysen. *Zeitschrift für Kinder- und Jugendpsychiatrie*, **17**, 150–7.

Kind, H. (1982). *Psychotherapie und Psychotherapeuten*. Stuttgart: Thieme.

Lehmkuhl, G., Lehmkuhl, U. and Döpfner, M. (1992). Psychotherapie mit Jugendlichen. *Zeitschrift für Kinder- und Jugendpsychiatrie*, **20**, 169–84.

Lippitt, R. (1961). Dimensions of the consultant's job. In *The planning of change*, ed. W. G. Bennis, K. D. Benne and R. Chin, pp. 156–62. New York: Holt, Rinehard & Winston.

Müller-Küppers, M. (1988). Kinderpsychotherapie. In *Psychiatrie der Gegenwart*, 3rd edn, vol. 7, ed. K. P. Kisker, H. Lauter, J-E. Meyer, C. Müller and E. Strömgren, pp. 429–54. Berlin: Springer.

Remschmidt, H. (1992). *Psychiatrie der Adoleszenz*. Stuttgart: Thieme.

Remschmidt, H. and Schmidt, M. H. (1988). *Alternative Behandlungsformen in der Kinder- und Jugendpsychiatrie. Stationäre Behandlung, tagesklinische Behandlung und home-treatment im Vergleich*. Stuttgart: Enke.

Riemann, F. (1961). *Grundformen der Angst*. München: Reinhardt.

Riemann, F. (1974). *Grundformen helfender Partnerschaft*. München: Pfeiffer.

Rogers, C. (1951). *Client-centered therapy*. Boston: Mifflin.

Schmidtchen, S. (1989). *Kinderpsychotherapie*. Stuttgart: Kohlhammer.

Seiffge-Krenke, I. (1986). *Psychoanalytische Therapie Jugendlicher*. Stuttgart: Kohlhammer.

Wolberg, L. R. (1969). *The technique of psychotherapy*. New York: Grune & Stratton.

11 Group psychotherapy and psychodrama

Gerhard Niebergall

Group psychotherapy

Introduction

Group psychotherapy is a psychotherapeutic method for treating several individuals simultaneously. The approach to this type of treatment depends on a wide range of factors, including:

- theoretical concept,
- concept of group applied to therapy,
- established group therapy,
- group interaction,
- the role of the individual in the group,
- treatment aims,
- criteria used for composing a group,
- treatment setting,
- duration of treatment,
- the role and tasks of the therapist,
- indications and contraindications applied,
- evaluation of group therapy,
- economical considerations and effectiveness.

At the onset of the group therapy movement (Moreno, 1964), economical issues were an important consideration. As one therapist can treat a greater number of patients than with individual psychotherapy, group therapy is more economical in terms of time and effort. It is important to bear in mind, however, that group sessions require careful preparation, and successful outcome depends to a considerable degree on the therapist's competence. Therapists should be well trained in a group therapy technique and have clinical experience with children and adolescents, especially when undertaking group therapy with severely disturbed patients.

There are several advantages to group psychotherapy with children and adolescents besides economical considerations. These are relevant both to specific theoretical concepts and to the practical relevance of groups in everyday life. Individuals constantly interact with one another in our society. This leads to the development of a variety of groups, each with common characteristics, e.g. families, school classes, groups of colleagues at work, clubs, political parties, etc. A group is not merely an association of individuals; it requires interpersonal relationships ('cohesion') and interaction between group members in order to function. Group relationships and the role of the individual in a group may be described in terms of 'social roles' (Remschmidt, 1992).

Groups often have a somewhat hierarchical structure, the nature of which depends on the common goals. Usually one group member has a leading role, whilst others are in an intermediate position, and a few individuals are in an 'omega position'. Although group structure may change as the group's goals change, common goals and the aims of individuals generally determine the group's specific and general behavioural standards. Thus, adolescents tend to adapt their own behaviour to resemble that of the peer group.

Group conflicts may occur when common goals are absent or unclear, when the group hierarchy is not clearly defined, and when individuals break behavioural standards. Conflicts between group members, e.g. rivalry or role conflicts may ensue (e.g. when conflicts occur between internalized behavioural norms and the group's behavioural standards). Such conflicts may result in social maladaption, behavioural disorder, and a variety of psychological symptoms.

Group therapy is particularly effective for treating adolescents who are struggling with conflicts in their peer group. In a group setting, patients tend to be confronted with situations which resemble those experienced in reality. Thus, disorders which manifest themselves in groups, such as disorders arising from interactional problems at school can be recognized and treated more easily in a group setting.

Approaches to group therapy

There are several possible approaches to group therapy (Stoiber and Kratchowill, 1998). Lehmkuhl (1990) has distinguished between group training, group work and group psychotherapy. Whilst group training aims to improve defined behavioural abnormalities and is extremely structured, e.g. specific training exercises, rigid treatment plan, group work is less structured and uses social experiences to bring about behavioural improvement. The aim of group psychotherapy, on the other hand, is to facilitate the experience of emotions and bring about psychological modifications. Group psychotherapy is moderately structured, and both the individual patient as well as the whole group is given the opportunity to open up and explore areas of conflict (Remschmidt, 1992).

Group psychotherapy techniques differ according to the way in which the individual patients relate within the group. Various specific techniques may be used in a group setting, e.g. relaxation training, hypnosis, and verbal interventions; in these, group dynamics usually play an insignificant role. Other techniques place great reliance on group interactions to bring about improvement in individual patients, e.g. psychodrama, psychoanalytically orientated group therapy, self-assertiveness training. Further approaches focus on treating the group as a whole, e.g. 'socio-drama'.

Both verbal interventions and behavioural measures may be used in all types of group therapy. However, it is important to undertake full assessment and diagnostic procedures and to define appropriate treatment steps before group therapy starts.

In practice, the boundaries between different types of group therapy are not always clear. Verbal interventions are generally more useful with adolescents (14 years or older) than with children. According to Siefen (1988), the aim of psychoanalytically orientated group therapy is to aid patients to become conscious of repressed conflicts, which are thought to contribute to abnormal behaviour and psychopathological symptoms. As in individual psychotherapy, psychoanalytically orientated group therapy is based on transference, counter-transference, and working through resistance, using confrontation, clarification and interpretation as interventions. According to psychoanalytical theory, the overcoming of resistance is a gradual process which eventually enables the patient to recognize his defence mechanisms and become conscious of repressed conflicts. This leads to improved self-knowledge and insight into the complicated connections between the patient's behaviour and the reactions of others. This process should be encouraged in every member of the group, enabling the patients to behave in a more appropriate way outside group sessions.

The therapist's attitude and role in psychoanalytically orientated group therapy with adolescents is slightly different from that with adults (Haar, 1980). Adolescents require more structuring (to reduce anxiety), playful interaction between group members, and active participation of the therapist (modelling), e.g. by talking about his own experiences in life. Adolescents who take part in group therapy emphasizing verbal expression (Slavson, 1966) generally respond positively when told that they are not alone and that other adolescents have similar problems. Such interventions facilitate discussions about previously secret personal difficulties and contribute to the development of a trusting atmosphere in the group.

Behavioural group therapy can usually be undertaken with children of 9 years old and above. Previous approaches to behaviour therapy were strictly based on the principles of learning theory (classical and operant conditioning, positive and negative reinforcement), and these have been revised and modified with the introduction of cognitive behaviour therapy. Emotional factors and the issue of introspection are also considered to be important with this approach. Several fairly structured treatment and training programmes have been introduced (Meichenbaum, 1977; Petermann, 1983; Mattejat and Jungmann, 1981). Such programmes would be suitable for systematic evaluation, however, in clinical practice inflexible 'treatment programmes' and rigid theoretical models may be difficult to follow. In contrast, when undertaking behaviour therapy, using principles of learning theory with children and adolescents, the therapist should approach the task with a flexible, active, friendly and benevolent attitude. Rogers (1951) identified the following important criteria: empathic understanding, a sense of genuinness, and unconditional positive regard.

In addition to existing methods based on verbal intervention and learning theory, a number approaches to group therapy have been introduced more recently, including action techniques. These techniques are based on the same principles as earlier methods, but particularly emphasize actions and training excercises in the group. The approach has been used successfully with children and adolescents, and the two most important techniques (psychodrama and therapeutic role play) are explained in more detail below.

The practice of group therapy

When planning group therapy, it is of paramount importance to consider the setting (inpatient or outpatient treatment). The younger the participants are, the more important it is to ensure that the age structure within the group is homogeneous. The psychiatric symptoms being treated in the group are likely to be variable, although some constraints may be necessary. Prior to commencing group treatment, it is important to determine whether the group will be 'open' or 'closed'. Participants need to know who will lead the group, how many patients will take part, and who the participants are. In group therapy with children and adolescents a group size of 6–8 participants is usually appropriate. Before commencing, it is advisable to undertake individual preparatory sessions with each prospective participant in order to assess motivation, answer any questions, and prepare the participants for therapy. This approach should dispel any unrealistic anxieties and help the participants overcome any reluctance to take part in therapy.

Initially, group therapy is often difficult for all involved; it becomes easier once the participants have merged to form a proper group. As groups form, they generally go through several specific phases, which apply to both therapeutic and non-therapeutic groups (Remschmidt, 1992):

Exploration

A general sense of insecurity usually prevails during the first phase of group formation. The individual tries to find out whether he can identify with the group's behavioural norms and whether cooperation with other group members is likely to be successful.

Identification

This phase is characterized by the development of a sense of cohesion and identification within the group. Specific group goals are still absent. Thus, identification is 'formal', i.e. individuals can feel secure within the group without the necessity of having to focus on specific aims. Such a feeling of security is the most important cohesive factor in the group.

Development of collective goals and norms

Collective goals generally develop in groups, even when they consist of very few individuals. The goals subsequently result in group cohesion. Groups, including therapeutic groups, break up easily in the absence of common goals.

As groups are formed, specific roles develop which will depend on the group's common goals, group stability, and the needs of individual group members. The process of group formation and the gradual appropriation of each individual's role will help the therapist to identify the status of individuals within the group and provide a working model of the group structure. The therapist can then utilize this knowledge in future sessions. Usually hierarchies, group cohesion and ranks develop in the group, regardless of which therapeutic method is used, reflecting the conflicts and social significance of individual group memebers. These issues should be addressed during sessions. Slavson (1977) has proposed several aims of group psychotherapy with adolescents:

- the development of positive aspects of the self,
- the building up of self-esteem,
- the encouragement of a more realistic attitude,
- positive interactions with other group members,
- improvement in social relationships,
- better interaction with other group members and the therapist,
- identification with the therapist and other group members,

- reduction of defence mechanisms if they are hampering positive development,
- maturation of psychological development,
- clarification of role behavior towards adults through improved interaction with the therapist.

With group psychotherapy focusing on behaviour, the process of 'clarification' can be followed by a practice phase, during which new insights are used to bring about modified behaviour, which can subsequently be practised within the group (e.g. psychodrama).

Psychodrama

Psychodrama is a group therapy technique developed by Moreno (1964). He wanted to utilize the positive effects that theatre performances were seen to have on both spectators and actors ('catharsis theory'), which had been known for centuries. Moreno applied his own experience with improvised plays to group psychotherapy settings.

Moreno developed an additional component of psychodrama which he designated 'sociometry'. Thus, the approach is characterized by three main aspects: group psychotherapy, psychodrama and sociometry. Sociometric studies can provide insight into the types of emotional bonds which exist within groups (Niebergall, 1987), and an assessment along sociometric lines is often used in the context of group psychotherapy. The sociometric position of the individual group members can subsequently be fed back to the participants during therapy sessions.

As psychodrama is not bound to any one specific theory, it allows the therapist to include a variety of theoretical developments, such as psychoanalysis (Ploeger, 1983), behaviour therapy (Petzold, 1978), and other types of therapy (Franzke, 1977). Today, a wide range of psychodramas have been developed (Yablonski, 1976). Any potential therapist should have appropriate training and clinical experience in order to be able to use the technique successfully and safely.

Psychological symptoms are considered to result from conflicting roles, fixed roles, inadequate flexibility in roles, and disturbed development of roles. Leutz (1974) considered symptoms to be the result of a 'creativity neurosis' and 'motivational inhibition'.

The practice of psychodrama

Psychodrama is a useful technique for treating children and adolescents, and has also been used successfully to support diagnostic appraisal and educational measures (Widlöcher, 1974). Role play is one approach to psychodrama. The technique may be used to improve the patients' perception of emotions and initiate a learning process which may otherwise be difficult to bring about with other methods.

Several different psychodrama 'techniques' are available for use in group therapy, one of which is group playing (Schützenberger, 1979). This technique facilitates enacting either fairy tales or typical situations from everyday life, e.g. going shopping or a situation at school, enabling the therapist to illustrate that 'we are all in one boat together'. Other techniques which can be used include 'monodrama' and 'autodrama'. However, the most important aspect of psychodrama is 'protagonist centred play', which closely resembles the form of the ancient Greek tragedies.

Petzold (1978) introduced a 'tetradic' system to distinguish between different phases in protagonist centred play: (i) initial phase, (ii) action phase, (iii) integration phase, and (iv) reorientation phase. These steps are summarized in Fig. 11.1. Several psychodrama techniques follow these four phases. Such techniques can be used to increase the emotional intensity in the course of the play, bringing about a cathartic climax, after which the protagonists are given the opportunity to reflect on their intrapsychical conflicts and behavioural difficulties.

In the terminology of psychodrama, participants who play a central role are called 'protagonists'. Assisted by the therapist, protagonists enact their conflicts and attempt to find solutions with the help of behavioural techniques. They are supported by the other group members who play the role of 'antagonists'.

The initial phase is characterized by group discussions, which help to clarify the conflicts of individual group members. During this phase, the patients' needs in terms of the protagonist centred play become increasingly clear. Patients' willingness to address their problems and conflicts tends to improve in this phase. Specific techniques, e.g. 'warm-up' techniques may be helpful in bringing about a positive therapeutic atmosphere and help potential 'protagonists' to overcome their inhibitions and participate fully (see Fig. 11.1.). Initially, the therapist may need to work at encouraging individual patients to participate. This, for example, may involve standing behind the unwilling patient, acting as his 'double', expressing his doubts, anxieties and ambivalent feelings. In this manner the therapist supports the patient in addressing his conflicts within the group. During the initial phase it is the therapist's task to recognize the level of motivation of individual group members, determine which conflicts can be addressed using role play, encourage potential protagonists to play a central role, and prepare for the action phase by involving the other group

Initial phase
Aims: history, diagnostic appraisal
Recall/stimulate

Warm-up | Contact | Cohesion

Analysis of movement, expression, behaviour, speech

From a psychodynamic perspective: appraisal of projections

From a gestalt theory perspective: context and pregnancy analysis

From a learning theory perspective: behavioural analysis

Conflict-centred or *experience-centred* approach

↓ ↓

Action phase
Psychocathartic aim
Repeat/explore

Serious play
conflict-orientated work with breathing, voice, expression and imaginative exercises
catharsis

Cheerful play
experience-orientated work with exercise, dance, encouraging fantasy and sensitivity
peak experience

Experience of opening and closing, pregnance experience
Emotional experience
Learning by experiencing (emotional learning)

↓ ↓

Integration phase
Analytical-communicational aim
Work through/integrate

Look back | Share | Feed back | Analyse

Clarify psychodynamic connections, transference

Analyse behaviour patterns and communication structures

Reflect about context, continuity and completeness
Rational insight
Insight learning

↓ ↓

Reorientation phase
Aim: behavioural modification
Modify/try out

Training of sensivity, expressivity, flexibility, relaxation training, etc.

Behavioural programmes, shaping, desensitization, modelling, behaviour drama, transfer training, etc.

Experimentation, new formation of shapes
Behavioural modification
Behavioural learning

Fig. 11.1. A 'tetradic' system of integrative psychodrama therapy (Petzold, 1978).

members. It is essential that the participants trust one another, including the therapist. In this context, transference and countertransference issues may be relevant.

Prior to the action phase the protagonist is asked to discuss his problem with the therapist ('exploration'). The therapist may use the technique of playing the patient's 'double' (Fig. 11.2). The therapist may need to persuade the protagonist to participate, addressing any resistance which may be present. The scene which is enacted often reflects a current problem or conflict, with other participants playing specific roles such as siblings according to the directions given by the protagonist regarding the traits of these individuals. Individual participants may not play their role in the way the protagonist wants, and he may then have to demonstrate how he would like a particular person to be enacted. It is often helpful to encourage the protagonist to exchange roles, demonstrating how the person being enacted might behave in specific situations. By switching from one role to another the protagonist has the opportunity to experience situations not only from his perspective, but also from that of the person being enacted.

It is often helpful to use a scene representing a current conflict to explore the development of the conflict and its influence on everyday life. During this process, the protagonist is confronted with 'repressed' conflicts originating in childhood. The regression involved in role play gives the protagonist the opportunity to recognize how conflicts have influenced his own personal development. During this phase of protagonist-centred play the patient usually experiences intense emotions, and the therapist has the difficult task of deciding whether further 'cathartic' experiences are likely to be helpful or whether they might excessively burden the patient. From a therapeutic point of view, 'cathartic abreaction' is usually beneficial; however, there is a small risk that confrontation with previous traumatic experiences may cause aggravation of symptoms in patients with a weak 'ego' or in those at risk of suicide or psychosis.

The action phase is followed by an integration phase, during which participants discuss their experiences with their role ('role feedback'). Frequently, participants spontaneously discuss their experiences with one another ('sharing'). It is also important, however, that the therapist analyses the process, explaining the internal logic of the play and the associated psychological and interpersonal conflicts. This is intended to develop better insight into the protagonist's behaviour ('interpretation and reflection').

A final reorientation phase may also be undertaken. In this phase, specific training sessions should be held, during which socially acceptable ways of

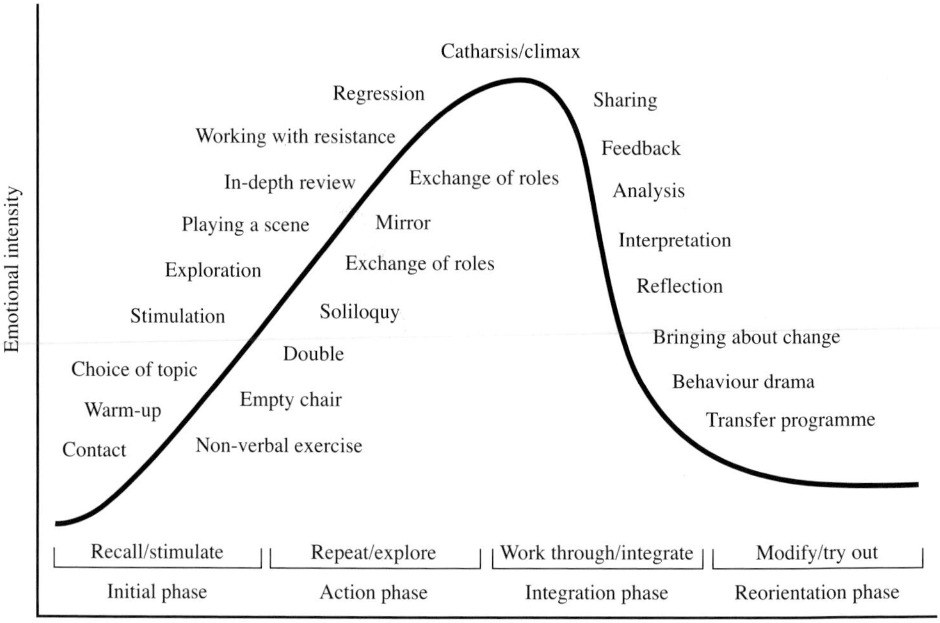

Fig. 11.2. Course of a psychodrama process within the tetradic system (Petzold, 1978).

behaviour can be practised.

Role play, exchange of roles and 'role feedback' are the basic elements constituting psychodrama. The following case report provides an example of psychodrama with adolescents.

Case report of psychodrama with adolescents in an inpatient setting

The group consisted of six inpatients, who had gained some experience with psychodrama over the course of several sessions: Peter (a 17-year-old boy with obsessional symptoms and a schizoid personality structure), Arne (a 15-year-old-boy with severe obsessive–compulsive disorder), Hans-Werner (a 16-year-old boy with anxiety disorder), Ute (a 14-year-old girl with school anxiety, low self-esteem and dysmorphophobia), Anna (a 16-year-old girl with reactive depression following the separation of her parents and disintegration of the family), and Christine (a 16-year-old girl with depressive and psychosomatic symptoms, who had made a suicide attempt).

During the initial phase of the sixth session, the therapist noted considerable resistance in the group against addressing personal problems. The therapist asked the adolescents to stand up and indicate by the distance between the patient and chair, their willingness to take part in protagonist centred role play. All the male participants immediatly moved away from their chairs, whilst the three girls remained seated, demonstrating their intense interest in role play. The three were subsequently asked to explain to the group why they so urgently wanted to take part in role play. Christine had the least difficulty, and described how she felt when she saw her brothers fight during a recent visit at home ('it was a dreadful shock').

Roles were subsequently delegated (Arne = elder brother, Hans-Werner = younger brother), and the scene was enacted in the action phase. As the fight was being enacted by the two 'brothers', Christine's expression froze. The therapist (Th.) stood behind her (P.), and attempted to verbalize and intensify her feelings ('doubling'):

Th.: 'When I have to see this sort of thing, I don't feel like going home either.'

P.: 'Yes, you are right, it doesn't make any sense, I don't want to live any more.'

Th.: 'I would like to be dead.'

P.: 'Yes, if only I knew how life after death was . . . I'm afraid of that.'

Th.: 'If this fear wasn't there . . .'

P.: 'Then I would like to disappear. That's what I wanted when I tried to kill myself.'

Th.: 'Shall we try to enact what it would be like in the life after?'

P.: 'Yes.'

Second scene: two worlds, one is the real world, the other the 'world beyond', after suicide. Transition and interview.

Th.: 'Where would you like to be?'

P.: 'I don't know, I'm in-between.'

Th.: 'In-between what?'

P.: 'Between my family, the psychiatric unit, school, and I have a stomach ache and feel dizzy, so I don't want to live any more.'

The 'dialogue' continued with the therapist playing the part of the patient's 'double'. The patient addressed her physical complaints, and in the course of the play she experienced her feelings with increasing intensity ('cathartic climax'). At this point she said: 'I don't want to live any longer, I want to die!' She subsequently 'passed on' into the 'life after', to live in 'paradise'. However, the 'eternal peace' she expected to experience there did not last long. She eventually became increasingly insecure in the face of a vaguely imagined God. She felt sinful, guilty for what she had 'done' and a sense of ambivalence about whether or not it had been correct.

During the integration phase the therapist said: 'You have enacted your problems. Now we have to return to reality.' After this change of scene the patient was once again confronted by the group, where a process of 'sharing' and role 'feedback' was undertaken and subsequently analysed. After the session, the patient returned to the ward.

In an individual therapy session the following day the patient continued to express depressive ideas. However, over the course of the session, the issue of a realistic perspective for the future was addressed and ways in which she could improve her present situation were raised, e.g. leaving the difficult situation at home, attending boarding school, the possibility of completing secondary school and going to university, the possibility of a temprorary return to the family, provided family therapy was undertaken, and continued individual and group psychotherapy.

Psychotherapeutic role play

Studies have shown that role play and practising social roles leads to positive psychological development in children and adolescents (Oerter and Montada, 1982). Taking on social roles, e.g. gender roles is a dynamic process, which may be associated with conflicts due to the contradictory expectations that are frequently associated with various roles in the family, at school, among peers, at work and in intimate relationships (Remschmidt, 1992). Severe and persistent conflicts may cause difficulties with social adaptation, behavioural problems in the family and at school, and psychological symptoms. In such situations, role play tends to be an effective method of treatment, both in a group and during individual sessions. In contrast to counselling, active participation and the systematic practice of specific behaviours are emphasized. Role play may be used as a therapeutic adjuvant together with other techniques, e.g. behaviour therapy, family therapy, counselling, or as an educational method, e.g. at school, during supervision. Role play can also be undertaken with children as a part of play therapy. Play techniques using toys may help the child to express specific conflicts, which can subsequently be discussed with the child, helping him to improve his understanding of the problem. Behavioural alternatives can be developed subsequently and practised during individual sessions or in a group setting in order to facilitate transfer to everyday situations (Müller-Küppers, 1988).

Types of role play

The following types of role play can be distinguished:

(i) group play
(ii) spontaneous play
(iii) conflict centred play
(iv) individually centred play
(v) theme centred play
(vi) role play in assertiveness training
(vii) role play in family therapy
(viii) role play in individual psychotherapy (play therapy)

Group play is especially appropriate at an early stage of group therapy, as it enables the group members to become familiar with the method, reducing any anxieties and inhibitions about taking on roles. The process of group integration is encouraged by including all group members in the role play. It is usually helpful to begin group play by enacting fairy tales which are usually well known and not associated with too much conflict. Initially, the participants are asked to choose a role to play and then proceed to enact the story, with as little help from the therapist as possible. The therapist can obtain valuable information about interaction amongst the participants ('group dynamics') and individual difficulties during the subsequent discussion of the play. Difficulties may include resistance to identifying with a specific person and playing the role of that person, whilst other participants may be particularly eager to play the roles associated with the most power and social status. In contrast to theatre plays, which are based on specific roles and a predefined text, role play offers the opportunity for spontaneous improvisation. This aspect may help individual group members to overcome inhibitions, become aware of their responsibilities and show consideration for other group members.

Spontaneous play may be undertaken in groups with some experience in role play, e.g. family or school scenes. In such cases the play generally develops without any formal supervision and follows the group's social hierarchy. However, intervention by the therapist may be necessary if serious disagreements occur, which threaten to escalate. This happens easily with children and adolescents. Many patients feel that spontaneous play provides a greater degree of emotional involvement and allows more intense involvement in the group process than more structured approaches to role play.

Other types of role play can be even more structured. For example, conflict centred play may be used to address the specific conflicts and issues which arise, for example, within the group, in the psychiatric unit, at school, and in families. Thus, a conflict which repeatedly occurs in a psychiatric unit may be addressed using conflict centred play. For example, patients may collectively refuse to get up in the morning, insisting that they have been woken too early in the morning or in an unfriendly way. Such situations can be enacted using conflict centred play. One member of the group is asked to play the role of the 'nurse', whose task it is to wake up the patients in the morning, whilst the other patients play themselves or other patients. In the play, the 'nurse' enters the room and shouts: 'Wake up, everyone!' The 'patients' subsequently refuse to comply. In the play, all participants re-experience a scene familiar to them, however, in contrast to the real situation, the participants have the opportunity to discuss their feelings and observations. The patients might feel treated unfairly, resulting in refusal. In turn, the patient in the role of the 'nurse' might express his feelings and observations while playing that role. He may say that he felt like he was doing his 'duty' without any unfriendly intentions, and was only trying to prevent delays of the 'ward routine', e.g. washing, dressing, breakfast, school. Such role plays and subsequent discussions may either bring about a greater understanding of the importance of keeping rules in a social setting such as hospital units, or may result in the patients expressing their wish to be woken up in a different manner in future. The scene can then be repeated, with the 'nurse' asking the 'patients' to get up in a more pleasant way (rather than shouting at them), in which the patients will probably comply without protest. The result of such a role play session can then be discussed with the nursing staff in order to negotiate any future changes.

Individually centred role play focuses on the members of the group as individuals. Role play is undertaken after a patient has outlined his problems. This approach enables the patient to re-experience conflicts in a sheltered therapeutic environment and analyse options for coping with the conflicts. It may be helpful to exchange roles, e.g. between the protagonist and the person, with whom he is in conflict. Exchanging roles can be very effective in improving understanding of the reciprocal point of view. For instance, enacting a family conflict using exchange of roles may be helpful for understanding the way family members interact the way they do.

When using theme centred role play, the group chooses a specific theme which is important for all participants. This approach has the advantage that individual group members are less exposed and tend to cope better with anxiety. For example, some individuals may feel anxious about interacting with peers in a group. The experience of individual group members with such anxieties can be enacted using role play, giving the patients the opportunity to consider the difficulties associated with the anxiety and subsequently develop coping mechanisms. Other group members or the therapist can support this process by suggesting ways of improving the patient's interaction with his peers. Modifications can subsequently be practised in specific training sessions.

Role play can also be used as a component of assertiveness training (Mattejat and Jungmann, 1981). Scenes and roles which the patient finds particularly distressing can be enacted quite easily using this approach. Role play may also be used as a specific training exercise (e.g. social rehabilitation training in patients with schizophrenia). In such programmes, patients are expected to practise everyday tasks such as going shopping, asking strangers the way, buying a train ticket, etc. (Bosselman et al., 1993).

Role play can also be used as part of family therapy (Innerhofer and Warnke, 1980; Warnke, 1988). It may, for example, be helpful to enact frequent conflicts and recurring family scenarios in order to facilitate access and reconsideration of problems. Often, the therapist observes a marked change in behaviour when family members exchange roles, e.g. when the 'disturbed' child takes on the role of his punishing father. This may help the father to recognize what punishment actually means for the child.

Role play may be useful in the course of individual psychotherapy, e.g. in patients with academic problems at school due to interactional difficulties between the patient and his teacher. Role play may be undertaken with the therapist in the teacher's role. The therapist gradually confronts the patient with increasingly anxious situations, constantly encourages him, and praises him when he copes appropriately with the anxious situations. The experience of being able to deal with situations previously associated with extreme anxiety improves the patient's self-esteem and reduces his future anxiety and avoidance.

The basics of role play

Role play in a group psychotherapy setting occurs in several phases:

(i) preliminary discussion (participants agree on themes and conflicts)
(ii) transition to role play
(iii) distribution of roles
(iv) role play
(v) 'role feedback'/sharing of experiences
(vi) verbal analysis of the play
(vii) develop insight into conflicts
(viii) develop and practise alternative ways of perception and behaviour

Sessions begin with a preliminary discussion, enabling the participants to agree to enact conflicts which seem suitable for role play. Following the preliminary discussion, the participants can begin the role play itself. An experienced group familiar with the rules will usually have little difficulty in distributing roles and commencing role play. The scene can then be enacted along the lines of a predetermined 'scenario'. Following this, the process of 'role feedback' is undertaken, during which the participants have the opportunity to share their experiences during the play. This may involve the presence of intense emotions. Because the participants do not usually have their actions fully under control, participants may unintentionally hurt one another's feelings. The therapist may under certain circumstances need to prevent the play or discussion from getting out of hand. During the analysis of the play, the experiences of individual participants are shared with the group to help patients gain a better understanding of their conflicts, modify their perception and develop alternative strategies for their behaviour.

The practice of role play

Role play with children should be untertaken in a group as homogeneous as possible in terms of age and developmental stage. A group size of six to eight children is generally considered appropriate. In an outpatient setting it may be difficult to find a sufficient number of patients, whereas in an inpatient setting this is usually not a problem. It may also be easier to assess the appropriateness of patients for role play and undertake treatment in an inpatient setting. Sessions usually last between 1 and 2 hours, depending on the stamina of the participants. Ideally, two therapists should run the group and they should have sufficient experience both with the treatment technique as well as with the disorders being treated. Therapists can increase their competence with role play through special training in psychodrama, play therapy, behaviour therapy and other types of group psychotherapy.

Indications and contraindications for group therapy, psychodrama and therapeutic role play

Prerequisites for participation in psychoanalytically orientated group therapy or group therapy based on the principles of counselling (Rogers, 1951) include adequate verbal skills, such that participants are able to express their experiences and emotions, and a willingness to cooperate with the group. In contrast to younger children, who generally do not meet these requirements and tend to benefit more from strictly behaviourally orientated group therapy, adolescents aged 13 and older are more promising candidates for this type of treatment.

Group psychotherapy and role play may contribute to improvement in children and adolescents with psychiatric disorders, e.g. conduct disorder, interpersonal anxieties, specific emotional disorders, introverted disorders, interactional difficulties, and can often be combined with other modes of treatment. The technique is also appropriate for treating disorders such as academic problems or speech disorders at school. Psychodrama tends to be more demanding than role play, especially when the classical approach is used, i.e. 'protagonist-centred play', and is more appropriate to an older age group.

Group psychotherapy is contraindicated if there is a significant risk of suicide and also in cases of acute psychosis, hyperkinetic syndrome, mental retardation, marked neurotic disorder and severe conduct disorder.

Evaluation

There is a paucity of studies on the outcome of group psychotherapy with children and adolescents (Dies and Riester, 1986). Findings reported in the literature should be regarded with caution because many studies have flaws, e.g. small sample size, no control group.

Group psychotherapy with children and adolescents has been shown to be effective in a study with delinquents (Goldstein et al., 1978). 'Social competency training' in groups (Döpfner et al., 1981) and 'group training with adolescents' (Petermann and Petermann, 1987) have also been shown to be effective. In a review article, Siefen (1988) concluded that psychoanalytically orientated group therapy in an in-patient setting did improve psychiatric symptoms in adolescents.

Very few systematic studies on the effectiveness of psychodrama with children and adolescents have been undertaken. Some positive reports in the literature support the view that psychodrama can be effective (Bosselmann et al., 1993; Holl, 1981; Widlöcher, 1974). Bender (1986) reported a beneficial effect when treating adult schizophrenic patients using psychodrama. Therapeutic role play can be used as a component of various types of group therapy, however, there is a lack of pertinent follow-up studies.

REFERENCES

Bender, W. (1986). Psychodrama mit Psychose-Patienten. *Gruppenpsychotherapie und Gruppendynamik*, **21**, 307–17.

Bosselmann, R., Kindschuh-van Roje, E. and Martin, M. (1993). Einige Einsatzmöglichkeiten des Psychodramas im therapeutischen Heim. In *Variationen des Psychodramas*, ed. R. Bosselmann, E. Lüffe-Leonhardt and M. Gellert, pp. 240–6. Meezen: Limmer.

Dies, R. R. and Riester, A. E. (1986). Research on child group therapy. Present status and future directions. In *Child group psychotherapy*, ed. A. E. Riester and J. A. Kraft, pp. 173–220. Madison, CT: International Universities Press.

Döpfner, M., Schlüter, S. and Rey, E. R. (1981). Evaluation eines sozialen Kompetenztrainings für selbstunsichere Kinder im Alter von neun bis zwölf Jahren. Ein Therapievergleich. *Zeitschrift für Kinder- und Jugendpsychiatrie*, **9**, 233–52.

Franzke, E. (1977). *Der Mensch und sein Gestaltungserleben. Psychotherapeutische Nutzung kreativer Arbeitsweisen*. Bern: Huber.

Goldstein, A. P., Sherman, M., Gershaw, N. J., Sprafkin, R. P. and Glick, B. (1978). Training of aggressive adolescents in prosocial behavior. *Journal of Youth and Adolescence*, **7**, 73–92.

Haar, R. (1980). Gruppentherapie mit Kindern und Jugendlichen in Klinik und Heim. *Praxis der Kinderpsychologie und Kinderpsychiatrie*, **5**, 182–94.

Holl, W. (1981). Erfahrungen mit einer Psychodrama-Jungengruppe. In *Psychodrama in der Praxis*, E. Engelke. München: Pfeiffer.

Innerhofer, P. and Warnke, A. (1980). Elterntrainingsprogramm nach dem Münchener

Trainingsmodell. Ein Erfahrungsbericht. In *Familiäre Sozialisation und Intervention*, ed. H. Lukesch, M. Perrez and K. Schneewind. Bern: Huber.

Lehmkuhl, G. (1990). Gruppenpsychotherapie mit Jugendlichen. In *Das Jugendalter. Entwicklung – Probleme – Hilfen*, ed. H. C. Steinhausen. Bern: Huber.

Leutz, G. (1974). *Das Klassische Psychodrama nach J. L. Moreno*. Berlin: Springer.

Mattejat, F. and Jungmann, J. (1981). Einübung sozialer Kompetenz. Erfahrungen bei der Entwicklung und Erprobung eines gruppentherapeutischen Programms für Kinder. *Praxis der Kinderpsychologie und Kinderpsychiatrie*, **30**, 62–70.

Meichenbaum, D. H. (1977). *Cognitive-behavior modification*. New York: Plenum Press.

Moreno, H. L. (1964). *Introduction to psychodrama*, vol. 1. Beacon, NY: Beacon House.

Müller-Küppers, M. (1988). Kinderpsychotherapie. In *Psychiatrie der Gegenwart*, vol 7, ed. K. P. Kisker, H. Lauter, J-E. Meyer, C. Müller and E. Strömgren, pp. 429–54. Berlin: Springer.

Niebergall, G. (1987). Soziometrische Erfassung von Stationsgruppen- und Familienstrukturen. In *Kinder- und Jugendpsychiatrie*, ed. H. Remschmidt, pp. 78–81. Stuttgart: Thieme.

Oerter, R. and Montada, L. (1982). *Entwicklungspsychologie*. München: Urban & Schwarzenberg.

Petermann, F. and Petermann, U. (1987). *Training mit Jugendlichen*. München: Psychologie Verlags Union.

Petermann, U. (1983). *Training mit sozial unsicheren Kindern. Einzeltraining, Kindergruppen, Elterntraining*. München: Urban & Schwarzenberg.

Petzold, H. (1978). Das Psychodrama als Methode der klinischen Psychotherapie. In *Klinische Psychologie*, vol. 2, ed. L. J. Pongratz, pp. 2751–84. Göttingen: Hogrefe.

Ploeger, A. (1983). *Tiefenpsychologisch fundierte Psychodramatherapie*. Stuttgart: Kohlhammer.

Remschmidt, H. (1992). *Psychiatrie der Adoleszenz*. Stuttgart: Thieme.

Rogers, C. (1951). *Client centred therapy in current practice. Implications and theory*. New York: Houghton Mifflin.

Schützenberger, A. (1979). *Psychodrama. Ein Abriss. Erläuterungen der Methoden*. Stuttgart: Hippokrates.

Siefen, R. G. (1988). Gruppentherapie. In *Kinder- und Jugendpsychiatrie in Klinik und Praxis*, vol. I, ed. H. Remschmidt and M. H. Schmidt, pp. 707–12. Stuttgart: Thieme.

Slavson, S. R. (1966). Unterschiedliche psychodynamische Prozesse der Aktivitäts- und Aussprachegruppen. In *Analytische Gruppenpsychotherapie. Grundlagen und Praxis*, ed. H. G. Preuss. München: Urban & Schwarzenberg.

Slavson, S. R. (1977). *Analytische Gruppentherapie. Theorie und Anwendung*. Frankfurt: Fischer.

Stoiber, K. C. and Kratchowill, T. R. (ed.) (1998). *Handbook of group intervention for children and families*. Boston, MA: Allyn & Bacon.

Warnke, A. (1988). Elternarbeit in der Kinder- und Jugendpsychiatrie. In *Kinder- und Jugendpsychiatrie in Klinik und Praxis*, vol. I, ed. H. Remschmidt and M. H. Schmidt, pp. 750–62. Stuttgart: Thieme.

Widlöcher, D. (1974). *Das Psychodrama bei Jugendlichen*. Olten: Walter.

Yablonski, L. (1976). *Psychodrama. Resolving emotional problems through role-playing*. New York: Basic Books.

12 Family therapy

Fritz Mattejat

Introduction

Family therapy is a commonly used approach to treat disorders in childhood and adolescence. An important impetus for the development of family therapy was the 'double-bind' theory of schizophrenia (Bateson et al., 1956) and other family theories of schizophrenia (Lidz, 1958; Wynne and Singer, 1963). Simultaneously, but independently family-orientated techniques were developed on the basis of clinical experience with families. Early pioneers of this development include Ackerman (1958), Bowen (1960), Haley (1963), and Satir (1964). Minuchin (1974) introduced family therapy techniques in the field of child and adolescent psychiatry. The 'Milan group' (Selvini-Palazzoli et al., 1978) had a great influence on family therapy, especially during the phase in which the technique became popular. This is reflected by the fact that the term 'systemic family therapy' is often used to refer to the approach developed by the Milan group, whose therapeutic techniques were based explicitly on the systems theory developed by Bateson (1972). However, systemic ideas have influenced all schools of family therapy, even where this is not so obvious. Madanes and Haley (1977) have proposed a way of distinguishing different family therapies.

(i) Strategic family therapy includes approaches developed by Watzlawick et al. (1974) and the 'Milan approach' developed by Selvini Palazzoli et al. (1978) Both approaches are based on the prinicples of systems theory initially introduced by Bateson (1972).

(ii) Structural family therapy relates to the approaches developed by Minuchin (Minuchin and Fishman, 1981). The approach emphasizes the importance of subsystems in families and boundaries between generations.

In addition to these, the traditional psychotherapy schools have developed their own particular approaches to family therapy, including:

(iii) Psychodynamic family therapy,

(iv) Experiential and person centred family therapy,

(v) Behavioural family therapy.

The theories on which the various approaches are based often differ considerably, and practical guidelines are commonly contradictory. Thus, the field of family therapy is manifold and Ackerman's (1971) remark still seems fitting today: 'Every family therapist is doing his own thing.' The aim of this chapter is not to discuss the various types of family therapy systematically, because such systematic discussions can be found elsewhere (Skynner, 1976; Textor, 1985; Gorell-Barnes, 1994). Here, the relevant issues for treating children and adolescents with psychiatric disorders in a clinical setting will be addressed, with particular emphasis on the approach which has been developed and used successfully in our Marburg unit.

Theoretical principles

Basic assumptions

Although the approaches to family therapy differ widely, they are usually based on the following basic assumptions, which are widely accepted.

The individual and the system

In order to understand the way an individual feels and behaves, it is necessary to consider his environment and the behaviour of persons with whom this individual has close relationships (attachment figures). Individual behaviour is always part of a system at a higher level, e.g. the family, social, economical and cultural environment, and can be understood from this perspective.

The family and psychiatric disorder

There are close relations between family processes and psychiatric disorders. Individual symptoms often disturb family interaction, whilst disturbed interaction tends to sustain or aggravate symptoms. Furthermore, psychiatric disorders in children and adolescents may indicate a disturbance of interpersonal relationships within the family. At the same time, symptoms can also be considered as important and helpful attempts to solve problems and stabilize the family system.

Family therapy

When treating children and adolescents, it is always important to consider the family situation and assess the relevance of all environmental factors, independent of their apparent relationship with aetiology. The term 'family therapy' is used when treatment aims to modify interpersonal relationships within the family system.

Systemic developmental orientation

Children and adolescents treated for psychiatric disorders frequently come from multiple-problem families (Mattejat, 1985a). However, conclusions should be drawn very carefully, and it is important always to distinguish facts from speculations. Family therapy should never be based on the assumption that psychiatric disorders in children and adolescents are caused by the family. Such a view would be too simplistic and inappropriate in clinical practice as it fails to address two important issues:

The systemic perspective

It is an oversimplified view to regard the family only as the cause, whilst the disorder is considered only to be the result. This view has led to the common misconception that the aim of family therapy is to find fault with the family. However, blaming the family is not only clinically unlikely to help the patient, but is invariably an oversimplification, because aetiological factors are usually very complex. Interpersonal relationships in the family are influenced by the child's disorder just as the child's behaviour is influenced by family interaction. Terms from systems theory such as 'circularity', 'network', 'interdependency' and 'co-evolution' have been used to refer to such complex interrelationships. Because family relationships and individual symptoms are codependent and both aspects are part of one single developmental process, it is therefore, always important to consider the principles of family therapy when treating children and adolescents.

Thus, systemic orientation is based on the assumption that psychological problems cannot be solved only at an individual level, but need to be considered at different levels, which include dyadic relationships and more complex interconnections, e.g. triadic relations, higher level systems.

Developmental orientation

Family therapy should focus on developing alternative strategies or solutions to the patient's problems rather than merely explaining symptoms. Family therapy should aim to bring about improvement of the patient's symptoms by encouraging the family to use its resources and to develop coping strategies. The family, especially the parents, may offer the best and most valuable support for the child. The family therapy approach is important in practice because the family usually is able to make significant contributions towards coping with psychiatric disorders in children and adolescents. Family therapy techniques are intended to support normal developmental processes, especially in providing help for developmental problems and assisting the child in coping with the demands of normal development.

The family as a developmental space

When this systemic developmental perspective is applied to the field of child and adolescent psychiatry, the family can be regarded as a specific environment in which the child develops under more or less favourable conditions (L'Abate, 1994). The child contributes to his own development by actively influencing his environment, as do all members of the family. Thus, the family can be regarded as a developmental space, i.e. system of developmental conditions, in which each individual family member as well as the family as a whole is in a state of flux. The system is 'self-referential', i.e. the system's characteristics are both the result of a development process and continue to influence the process. A family usually requires the help of a therapist when coping strategies are not sufficient in relation to the stress the family has to endure. In this case, the aim of family therapy would be to help the family to develop coping strategies to deal with the stress. Thus, what was previously considered 'stress' is transformed into a 'developmental stimulus' (Olbrich, 1984, 1985). When a family decides to seek professional help, the therapist becomes involved in this complex process. Specific patterns of interaction rapidly develop between individual family members and the therapist, which reflect both 'professional' assumptions and the structure of interaction in the family, including defence and coping strategies.

Cooperation with the family: a working model

When a child or adolescent is referred for treatment, we should not automatically consider the entire family the 'true patient'. Such an attitude can seriously impair cooperation between the family and the therapists. The focus of treatment should be determined in agreement with the family.

In practice, all families can be offered professional advice. In a considerable number of cases, counselling alone is insufficient and it may become necessary to undertake a supportive family therapy or psychoeducative interventions. In a smaller proportion of these families, fundamental family conflicts can be addressed in order to change patterns of interaction. So cooperation with families can be undertaken at three interventional levels, which can be distinguished by the degree to which parents participate in therapy (see Fig. 12.1). The specific methods which can be used to approach treatment goals at each level are summarized in Fig. 12.2. and explained below.

1. Consultation /counselling for parents and families	**Typical situation:** Treatment focusses on individual psychotherapy of the child/adolescent; intensive work with parents is not essential at this level **Aims:** Individual psychotherapy should be accompanied by sessions with parents, during which they have the opportunity to exchange information with the therapist. Sessions with parents should enable them to understand and support treatment (therapeutic rapport). Such sessions can help to prevent dropout from treatment
⇩	
2. Supportive family therapy (psycho-educative interventions)	**Typical situation:** Issues discussed include how parents can support their disturbed child, and the interaction between the child's symptoms and parents' reactions to symptoms. This interaction may sustain or even aggravate symptoms, and should therefore be addressed within the family **Aims:** Working with families should enable the parents (and other care-givers) to better understand the child's problems, recognize their reactions to the child's behaviour, and support the child in coping with difficulties
⇩	
3. Relationship-orientated family therapy	**Typical situation:** Family members are expected to discuss conflicts or difficult family relationships, rather than only the child's symptoms **Aims:** Patterns of family interaction should be addressed, aimed at solving conflicts, and overcoming problems which prevent normal child development. Family relationships should be modified in order to allow all family members to satisfy their needs and take up new opportunities for personal development

Fig. 12.1. Levels of cooperation with parents and families: typical situations and aims of treatment.

Consultation and counselling for parents and families

Regardless of the type of therapy being undertaken, parents and families need to be offered information and advice about all aspects of their child's disorder. Parents and families also need to be provided with information when individual psychotherapy is being undertaken with the patient, in order to ensure family support for any changes which occur over the course of treatment and to prevent early discontinuation of treatment. Advice to parents and families is the basis for cooperation between them and the therapist. The mere fact that a child has a psychiatric disorder often results in destabilization of the family. Parents tend to feel guilty and helpless, especially when previous coping strategies have failed, reducing their own self-confidence and self-esteem. Thus, in liaison with families it is important to provide sufficient information, convey a sense of orientation and security, and encourage the family members' motivation for change (develop a trusting relationship for cooperation).

Supportive family therapy and psychoeducative interventions

This approach focuses not only on the individual patient's behaviour, but also takes into account other family members. This type of therapy is appropriate

Level	Principal methods
1. Consultation /counselling for parents and families	· Provision of detailed information and advice · Drawing up of clear agreements · Use of techniques to improve the relationship, e.g. acceptance, positive acknowledgement, support
⇩	
2. Supportive family therapy (psycho-educative interventions)	· Observation and discussion of interactions · Development of coping strategies with the family · Encouragement of structured problem solutions · Parent training sessions and educational family therapy · Behavoural therapy methods, e.g. contracts, behavioural tasks, cognitive techniques · All methods used at level 1
⇩	
3. Relationship-orientated family therapy	· Clarify the family relationships in sessions using verbal, non-verbal and actional techniques, e.g. family sculpture, psychodrama · Uncover conflicts and reveal individual and family factors which may have contributed to the disorder · Various interview techniques, e.g. circular or hypothetical questioning · Reframing · All methods used at levels 1 and 2

Fig. 12.2. Levels of cooperation with parents and families: principal methods.

when individual symptoms are aggravated by family members, or when the entire family is going through a crisis because of the patient's disturbance. The aim is to neuralize the effect of specific symptoms on family life, i.e. break up interactional patterns which are repeatedly triggered and reinforced by the symptoms, and support the family in developing patterns of interaction which facilitate the coping with symptoms. In this context, methods aimed at modifying symptoms directly, i.e. coping strategies are of great importance. Various methods may be effective, and the most widely used include educational and behavioural approaches (e.g. self-observation, self-control techniqes, behavioural contracts), complemented by video feed-back and role-play.

Relationship orientated family therapy

In some cases, e.g. generational conflicts, interactional problems form the presenting symptoms, whilst individual symptoms play a secondary role and the families wish to address their interactional conflicts. In other cases with a severely disorderd child or adolescent, such conflicts become manifest only when individual symptoms have decreased. The emphasis of sessions then may shift from individual symptoms to more complex problems, which may to some extent comprise the difficulties which almost all families with adolescents have to deal with. Relationship-orientated family therapy should be considered when symptoms reflect interpersonal difficulties within the family, or when roles in the family and patterns of interaction prevent the child from dealing appropriately with symptoms, e.g. if 'healthy' behaviour does not 'fit' a family's disturbed interactional patterns. The aim is to support the family to develop ways of relating to one another which allow individual family members to satisfy their needs. The therapist should encourage family members to discuss openly conflicting opinions, a process which often results in the development of resistance. Such resistance is usually based on an understandable anxiety about change. In such situations, the therapist can question rigid beliefs and attitudes by confronting the family directly, or may 'go with the resistance', in advising the family to avoid excessively rapid or fundamental changes. Interventions should be undertaken with care, as the therapist is dealing with extremely private family issues, which can be decided only by the family members themselves.

Psychiatric disorders in childhood and adolescence are frequently associated with marital discord, and in a considerable number of cases one or both parents themselves also suffer from a psychiatric disorder. In such cases, individual or marital therapy should be considered. Parental disorder may be obvious from the beginning, and in some cases parents may present their child as a pretext to addressing their own problems. Help should then be offered to the parents immediately. However, usually parents can only address their own problems after treatment of their child and a trusting relationship with the therapist has been established.

The levels or phases shown in Fig. 12.1 show the main issues which the therapist needs to address when deciding upon cooperation with the family. However, these levels should not be considered strictly independently of one another. The issue of motivation for change is relevant in all phases of treatment: simple information may influence relationships within the family to a significant degree, and the transition from interventions directed at the child and to those addressing family interaction is usually gradual. The levels of cooperation are not intended to reflect on their value. Offering information and support with structuring behaviour are just as important as relationship-orientated therapy, and also require considerable professional competence.

The most important aspects of the approach to family theapy proposed here include the following.

(i) Therapy should be impartial and based on cooperation with the whole family. The nature of this cooperation needs to be determined by the family and therapist together.

(ii) Cooperation with families should be problem orientated. The therapist should focus on the problems addressed by the family. Cooperation with families is not always aimed at bringing about major changes of family structure, nor does cooperation mean continuous help with everyday life. Cooperation with families implies offering support for a limited period of time.

(iii) Cooperation with families should support normal coping strategies and normal development, i.e. focus on problem solution. Cooperation with families is important because the family can make an essential contribution to coping with psychiatric problems of individual family members.

(iv) It is the therapist's task to adapt therapy to the problems being addressed. Thus, treatment should be undertaken differentially, i.e. the method should be adapted to the specific needs of the family and coordinated with all other treatment steps. Often family therapy is combined with other kinds of interventions, e.g. the Marburg 'component model of therapy'.

(v) The approach to family therapy proposed here is guided by the idea of evidence-based practice. This also involves constantly appraising one's work critically, in order to offer patients and their families the best possible help.

Indications

When considering family therapy (Strunk, 1987), two questions have to be answered:

- first, is family therapy indicated at all?
- secondly, if family therapy is thought to be indicated: what is the most appropriate setting, participant constellation, session intervals, interventional level (Fig. 12.1 and 12.2) and technique?

The first issue can usually be decided on the theoretical principles explained above. The provision of information and advice to parents and families is always appropriate. Supportive family therapy and psychoeducational interventions should be considered when family problems play a significant role in the aetiology and maintenance of symptoms, or when family members can help with problem-solving or motivating the child to use self-help techniques. The decision as to the more specific issues, e.g. treatment setting and techniques can be considered under three headings.

Institutional conditions and the therapist's personal characteristics

This includes the issue of opportunities and limitations of family therapy in specific institutions. The therapist's training and clinical experience is also important. The therapist should be aware of his capabilities and limits of expertise and should consider the value of having a co-therapist or supervisor.

Family characteristics (the characteristics of individual patients and those of family members)

The patient's age, developmental stage, type of disorder, severity of symptoms, previous course, prognosis and coping strategies should be taken into account. Relevant family characteristics include all factors detrimental to the family, e.g. social stress, psychiatric disorder, abnormal family interaction, abnormal family structure, abnormal developmental family history, lack of coping strategies.

Relationship during therapy

The relationship between family and therapist is another relevant factor.

The following guidelines may be helpful when deciding on treatment settings. Sessions with the entire family can be recommended when the family itself considers individual problems a result of disturbed familial relationships, or when the family feels that individual symptoms reflect in fact the entire family's problem. Sessions with the whole family are likely to be successful when all involved are motivated towards change and willing to cooperate with the therapist (Martin, 1981). Crises tend to improve family cohesion. Family sessions tend to be especially helpful following suicide attempts. Family therapy has been used frequently with families characterized by close relationships and strong cohesion. The approach has been shown to be significantly more successful in such families than in less cohesive families (Aponte and Vandeusen, 1981; Heekerens, 1989).

The patient's diagnosis is also important when deciding on a treatment setting. Family therapy has been shown to be effective in psychosomatic and internalizing disorders, separation anxiety, and autonomy conflicts in adolescence (Gurman and Kniskern, 1981a; Aponte and Vandeusen, 1981). However, it may be more difficult with aggressive and antisocial patients who tend to act out. Family sessions may be even more difficult in psychosis, although such sessions may be useful in the rehabilitation phase to support the patient's reintegration in the family after discharge from hospital. Although family work may help to reduce expressed emotions (EE) in the interaction with schizophrenic patients, family sessions are not recommended if they prove too stressful or cause considerable anxiety, e.g. in severe anxiety or obsessional disorders or in acute psychoses. Sessions with all family members are also contraindicated when abnormal patterns of behaviour recur often during sessions, e.g. marked hysterical symptoms, aggressive behaviour. Such sessions may escalate and get out of hand, resulting in an aggravation of problems. Family sessions are also contraindicated in the presence of severe conflicts between parents, such as severe marital discord or sexual problems. Reports in the literature suggest that the success of family therapy depends to a significant degree on the relationship between the parents (Gurman and Kniskern, 1981b). Thus, in cases of severe conflict between parents, marital therapy is more appropriate than family therapy.

The therapy technique used also depends on the severity of the disorder and the extent to which the family is likely to be able to tolerate the stress which is associated with some techniques. Whilst supportive family therapy with particular emphasis on structuring is appropriate for families with psychotic patients, more demanding changes may be expected of families when the adolescent has only mild or moderate symptoms. In addition, it is important to consider the type of family: neurotically overinvolved families frequently are able to profit from psychodynamic and systemic methods. Paradoxical intervention techniques and non-verbal methods may be used to bring about modifications, especially in inflexible families which tend to intellectualize. In contrast, disorganized and chaotic families usually require more structuring, e.g. behavioural tasks and contracts. The same is often true of therapy with underprivileged families from a poor social background. In these cases, supplementary social work may also be required. When choosing techniques, the child's developmental level must be considered. The younger or mentally retarded child is less likely to be able to control his behaviour. In these cases, treatment techniques which address the child's behaviour directly, e.g. reinforcement schedules, behavioural parent training programmes are more likely to be successful. In contrast, verbal methods are more appropriate when treating adolescents.

Initial diagnostic appraisal is essential prior to deciding on an approach to treatment. Moreover family therapy generally requires ongoing assessment of the therapeutic process. This assessment helps the therapist to decide on the main issue: 'Can the family utilize the therapeutic support offered?'. Therapists need to be flexible and willing to reconsider their own attitudes and decisions in order to expand the family's range of developmental options.

Diagnostic assessment of families

Aims of family diagnostic assessment

The aim of family diagnostic assessment is to identify psychosocial factors which influence the development and sustenance of psychiatric disorders, and factors which might be useful for improving psychopathology and coping processes. Family diagnostic assessment can be undertaken at two levels:

The level of the family system

It is important to consider the contribution of family interaction to individual psychopathology and how the patient's symptoms influence the family. The aim of family diagnostic assessment at this level is to lead to a better understanding of the family problems.

The level of the therapy system

It is equally important to uncover the types of assistance the family is willing to accept (or reject), and to discover in which respect the family's and therapist's ideas correspond. The aim of the assessment at this level is find out the most appropriate way of working with the family.

Methods of diagnostic assessment with families

Two major approaches to family diagnostic assessment can be distinguished. Observation techniques include methods based on direct observation of family situations, whilst self report techniques usually comprise questionnaires, in which individual family members are expected to describe and to evaluate aspects of family life (Kaslow, 1996). Thus, with observation techniques, information is gathered by an 'external' observer, whilst self-appraisal techniques are based on an 'internal' perspective. A pragmatic classification of methods is shown in Fig. 12.3. The most commonly used family diagnostic assesment technique by far is the family interview, which may be complemented by interactional tasks or individual assessment of each family member. Because of its paramount importance, the family interview is discussed in detail below.

Family interview

An approach for undertaking initial family diagnostic interviews has been developed in the Family Therapy Clinic at the Hospital for Child and Adolescent Psychiatry, University of Marburg, Germany. In this, both the patient and parents are asked to attend the initial session, and when necessary, other family

Diagnostic setting:	Diagnostic methods:		
	Interview	Questionnaries/other techniques	
Together with the whole family	Conjoint family interview	Interactional tasks, e.g. family Rorschach test	
Individually with one child / adolescent or other family members	Family-orientated individual interviews	Questionnaires, e.g. FACES*	Other assessment techniques, e.g. projective tests

Fig. 12.3. Classification of family diagnostic assessment methods. *Family adaptability and cohesion evaluation scales (Olson et al., 1985).

members are also included. The initial interview involves two therapists: one conducts the interview, the other observes the session by means of a video link-up. Normally, the session is videotaped.

Principles for performing the family interview
The following principles should be borne in mind.

Transparency
For a family to feel at ease with the therapist, the therapeutic situation should be clear and the family should be fully informed. The therapist should reveal all the information he has about the family. In addition, he should explain the purpose of the session and the methods used in therapy, address the issue of who is to have what information, and obtain the consent of all involved.

Perspectivity
The therapist should be impartial and emphasize that the perspectives of all family members are equally important, and the entire family can contribute to the therapeutic process by expressing their views. Thus, the therapist should ask each family member in turn about their opinions, and offer an empathic response to each person. This requires the therapist to 'switch' from one perspective to another rather quickly.

Diagnostic-empathic attitude

It is important to listen and accept everything the family wishes to say. Thus, judgements and interpretations are inappropriate; instead, the therapist should strictly adhere to listening and trying to understand. Questions about treatment should be temporarily deferred by stating that the problem needs to be better understood before advice can be offered. The interview should not include interventions with the intention of altering or changing the family, nor should the therapist immediately redefine the patient's symptoms as a family problem.

Developmental orientation

The therapist should honour the trust that the family places in him. He should emphasize points and opportunities for positive development. The interviewer's questions and final comment should focus on the family's goals and emphasize their resources and self-help capacities. Increasing emphasis on developmental aspects indicates the transition from diagnostics to family therapy.

Structure and thematic sequence

The initial family interview need not be structured as rigidly as is required for research purposes. The family should be permitted to lead the conversation, although the issues in Fig. 12.4. should be addressed over the course of the interview. The idea of the Marburg Family Interview involves some careful structuring, without preventing diagnostically important information from being brought up. Usually, the family addresses important topics automatically, and this process should not be inhibited. But, usually the following issues should be discussed.

Initial contact and general information

The interviewer should introduce him/herself, address each family member and ask their name. The family should be informed about the video recording and the other therapist(s) behind the one-way mirror or at the video screen, and consent should be obtained for this and any other recordings to be made. The interviewer should inform them about the aims and duration of the session, and emphasize the interest in the family.

Previous experience, mode of referal, decision to seek consultation

The interview should continue with the issue of what caused the family to seek consultation and how they came to seek help. They should be given the

1. Initial contact and general information

⇩

2. Previous experience, mode of referral, decision to seek consultation

⇩

3. Discussing the patient's individual problems

⇩

4. The family: problems and resources

- Reactions to the child's problems
- Interpersonal relationships and coping strategies in the family
- General family situation and extrafamilial relationships

⇩

5. Expectations regarding treatment

- General ideas towards problem solutions (How can problems be solved?)
- Specific therapeutic ideas (How can therapists help?)

⇩

6. Final agreement

Fig. 12.4. Structure of topics in an initial family diagnostic interview.

opportunity to discuss the child's role as a 'patient', and discuss any previous attempts at treatment.

Discussing the patient's individual problems

This part of the discussion may be introduced by questions such as: 'Could you tell me the reason you've come here?', or 'Exactly what problems are we talking about?' Such open questions can be followed by circular questions in order to encourage discussion.

The family

The broad issue of 'the family' often takes the most time to discuss, and usually includes three aspects: (i) how the family perceives the child's disorder, reacts at a cognitive and emotional level, and what attempts they have made to cope with the problem; (ii) interpersonal relationships within the family and coping strategies developed; (iii) the general family situation (problems, stress factors, resources) and other important relationships.

Expectations concerning treatment

Typical questions might be: 'How do you think can we help you to find solutions to these problems?' or 'Do you have specific ideas about what treatment you think would help?' or 'Do you have any concerns in connection with treatment?'

Final agreement

Before the session is brought to an end the interviewer should ask whether the family has any further questions. Finally, the therapist should thank the family and emphasize that he has received helpful information with respect to therapy planning. He may comment further on the session, and begin to make plans of any further steps, e.g. additional diagnostic investigations or family therapy session.

Family interview sessions generally last about 45–60 minutes. In most cases all topics can be addressed in this time. Usually, the therapist does not need to bring up the topics himself, as families usually do so automatically. However, the therapist needs to make sure that family members have the opportunity to express their view on all the issues. In some cases a family may not address one or two topics, even with encouragement. In extreme cases, the family may only discuss the issue of consultation and spend all their time complaining vehemently about previous treatments. Even such interviews can contribute significantly to diagnostic appraisal. The structure of the interview serves as a basic pattern, allowing comparisons to be made. Those interviews which do not follow the basic pattern are often particularly revealing from a diagnostic point of view.

Analysing and evaluating the interview

When gathering diagnostic information by means of family interviews, it is important to be aware of two important aims:

Subjective perspectives
During the interview the therapist should attempt to understand each family member's point of view and recognize differences between the various subjective perspectives. In contrast to taking a history, the aim is not to collect objective data, but to understand the subjective views and attitudes of the individual family members.

Objective interactional behaviour
Observing the family's interactions is just as important as obtaining verbal information. This includes both intrafamilial interactions and interactions with the therapist.

When analysing the interview, it is helpful to compare the impression of the therapist who led the session with the opinion of the second observing therapist. The 'interviewer' is usually more involved and should have a diagnostic-empathic attitude, whilst the 'observer' tends to be able to adopt a more detatched point of view. In this context, Bateson's (1972) definition of information holds true: 'Information is the difference that makes a difference'. It can be both informative and stimulating when the two observers arrive at different opinions. These differences require discussion and reconsideration to arrive at a congruent assessment. The result of such discussions should be recorded as part of the family diagnostic procedure. Clinical rating scales can be used to evaluate sessions systematically. Interactional microanalysis can also be utilized. Such techniques include chronological analysis of interaction, assessment of interaction by means of specific predefined categories, or analysis of content. However, such techniques are impractical in a clinical setting and only appropriate for research purposes. The issues which should be addressed when assessing family diagnostic interviews are summarized in Fig. 12.5.

Methods for family therapy

The therapeutic attitude

The principles that apply to initial family diagnostic assessment also apply to treatment. The therapist should demonstrate an empathic attitude, listen carefully to what the family has to say, and try to perceive as much as possible in order to obtain an understanding of the situation of each family member. This is important both for individual and family therapy sessions.

Ideally, the therapist should aim to show equal empathy to each family member. He can demonstrate this by dividing his attention equally between the participants during family therapy sessions. This does not necessarily refer

Issues of the family system

Problem description	• What are the most important individual, familial and social difficulties and how serious are they?
Conditional hypotheses	• How do problems interrelate? • What function do the problems have in the family system? • How can the symptoms be explained (hypotheses)?
Coping strategies	• What coping strategies do individual family members favour? • How do the various coping strategies interrelate? • What capabilities and resources are available to the family that have not been used yet but may be put to use in order to cope with the problems?

Issues of the therapeutic system

Preconditions with the family	• Who sought contact with the institution? • What are the aims of individual family members? • What ideas about treatment do the family members have, and what hopes and anxieties do they associate with therapy?
Preconditions with the therapist	• What personal and institutional resources are available to help the family?
Opportunities for cooperation	• How does the family react to being offered an interview and interventions ('rapport')? • How does the therapist react to the individual family members? • Are the family's wishes congruent with the therapist's ideas? • Which aspects of cooperation require special attention, which positive opportunities can be used, and which risks should be observed?

Fig. 12.5. Important issues when assessing family diagnostic interviews.

to measurable time. It is important to listen to all opinions on a topic with equal acceptance. This requires a considerable amount of flexibility, i.e. constant 'switching', especially when opinions are contrary. The ideas of empathy and multiple perspectives are closely linked in family therapy, and it is important to develop the skill of showing empathy to one family member without automatically rejecting the others' opinions. This may require avoiding giving a 'verdict' on the validity of a specific opinion. Thus, if confronted with issues of right or wrong or whether a behaviour reflects disorder or misbehaviour ('mad' or 'bad'), he should emphasize the importance of each individual's point of view. As the therapist demonstrates his effort to understand each individual, the family members often become more inclined to accept one another's opinion (modelling).

The success of family sessions depends to a considerable degree on whether the therapist is able to demonstrate empathy for different views ('multiple perspectives') and whether the family is willing to follow this type of communication. This is not always the case. Occasionally, even the attempt to undertake a session during which each participant has the opportunity to say something fails. Difficulties may also occur when participants are unable or lack the courage to explain their opinion, or when members of the family prevent one another from openly expressing their views. In such cases, family sessions may be stressful and have a detrimental effect on the family. The same is true when families fail to understand the aim of family sessions or misunderstand the therapist's behaviour. This, for example, may be the case when a father feels his authority is being undermined as a result of his son being given the opportunity to express his own views, or when the therapist is inextricably manoeuvred into a judgemental role. In such situations, the appropriateness of family therapy should be questioned. Bringing about an appropriate attitude in all participants towards family therapy constitutes the first step towards success. Improved understanding of oneself and others enables the development of an accepting attitude, which is important to enable family members to expand their behavioural repertoire and try out new behavioural options. In successful cases, families can develop this positive developmental attitude with a minimum of therapeutic assistance. Whilst specific techniques can be used to support the family in modifying behaviour, this is not always necessary. Often, simply providing the family with space to change and occasional encouragement, reinforcement and critical appraisal is all the family requires.

Specific family therapy techniques

Interventions in family therapy should generally be based on the principles mentioned above. A pragmatic classification system for intervention techniques is shown in Fig. 12.6. Techniques related to interaction during family therapy sessions are distinguished from those related to interaction in-between sessions. The four different methods are explained below, using one technique from each category to illustrate the method.

Techniques related to interaction during sessions		Techniques related to interaction between sessions	
Verbal techniques	Actional techniques	Direct interventions	Complex (paradoxical) interventions
• Control of the sequence of communication • Circular questioning • Reinterpretation • Family pedigree • Suggestive and metaphorical communication	• Use of the space, e.g order of sitting • Family sculpturing • Role play and psychodrama	• Observational techniques, e.g. self-observation, observing another person • Behavioural tasks • Family contracts	• Symptom prescriptions • Rule prescriptions • Ritual and metaphorical prescriptions

Fig. 12.6. Classification and examples of family therapy techniques.

Reframing

The technique referred to as 'reframing' is based on the assumption that the meaning and significance which is attributed to individual behaviour is determined by the social and individual context in which it occurs and by the frame of reference, which is used to interpret the behaviour. This can be illustrated using an adolescent conflict. Whilst an adolescent boy's parents considered the frequent disobedience of their son inacceptable and dangerous, the boy felt his parents were becoming more and more restrictive without any reason. In situations such as this, the therapist can 'reframe' the behaviour in order to facilitate a useful discussion and clarify the different views. A useful frame for the parents' view might be: 'You take the responsibility for your son very seriously and would go to great lengths to protect him.' A helpful frame for the boy might be: 'You would like to show that you are capable of acting independently and responsibly.' If the parents and the boy accept such positive reframing, it may be possible to overcome the reciprocal accusations and address the issue in a more matter-of-fact way. The therapist might continue the session by asking the parents: 'Are you capable of protecting your son? Are there any better alternatives?'. And he might ask the boy: 'How can you best develop your independence? Can you do so in such a way that your parents realize that you aren't a child anymore?' So problems can be redefined and made more accessible by viewing them in a different context. It is the therapist's task to redefine the participants' problems in such a way as to enable them to provide an alternative interpretation, which allows them to respond in a more constructive way. The therapist should refrain from offering his own solutions, because the best problem solution strategies are usually those developed by the family itself.

Family sculpture

Non-verbal and actional therapy techniques are particularly appropriate when verbal techniques fail, when much is spoken but little said, e.g. in individuals who tend to intellectualize, or when participants lack adequate verbal skills.

Families can literally demonstrate the relationship between family members using family sculpture. With this techniqe one family member (the 'protagonist') is chosen and asked to assemble the family in such a way as to illustrate the relationship of family members by means of spatial arrangement, position, gestures, etc. The protagonst's task resembles that of a sculptor, who has to create a statue consisting of a group of individuals, and express the 'relationships' which the sculptor sees them as having towards each other. Thus, the family situation becomes literally 'palpable'. As a result, arguments and fruitless discussions may abate. The technique has the advantage that the protagonist can express himself without being interrupted, the other family members cease to be opponents for him, and become 'wax in his hands'. The transition from intellectual discussion of problems to careful physical contact between family members often changes the atmosphere of family sessions, helping to reveal the true nature of interpersonal relationships within the family.

The therapist's task is to supervise the creation of a family sculpture by explaining the method, obtaining the family's consent, and assisting the protagonist by telling and demonstrating how to go about making the sculpture. The therapist should give the protagonist time and offer any necesary support. Ideally, all family members should have the opportunity to experience themselves as protagonist. The therapist also has the task of protecting the participants, who may not always realize exactly what they are involved in. Thus, the therapist should ensure the continuing willingness of family members to participate. The therapist should never press families to participate. Family sculpture should only be used if the therapist is familiar with the family and can assess each individual's psychological tolerance.

Following the creation of the sculpture, all participants should have the opportuninty to discuss how they felt whilst work was in progress. This may take an entire session. The technique may be extended to include 'ideal sculptures' which can be used to express the interactional situation the participants would like in reality, or 'moving sculptures' which may change as the participants modify their positions. Thus, family sculpture, role play and psychodrama can overlap.

Family contracts

Every type of psychotherapy relies on implicit agreements or 'contracts'. Therapeutic rapport is the basis of all treatment, regardless of the technique used. The use of written contracts originated from behaviour therapy. Such written contracts help to define specific behaviours and focus on treatment aims. In addition to these explicit aspects, the implicit aspects of using contracts are also important, especially the implication that the therapist is dealing with responsible individuals.

In addition to being aware of the explicit and implicit aspects of contracts, the therapist should consider the dynamics of external control and self-responsibility, and balance the family's need of psychological support against the demands of therapy. Whilst contracts generally confront the patient (and/or the parents) with specific demands and a considerable amount of external control, they also aim to give the patient (and/or the parents) support and confer responsibility. A contract may address interpersonal behaviour within the family, e.g. rules for communication and interaction, etc. However, from a family dynamic perspective, the most interesting contracts are those which address individual symptoms indirectly by focusing on modification of intrafamilial relationships. Therefore, it is important to bear in mind two levels when drawing up a contract: (i) the individual level, and (ii) the covert content of the contract, which affects interpersonal relationships. For example, observational tasks may affect family interaction to a considerable degree, such as when a father who has never been concerned with 'symptom management' is given the task of recording the child's symptoms. This new role may provoke interactional difficulties between father and child, which may also result in new interaction between father and mother. Thus, family interaction may be influenced to a considerable degree, although the contract does not directly refer to interaction.

Several principles should be observed when using contracts in family therapy. Contracts should always be orientated towards success. Thus, all involved should have the capacity to fulfil the contract in order to avoid demoralization. This means that contracts should be tailored to meet the needs of each individual. As contracts are especially useful when motivation is high, they should never be pushed on a family. The content of an agreement should be developed in sessions, taking into account suggestions from all individual family members. Family contracts tend to be especially useful in cases when therapy seems to lack adequate structure and orientation and when family interaction requires more external control, e.g. in order to avoid escalation of conflicts or deterioration of symptoms. Such contracts may also be useful to encourage structure and boundaries within the family and make clear to family members the distribution of responsibility.

Symptom prescription

In contrast to techniques which are directly aimed at changing behaviours, e.g. general advice or behavioural tasks, paradoxical interventions require particular caution. This technique should be considered when direct interventions threaten to make problems worse rather than better. This may be the case when problems are maintained by the very attempts undertaken to solve them. For example, the attempt to speak fluently by an individual who stutters is likely to result in aggravation of stuttering. Direct interventions are also unlikely to be successful when family members are stuck in a paradoxical situation. Paradoxical therapeutic situations can occur, for example, when the patient thinks: 'I would like to find my way out of the difficulties on my own, but I haven't managed to do so. That is why I feel incapable of anything. But if therapy works and brings about improvement, I will have proof that I am incapable, so I won't cooperate with the therapist.' Another well-known paradox is this statement: 'I would like the therapist to remove the symptoms, but I don't want to change.'

In such situations the therapist can attempt to respond to the paradox with a 'therapeutic paradox'. For example, the therapist might emphasize the importance of keeping things as they are and avoiding any change, or he might advise the patient to keep his symptoms or even increase them. Thus the patient doesn't feel discouraged if therapy fails to bring about any improvement initially, and can continue to follow the therapist's advice and cooperate with therapy. However, when the symptoms disappear, the patient will have achieved exactly what was wanted from the start, and will seem to have overcome his problems against the therapist's explicit advice.

This mechanism is best illustrated using an example. A family came for consultation because of the long and severe quarrels between the parents and their daughter. The quarrels occurred every day, and usually resulted in secondary disagreements between the parents. Even when all family members went to great lengths to avoid one another, quarrels continued to occur at the slightest provocation. This situation had become very stressful for the entire family. The quarrels continued during family therapy sessions, and because the therapist had great difficulty interrupting sessions to prevent escalation, the continuation of family therapy was in jeopardy. In a situation such as this, symptom prescripition focusing directly on the participants' behaviour might be a useful option: 'You have just demonstrated how your quarrels begin, and I think I have some idea of what they are like. Perhaps you could continue quarrelling for a few minutes so that I can obtain a better impression. We can discuss the quarrel later.' Thus, the family is asked to consciously do something, which usually 'happens' of its own accord. If the family continues to argue, this can be considered cooperation with the therapist as they are following instructions. However, if the argument abates, more productive discussion is possible. In the past, symptom prescription and redefiniton have been used in ways suggesting that therapists generally use therapeutic 'tricks' in order to manipulate families behind their backs. It should be emphasized, however, that clandestine interventions are inappropriate and unlikely to contribute to improvement. Although psychotherapeutic communication often includes unavoidable paradoxical aspects, paradoxical techniques are justified only as part of a serious attempt to help the family. Any deceit in dealing with patients and their families is clearly unethical.

Case reports

The following two examples intend to give an impression of the range of cases encountered in family therapy. The reports are anecdotal and should not be considered to be complete case studies.

Family therapy in a case of separation anxiety (18 sessions)

A 12-year-old boy, George, presented for assessment because of school refusal. George tended to worry about his achievement at school, which he considered poor. He was very concerned about a recent bad result and had considered suicide. George's anxieties were frequently associated with stomach aches and palpitations. Over the 2 weeks prior to consultation, his symptoms had become worse, and he had been unable to remain at home alone because of anxiety. A diagnosis of separation anxiety disorder was considered, and inpatient treatment recommended. As the parents refused hospitalization, the therapist agreed to attempt outpatient treatment. As this treatment resulted in improvement, subsequent admission for inpatient treatment was considered unnecessary.

Therapy lasted 18 sessions, which were undertaken once a week initially with greater intervals as treatment progressed. Both George and his mother attended all sessions, whilst the father was only able to participate in five sessions as a result of work commitments. Initially, therapy focused on the boy's symptoms. When the conversation shifted away from the symptoms, the parents appeared insecure and defensive. Interpersonal relationships within the family were addressed in a later phase of treatment after the resolution of symptoms.

Therapy contract

We agree to keep the following rules:

1. George's parents have the task of discussing this contract with his teachers in order to make sure that no difficulties arise with the school.

2. George has the task of attending school for at least two lessons every day (specifically the first two lessons). Next week he has the task of gradually increasing school attendance to about four lessons per day.

3. George has the task of recording school attendance (duration), anxiety (evening, morning, noon) and any physical symptoms in the prepared record sheet.

4. As long as George fulfils the task of school attendance for two lessons every day, treatment will continue on an outpatient basis. If George fails to achieve this goal, treatment will continue on an inpatient basis after admission on *[date]*.

Signatures:

[mother] *[father]* *George*

[therapist] *[co-therapist]*

Fig. 12.7. Example for a contract used in family therapy.

During the initial $5\frac{1}{2}$ months, treatment was based on a therapeutic contract. During essions, the contract, George's psychological state and the general family situation were discussed. The final $2\frac{1}{2}$ months of therapy were undertaken as family therapy without any formal contract.

It was clear from the start that outpatient treatment would be successful only if George could be persuaded to resume school. The therapist was able to rely on a suggestion the patient himself had previously made: George felt sure that he could attend school for two lessons a day because he attributed the anxiety to longer school attendance. The first contract is shown in Fig. 12.7. Both the patient and his parents considered the contract a great help because it defined a specific goal and opened up new perspectives, although the contract also exerted considerable psychological pressure because it included the option of hospital admission. The contract was modified over the course of therapy (almost every session). The following modifications were made.

(i) Initially, the option of admission was intended as a consequence in case George was unable to fulfil the contract. Later, this option was replaced by the requirement to call the therapist immediately if he was unable to fulfil the agreement.

(ii) The duration of required school attendance was increased only when George was able to fulfil all 'compulsory' requirements and he was close to fulfilling the new 'additional' requirement. All further steps were undertaken only with George's consent.

(iii) After having emphasized the issue of school attendance at the onset of therapy, later other aspects of therapy were emphasized. Over the course of treatment it became clear that George exerted considerable pressure on his mother to let him stay at home by pleading, crying and complaining. This behaviour was later also integrated in the contract. Eventually other issues were also included, e.g. visiting friends.

(iv) Prior to the inclusion of any new issue, e.g. the issue of pressuring his mother, George was given the task of observing and recording his own behaviour.

(v) The contract also defined the degree to which the parents should assist George. They were expected to stop accompanying him to school. This issue and others, e.g. the parents' assertiveness, and boundaries between George and his parents were addressed in a second contract with the parents. The father was expected to take on tasks which had previously been undertaken by the mother.

Family therapy in a case of acute adolescent conflict (three sessions)

The mother of the 17-year-old boy Marcus requested an appointment for her son in the outpatient clinic, adding that whilst her husband was willing to come for consultation, Marcus was very reluctant. The reason for consultation was that Marcus had started stealing money from his parents, and the problem had become increasingly serious in the course of the past few months. The parents were concerned about Marcus becoming criminal.

All three presented for consultation. The father was a white-collar employee, the mother working part-time as a secretary. Marcus had a 12-year-old sister whom the parents had not brought with them in order to 'keep her out of the whole thing'. Later on, the mother admitted that she did not want anyone to 'mess about psychologically' with the girl.

Marcus was attending secondary school and achievement was considerably high. He was especially good at sports. The reason for consultation was that Marcus had stolen money from his parents and secretly consumed food intended for the whole family, e.g. beverages, rolls, tinned food. The parents only realized that Marcus had consumed the food when they found food remains and empty wrappings under his bed or in his cupboard.

Both parents emphasized that Marcus is allowed to eat as much as he likes, and wondered why he should eat in secret. They felt Marcus should ask first, but that was precisely what he refused to do. Whilst the parents were concerned but not alarmed about the issue of food, they were more worried about the stealing. Marcus has stolen about £300 from his parents in the past month. The parents were concerned for two main reasons: first, the quality of family life was seriously vitiated by the stealing because the parents constantly had to watch out for their money, and secondly, they were anxious about Marcus stealing outside the family setting and beginnig a criminal career. Finally, the parents were concerned that Marcus might be psychiatrically ill, because they could not explain his behaviour.

When asked why he behaved in this way, Marcus either refused to answer or gave terse answers such as: 'Because I need money' or 'Because I felt hungry' when food was the issue. When asked why he did not ask for the money or food ('You can't just take things without asking') he would give replies such as: 'I didn't feel like it', and when asked 'Why do you let us find you out?', he would answer: 'I haven't thought about it'.

Marcus was a tall and athletic boy who looked more like 20 years of age. As his parents explained the situation, he looked rather shamefaced and appeared to be thoroughly embarrassed by the revelation of his misbehaviour. At the same time he made an uncomfortable and obstinate impression, and seemed to feel threatened. He had obviously required a considerable amount of persuasion to come for consultation.

During the session his mother spoke mostly with the therapist, but frequently addressed Marcus. She gave the impression of being an extremely concerned and insecure person, saddened by the current difficulties. She wanted the therapist to 'find out the reason' for Marcus' behaviour, and expressed great concern that she and her husband may have made mistakes in dealing with the boy (without being specific), and that something might be wrong with the family. She proceeded to wonder what she could do to make up for the mistakes she was convinced she had made. In contrast, her husband was sullen and withdrawn and appeared uncomfortable. When his wife expressed concern, he appeared angry. He considered his son's behaviour inappropriate, and wondered whether the problems was related to upbringing or constituted a psychiatric disorder. If the former, he felt he should react with disciplinary steps, e.g. stop pocket money, house arrest, etc., if the latter, he accepted that professional help would be required. Thus, he was more or less asking the therapist to make a decision as to whether Marcus was 'bad' or 'mad'.

The conversation improved as other problems and conflicts were discussed. When asked what changes Marcus would like to see at home, he replied that did not want his mother to listen in on his telephone conversations. His mother was dumbfounded when she heard this, whilst his father appeared irritated. He considered Marcus' complaint an inappropriate distraction, and demanded that Marcus answer the therapist's questions properly. However, the therapist continued with this topic, and the family eventually explained that they had two telephones in the house and Marcus' mother had indeed overheard telephone conversations in the past (whether intentionally or not remained unclear). Markus explained that he felt observed and patronized by his parents. Whilst saying this, he seemed on the verge of bursting into tears and appeared much younger. In the following discussion, Marcus managed to give further examples, e.g. that his mother would tidy up his room without asking, and that he was not allowed to visit discos. Again, his parents were stunned and maintained that Marcus had never raised these issues. Subsequently Marcus remembered an occurrence several years ago, when he had wanted to accompany friends of the family, but his parents had been reluctant to let him go, and asked him to stay at home. Marcus tended to give up quickly if he saw no chance of succeeding against his parents, whatever the reason might be.

In the therapist's opinion the main issue was one of appropriate distance and individual boundaries in the family. Whilst Marcus' parents complained that their son was infringing on their private life by stealing money, Marcus complained that his parents would not let him live his own life. Thus, the most important family issues seemed to be 'personal property' and 'personal territory'. The parents' reactions to this interpretation of the therapist were interesting. The mother immediately took on board her son's criticism and thought about ways to modify her behaviour in future. She said she would never listen to telephone conversations again and still seemed shocked by her son's complaint. She also considered the issue of tidying Marcus' room, and asked the therapist for advice. In contrast, the father said that the family had not sought consultation to discuss the issue of tidying up, but to address more serious matters. He thought the session was not getting anywhere, and again raised the issue of whether his son simply required stricter management or did in fact need psychotherapy.

The therapist told Marcus and his mother: 'It is a good thing to be self-critical, but I don't think you [the mother] should modify your behaviour. Perhaps Marcus should try to change his behaviour. After all, he is old enough to express his views to his parents, don't you think so?.' And he addressed the father, saying something like this: 'At the moment I can only give you my personal opinion. I don't think issues of upbringing are the problem here, and you are unlikely to get anywhere being stricter with Marcus – that is what you have tried in the past. At the moment I don't know whether psychotherapy is appropriate.' The way the session ended is not surprising. Marcus was almost cheerful and said he would like to return for another session. Whilst his mother was satisfied with the result of the session, his father seemed irritated and frustrated, because he had not received 'proper' answers to his questions. The family agreed to return for a second session 2 weeks later, but because symptoms had disappeared immediately after the first session, an additional session was deemed unnecessary at this point.

Obviously, the course of family therapy and the effect is difficult to predict. Marcus suffered a brief relapse about 3 months later, and two additional family sessions were undertaken. However, they focused on issues such as sibling rivalry, quarrels over going out in the evening, helping at home, and the fact that Marcus had started smoking. This particularly exasperated his parents, because Marcus was so keen on sport. Disagreements also ensued when Marcus acquired a girlfriend. Thus, the sessions addressed the usual problems that arise between adolescents and their parents. The results of family diagnostic appraisal were confirmed in the course of the two additional sessions: The mother tended towards depression and had difficulties detatching from her own parents, resulting in marital discord. However, this issue was not discussed in detail because the couple did not feel that they wanted professional help.

These two cases were chosen because they are typical for outpatient child and adolescent family therapy settings. The first example is a case of long-term family therapy (with gradual modifications). The emphasis of therapy was to support and structure the family using therapeutic contracts. One aim was to bring symptoms under control (preventing escalation), and an additional aim was to encourage the parents' competence in dealing with their son. The second example summarizes a very brief family therapy of only three sessions. The most important changes were probably actuated by the first session. The approach was largely interpretational, and no direct suggestions regarding behaviour modification were given. The aim of therapy was to question rigid patterns of family interaction and unflexible attitudes in order to open up developmental options, lift excessive parental control, and strenghten the adolescent's sense of responsibility. Although the treatments differ considerably, there are several similarities. Both were outpatient family therapies focusing on the issue of cohesion, and in both cases the index patient would be considered 'neurotic' in traditional terminology. In contrast to these two examples, family therapy with severely disturbed antisocial or psychotic patients may be more difficult. Furthermore, treatment is not always as successful as in these two examples. In practice, therapy does not always follow the ideal course and the examples found in psychotherapy textbooks.

Effectiveness

The effectiveness of interventions based on family therapy techniques is empirically well established and documented in the literature. Table 12.1 shows the most important meta-analyses on family therapy (see also Shadish et al., 1993, 1997b). The average effect size of family therapy is between 0.36 and 0.70, somewhat less impressive than that for interventions in child and adolescent

Table 12.1. Important meta-analysis on family therapy techniques

	Number of studies	Median effect size
General family therapy (Hazelrigg et al., 1987)	20	0.36
Family therapy (conjoint) (Marcus et al., 1990)	19	0.57
Family therapy with problem children (Montgomery, 1991)	43	0.61
Behavioural family and couple therapy (Shadish et al., 1997a)	58	0.70
Couple and family therapy compared with untreated control groups (Shadish et al., 1997a)	71	0.51
General parent training (Cedar and Levant, 1990)	26	0.33

psychotherapy in general. Although these values appear to reflect well on the value of family therapeutic interventions, they need to be interpreted with caution because there are a number of methodological problems to take into consideration when evaluating family therapy.

The effectiveness of behavioural systemic techniques has been particularly well established (Henggeler et al., 1998), as has that of behaviourally orientated family therapy (see Heekerens, 1993) and psycho-educative techniques (see Buchkremer and Rath, 1989). The studies mentioned above also testify to the effectiveness of other family therapy techniques. Grawe et al. (1994) make the point, however, that there is still a significant discrepancy between the claimed or assumed value of family therapy and its empirically proven benefit. Therefore, it is important to undertake further research in this area in order to arrive at a more scientifically based assessment of the value of the different techniques used in family therapy, e.g. systemic, psychodynamic, humanistic (Grawe, 1997).

For practical purposes, those studies derived from clinical therapeutic work and assessments about the indications for family therapy are particularly useful (see Roth et al., 1996). For example, Russel et al. (1987) have demonstrated that in young anorexic patients at a relatively acute stage of their illness, family therapy is more effective than individual therapy, whereas older patients with a more chronic illness pattern are more likely to benefit from individual therapy. Our group has also undertaken research to look at which familial characteristics are of prognostic value and should be considered of particular importance in family therapy (Mattejat and Remschmidt, 1997).

Quality assurance

Quality assurance in family therapy shares many of the features that are generally appropriate in child and adolescent psychotherapy (see Mattejat, 1997b; Schmeck and Poustka, 1998). The following aspects of quality assurance are of particular importance in the field of family therapy.

Transparent cooperation

The most important and basic aspect of quality assurance involves the provision of comprehensive information about the nature of therapy to all family members and their inclusion in the therapy planning, implementation and assessment processes. Of particular importance is the setting of therapeutic goals, continual assessment of the way in which different family members are experiencing the therapeutic process, and their general satisfaction with, therapy. It can, for example, be helpful to state at the onset of therapy how long or how often a particular issue will be covered and also when an assessment will be made as to how helpful this has been. If, for example, it has been agreed that a series of family sessions will be held, it is usually sensible to specify that, after a certain number of sessions, the situation will be assessed and the desirability of further sessions reviewed.

Professional qualifications

A second, but equally important basic aspect of quality assurance concerns professional qualification and supervision. The therapist should have acquired appropriate qualifications and be a member of a professional body. He can also be expected to participate in ongoing professional education looking at the quality of his work and to undergo regular supervision by a qualified professional, either individually or as part of a supervision group.

Standardized documentation

A further important aspect of quality assurance is the keeping of clinical records. These should record important personal details, the results of any relevant tests and brief details about the sessions held. These details should be documented in a standardized form such that they would be meaningful to other professionals should the need arise.

Systematic evaluation

Finally, diagnostic and therapeutic activities should be evaluated in a systematic and standardized manner. The actual way in which this is undertaken may be more or less detailed. One possibility is to utilize a standardized instrument such as the Goal Attainment Scale (GAS), first proposed by Kiresuk and Sherman (Kiresuk et al., 1994). This allows an accurate assessment of the degree to which goals set at the onset of therapy have been achieved. It is not particularly time-consuming and can be used at the end of therapy to act as a marker of therapeutic success. Another well-established instrument, which can be used in this setting, is the Child Behaviour Check List (Achenbach and Edelbrock, 1983; Remschmidt and Walter, 1990). In recent years, a number of new instruments have been developed, which look not only at symptomatology or psychopathology, but attempt to make an assessment of the whole therapeutic process and therapeutic satisfaction (see Mattejat and Remschmidt, 1998). Although this type of therapeutic evaluation is still perceived with scepticism and concern by some therapists, there is now a general movement towards transparency, which means that professionals must be prepared to accept external evaluation and constructive criticism.

REFERENCES

Achenbach, T. M. and Edelbrock, C. S. (1983). *Manual for the child behavior checklist and revised child behavior profile*. Burlington, VT: University of Vermont.

Ackerman, N. W. (1971). The growing edge of family therapy. *Process*, **10**, 143–56.

Ackerman, N. W. (1958). *The psychodynamics of family life*. New York: Basic Books.

Aponte, H. J. and Vandeusen, J. M. (1981). Structural family therapy. In *Handbook of family therapy*, ed. A. S. Gurman and D. P. Kniskern, pp. 310–60. New York: Brunner/Mazel.

Bateson, G. (1972). *Steps to an ecology of the mind*. New York: Ballantine.

Bateson, G., Haley, J. and Weakland, J. (1956). Toward a theory of schizophrenia. *Behavioral Science*, **1**, 251–64.

Bowen, M. (1960). A family concept of schizophrenia. In *The etiology of schizophrenia*, ed. D. D. Jackson. New York: Basic Books.

Buchkremer, G. and Rath, N. (ed.) (1989). *Therapeutische Arbeit mit Angehörigen schizophrener Patienten*. Bern: Huber.

Cedar, B. and Levant, R.F. (1990). A meta-analysis of the effects of parent effectiveness training. *The American Journal of Family Therapy*, **18**, 373–84.

Gorell-Barnes, G. (1994). Family therapy. In *Child and adolescent psychiatry. Modern approaches*, ed. M. Rutter, E. Taylor and L. Hersov. Oxford: Blackwell Science.

Grawe, K. (1997). Research-informed psychotherapy. *Psychotherapy Research*, **7**, 1–19.

Grawe, K., Donati, R. and Bernauer, F. (1994). *Psychotherapie im Wandel. Von der Konfession zur Profession*, 3rd edn. Göttingen: Hogrefe.

Gurman, A. S. and Kniskern, D. P. (eds.) (1981a). *Handbook of family therapy*. New York: Brunner/Mazel.

Gurman, A. S. and Kniskern, D. P. (1981*b*). Family therapy outcome research. Knowns and unknowns. In *Handbook of family therapy*, ed. A. S. Gurman and D. P. Kniskern, pp. 742–76. New York: Brunner/Mazel.

Haley, J. (1963). *Strategies in psychotherapy*. New York: Grune & Stratton.

Hazelrigg, M. D., Cooper, H. M. and Borduin, C. M. (1987). Evaluating the effectiveness of family therapies. An integrative review and analysis. *Psychological Bulletin*, **101**, 428–42.

Heekerens, H-P. (1989). *Familientherapie und Erziehungsberatung*. Heidelberg: Asanger.

Heekerens, H-P. (1993). Verhaltensorientierte Familientherapie. In *Handbuch Verhaltenstherapie und Verhaltensmedizin bei Kindern und Jugendlichen*, ed. Steinhausen, H-C. and M. v. Aster, pp. 601–25. Weinheim: Belz/Psychologie Verlags Union.

Henggeler, S. W., Schoenwald, S. K., Borduin, C. M., Rowland, M. D. and Cunningham, P. B. (1998). *Multisystemic treatment of antisocial behavior in children and adolescents*. New York, London: Guilford Press.

Kaslow, F. W. (ed.) (1996). *Handbook of relational diagnosis and dysfunctional family patterns*. New York: Wiley.

Kiresuk, T. J., Smith, A. and Cardillo, J. E. (eds.) (1994). *Goal attainment scaling: applications, theory, and measurement*. Hillsdale: Lawrence Erlbaum Associates.

L'Abate, L. (ed.) (1994). *Handbook of developmental family psychology and psychopathology*. New York: Wiley.

Lidz, T. (1958). Schizophrenia and the family. *Psychiatry*, **21**, 21–7.

Madanes, C. and Haley, J. (1977). Dimensions of family therapy. *Journal of Nervous and Mental Disease*, **165**, 88.

Marcus, E., Lange, A. and Pettigrew, T. F. (1990). Effectiveness of family therapy. A meta analysis. *Journal of Family Therapy*, **12**, 205–21.

Martin, P. A. (1981). No treatment as the treatment of choice. In *Questions and answers in the practice of family therapy*, ed. A. S. Gurman and D. P. Kniskern, pp. 67–9. New York: Brunner/Mazel.

Mattejat, F. (1985a). *Familie und psychische Störungen*. Stuttgart: Enke.

Mattejat, F. (1997b). Qualitätssicherung. In *Psychotherapie im Kindes- und Jugendalter*, ed. H. Remschmidt, pp. 69–77. Stuttgart, New York: Thieme.

Mattejat, F. and Remschmidt, H. (1997). Die Bedeutung der Familienbeziehungen für die Bewältigung von psychischen Störungen – Ergebnisse aus empirischen Untersuchungen zur Therapieprognose bei psychisch gestörten Kindern und Jugendlichen. *Praxis der Kinderpsychologie und Kinderpsychiatrie*, **46**, 371–92.

Mattejat, F. and Remschmidt, H. (1998). *Fragebogen zur Beurteilung der Behandlung (FBB)*. Göttingen: Hogrefe.

Minuchin, S. (1974). *Families and family therapy*. London: Tavistock.

Minuchin, S. and Fishman, H. C. (1981). *Family therapy techniques*. Cambridge, MA: Harvard

University Press.

Montgomery, L. M. (1991). *The effects of family therapy for treatment of child identified problems. A meta-analysis* (Doctoral Dissertation, Memphis State University 1990). *Dissertation Abstracts International*, **51**, 6115B.

Olbrich, E. (1984). Jugendalter. Zeit der Krise oder der produktiven Anpassung? In *Probleme des Jugendalters. Neuere Sichtweisen*, ed. E. Olbrich and E. Todt, pp. 1–48. Berlin: Springer.

Olbrich, E. (1985). Konstruktive Auseinandersetzung im Jugendalter. Entwicklung, Förderung und Verhaltenseffekte. In *Lebensbewältigung im Jugendalter*, ed. R. Oerter, pp. 7–29. Weinheim: VCH Verlagsgesellschaft.

Olson, D. H., Portner, J. and Lavee, Y. (1985). *FACES III – family adaptability and cohesion evaluation scales*. St. Paul: University of Minnesota.

Remschmidt, H. and Walter, R. (1990). *Psychische Auffälligkeiten bei Schulkindern. Mit deutschen Normen für die Child Behavior Checklist*. Göttingen: Hogrefe.

Roth, A., Fonagy, P., Parry, G., Target, M. and Woods, R. (1996). *What works for whom? A critical review of psychotherapy research*. New York: Guilford.

Russel, G. F. M., Szmukler, G. I., Dare, C. and Eisler, I. (1987). An evaluation of family therapy in anorexia nervosa and bulimia nervosa. *Archives of General Psychiatry*, **44**, 1047–56.

Satir, V. (1964). *Conjoint family therapy. A guide to theory and technique*. Palo Alto: Science and Behavior Books.

Schmeck, K. and Poustka, F. (ed.) (1998). *Qualitätssicherung und Lebensqualität in der Kinder- und Jugendpsychiatrie*. Wien, New York: Springer.

Selvini-Palazzoli, M., Boscolo, L., Cecchin, G. and Prata, G. (1978). *Paradox and counterparadox*. New York: Aronson.

Shadish, W. R., Matt, G. E., Navarro, A. M. et al. (1997a). Evidence that therapy works in clinically representative conditions. *Journal of Consulting and Clinical Psychology*, **65**, 355–65.

Shadish, W. R., Montgomery, L. M., Wilson, P., Wilson, M. R., Bright, I. and Okwumabua, T. (1993). Effect of family and marital psychotherapies: a meta-analysis. *Journal of Consulting and Clinical Psychology*, **61**, 992–1002.

Shadish, W. R., Ragsdale, K., Glaser, R. R. and Montgomery, L. M. (1997b). Effektivität und Effizienz von Paar- und Familientherapie. Eine metaanalytische Perspektive. *Familiendynamik*, **22**, 5–33.

Skynner, A. C. R. (1976). *One flesh, separate persons: principles of family and marital psychotherapy*. London: Constable.

Strunk, P. (1987). Möglichkeiten und Grenzen der Familientherapie bei psychiatrischen Störungen im Kindes- und Jugendalter. *Zeitschrift für Kinder- und Jugendpsychiatrie*, **15**, 245–56.

Textor, M. R. (1985). *Integrative Familientherapie*. Berlin: Springer.

Watzlawick, P., Weakland, J. H. and Fisch, R. (1974). *Change. Principles of problem formation and problem resolution*. New York: Norton.

Wynne, L. C. and Singer, M. (1963). Thought disorder and family relations of schizophrenics. I: Research strategy. *Archives of General Psychiatry*, **9**, 191–8.

13 Parent training

Andreas Warnke

Parent training is a specific and systematic approach to cooperating with parents. Cooperation with parents is an essential part of treatment in child and adolescent psychiatry and should not be neglected (Briesmeister and Schaefer, 1998).

Parent training requires a positive therapeutic attitude. It has been shown that psychotherapy is most effective when the family's psychosocial situation is promising and the family is willing to support treatment (Mattejat and Remschmidt, 1991).

A normal family is a protective factor for a child's psychological development. This beneficial effect can be used to support therapy. However, parents also bear the responsibility of directing treatment when problems arise. As long as the child lives in a family, the family will influence the child's development to a greater extent than any other care-givers or educators. Parents are an integral part of a child's environment, and changes in parental behaviour have a significant influence on the way the child experiences his environment.

Parents who are concerned about abnormal behaviour in their child will usually seek professional help. Simultaneously, parents will be grateful if their competence as parents is acknowledged by professionals. As professionals, we usually rely on parents' competence in child raising and request their cooperation when we undertake psychotherapy. Studies looking at parent training have shown that many parents are able to acquire some psychotherapeutic techniques and use them effectively to support their child's development (Innerhofer, 1977; Warnke and Innerhofer, 1978; Briesmeister and Schaefer, 1998).

The interaction between the therapist and parents should be considerate, tolerant, empathic, supportive and without reproach. The family's need for help may be understood as an opportunity to give up outdated and superfluous values and attitudes in order to improve outlook on life, develop new interests, aims, skills and options. Ideally, the attitude towards parents should be that of empathic understanding, unconditional positive regard, and genuinness as suggested by Rogers (1951). More specifically, a helpful attitude towards parents will include the following points (Dührssen, 1988): an interest in the family's capacity to cope; diagnostic appraisal of the family system; help and emotional support for the patient's parents. The therapist should avoid blaming the family, should not identify with the child and take up a stance against the family, and should also attempt to appreciate the parents' standards or goals.

Cooperation with parents is an essential and integral part of both psychotherapy and medical treatment of children and adolescents, and such cooperation should not primarily focus on educating parents or excluding them if they fail to bring up their child appropriately. It should rather be seen as an opportunity to improve the emotional relationship between the patient and his parents and incorporate the family's educational competency and other family resources in order to complement other treatments. The family's own self-help competency should be included in treatment planning from the start. The form and content of cooperation with parents needs to be adapted to suit the family's resources in terms of available time, personnel, competency, needs, values, and treatment goals. Adaptation does not imply 'fraternization' between therapists and non-professionals, but suggests a linkage of family resources with professional expertise ('linking competencies'). Parents should also be given sufficient time to discuss their own personal issues. They will expect to receive information and assistance for the future ('parent orientated cooperation'). Cooperation with parents aims to improve the family's cohesion and should encourage the seeking of external sources of help such as self-help groups and parents' associations. Parent training is a form of parental cooperation in which parents are encouraged actively to participate in the psychotherapy of their child, thus taking an active positive role for the benefit of their child (Warnke, 1999).

The term 'parent training'

The term parent training may be considered synonymous with co-therapy by parents and professional advice to parents. The idea of parent training is based on ideas from behavioural therapy (Briesmeister and Schaefer, 1998). Over the course of time, ideas from communication theory, theory of action, client-centered psychotherapy and family therapy have been incorporated into the concept (Innerhofer, 1977; Innerhofer and Warnke, 1989; Warnke, 1993). Parent training has been evaluated (Graziano and Diament, 1992).

Parent training is an indirect psychotherapeutic approach. Interventions are based on cooperation with parents and do not necessarily require the patient's presence.

Parent training was initially introduced to enable parents to participate in specific treatment programmes, much like teaching parents to undertake physical therapy in a child suffering from cerebral palsy.

Today, parent training programmes have a much wider scope. Cooperation with parents aims to modify value systems, ability to experience emotions, competency to act, and capacity to utilize coping mechanisms. Psychotherapeutic goals such as supporting the child's development and improving psychological symptoms are addressed via improving parent's child-raising skills, facilitating interaction between parents and the child, reducing parents' emotional stress, and helping them to develop coping strategies.

The approach is based on an assumption that most parents are competent in child rearing, exercise influence over their child's social experiences, react to changing developmental stages and determine external living conditions, e.g. the home environment and the child's daily schedule. The approach does not go as far as to attribute 'psychotherapeutic skills' to parents; however, it is based on the assumption that the entire family may make a significant contribution towards establishing such conditions in the patient's normal environment which support psychotherapy and improve its effectiveness. Parents are included in treatment as 'advisors' and 'assistants', depending on their individual resources. The therapist's role is one of 'trainer', who encourages parents to make use of their own competencies.

Thus, mutual support is an important issue in parent training. Parents should learn how to:

- observe interaction in order to perceive issues relevant for problem-solving;
- interpret interrelations, i.e. explain, understand and assess;
- understand problems, identify values and aims, modify the child's environment and their child-raising practice, so that the child's and the family's further development is optimized.

Approaches to parent training

Three different concepts or approaches to parent training may be distinguished.

Symptom-orientated training programmes

This approach educates parents about specific behavioural disorders or deficits in children and adolescents. Direct interactional training is used to instruct parents how to use behavioural therapy techniques (Schmitz, 1976; Kane et al.,

1974). For example, parents of a mentally handicapped child would be instructed to help the child put on a coat in such a way that the child can eventually put on the coat without help (Kane and Kane, 1976).

Instruction in psychological theories

Training programmes in which various styles of upbringing are discussed in the light of psychological theories, e.g. principles of behavioural therapy (Perrez et al., 1974), or communication theory may be helpful. In this approach, the family's own specific problem is not addressed. The parents will have to decide for themselves which conclusions to draw and how to apply their knowledge to solve current problems.

Training in problem-solving strategies

This approach gives parents the opportunity to develop psychotherapeutically helpful problem-solving strategies. Training goals are not abstract, but defined by actual problems suggested by parents, e.g. how to deal with a daughter suffering from anorexia nervosa (Innerhofer, 1977; Warnke, 1988). This approach, like the first, is symptom orientated, and, like the second, guided by theoretical considerations, rather than by any single therapeutic or educational approach. Most importantly, the resulting problem-solving strategy is appropriate for the given problem, the family's situation and its coping capacity.

General characteristics of parent training

The basic issues of problem-solving training

Task-orientated treatment goals

Therapy is defined by a specific educational task, e.g. getting a patient with hyperkinetic syndrome to go to bed, psychiatric symptom, e.g. bed-wetting or conflict, e.g. an argument between siblings. Parents use role play to demonstrate the issue with which they need help.

Conflict-orientated approach

The problem which is addressed in parent training sessions needs to reflect an important conflict or a specific symptom. How to deal with a hyperactive child taken out to a restaurant for lunch can be addressed neither by showing a film on conditioning techniques with rats nor discussing interactional difficulties in early childhood. The problem is much better addressed by demonstrating a visit to a restaurant using role play.

Motivational teaching
Cooperation with parents should enable and encourage parents to actively participate in treating their child.

Resource-orientated learning
Sessions should emphasize personal strengths and resources that parents can mobilize rather than their deficits.

Situation-appropriate learning
The situational resources which are available to parents need to be incorporated in treatment, e.g. parental availability, environmental conditions, etc.

Augmenting the repertoire of appraisal and action
Alternative ways of appraising situations and acting upon them need to be developed and tried out. New ways of explanatory models are less important, as these do not necessarily translate into different behaviour.

Generalization
The focus of the training session should enable parents to develop a coping strategy which will be likely to generalize to other situations.

Effective learning
Parent training aims to achieve improvement in an effective way, which also makes the lightest possible demands on the family in terms of time and personnel.

Assessment
The outcome of therapy, i.e. problem-solving ability needs to be fully assessed. Behavioural observation schedules can be helpful in this, and follow-up treatment may help to stabilize and generalize improvements.

Interactional analysis as a diagnostic principle

Interactional analysis is the most important diagnostic technique in parent training (Innerhofer, 1974, 1980). This technique identifies the functional connections of interaction between parents and children, thus making possible an appraisal of child raising practice. Interactional analysis is undertaken following a standard child and adolescent psychiatric assessment including history, physical examination, neurological assessment, a psychiatric interview and standardized psychological tests. The ultimate aim of parent training is to modify the interaction between parents and children.

Parent training as 'educational space'

Parent training may be regarded as a systematic technique for helping parents to understand how coping strategies develop. They are taught to perceive situational interactions, develop their capacity for self-help in difficult situations, seek solutions to problems and attempt to bring these about. Parents are also given the opportunity to practise solutions which they find helpful. The therapist's task is to facilitate a setting in which parents can learn to perceive and modify their behaviour. The therapist needs to organize appropriate facilities, teaching aids, and technological aids, e.g. a video system, and use his experience to go through a range of training exercises. Parents are expected to develop the ability to appraise, experience and interact in an appropriate way, thus supporting therapy. The following techniques are often used in parent training.

Educational aids and self-help manuals

These can help parents to address co-existent emotional difficulties as well as educating them about specific therapeutic techniques. A number of manuals have been developed for this purpose (Boggs, 1981; McMahon and Forehand, 1980; Bernal and North, 1978; Clarke-Stewart, 1978; Glasgow and Rosen, 1978).

Systematic behavioural observation

This technique usually forms part of diagnostic appraisal, but may in itself have the effect of modifying attitudes and behaviour. The technique is used to assess treatment progress, by keeping a daily behavioural diary, e.g. to record the nights during which a child with enuresis did not wet his bed. Fig. 13.1 shows a 'sleep diary' which can be used to treat children with sleep problems (Douglas, 1989).

Training exercises and feedback techniques

This approach encourages parents to practise specific techniques using role play, either with or without their children. Modelling techniques may also be used. Using this approach, the therapist might demonstrate to parents how to teach a mentally retarded child, how to put on a shirt without help (Kane and Kane, 1976). When parents begin to undertake such training programmes with their children, the therapist switches to supervising the parents. This may be undertaken either directly, i.e. with the therapist's participation and direct

Sleep behaviour	Mon	Tue	Wed	Thu	Fri	Sat	Sun
Waking up time							
Length and duration of sleep during the day							
Going to bed time							
Going to sleep time							
Length of wakefulness in the evening and educational measures							
Length of wakefulness at night and educational measures							

Fig. 13.1. 'Sleep diary' for children with sleep problems.

support, or indirectly, i.e. by means of video observation and instruction by an ear microphone (so called 'bug in the ear technique'). Video recordings can also be used retrospectively to analyse interactions at a later stage and review progress.

Modelling is a relatively straightforward technique, which is usually not difficult to undertake in straightforward situations, e.g. demonstrating how to use a night alarm to treat a child with enuresis. However, modelling is unsuitable in more complicated psychotherapeutic interventions. Demonstrating 'ideal' child-raising is likely to make parents feel insecure, particularly as children will inevitably behave differently towards their parents than towards the therapist. In these circumstances, role play, video feed-back and group sessions are likely to be more helpful.

Video recording

In this technique the therapist has the opportunity of observing and analysing situational conflicts systematically. Parents can observe their problem-solving behaviour much like 'television spectators' and analyse the flow of their interactions in a more objective manner. They can focus on those sequences which show particular difficulties and analyse these in detail. Perceptions and interpretations are then discussed with one another and the therapist. This transparent way of working enables parents to assess the therapist's work constantly, and he will be encouraged to be careful and realistic in his interpretations. Working with video recordings usually helps the therapist to focus on actual problems and discuss difficulties in family interaction in everyday words, thus avoiding problems in communication with the family (Innerhofer, 1977; Innerhofer and Warnke, 1989).

Parent groups

Such groups help parents to share their experience with fellow sufferers and may relieve them of their difficulties to some degree. Parent groups may also help cooperation with individual therapists. However, successful cooperation usually requires leadership by someone with experience in group dynamics (Innerhofer, 1977). Discussions, 'brain-storming' sessions and games may be undertaken, and the outcomes may subsequently be incorporated into role play and behaviour modification exercises.

The 'Munich parent training programme'

The 'Munich parent training programme', initially developed by Innerhofer (1977), has been used successfully to supplement the treatment of children and adolescents with psychiatric symptoms. It is also an integral part of work with parents in child guidance centres, residential homes and other child care facilities. It is a standardized approach, which has been evaluated, and has become an integral part of psychotherapy training programmes as well as social science and clinical psychology courses at university.

Consultation and diagnostic appraisal

Parents are invited to attend an introductory session 3–4 weeks before training sessions commence. They are informed about treatment planning, the approach to treatment (including role play and video sessions together with other parents), and the aims of the parent training course. It is important to address difficulties which might put treatment at risk, such as unreliable attendance because of work or home committments. These can be overcome by providing child-minding services during sessions or undertaking training sessions out of working hours (Innerhofer and Warnke, 1978).

It is important to find a way of describing the child's behavioural abnormality or symptom in such a way that it can be addressed by parent training. The issue for a particular child, e.g. quarrel about homework with a hyperkinetic child needs to be discussed in great detail and relevant situational factors must be determined, e.g. specific situations, individuals involved, the time of day, situational demands. Visit to places where symptoms occur or become severe, e.g. kindergarten, school, home may be useful. All individuals who usually deal with the child, e.g. kindergarten personnel or school teachers should be included in the work with parents if possible. Video recordings of conflicts may provide important additional information and are usually very helpful when undertaking parent training (Innerhofer and Warnke, 1989).

Preparing and organizing parent training

Full preparation of parent training sessions requires the development of working hypotheses, which determine the specific content and aims of training sessions. The following aims and contents of parent training need to be clarified:

- the presenting problem, for which a solution is being sought;
- preliminary suggestions on how to modify situations;
- preliminary suggestions on how the individuals involved in a conflict can modify their behaviour;
- the order in which modifications would be best undertaken;
- the method by which modifications can be brought about.

A parent training group usually includes the parents of three to four families. Obviously, all parents involved in parent training are confronted with similar problems and therefore have much in common. However, initially it may be helpful to invite only one parent per child rather than couples, in order to prevent family conflicts from disrupting the group setting. As treatment proceeds, spouses may be included and couples invited together, allowing the therapist to address particular family conflicts.

Training sessions are usually led by two therapists, who will divide the different tasks of therapy between them, e.g. explain the hypothesis behind parent training, inform them about the use of video recordings, operate the equipment, give instructions, direct role-play and analyse participant behaviour (Innerhofer, 1977).

Introducing the general rules and role play

The room in which sessions are to be undertaken should be pleasant and relaxing to put participants at ease. Initially, the participants should introduce themselves. A brief role play session may help to demonstrate the parent training approach, and the therapist should explain the rules:

- Role play sessions are brief, lasting about 2–3 minutes.
- The role play area should be used exclusively for role play and not discussion.
- Likewise, the discussion area should not be used for role play.
- Anyone may interrupt role play at any time.

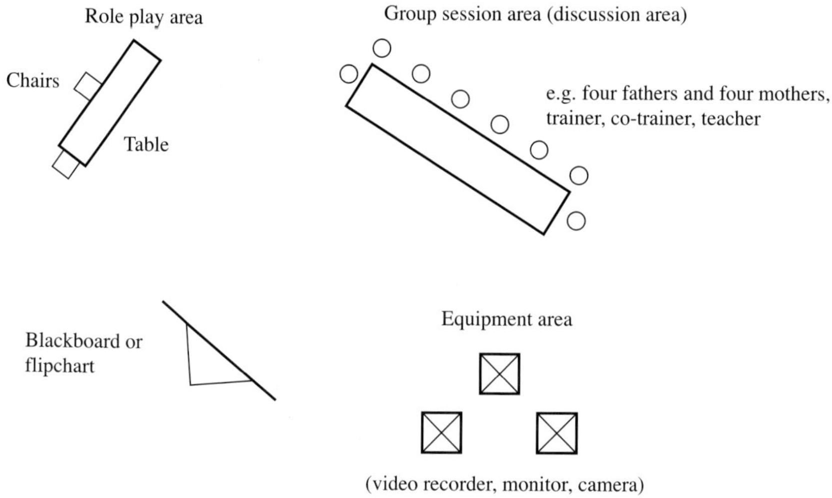

Fig. 13.2. Possible arrangement of the room for parent training sessions.

- Anyone may request a break.
- Everyone is responsible for ensuring that the rules are kept.

These guidelines illustrate the importance of making clear agreements with parents prior to beginning parent training. Rules apply to the room, time schedule and content of sessions, and it is common responsibility to ensure that rules are kept. Fig. 13.2 illustrates the way in which a room for parent training sessions may be set up.

First interventional step: description of behaviour – learning to observe

The first step comprises three parts:

(i) One parent is asked to describe a particular problem which is subsequently addressed in training sessions ('stage directions').

(ii) The problem is enacted in role play by the participants. The play is recorded on video ('role play').

(iii) Video sequences of the enacted problem are evaluated systematically ('systematic observation').

Behaviour is systematically evaluated according to specific guidelines. Initially, one particular video sequence is selected for evaluation. Usually, the following actions or events need to be described in detail:

- the onset of the conflict;
- a sequence in which the conflict escalates and is maintained;
- the end of the conflict;
- sequences which contain interactions facilitating problem solution;

- sequences which illustrate the (frustrated) expectations and aims of those involved.

  The sequences discussed in more detail typically last for about 1–2 minutes. Interaction is described precisely second by second, and pertinent observations are written down. The following questions need to be answered.

Situational appraisal

- What types of situations can be identified? (This includes the room itself including furniture and other objects, the situational content, individuals involved and their location in the room.)

Behavioural appraisal

- What is literally said? (speech)
- What actions are undertaken? (gross motor behaviour)
- Where do the participants look? (eye contact)
- What facial expressions, gestures and modulations of voice can be observed? (emotional behaviour)
- What is the sequence of actions? (time scale)

  Ideally, the learning process leads to the formation of a common view of the problem and a better understanding of both situations and interactions. The parents themselves should attempt to evaluate their behaviour. It is important for the therapist to refrain from interpreting and appraising behaviour in order to prevent demoralizing any individual in the group. The role-play should, on the contrary, improve the participants' self-esteem and confidence.

Second interventional step: understanding interactions during child-raising – learning to interpret and appraise

In this context, describing behaviour means appraising and interpreting interactions according to defined guidelines. Only when interactions are observed carefully and assessed systematically can interactions be interpreted appropriately. Likewise, the appropriate interpretation of interactions is a precondition for understanding them, whilst comprehension is important for modifying behaviour. Only when parents understand the interactions between them and their child will they be able to modify their behaviour and expect to see behavioural improvement in their child.

In order to encourage the systematic appraisal of interactions, a variety of educational aids such as training manuals and video films have been developed. However, the effectiveness of such educational material remains controversial. The 'Munich parent training programme' emphasizes a somewhat different approach. Parents are expected to learn by means of experimental demonstration of interactions using role play. The guidelines by which interactions are interpreted and appraised are gradually developed by means of self-awareness during role play and feedback of video recordings. This aim is achieved in two steps.

(i) Experimental demonstration of interactions (role play) using video recordings, e.g. the 'assistance game'.

(ii) Systematic observation and assessment of role play using video recordings, e.g. 'What is appropriate assistance and how does it work?'.

The 'assistance game'

The 'assistance game' may be helpful in learning to distinguish appropriate from inappropriate help. The game is carried out in two steps.

(i) One member of the group of parents is asked to solve a difficult task (but one that can be solved) under two conditions: first, with appropriate assistance, and second, with inappropriate assistance.

(ii) Different manners of behaving towards the person solving the task and the resulting interactions are demonstrated and recorded on video film. Subsequently, the recording is assessed by the group.

The group of parents is given the following instructions: 'The next task is to try to understand the child's behaviour and the way he/she depends on his surroundings. I'd like us to do two role-plays to learn which options are available to us to help the child make progress and learn. We will call this type of help "appropriate assistance". We will also encounter educational steps which are more likely to hinder the child's progress. We will call this type of help "inappropriate assistance".'

One parent is asked to sit down at the table, with several pieces of a puzzle in front of him. The puzzle consists of seven pieces of different shapes (triangles, squares, a parallelogram). Using these pieces, a variety of shapes can be made up.

The initial instruction is: 'I am now going to "help" you in an inappropriate way. You can see the seven pieces in front of you. If you do it properly, you can put all the pieces together to make up a square. Now, please try, you have 2 minutes.'

The parent then starts on the task, whilst the therapist gives 'inappropriate assistance'. For example, he may address the parent in a polite but unhelpful manner: 'As I said, you have 2 minutes to solve the task. But don't let me put you under any pressure. The task is very simple' (although it is actually quite difficult). 'You are doing very well' (although not a single piece has been placed properly). 'Remember the motto: "look before you leap". You must approach the problem systematically and concentrate on what you are doing. There is no need to get nervous . . .'. The therapist behaves in a generally restless way, fidgets with his watch, moves his chair back and forth, etc. Eventually, after about 2 minutes, he interrupts the task.

The same task is then repeated, this time with 'appropriate assistance' from the therapist. He explains how difficult the task really is, encourages the right moves, refrains from making any unnecessary and inappropriate comments and avoids restlessness.

The two sessions are then evaluated using video recordings. Parents are asked to consider What are inappropriate and appropriate assistance and how do they work? Comments on personal feelings, interpretations and views can be encouraged during the session.

The 'assistance game' should always be related in some way to a problem demonstrated by a parent during role play in the first interventional step. Tables 13.1 and 13.2 show how the game may be evaluated. The following points can be explained using experimental demonstration of interactions and role play:

- understanding how behaviour, self-perception, perception of others and perception of emotions depend upon environmental conditions;
- learning how to distinguish between intended effects and the actual results of one's own child-raising behaviour and learning how to control the effectiveness of one's behaviour;
- understanding how child-raising behaviour directly affects the child's perceptions and behaviour;
- learning how to distinguish between appropriate and inappropriate assistance in the context of actions and effects; appraising and controlling behaviour with respect to specific aims.

This learning process will ultimately result in a better understanding of the 'functional anatomy' of behavioural difficulties or interactional problems occurring in families.

Case vignette

The parents of a child with a specific developmental disorder and behavioural difficulties habitually discussed these problems in a depreciating way. They did not include the child in discussions nor show any empathy with him. Consequently, the child became increasingly restless and suspicious when his parents spoke together. The following task was developed to improve the parents' understanding of how to communicate in a child-appropriate way.

Table 13.1. 'Appropriate assistance' whilst supervising homework. Results of appraisal by a parent training group

How can we assist appropriately? e.g. whilst supervising homework (i) Prevent distraction Provide a quiet place to work Provide only the necessary material Avoid interruptions Observe quietly (ii) Appropriate assistance Give clear instructions Adapt tasks to the child's capacity Explain the tasks Correct mistakes in a matter-of-fact manner Answer pertinent questions Avoid excessive encouragement Ignore refusal and attempts to argue Be accommodating and cooperative *How does appropriate assistance affect others?* Appropriate assistance generally helps others to achieve aims. Thus, appropriate assistance to some extent resembles reinforcement, and may replace material or social rewards in some cases. Punishments such as criticism, admonitions or complaints can be avoided by appropriate assistance.	*How does appropriate assistance affect self-esteem?* Increases self-confidence Increases willingness to accept challenges Reduces initial anxieties Reduces feeling of responsibility for problems *How does appropriate assistance affect achievement?* Makes it easier to: concentrate be independent commit oneself Helps to avoid mistakes Makes it easier to work effectively Reduces the risk of failures Reduces stress Improves achievment *How does appropriate assistance affect social behaviour?* Makes it is easier to listen Improves cooperation Avoids or solves conflicts Prevents misunderstandings Replaces material rewards Reduces criticism, admonitions and complaints Improves others' willingness to help

From Innerhofer (1977).

One parent was asked to take on the role of the child, whilst the other parent took over the role of the child's mother. The therapist's role was that of a 'tester'. The 'child' was confronted with a task. The child's progress in solving the task was described to the 'mother' by the 'tester'. Initially, the 'tester' emphasized the 'difficulties' and 'problems' the child was having with the task. ('As you can see, your child has to think very hard even about easy tasks. That's why you consider him slow. He is listening to what I'm saying rather than concentrating on his task. This is a sign of distraction . . .').

Table 13.2. **'Inappropriate assistance' whilst supervising homework. Results of appraisal by a parent training group**

How do we impair someone by inappropriate assistance? e.g. whilst supervising homework (i) Through distraction Disturbing quiet work Asking questions in an emotional way Making irrelevant comments Being impatient Interrupting work (ii) Through inappropriate assistance Repeating instructions unnecessarily Giving information which is already known Asking someone to try harder Suggesting a task is easy Making thoughtless comments ('Oh, I'm sure you will manage') (iii) Through unnecessary assistance Handing the pen or pencil Opening the book Arranging the chair Repeating instructions in a stereotyped way Making superfluous comments *How does inappropriate assistance affect others?* Inappropriate assistance prevents others from achieving their aims or makes it difficult.	*How does inappropriate assistance affect self-esteem?* Reduces self-confidence Causes nervousness and restlessness Causes one to consider problems a result of personal failure Increases anxiousness of any demands Decreases independence *How does inappropriate assistance affect achievement?* Causes a decline in achievement Impedes progress Results in excessive demands being made Increases stress Causes conflicts *How does inappropriate assistance affect social behaviour?* Increases dependence on others Causes refusal Causes defiant behaviour Causes taciturn behaviour Results in impatience Results in aggression

From Innerhofer (1977).

In the second phase the 'tester' refrains from making any depreciating comments and addresses the 'child' in an appropriate way, whilst explaining his observations to the 'mother'. Comparing video recordings of the two made it clear to the parents how the 'child' became so insecure during the first phase that he was unable to address the task, whereas in the second phase, the 'child's' confidence progressively increased with child-orientated communication and appropriate assistance, so that the 'child' was eventually able to solve the task (Innerhofer and Warnke, 1980).

Third interventional step: problem-solving – improving the behavioural repertoire

The process of problem-solving can be divided into a series of smaller steps:

- analysing problematic behaviour,
- collecting options by which the problem may be solved,
- testing options by trial and error using role play,
- using the problem-solving options favoured by one family for another family,
- the preparation and practice of problems likely to be encountered at home.

The following guidelines are important in the problem-solving process.

- The variety of options available to the family need to be discussed.
- Parents' should be encouraged and their own confidence built up.
- The personal history of parents is discussed only if personal experiences are preventing parents from modifying their behaviour.
- Obstructive, unethical or demeaning attempts at problem-solving are always contraindicated. The therapist should always encourage positive problem-solving strategies during parent training.

Assessing problems – behavioural analysis

The assessment determines the aims, situational factors, options for action and biographical factors which may have some influence on the problem and the individual coping strategies.

(i) Analysis of aims focuses on the goals, intentions and wishes expressed. For example, analysis of aims may address a number of issues such as: (a) hyperkinetic behaviour in a child with sibling rivalry, (b) specific learning problems and conduct disorder at school in a child of normal intelligence, (c) daily encopresis. The aims may be viewed differently by different members of the family. In this case, the mother was keen to initially concentrate on the learning difficulties and hyperactivity, whereas for the child, the main issue was the relationship with his sibling.

(ii) The situational analysis determines the personal, temporal, spatial and material conditions which contribute significantly to the problem. For example, situational analysis of the above mentioned case revealed that: (a) residential conditions were good and the rural environment in which the family lived provided enough space for the child. (b) The child was well integrated in various local clubs, and (c) attended a school and class appropriate for his intellectual capacity. (d) The fact that the child had to share one room with his brother whom he experienced as a rival was considered to be relevant from the child's point of view. (e) In addition, there was no clear agreement about who was to use the room at what time to do homework.

(iii) The analysis of events attempts to discover potential alternatives in reacting to difficult situations. It should be restricted to those interactions which are likely to be helpful for developing problem-solving strategies. The interactions which take place during conflict need to be analysed carefully in order to identify strengths and weaknesses relevant to developing problem-solving strategies. For example, in the case mentioned above: (a) the child was capable of bringing his school bag to his desk and preparing his homework. Thus it was no longer necessary for his mother to get his books ready, although she generally did so. (b) The child's mother demonstrated that she was able to assist the child appropriately and applied this skill systematically to help the child with his homework, e.g. structuring homework by dividing tasks into short work phases and praising correct results rather than criticizing mistakes.

(iv) The biographical analysis focuses on details of an individual's history relevant to the current problem. The aim here is also to discover appropriate coping strategies and assess whether particular behavioural options are likely to be successful. Thus biographical analysis may be undertaken when a particular approach to problem-solving 'theoretically' seems promising, but parents have difficulties in developing coping strategies in practice.

Discovering options of action

During parent training, parents learn to develop alternative ways of acting which may help them to develop new problem-solving strategies. This process of discovery and learning is often better achieved in a group setting where new ideas can be developed in several ways.

'Brain-storming'

Initially, a parent is asked to define the aim of a particular child-raising behaviour, e.g. action to prevent school avoidance. The group subsequently develops a range of novel situational or behavioural alternatives.

Collecting ideas by trial and error (using role play and video recordings)

Parents are given the opportunity to suggest problem-solving strategies, which are then tried out using role play. During role play, further problem-solving strategies may become apparent. Thus, alternative ways of action can be sought by trial and error, self-experience and video-supported observation. It is important to emphasize those sequences which show individuals' resources rather than deficits, and effective problem-solving strategies rather than inappropriate behaviour.

Each solution is characterized by a number of specific steps which need to be undertaken.

Solution by objectives

This emphasizes the need for specific behavioural aims in order to arrive at a solution. This is present when a conflict could be solved by behavioural modification or modified appraisal of behaviour. For example, in the case of the hyperkinetic behaviour mentioned above, the child's scholastic difficulties and behavioural problems were considered to be of particular importance. Parent training focused on these issues, whilst issues such as sibling rivalry and encopresis were not initially addressed. The behavioural disturbance associated with the task of homework was identified as a particular issue. The aim was to enable the child to do his homework alone, avoiding disagreements.

Situational solution or prevention

This type of solution is characterized by modifications in the spatial, temporal, or material conditions to which the child is exposed, in order to improve behaviour and enable the child to develop normally. Such modifications include changing school, e.g. to a more appropriate school in a child with a learning disability, organizing appropriate child-care, e.g. if a single parent is at work, modifying the visiting hours of separated parents, or opting for an out-of-home placement. For example, in the case mentioned above, the following situational modifications were agreed upon: (a) a specific time for homework, (b) the regular and reliable presence of the child's mother to supervise homework, (c) installing a suitable desk, (d) ensuring that the television set in the room was not on, (e) medication with methylphenidate (Ritalin).

Interactional solution

This type of solution is recommended when interactional conflicts are present and it is desirable that parents modify their behaviour. For example, in the case mentioned above: (a) rules for how to begin homework were agreed upon (the child was expected to write down the day's homework, unpack his school bag, and get his books ready). (b) Specific rules were established with regard to how to deal with the child, such as ignoring inappropriate behaviour, avoiding superfluous assistance, helping the child appropriately with actual mistakes (Tables 13.1 and 13.2), and agreeing on activities as a reward after the child had completed his homework.

Biographical solution

This type of solution is rarely achieved during parent training. If a parent requires more in-depth psychotherapeutic help, this will usually be undertaken in another setting. For example, a child's mother refused to cooperate during interactional analysis. She refused to watch the video recording of her interactions with the child and left the room during this first phase of parent training. However, she was keen to participate in the analysis of other parents' behaviour. During a subsequent individual session, she admitted to having low self-esteem. She had been unwilling to cooperate during the first phase because of concerns over her body image: she generally felt too fat and had been unable to tolerate the sight of herself in the video recording. Individual therapy sessions focussed on this problem. Depression was diagnosed and treated, after which she was able to tolerate viewing video recordings of herself. She later became a keen member of the parent training group, took an active interest in local politics and eventually became a member of the town council. Her son, who suffered from severe dyslexia, ultimately completed school and successfully took up an occupation as a technician.

Follow-up

Problem-solving strategies developed by parents during parent training sessions are recorded in writing and can be taken home by the individual. Towards the end of parent training the therapist will need to discuss with participants how to inform other family members about the new problem-solving strategies which have been developed in the course of parent training. Here, also, role play may be helpful, as it gives parents the opportunity of practising a family discussion situation. Subsequent therapy sessions may, perhaps, include the participant's spouse, and role play and video feedback techniques may be used to explain the problem-solving strategies developed. These techniques need not be restricted to group settings, but may also be effective when used in an individual setting on an outpatient basis, e.g. helping a mother to improve the way she supervises homework.

Indications for parent training

Parent training is a psychotherapeutic approach which may be appropriate when parents are able to utilize situational options and individual child-raising skills to encourage the normal development of the child. The spectrum of symptoms which can be treated by this approach is broad, including excessive crying, sleep disorder, stereotypical behaviour, interactional disorder, conduct disorder, hyperkinetic syndrome, emotional disorder, eating disorder, enuresis, encopresis, self-harming behaviour, mutism, obsessional disorder, aggressive behaviour, chronic constipation, pyromania, tics, anorexia nervosa, difficulties with homework in children with specific developmental disorder, kleptomania, stuttering and the behavioural problems associated with mental retardation and autism.

Parent training techniques have been shown to be effective in numerous studies (Innerhofer and Müller, 1974; Innerhofer and Warnke, 1980; Minsel, 1984; Schmitz, 1976; Briesmeister and Schaefer, 1998; Kane et al., 1974; Warnke and Innerhofer, 1978); however, as with any therapy one should always bear in mind potential unwanted effects. Modifications of child-raising behaviour usually result in a phase during which feelings of insecurity may occur in the child. Such insecurity may cause a temporary aggravation of symptoms. In many cases improvement occurs only after a latency period ('sleeper effect'). This phenomenon must be explained to parents and they should be offered additional sessions to support them and their child during this phase. Additional difficulties may result in feelings of guilt in parents and in some cases parents may discontinue treatment. Compliance may be improved in several ways:

- by demonstrating a positive attitude in the cooperation with parents from the start;
- by being fully prepared so that the risk of inappropriate decisions is reduced;
- by choosing interventions which meet the family's needs, avoiding unnecessary stress;
- by bearing in mind the child's interests and aims as well as parents' needs, living conditions and their capacity for cooperation;
- by keeping parents fully informed about the disorder and therapeutic options; scientific lectures and technical terms should be avoided; parents should learn by self-experience, observation and techniques such as video-recordings, role-play, group sessions and relaxation training (Innerhofer and Warnke, 1978);
- by emphasizing parents' own competency and resources;
- by concentrating on those conflicts which pose the greatest problem for parents;
- by keeping the demands in terms of time and effort on the family as low as possible;
- by providing additional help to families who live in difficult social conditions such as finanical aid, assistance with bureaucratic affairs, finding work, planning their daily routine, etc. prior to commencing parent training.

The therapist will need to find an equilibrium between therapeutic possibilities and the child's needs, always keeping in mind the needs of the family as a whole.

REFERENCES

Bernal, M. E. and North, J. A. (1978). A survey of parent training manuals. *Journal of Applied Behavior Analysis*, **11**, 533–44.

Boggs, C. J. (1981). Train up a parent. A review of the research in child rearing literature. *Child Study Journal*, **10**(4), 261–84.

Briesmeister, J. M. and Schaefer, C. E. (ed.) (1998). *Handbook of parent training. Parents as co-therapists for children's behavior problems*, 2nd edn. New York: Wiley.

Clarke-Stewart, K. A. (1978). Popular primers for parents. *American Psychologist*, **33**, 359–69.

Douglas, J. (1989). Training parents to manage their child's sleep problem. In *Handbook of parent training. Parents as co-therapists for children's behavior problems*, ed. C. E. Schaefer and J. M. Briesmeister, pp. 13–37. New York: Wiley & Sons.

Dührssen, A. (1988). Analytische Psychotherapie bei Kindern und Jugendlichen. In *Kinder- und Jugendpsychiatrie in Klinik und Praxis*, vol. I, ed. H. Remschmidt and M. H. Schmidt, pp. 672–85. Stuttgart: Thieme.

Glasgow, R. E. and Rosen, G. M. (1978). A behavioral bibliography. A review of self-help behaviour therapy manuals. *Psychological Bulletin*, **85**, 1–23.

Graziano, A. M. and Diament, D. M. (1992). Parent behavioral training. An examination of the paradigm. *Behavior Modification*, **16**, 3–38.

Innerhofer, P. (1974). Ein Regelmodell zur Analyse und Intervention in Familie und Schule. Abänderung und Erweiterung des S-R-K-Modells. *Zeitschrift für Klinische Psychologie*, **3**, 1–29.

Innerhofer, P. (1977). *Das Münchner Trainingsmodell. Beobachtung, Interaktionsanalyse, Verhaltensänderung*. Heidelberg: Springer.

Innerhofer, P. (1980). Soziale Interaktionen zwischen Mutter und Kind. In *Entwicklung der Verhaltenstherapie in der Praxis*, ed. J. C. Brengelmann. München: Röttger.

Innerhofer, P. and Müller, G. F. (1974). *Elternarbeit in der Verhaltenstherapie*. Sonderheft I. Mitteilungen der Gesellschaft für Verhaltenstherapie. München: Gesellschaft für Verhaltenstherapie.

Innerhofer, P. and Warnke, A. (1978). *Eltern als Co-Therapeuten. Analyse der Bereitschaft von Müttern zur Mitarbeit bei der Durchführung therapeutischer Programme ihrer Kinder*. Heidelberg: Springer.

Innerhofer, P. and Warnke, A. (1980). Elterntrainingsprogramm nach dem Münchner Trainingsmodell. Ein Erfahrungsbericht. In *Familiäre Sozialisation und Intervention*, ed. H. Lukesch, M. Perrez and K. Schneewind, pp. 417–39. Bern: Huber.

Innerhofer, P. and Warnke, A. (1989). Die Zusammenarbeit mit Eltern nach dem Münchner Trainingsmodell in der Praxis der Frühförderung. In *Frühförderung mit den Eltern*, ed. O. Speck and A. Warnke, pp. 151–84. München: Reinhardt.

Kane, J. F. and Kane, G. (1976). *Geistig schwer Behinderte lernen lebenspraktische Fertigkeiten*. Bern: Huber.

Kane, G., Kane, J. F., Amorosa, H. and Kumpmann, S. (1974). Einweisung von Eltern in die Verhaltenstherapie ihrer geistig behinderten Kinder. *Zeitschrift für Kinder- und Jungendpsychiatrie*, **2**, 87–110.

Mattejat, F. and Remschmidt, H. (1991). Die Bedeutung der familialen Beziehungsdynamik für den Erfolg stationärer Behandlungen in der Kinder- und Jugendpsychiatrie. *Zeitschrift für Kinder- und Jugendpsychiatrie*, **19**, 139–50.

McMahon, R. J. and Forehand, R. (1980). Self-help behaviour therapies in parent training. In *advances in clinical child psychology*, vol. 3, ed. B. B. Lahey and A. E. Kazdin, pp. 149–76.

Minsel, B. (1984). Elterntraining. *Zeitschrift für personenzentrierte Psychologie und Psychotherapie*, **3**, 55–66.

Perrez, M., Minsel, B. and Wimmer, H. (1974). *Eltern-Verhaltenstraining*. Salzburg: Müller.

Rogers, C. (1951). *Client centered therapy in current practice. Implications and theory*. New York: Houghton Mifflin.

Schmitz, E. (1976). *Co-Therapeuten in der Verhaltenstherapie*. Weinheim: Beltz.

Warnke, A. (1988). Elternarbeit in der Kinder- u. Jugendpsychiatrie. In *Kinder- und Jugendpsychiatrie in Klinik und Praxis*, vol. I, ed. H. Remschmidt and M. H. Schmidt, pp. 750–63. Stuttgart: Thieme.

Warnke, A. (1993). Grundzüge der Elternberatung und Elterntherapie. In *Psychotherapie und Psychopharmakotherapie*, ed. G. Nissen, pp. 82–100. Bern: Huber.

Warnke, A. (1999). Elterntraining. In *Verhaltenstherapie und Verhaltensmedizin bei Kindern und Jugendlichen*, 2nd edn, ed. H-C. Steinhausen and M. von Aster, pp. 621–37. Weinheim: Beltz.

Warnke, A. and Innerhofer, P. (1978). Ein standardisiertes Elterntraining zur Therapie des Kindes und zur Erforschung von Erziehungsvorgängen. In *Familiale Sozialisation*, ed. K. Schneewind and H. Lukesch, pp. 294–312. Stuttgart: Klett-Cotta.

14 Combination of treatment methods

Helmut Remschmidt

Combining several therapeutic techniques

Combination treatment is the simultaneous use of several therapeutic methods in psychotherapy, or a concomitant use of psychotherapy with non-psychotherapeutic treatments, e.g. medication or physical therapy.

Much like psychotherapy, three basic prinicples need to be considered when undertaking combined treatment: the psychotherapeutic method, the setting in which treatment is undertaken, and the disorder which is to be treated (Remschmidt and Schmidt, 1986). The three dimensions of this approach are explained in Chapter 1 and shown in Fig. 1.1.

Usually several methods, e.g. behaviour therapy, relaxation training, psychodynamic therapy, behaviour therapy, family therapy can be used together, as can several different settings, e.g. individual and group therapy or day-patient treatment followed by outpatient treatment.

However, treatment methods should never pursue incompatible goals and should work towards similar treatment aims. Thus, a very structured approach, e.g. operant conditioning techniques is considered incompatible with a *laissez-faire* approach, in which behaviour is left entirely up to the patient, e.g. non-directive play therapy. The aims of the two approaches are contradictory: on the one hand, strict behavioural rules are drawn up with the aim of modifying behaviour, whilst on the other hand, treatment is based on the idea that the patient can expand his behavioural repertoire through his own creativity, resulting in improvement of symptoms.

Although it is generally up to the therapist to choose appropriate techniques, the following guidelines may be helpful:

(i) All techniques used should be clinically and empirically evaluated (research-informed psychotherapy). Clinical experience has shown that many techniques are reliable, but not all techniques have been empirically evaluated, especially with children and adolescents. Therefore, in many cases one will have to use psychotherapeutic techniques whose effectiveness has not yet been empirically evaluated.

(ii) The techniques need to be compatible with the specific aims of treatment.

(iii) The techniques need to be part of a larger treatment plan and compatible in every detail.

(iv) The techniques need to be age appropriate and suit the individual patient.

(v) The techniques need to be used in an appropriate setting.

(vi) Cooperation between the patient and his environment (parents and peers in kindergarten or school) is essential.

The following examples illustrate the use of a combination of several techniques in clinical practice.

Individual psychotherapy, group psychotheray and family therapy

The combination of individual psychotherapy, group psychotheray and family therapy is particularly useful during inpatient or day-hospital treatment. In both settings the patient is available for extended periods of time (24 or 8 hours per day), allowing intensive treatment.

Special emphasis can be placed on one of the three techniques, depending on the disorder being treated. This difference of emphasis is illustrated in the following two examples.

Hyperkinetic syndrome

When severe, this disorder often requires both medication and an individually structured behaviour therapy programme including specific training and self-instruction training steps. Both techniques are initially applied in an individual setting. In the next step, treatment may be undertaken in a group setting including school attendance, during which behavioural improvements are put to the test. Whilst offering advice to parents is part of treatment from the start, strict family therapy is usually not undertaken. This type of cooperation with families is usually continued over the course of treatment and intensified as the time of discharge approaches in order to prepare the way for outpatient treatment. This may be helped by home visits or home treatment.

Anorexia nervosa

In its initial phase, anorexia nervosa requires individual treatment. Ongoing cooperation with the patient's family is also important. Following adequate weight gain, and as the patient is increasingly able to cope with the demands of psychotherapy, group sessions can be introduced. Such groups should generally include patients with a similar diagnosis, in order to give them the opportunity of openly discussing individual experience with the disorder. Subsequently, family therapy is introduced, especially if patients are still young. The aim here is to identify factors which may have contributed to the precipitation of the disorder or which have helped to maintain it. Once these factors have been identified, they can be addressed appropriately.

Individual psychotherapy and relaxation training

Frequently individual psychotherapy, e.g. psychodynamic therapy or behaviour therapy may be combined with relaxation training techniques to treat a variety of disorders. Some techniques, e.g. systematic desensitization have to be combined with relaxation training.

Psychodynamic therapy and behaviour therapy

The issue whether psychodynamic and behaviour therapy can be combined is more controversial. The methods contradict one another fundamentally in terms of treatment goals and the approach to treatment. They would, therefore, seem to be incompatible. However, the rather stark contrast between the two approaches has been tempered somewhat in past years, as proponents of psychodynamic therapy have realized that the therapeutic changes they achieve are based on learning processes and congitive restructuring. Likewise, behaviour therapists have realized that behaviour therapy always takes place in the context of a relationship between patient and therapist, and have come to regard the therapeutic relationship as an important variable, which significantly influences therapy.

Thus the behavioural techniques used today to improve specific competencies are not generally considered incompatible with psychodynamic or psychoanalytical treatment. Likewise, most proponents of behaviour therapy realize that interaction between patient and therapist plays a significant role in therapy, although the idea of transference and countertransference is not universally accepted.

Integrated approach to therapy

Today, several approaches exist to psychotherapy, based on combining two or more distinct psychotherapeutic techniques. These usually feature treatment programmes which have been developed in institutions or outpatient treatment facilities. Several distinct therapeutic components are usually combined to make up a structured treatment plan (Knoblauch and Knoblauch, 1983).

Combination of psychotherapeutic methods with other treatment techniques

Combinations of psychotherapeutic methods with other (non-psychotherapeutic) treatment techniques are commonly used and have been shown to be effective in a variety of settings. Usually several methods are put together in a treatment plan. Treatment plans generally comprise a variety of therapeutic components, e.g. medication + behaviour therapy + family therapy, either as in- or outpatient treatment). The components are integrated and applied in a structured way. The therapeutic plan needs to include treatment goals, the necessary steps and a time schedule. However, the plan should be flexible enough to allow modifications should additional information make this necessary. The treatment plan and all modifications need to be recorded precisely in writing.

Various non-psychotherapeutic steps can be combined with psychotherapeutic techniques. The combination of medication or physical therapy with psychotherapy is the most common.

The following three examples illustrate the use of treatment plans. Two plans focus on specific disorders (hyperkinetic syndrome, schizophrenia in adolescence), the third one on a comparison of different treatment modalities.

Treatment programme for hyperkinetic syndrome

Many studies on the treatment of the hyperkinetic syndrome have shown that 'multimodal' treatment programmes have a better outcome than one type of treatment alone, e.g. play therapy, medication, behaviour therapy. Treatment programmes usually comprise a combination of several distinct techniques: structuring everyday life (improving general coping skills, keeping social rules), steps focusing directly on the patient (stimulant medication, behavioural contingency management, occupational therapy, motor control training), and steps focusing on the patient's environment (parental education, joint work with the patient's school and other facilites involved). Although the effect depends on dosage, stimulant medication generally helps to improve hyperactive symptoms, cognitive parameters and social adaption. Attention improves as determined by vigilance tests and reaction time, and interaction between mother and patient also improves with medication (Mash and Johnston, 1982; Barkley, 1988). These results have been confirmed repeatedly. As the patient's behaviour improves, parents feel less helpless and are motivated to respond to their child in a positive way. Thus normal interaction can gradually redevelop between the patient and his parents.

Treatment programme for adolescents with schizophrenia

Structured treatment programmes have been useful for adolescents with schizophrenia. Such programmes usually include a combination of neurolepic medication, supportive psychotherapy, occupational therapy and family therapy. The most effective treatment programmes have combined neuroleptic medication with supportive participation of the family (Goldstein et al., 1978; King and Goldstein, 1979). The combination of these two modalities has revealed two important results: (i) allowing the family to participate in the structured therapy programme prevented the patient from being exposed to excessive and hostile emotions; (ii) neuroleptic medication acted as protection to the patient preventing him from suffering from emotions expressed. These results suggest that treatments programmes have better outcomes than one type of treatment alone, e.g. psychotherapy or medication.

Comparing different treatment modalities: inpatient treatment, day-hospital treatment and home treatment

Remschmidt and Schmidt (1988) undertook a follow-up study to compare the outcomes of inpatient, day-hospital and outpatient treatment. The study included a total of 109 patients with disorders from ten different diagnostic groups. The patients came from two child and adolescent psychiatric university hospitals. The sample constituted 10–15% of the total number of patients who presented to the two hospitals. Patients were randomly assigned to one of the three treatment modalities. Similar methods were used with all three treatment modalities and adapted to the specific setting in which they were used. The choice of treatment techniques largely depended on the type of disorder being addressed: disorders with clearly defined symptoms or one single symptom were treated with behavioural techniques, whereas more complex disorders were treated with a combination of several treatment techniques such as behaviour, psychodynamic and family therapy This approach was regarded as appropriate, particularly considering the multifactorial aetiology of most psychiatric disorders in childhood and adolescence. The study revealed the following results.

- There were no significant differences in outcome in the three groups, although outcome differed between the various diagnostic groups. As expected, neurotic and emotional disorders had the best outcome with all three treatment modalities, whilst treatment of conduct disorders and antisocial behaviour was the least successful.
- There were no significant differences between the three groups regarding the duration of treatment.

This study shows that home treatment, day-hospital treatment and inpatient treatment are equally effective for a small selection of patients. For practical purposes this means that about 10–15% of patients who are admitted for inpatient treatment would benefit to the same degree if day-hospital or home treatment were undertaken. Such treatment would probably result in a reduction of treatment cost. With this approach to treatment the choice of an appropriate technique is obviously particularly important.

REFERENCES

Barkley, R. A. (1988). The effects of methylphenidate on the interaction of preschool ADHD children with their mothers. *Journal of the American Academy of Child and Adolescent Psychiatry*, **27**, 336–41.

Goldstein, M. J., Rodnick, E. H. and Evans, J. R. (1978). Drug and family therapy in the aftercare of acute schizophrenics. *Archives of General Psychiatry*, **35**, 1169–77.

King, C. E. and Goldstein, M. J. (1979). Therapist ratings of achievement of objectives in psychotherapy with acute schizophrenics. *Schizophrenia Bulletin*, **5**, 118–29.

Knoblauch, F. and Knoblauch, J. (1983). *Integrierte Psychotherapie*. Stuttgart: Enke.

Mash, E. J. and Johnston, C. (1982). A comparison of the mother–child interaction of younger and older hyperactive and normal children. *Child Development*, **53**, 1371–81.

Remschmidt, H. and Schmidt, M. H. (ed.) (1986). *Therapieevaluation in der Kinder- und Jugendpsychiatrie*. Stuttgart: Enke.

Remschmidt, H. and Schmidt, M. H. (1988). *Alternative Behandlungsformen in der Kinder- und Jugendpsychiatrie. Stationäre Behandlung, tagesklinische Behandlung und home treatment im Vergleich*. Stuttgart: Enke.

Part III

The practice of psychotherapy for specific disorders in childhood and adolescence

15 Anxiety disorders

Helmut Remschmidt

General considerations, definition and classification

The term anxiety disorder comprises a number of different clinical disorders, each of which is characterized by two features: overwhelming and inappropriate anxiety and avoidant behaviour. The avoidance of specific objects or situations is usually distinguished from generalised or nonspecific ('free-floating') anxiety. The former is associated with phobic disorders, the second with anxiety neuroses. In the last few years attempts have been made to refine this distinction, but these efforts have still failed to produce unambiguous classification of anxiety disorders. Table 15.1 shows the classification of anxiety disorders in ICD-10 (WHO, 1992). Phobic disorders are distinguished from other anxiety disorders. Two types of agoraphobia are distinguished (both with and without panic attacks).

This attempt at classification (Table 15.1) illustrates the difficulty in clearly discriminating between various anxiety disorders. In some cases classification is almost impossible, because a combination of phobic symptoms may be present simultaneously. An alternative is to split the disorder into a component defining the situation and temporal characteristics of the anxiety which may be one or more of the following:

(i) phobic anxieties, i.e. fear of specific objects or situations, including agoraphobia, social and monosymptomatic phobias (also called simple phobias);

(ii) acute attacks of anxiety, which are not associated with a specific object or situation and occur as sudden attacks of anxiety in which physical symptoms predominate (panic disorders);

(iii) generalized anxieties, which last longer, i.e. days, weeks or months. They do not depend on specific objects or situations. This type of anxiety is also called 'free-floating anxiety'.

Then the symptomatic characteristics of the anxiety can be considered, which may include aspects on one or more of the following planes.

Table 15.1. Classification of phobic anxiety disorders in ICD-10

F40	*Phobic anxiety disorders*
F40.0	Agoraphobia
F40.00	Without panic disorder
F40.01	With panic disorder
F40.1	Social phobias
F40.2	Specific (isolated) phobias
F40.8	Other phobic anxiety disorder
F40.9	Other phobic anxiety disorder
F41	*Other anxiety disorders*
F41.0	Panic disorder [episodic paroxysmal anxiety]
F41.1	Generalized anxiety disorder
F41.2	Mixed anxiety and depressive disorder
F41.3	Other mixed anxiety disorder
F41.3	Other specified anxiety disorder
F41.9	Anxiety disorder, unspecified

The cognitive plane

This includes apprehensions, feelings of impairment and thoughts to avoid situations which might cause anxiety.

The behavioural plane

This includes avoidance strategies such as flight, evasion, running away or avoiding the situation. Avoidance strategies may include 'security-signs' that represent safety, i.e. objects or situations that make the occurrence of anxiety less probable because they signify the prospect of immediate help, e.g. a telephone to call the therapist, the presence of a particular person, medication in a coat pocket.

The physical plane

This includes the well-known physical signs and symptoms of anxiety such as tachycardia, sweating, shortness of breath, etc.

Distinction between the three planes on which symptoms of anxiety appear is of great help in diagnosis and planning treatment of the disorder. By breaking down the syndrome in this way, an accurate diagnosis can be made, and treatment coordinated accordingly within these three areas.

It is important for the clinician to establish first whether an anxiety attack represents a disorder or whether it is an appropriate physical reaction. It is rarely possible, however, to draw a sharp line between these two states. Anxiety can be considered abnormal when the following criteria are fulfilled (Remschmidt, 1992):

(i) excessive anxiety (quantitative aspect);
(ii) unusual content or object of the anxious state (qualitative aspect);
(iii) inappropriate anxiety reaction, entirely out of proportion to the situation in which it appears;
(iv) chronification of anxiety reactions;
(v) lack of mechanisms to reduce or cope with anxiety;
(vi) marked impairment in the ability to take part in age-appropriate activities of daily life.

It is important to appreciate the age-related changes in anxiety that take place in the normal course of human development. As potential dangers evolve and change in the course of childhood and adolescence, so do the objects of anxiety. While younger children (up to the age of 8) are most commonly afraid of imaginary objects, e.g. witches, goblins, ghosts and have relatively few realistic anxieties, adolescents principally express a fear of people in authority, social situations and tests of performance (Remschmidt, 1973).

There is high correlation between parental anxiety and anxiety in their children. Furthermore, certain family attitudes, e.g. overprotective behaviour, a symbiotic bond between mother and child seem to facilitate the development of anxiety disorders.

There is a preponderence of anxiety disorders amongst females. This is true of children, adolescents and adults, but is particularly marked after puberty.

Many monosymptomatic (specific) phobias begin in childhood (especially animal phobias). On the other hand, social phobias most frequently begin at puberty and in early adolescence. This probably reflects the changing content of anxieties, with a strong trend towards the involvement of social situations.

A clinically useful distincion, reflected in the classification systems, distinguishes between four groups. The systems of classification commonly in use also distinguish between these groups. They include: (i) separation anxiety and school phobia, (ii) phobic anxiety disorders, (iii) panic attacks and agoraphobia and (iv) generalized anxiety disorder (formerly: anxiety neurosis).

Separation anxiety and school phobia

The term separation anxiety describes the anxiety which may occur as a result of the separation or anticipation of separation from a significant person in the child's life. In the course of development, a certain amount of separation anxiety in infants and preschool children is normal. A disorder is said to be present only if the anxiety is inappropriately severe, persists for an unusually long time or is occurring at an age by which the child should have outgrown such anxiety, e.g. in adolescence. In addition, it must interfere with the activities of daily life.

School phobia is a special form of separation anxiety and may occur either in children with a predisposition or in generally anxious children. The disorder peaks at several different ages: first preschool, secondly on beginning school and thirdly during adolescence, when increased detatchment from parents is viewed as desirable. These peaks reflect stages of increasing independence, which is generally required of children and adolescents in western society. However, children with an excessively strong bond towards an attachment figure (in most cases their mother), may not be able to tolerate these separations.

Characteristics of the disorder

Clinical picture

The clinical picture is dominated by school refusal, usually accompanied by physical complaints, e.g. morning nausea, headache, abdominal pain particularly prior to leaving for school, and an excessively strong bond towards an attachment figure (usually the mother). Frequently, the child or adolescent expresses great concern about that person's well-being. Although the disorder is called 'school phobia', the main problem does in fact not lie in school, but at home.

Often physical complaints are the first symptoms of the disorder, and physical illness is often initially suspected. Frequently this leads to a series of referrals and investigations. The parents of affected children or adolescents frequently are quite convinced that there must be a clear 'physical' cause for symptoms

School refusal is often the secondary consequence of physical complaints. Anxiety regarding school is only rarely an initial feature, rather physical symptoms form the 'plausible' reason for the child not to go to school, in order that doctor's appointments can be arranged or attended. School phobia therefore, often initially presents to the family physician, general practitioner or paediatrician.

Severe anxiety usually only occurs when parents attempt to force their child into school attendance, after results of physical examination prove to be negative. States of anxiety similar to panic attacks and severe quarrels with parents or other care-givers may occur. Typically, physical symptoms are at their worst in the morning prior to the child leaving for school and also at the beginning of the week. Symptoms are usually absent during school holidays.

ICD-10 contains detailed diagnostic criteria for separation anxiety/school phobia. The criteria emphasize the unrealistic concern for an attachment figure, fear of separation from that person, tendency to avoid attending school, inability to remain at home alone and the presence of associated physical symptoms, which tend to be especially severe before an actual or anticipated separation. Additional symptoms of the syndrome include unhappiness and withdrawal, extreme anxiety, tantrums, crying and clinging tightly to an attachment figure immediately before separation.

Epidemiology

There is a paucity of data on the epidemiology of separation anxiety or school phobia. Available studies suggest prevalence rates of 1–2% of school children. Boys and girls are equally often affected.

In the differential diagnosis one must distinguish between school phobia, i.e. separation anxiety, school avoidance and truancy. The general term for all three of these syndromes is 'school refusal'. The three types of disorder have significant differences, as indicated in Table 15.2. Whereas in school phobia there is no antisocial behaviour, this tends to be marked in cases of truancy. Children and adolescents with school phobia are usually of normal intelligence and generally do not have problems with achievement at school. When questioned carefully, these children do not express a fear of people or situations at school, e.g. particular teachers or specific school subjects. However, adolescents showing school avoidance express marked anxieties concerning topics associated with school, such as anxiety of failure, fear of teachers or dread of other pupils.

Organic disorders must also be distinguished from school phobia, particularly since physical symptoms initially mask school phobia.

Aetiology and pathogenesis

An excessively close bond between the child or adolescent and his attachment figure (usually the mother) is characteristic of school phobia. The excessively close relationship usually develops early in the course of childhood. These anxious children or adolescents, whose social contacts are often restricted, frequently have overanxious mothers, who cannot permit their child's detachment. This kind of close, symbiotic relationship between mother and child may have been reinforced by tragic occurences within the family, e.g. the death of family members. An excessively close bond between mother and child prevents

Table 15.2. Types of school refusal

	School phobia	School avoidance	Truancy
Pathogenesis	Repression of separation anxiety from the mother (fear of loss) and displacement to the object	Evasion of school due to fear of humiliation (failure in school) or insult ('dunce')	Avoiding aversive situations in school by means of switching to pleasurable behaviour
Pathogenic factors	Abnormal bond between mother and child or justified anxiety of being abandoned	Mental or physical problems (learning difficulties or disorder of scholastic skills/physical weakness or disability)	Inadequate development of a conscience (weakness of the superego) or weakness of the ego (due to frustration in early childhood)
Effect	Infantile association with the mother is maintained for the time being – danger of separation remains	Instant emotional relief by means of evasive behaviour – fear that parents may break off contact	Ambivalent approval of school refusal and risk of redirection activity (day dreaming, antisocial behaviour) – fear of punishment

From Harbauer et al. (1980).

development of independence and detachment from the parents. These mothers frequently over-idealize their child and experience feelings of great guilt if they have critical thoughts regarding their child. Subsequently they intensify their caring behaviour (Mattejat, 1981). In these families the father often plays a minor part, tending to be passive and less involved with upbringing. He is thus unable to counterbalance the mother's excessively caring behaviour. This leads to the child or adolescent being unable to accept order, boundaries and guidance within the family system. There is also often a lack of clarity with regard to the roles of the different generations. Children may therefore already be excessively anxious at preschool age and may have difficulties attending both kindergarten and then school.

Physical symptoms play an important part in the process, due to the fact that they suggest a physical cause of the disorder to both the patient and the family. With increasing duration of absence from school, secondary problems increasingly take effect. The child or adolescent, who is usually depressed to begin with, experiences an increase in social isolation. He falls behind at school and develops a secondary anxiety of returning to school. Many children are concerned about being perceived as abnormal, truants or considered merely lazy. In this way a vicious circle ensues, that cannot be interrupted by either the patient or the family.

Family interactions are characterized by the fact that mothers freqently have as much difficulty separating from their child as the child does from the mother. Mothers often cannot permit detachment by the child and react with irritation when the child expresses these demands. The family situation is also often characterized by the fact that the child is more important to the mother than the father.

From the point of view of behavioural therapy, the symptoms of a child or adolescent with school phobia represents an avoidance reaction. It is triggered by an anxious situation and is reinforced by the mother's or both parents' behaviour (operant conditioning).

From a family-orientated perspective, school phobia is regarded as a disorder of the whole family system, going far beyond an abnormal dyadic relationship between mother and child. According to this point of view, families with a school phobic child or adolescent are characterized by an inadequate marital union, inadequate disengangement of parents and child and inability of the parents to confront their child with realistic demands (Skynner, 1976; Mattejat, 1981).

Psychotherapy and psychiatric guidance

A large number of methods have been tried in the treatment of separation anxiety. Psychoanalytical treatment of children and adolescents, counselling or treatment of parents, behavioural methods, e.g. systematic desensitization, parents' training and medication with tricyclic antidepressants have all been advocated. Since 1990, several different approaches to family therapy have also been pursued.

Aims and principles of treatment

The most important goals in the treatment of school phobia are shown in Table 15.3. It illustrates that treatment goals can be classified into three groups: the patient's symptoms, the patient's personality as well as his social behaviour and family interaction and the parents' attitude. This approach to classification

Table 15.3. Aims of treatment for school phobia

Area of intervention	Aims of treatment
The child's individual symptoms	(i) Achieving steady school attendance (ii) Reducing psychosomatic symptoms (iii) Reducing depressed and anxious symptoms
The child's personality and social behaviour	(i) Reducing dependency on parents (ii) Reducing social anxieties (iii) Improving the child's self-confidence and autonomy
Family interaction and parents' attitude	(i) Improving detachment within the family (ii) Reducing overprotective and symbiotic tendencies

From Remschmidt and Mattejat (1990).

emphasizes the importance of multidimensional psychotherapeutic treatment including the patient and his family.

The aims of treatment shown in Table 15.3 can usually be realized if the following general principles are observed (Mattejat, 1981; Remschmidt and Mattejat, 1990).

(i) An attempt should be made to reintroduce the patient to school as soon as possible. The longer school refusal continues, the greater is the risk of a secondary pathogenetic cycle developing within the family system, which may precipitate further symptoms and anxieties. However, this does not mean that patients should be forced by all means to attend school. Their willingness to comply and attend school should be attained or facilitated by means of supportive measures, e.g. accompanying the child to school.

(ii) The fact that no physical disorder is present must be explained clearly to parents and patient. This does not imply, that physical symptoms should be neglected. They should be accepted as real complaints and addressed in the course of treatment.

(iii) Parents should be supported in making clear and appropriate decisions regarding the child's school attendance. Parents should insist on their demands being met and work together to ensure that they are brought about. Children and adolescents should be included in the making of contracts as much as possible.

(iv) All measures should be carefully coordinated with those individuals involved in treatment, e.g. school teachers, general practitioner, in order to avoid mishaps, e.g. that the child is sent home from school or the physician provides a sick note for presumed physical illness.

These general principles are usually sufficient for the treatment of mild cases of school phobia. This may not be the case if school phobia is severe or has persisted over any significant length of time. In these cases treatment over a longer period of time may be necessary. Therapy may take place on an outpatient basis, as day-hospital treatment or may even require admission to hospital.

Different theoretical models and different ways of understanding school phobia have led to a number of different approaches to therapy (Eisen et al., 1995). Besides medication, these approaches include behavioural methods, psychoanalytically orientated psychotherapy and family therapy. In our experience, an integrative approach has proved effective. Specific methods are used depending on the course and the progress the patient is making. Thus behavioural methods and medication, on the one hand, and psychoanalytically orientated psychotherapy and family therapy, on the other, may be used together. The approach, according to which these techniques are coordinated, involves a gradual shift from simple methods and goals towards more and more complicated ones. A treatment strategy is usually developed stepwise and can be applied in the following manner.

- At first the therapist is largely responsible for treatment. He gives both support and extends control over both the patient and his parents. In the course of treatment these functions are gradually taken over by the patient and his parents. Thus the demands on the patient and his parents are gradually increased during the course of psychotherapy.
- A supportive and directive approach is usually advisable. Methods of addressing conflicts and uncovering unconscious motives may be applied once the family is more familiar with the situation, has gained confidence and feels more secure. At this point the family should be able to bear any resulting stress. Treatment should therefore initially be based on behavioural principles. Complementary medication with an antidepressant may help to stabilize the patient in this phase. At later stages of therapy, attention may be directed at the conflicts and dynamics of family interaction.

Indication for different therapeutic methods

Both outpatient treatment and admission to hospital can be effective in treating school phobia. If available, other methods of treatment can also be used, e.g. day-hospital. The following criteria should be considered in deciding whether outpatient treatment is sufficient or whether admission to hospital is necessary.

The child's age

In general, the younger a child is, the better are the chances for a good outcome. Thus in younger children, outpatient treatment is likely to succeed. In addition, inpatient treatment in young children is accompanied by negative consequences. Therefore, it is likely that inpatient treatment will usually be appropriate in adolescents. School phobia is quite common in adolescence and tends to be particularly persistent at that age. Affected patients have often already experienced phases of separation anxiety in their earlier childhood.

Severity of school phobia

The severity of the disorder is even more important for deciding on the method of treatment than the patient's age. The longer the symptoms have persisted, the greater is the risk of treatment being unsuccessful. This applies both to treatment in general but particularly to outpatient treatment. In chronic school phobia, inpatient treatment is usually unavoidable, particularly if one or more attempts at outpatient treatment have failed. In assessing school phobia, a number of criteria should be considered in addition to school refusal, e.g. severity of psychosomatic symptoms, depressive mood, anxieties and frequency of contacts with children of similar age (risk of social isolation).

Severity and extent of contributing factors in the family

This includes all factors of family life relevant for pathogenesis. A number of different contributing factors need to be considered:

- material living conditions, family structure, integration of the family in the local community;
- physical and mental health of the parents;
- possible marital or family conflicts;
- an abnormal or unusual attitude to the upbringing of the child.

In addition to assessing these general contributing factors in the family, the role of symptoms in the family system should be addressed. In most cases, symptoms of school phobia generally do not arise from the patient alone, but represent a pattern of interaction, in which the parents are also involved. In some cases, the parents have the problems with separation and not the child. Even when this is not the case, however, over-protective behaviour, an excessively close bond or parental anxieties may reinforce a child's symptoms. The difficulty some parents have when confronting the child may also aggravate symptoms. Parents who have problems with assertion and confrontation often experience feelings of guilt and frequently have an ambivalent attitude towards the child.

The way in which parents have learned to deal with symptoms illustrates how extensively school phobia pervades family life. If contributing family factors are severe, symptoms of school phobia are likely to continue to pervade family life and parents will reinforce symptoms through their behaviour. In such cases, the chances of outpatient treatment succeeding are small and inpatient treatment is advisable.

Cooperation

External circumstances and chances of success are largely determined by the family's ability to cooperate. There are three aspects of cooperation.

Objective circumstances of treatment

In order to determine whether outpatient treatment is advisable, answers must be found to the following questions. How often is the family able to attend appointments? Which family members will regularly attend appointments? Is at least one parent present at home to ensure that the child attends school?

Ability to cooperate

For example, intelligence and introspective abilities of parents and patient.

Willingness to cooperate

The willingness of family members to cooperate frequently depends on the degree of their distress. The extent of this distress is often influenced by the stage at which the family have sought help. The starting point of any therapy will, to some extent, be dependent on their current view of the problem. There are favourable and less favourable conditions at the onset of therapy. These conditions are shown in Table 15.4. The degree of distress and the level of desperation of the family will largely determine their attitude towards treatment.

Outpatient treatment

In mild cases of school phobia (especially in children under 10 years of age, living in a favourable family environment) symptoms may suggest an acute crisis. In these cases it is often possible to persuade the child to attend school again after giving simple advice to the parents. One should emphasize that the child is not physically ill and give appropriate direction as to how parents should proceed. However, in most cases merely advising parents is unsuccessful and more protratcted treatment is required. Our outpatient approach, which has proved successful, is based on three components:

- a behavioural therapy contract,
- pharmacotherapy, and
- in-depth psychotherapy or family therapy.

Table 15.4. Problem definition by parents of children with school avoidance as indicator for favourable or unfavourable circumstances for therapy

Content of problem definition	Example	Treatment or support expected by parents	
			Favourable conditions for therapy ↑
Interactional	Parents speak about their problem of asserting themselves or their own problem with separation	Family therapy or advice concerning the patient	
Symptomatic			
Psychological symptoms and missing school	Parents are concerned about their child missing school or about their child's anxiety and depression	Psychiatric or psychological treatment for the child	
Physical symptoms	Parents are anxious their child may be physically ill	Medical treatment for the child	
Induced by secondary means	Parents complain about unjustified pressure put upon them by the school or official authorities; struggle against external authorities	Support in confrontation with school authorities or other official authorities	
			↓ Unfavourable conditions for therapy

From Remschmidt and Mattejat, 1990.

Therapeutic contract

A therapeutic contract is an agreement between the therapist on one hand and both the patient and his parents on the other. In making a contract, we generally follow the principles of behavioural therapy. Aspects of interaction in the family are also incorporated.

In the therapeutic contract both patient and parents make certain pledges. The contract is intended to guide the child's (and sometimes the parents') behaviour. This is not, however, the sole purpose of the contract. The importance of implied factors is just as great as those explicitly stated in the contract ('implicit effect'). For example, all the individuals included in the contract are taken seriously and viewed as mature partners. In this manner, both the motivation and the ability to change behaviour is attributed to the patient. From a psychological point of view, the crucial influence of therapeutic contracts is achieved in the interrelationship between external control, on one hand (by the therapist) and internal control on the other (by the patient). A detailed discussion of therapeutic contracts can be found in Chapter 12.

In-depth individual psychotherapy or family therapy

Usually, all matters concerning the contract and problems which may occur in the course of outpatient family therapy are discussed. It is important not only to discuss ways of coping with symptoms, but also other relevant topics, e.g. conflicts in family relations. If symptoms of school phobia can be brought under control by means of the agreements laid down in the contract, time within the family therapy sessions can be freed for the therapeutic work such as problem-solving and communication. In this way, a gradual transition to more in-depth family psychotherapy is made. In other cases psychoanalytically orientated individual psychotherapy for the patient or parents may be the most effective way forward.

Supplementary pharmacotherapy

If the child has a depressive disorder, supplementary pharmacotherapy with an antidepressant may be helpful, e.g. SSRI, which may also have a positive effect on accompanying physical symptoms. Pharmacotherapy is rarely required after the first 2–3 months of treatment.

Inpatient treatment

Based on similar principles, we have also developed and evaluated an inpatient treatment programme for patients with severe school phobia. This programme uses a problem-orientated approach and is not bound to any particular school of pychotherapy. The basic principles are fixed, while details are flexible in order to take account of the special features of each individual case. The programme is composed of five phases (Mattejat, 1981; Remschmidt and Mattejat, 1990).

Preparing the family, making a therapeutic contract, admission

Admission to hospital should be carefully prepared, because the child or adolescent with school phobia will usually resist this step. Frequently outpatient treatment is an essential prerequisite in order to develop a good rapport with the patient and his parents. Once this has been achieved, admission is more likely to be accepted by the patient. When treatment must take place on an inpatient basis from the onset, admission should be discussed both with the family and the patient. The patient should be given the opportunity to see the ward prior to admission and speak to other children or adolescents there.

Inpatient psychotherapy (average duration: $1\frac{1}{2}$–2 months)

This is the longest phase of inpatient therapy and concentrates on underlying problems in the family. Regular in-depth conversations with the parents are held, whilst the child is supported by means of a number of therapeutic measures including reducing dependence on parents, improving self-esteem, reducing anxieties and improving assertiveness with the peer group. If progress can be achieved in this manner, frequently the patient's emotional situation improves, including his sense of self-worth and the depressive symptoms, which often accompany the disorder. Administration of an antidepressant drug may be a useful adjuvant during this stage. During the second phase of therapy, the patient should make an attempt to attend hospital school. This is usually located in the same building as the wards and differs significantly from ordinary schools, e.g. one-to-one teaching, small classes, sufficient attention given to the individual, similarly affected peer group. In this way any fear related to specific situations in school can be significantly reduced.

Reintegration in normal school (average duration: 3–4 weeks)

In this phase of treatment, the child or adolescent is gradually integrated at his local school.This must be prepared very carefully. Initially, the child attends school for just a few hours with the help of the therapist or other care-givers (nursing staff, social workers). This support is gradually reduced until the patient is able to go to school alone and cope with other aspects of school attendance.

Re-integration in the home environment

After a phase of continued school attendance without any accompanying physical symptoms or significant anxiety, the patient is discharged from hospital. This is clearly a critical step with regard to school attendance. Responsibility for the patient's well-being and attendance no longer resides with the hospital, but has been delegated back to the parents, and consequently the family must be offered even more support in order to prevent a relapse at this stage. In this context structural family therapy (Minuchin, 1974) is often helpful.

Outpatient follow-up

After discharge, follow-up on an outpatient basis is critical. The nature of this in terms of intensity and duration will depend on the family resources and expectations. If the patient attends school regularly and if therapy has led to a degree of 'reorganization' of family structure, such as disengagement of excessively close bonds between mother and child, follow-up will not need to be intense. However, if school attendance remains a problem and the bond between mother and child remains an issue, follow-up should take place at short intervals (weekly or fortnightly).

Evaluation, course and prognosis

Kammerer and Mattejat (1981) have evaluated the results of the above treatment approach in a sample of 20 children and adolescents (average age: 13.2 years; range: 9.2–17.2 years). Average follow-up was 19 months. Their results showed that age is a significant indicator for prognosis. All children admitted before their 13th year continued to attend school. In 78% therapy was completely successful in that continuous school attendance was achieved post-discharge. Duration of absence from school before admission was another important indicator for prognosis. The longer a patient had been absent from school, the smaller was the chance of successful therapy. Two patients in whom therapy was ineffective were among the oldest adolescents and had been absent from school for the longest duration. With respect to the whole cohort, therapy was totally successful in 44%, was successful to a large extent in 44% (successful upon evaluation, but not entirely successful at the time of home reintegration) and was unsuccessful in 12%.

These results and our experience in the treatment of school phobia allow the following conclusions to be drawn.

(i) The earlier school phobia is recognized and treated, the better are the chances of success. Almost all school phobias recognized early on can be treated successfully. With older patients and chronic school phobia therapy is likely to be unsuccessful and the long-term prognosis is poor. Parents should therefore receive help and school phobia should be treated as soon as possible. It is clearly important that professionals in contact with children (teachers, social workers, youth welfare services, general practitioners, pediatricians) need to be fully informed about the nature and treatment options in this disorder.

(ii) Successful therapy also depends to a large degree on working with the parents. Those patients who discontinue therapy represent the most important problem. We have achieved some encouraging results with our concept of 'temporary outpatient treatment contracts'. Experiences with other methods (day-hospital, mobile treatment services, outreach, home treatment) have also shown encouraging results. By these means, families who would otherwise be unable or unwilling to accept ordinary inpatient or outpatient treatment can be assessed.

Phobic anxiety syndromes

Characteristics of the disorder

Clinical pictures

Monosymptomatic (specific) phobias

In monosymptomatic (specific) phobias, in contrast to social phobias, symptoms are directed at specific objects and situations. Zoophobias such as fear of spiders, dogs, horses, etc. are quite common, but fear of closed spaces (claustrophobia), populated open spaces (agoraphobia), darkness and other specific situations are also examples of monosymptomatic phobias. Agoraphobia together with panic attacks is discussed in the following section, because most classification systems assume a connetion between these disorders.

Children and adolescents with specific phobias experience severe anxiety attacks when confronted with their phobic stimuli (dogs, spiders, etc.). In addition, they make every possible attempt to avoid such situations. Anxiety attacks are accompanied by somatic symptoms as a result of activation of the autonomic nervous system (sweating, urge to urinate, tachycardia, light-headedness). The personality of such children and adolescents has often introverted and anxious traits. Frequently, they lack assertiveness and have an excessively close bond to a particular person. Family members often have similar personality structures.

Monosymptomatic phobias typically occur during childhood and early adolescence, but may also emerge during early adulthood.

Social phobias

Social phobia is a common manifestation of anxiety in adolescence. Social situations are of increasing importance for adolescents and fear of social situations is often great. Symptoms tend to occur in challenging situations, such as eating or speaking in public, the presence of persons of the opposite sex and all types of public performances. They also fear the consequences of exposure, such as dizziness, nausea, or of being laughed at. Anticipation may also be accompanied by the physical reaction experienced in anxious situations, such as tachycardia, trembling of the hands, nausea, the urge to urinate and avoidance of visual contact.

In most cases, patients are unable to distinguish between the physical symptoms of anxiety and those situations precipitating anxiety. Patients frequently consider symptoms and not the situation or anticipation the primary problem. Symptoms may intensify and become regular panic attacks. As patients attempt to avoid these situations, they increasingly isolate themselves and often lose contact with peers or avoid joining in peer group activities.

Unlike other phobias, social phobias occur equally commonly in both sexes. The personality of affected children and adolescents is characterized by withdrawal, shyness, low self-esteem and fear of failure and criticism.

Despite the fact that terms used to name types of social phobias are largely descriptive, they are nevertheless useful to characterize phobic situations. Examples of social phobias include: examination phobia, illness phobia (nosophobia), sexual phobia, i.e. anxiety connected with sexuality, school phobia (usually based on sepration anxiety), claustrophobia, fear of flying, etc. Cardiac phobia is a particular case of phobia, which can be classified either under 'illness phobias' or under 'panic attacks'.

Aetiology and pathogenesis

Relevant factors in the aetiology and pathogenesis of social (specific) phobias include predisposition, conditioning and negative experiences in coping with anxiety. In this context, the theory of 'preparedness' (Seligman, 1970, 1971) is of special interest. This theory proposes that the anxieties of phobic patients have an evolutionary basis. Anxieties are exclusively directed at objects which have represented real dangers in the course of evolution, e.g. dangerous animals, great heights or sharp objects, whereas anxieties are rarely directed at the achievements of modern technology, e.g. washing machines, cars, radios or television sets. According to this theory, the objects of phobic disorders were previously inherent triggers of normal anxiety and flight reaction in the course of human development, which ensured the survival of the species. Anxious symptoms can therefore be understood as remnants of the evolutionary process.

The theory of conditioning has been extended in the course of the past few years. New theories have been developed, of which modelling is particularly significant. Modelling implies that the patient acquires symptoms from another person, who functions as model for a specific type of behaviour, e.g. taking on the mother's snake phobia.

Psychotherapy and guidance

Psychoanalytically orientated methods are less successful than behavioural methods in the treatment of monosymptomatic and social phobias. However, such methods have been applied successfully, such as in the therapy of 'little Hans', whom Freud (1909) treated for his phobia of horses.

In both monosymptomatic and social phobias behavioural methods are the treatment of choice and have shown superior results compared to other treatment methods (Lindemann, 1996). The following approaches have proved to be effective.

Systematic desensitization

This is a method developed by Wolpe (1958), which is of considerable historical importance and is still in use as an effective method of treating phobias. In this method, the patient is confronted with the phobic object in graded steps: first imagination is used ('exposure in imagination'), followed by actual situations ('exposure in practice'). In combining this method with relaxation training, the patient learns to tolerate first the thought of the phobic object or situation and later its actual presence. Compiling an hierarchy of anxieties with the patient is a prerequisite for this approach. In the course of time this method has been refined.

Flooding

This method contains elements of systematic desensitization but differs in that patients are exposed to a situation or object much earlier. In early phases of treatment, habitual reactions (running away, different ways of avoidance) are prevented. In using this technique, it is important to consider a number of points:

Analysis and understanding of objects or situations which cause anxiety

The triggers and the patient's avoidance strategies need to be precisely identified. An attempt should also be made to understand the patient's coping strategies. In most cases, phobia patients have developed not only avoidance strategies, but also techniques of coping with phobic situations. In order to be successful, therapy must also address these issues.

Careful and detailed explanation of approach

It is very important to explain the aims and objectives of the method to the child or adolescent. The patient must understand that success can only be achieved with exposure, which will without doubt be very stressful. Insight is a necessary prerequisite and can normally only be achieved in one to one sessions. A well-tried approach with children and adolescents is to explain that anxiety regularly subsides after exposure and that the method is tried and tested and will be effective again in them. Explanations such as these can only be made in the context of a trusting relationship when the patient is more likely to bear the discomfort involved in exposure.

Flooding in practice (exposure and reaction prevention)

As opposed to systematic desensitization, during which a phobic situation is imagined, in this approach the patient is exposed to a real situation. Confrontation with a phobic stimulus can be achieved by bringing about a phobic situation, e.g. in hospital.

It is important to remember three things while undertaking flooding.

- Duration of exposure should not be too short. If exposure is stopped before anxiety has substantially subsided, e.g. after a few minutes, exiting the situation may represent an alternative avoidance strategy. Depending on type and intensity of phobia, exposure for more than 60 minutes is normally required.
- The patient should be told that nothing can happen to him and that enduring the anxiety will definitely lead to reduction of anxiety.
- The therapist should assist the patient during the difficult time of exposure, reassuring him verbally and physically, e.g. touching the patient, holding hands.

A number of techniques can be combined with this approach. Because phobic patients tend to be anxious, shy and withdrawn, a combination with assertiveness training is often recommended (Kanfer et al., 1975; Kendall et al., 1988). Social skills can also be taught in other ways, e.g. role reversal, modelling. A number of group therapy methods are also useful, e.g. training groups, enunciation groups. Flooding is the most effective method for treating phobic syndromes.

Differences between systematic desensitization and flooding are given in Table 15.5.

Table 15.5. Differences of exposure techniques for the treatment of anxiety disorders

Anxiety avoidance training (desensitization model)	Anxiety management training (flooding model)
Confrontation in steps (maxim: 'small steps')	Quick and intense exposure (maxim: 'nothing ventured, nothing gained')
Avoidance of anxiety / panic	Induction of anxiety / panic
Relaxation training to reduce anxiety	Training to cope with induced anxiety / panic indirectly leads to relaxation
Antidepressants, tranquillizers or β-blockers may facilitate beginning self-help exercises	Tranquilizers prevent progress; antidepressants are sometimes helpful at the beginning of treatment; frequently they are unnecessary and occasionally even obstruct therapy
Usually performed as supervised self-help	Usually performed by therapist (usually in groups)

From Hand (1993).

Cognitive strategies

The use of cognitive treatment methods (with or without relaxation techniques) can be helpful. These include different methods of problem-solving and self-instruction, combined with assertiveness training. Cognitive methods do not, however, seem to be superior to flooding.

Psychopharmacologic treatment

Two groups of substances have been used most: antidepressants and benzodiazepines. Patients with panic disorder respond to treatment with antidepressants better than patients with monosymptomatic phobias. Otherwise the application of antidepressants depends largely on the presence of accompanying depression.

Benzodiazepines are generally regarded as anxiolytic. Although the temporary administration of benzodiazepines can be recommended for the treatment of children and adolescents with severe anxiety attacks, benzodiazepines should not be taken for a long period of time (more than 6 weeks) because of the risk of addiction.

Case report

Treatment of an adolescent with phobic–obsessional syndrome. The 18-year-old patient was seen because of obsessional symptoms. According to his parents, he washed his hands dozens of times a day and avoided touching a number of objects and places in the family home. As well as the parents, the patient's sister was involved, who induced severe anxiety in the patient merely by her presence. Due to these symptoms, frequent conflicts with other family members ensued, which were quite stressful for all concerned. The father had cardiac and gastric symptoms as well as depressive episodes, all of which he attributed to the patient's severe disorder. He commented on the many months of irritation and conflict in the family with the words: 'It was like hell.'

According to the patient, the disorder developed in the following stages: $4\frac{1}{2}$ years previously he had been ill with influenza. In order to take his temperature, whilst shaking the mercury down into the bulb, he broke the thermometer. The mercury spread all over the floor and was cleaned up by the parents. The mercury was kept in a rubbish bin until final disposure. During these proceedings, the patient did not experience any anxiety.

Two years later, a chemistry teacher cut open a battery in order to explain its function. The battery, which also contained mercury, was put by the teacher on a plate, which was eventually placed on the school bag of a friend who was sitting next to the patient. Anxiety was triggered and increased over a period of months, expanding to include more and more places. The patient was afraid he may have been poisoned or might be poisoned in the future. As he explained, symptoms are known to appear only years after exposure. (Patient: 'AIDS was there years before it was discovered.') He immediately developed coping strategies, such as washing his hands, avoiding contact with 'contaminated' pieces of clothing etc. He did not believe other family members would suffer in any way. He subjectively recognized his anxieties and coping mechanisms (compulsions) were senseless; however, he was unable to resist them. The diagnosis was phobic-obsessional syndrome ('mercury phobia').

Note on the approach to treatment

Seeing the close association between anxious and obsessional symptoms, it seemed advisable to concentrate on the phobic anxieties in treatment, because the obsessional ways of behaviour appeared to result directly from anxiety.

Phases of therapy and interventions by the therapist

Behavioural techniques were mainly used, such as systematic desensitization, exposure and cognitive restructuring. Homework was also prescribed. In addition, sessions were held with the patient and occasionally with the parents. For a while these

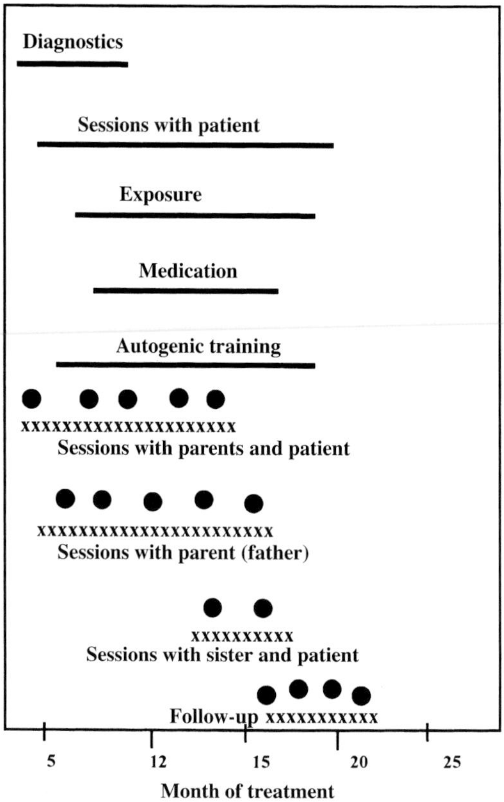

Fig. 15.1. Course of treatment in a case of phobic–obsessional syndrome (therapy with patient: 66 sessions; conversation with parents and patient: 5 sessions; conversation with parents only: 4 sessions; conversation with sister: 2 sessions).

measures were supported by medication with clomipramine. The sequence of these steps are shown in Fig. 15.1.

It became apparent that anxious situations depended on a number of variables. These included: mercury (or 'substitute for mercury'), objects such as shoes and pieces of clothing, that had come into contact with mercury at the time the thermometer was broken or had come near to the mercury, the distance from these objects, the duration of exposure to 'radiation' emanating from these objects, the height at which these objects were situated (the nearer to the head, the more dangerous), the stability with which these objects are placed and skin contact with family members and fellow pupils. The patient avoided shaking hands until the end of therapy. Anxiety was most severe when the patient was asked to imagine touching the end of a thermometer containing mercury. However, the aim of exposure treatment was to enable him to do so.

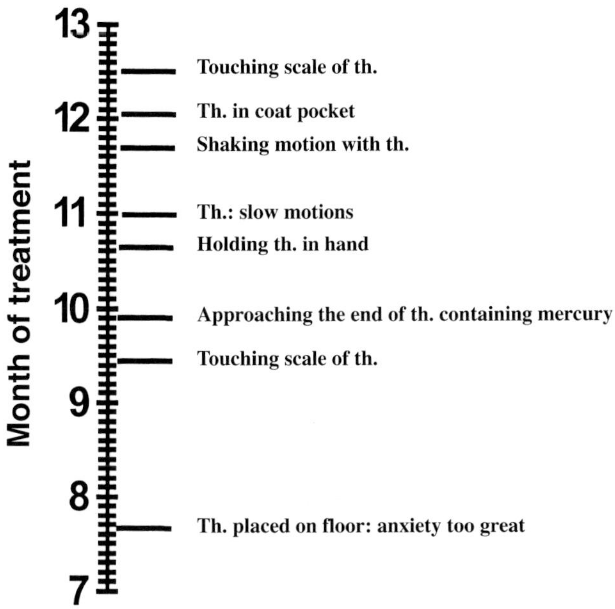

Fig. 15.2. Course of treatment in 'mercury phobia': point of time when anxiety is overcome and the thermometer (th.) is approached.

During the first stage of exposure, the patient was requested to approach a thermometer containing no mercury. He was subsequently exposed to an ordinary thermometer. The thermometer was put in a safe place (on a window ledge), far away from the door of a large room. The patient was encouraged to approach the thermometer as closely as he was able to. During the initial exposure, he was able to approach within 6 metres of the thermometer (see Fig. 15.2 and 15.3). During the following exposure sessions, he was able to approach to within 2 metres.

During the second stage of exposure, placement of the thermometer was varied, e.g. it was placed on a table, then on a chair and finally on the floor. The manner of approaching the thermometer and the duration of exposure were also varied. The quicker the patient approached the thermometer and the longer he remained in its vicinity, the more severe anxiety was. The therapist's 'part' at this stage was to constantly reassure and accompany the patient during exposure, observe the treatment process, recognize the constellation of conditions which triggered anxiety and vary the conditions accordingly.

During the next stage of treatment, the patient was able to come close to the thermometer with his hands and was finally able to touch it, shake it and put it into his own coat pocket. However, these steps were associated with some significant

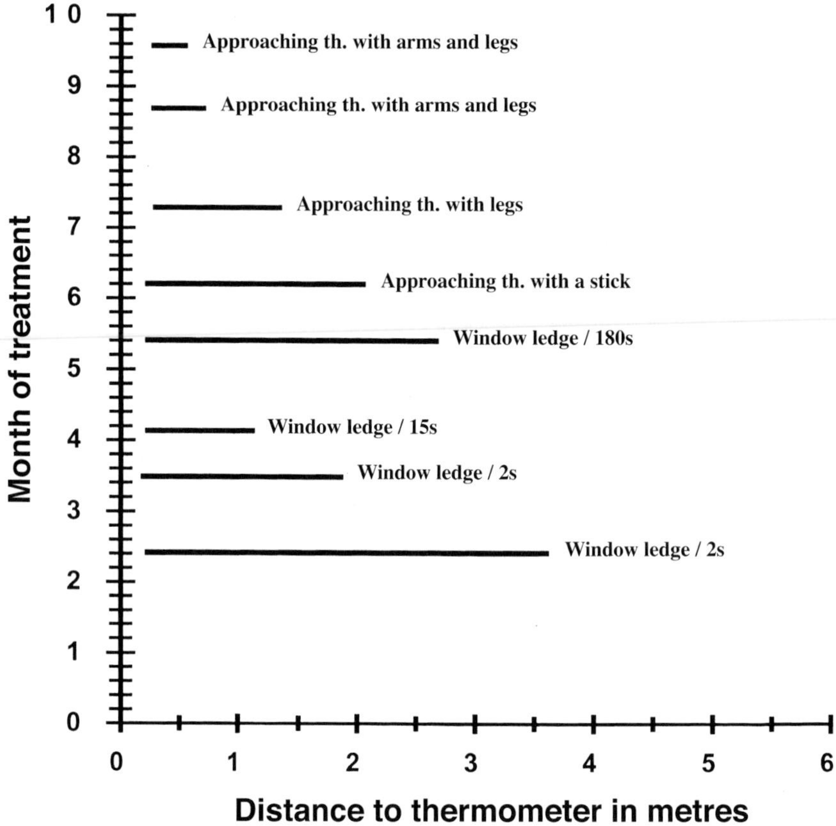

Fig. 15.3. Course of treatment in 'mercury phobia'. th. = thermometer, — = distance at which anxiety is subjectively tolerable / duration of exposure, s = seconds.

complications. The patient's parents reported that he changed his clothes completely after the first session because he was anxious about having 'contaminated' himself. For quite a while afterwards, he came to appointments in his 'therapy clothes'. Family sessions led to greater mutual understanding and gradually eased the enormous tension at home. The patient also made his contribution to decrease the stressful situation at home by continuing his exposure at home. This was carefully planned in conjunction with the therapist beforehand. He gradually became able to enter an increasing number of rooms he had previously considered 'contaminated'. Finally, he was no longer afraid that other family members would thoughtlessly force him into difficult situations. One source of anxiety, however, prevailed: he remained unable to deal with his friend's school bag, onto which the teacher had placed the plate with the battery 1 year earlier. Two years after the end of treatment the situation remained.

Panic attacks and agoraphobia are discussed together because they often occur simultaneously. They are classified under the same category in the commonly used systems of classification.

Panic attacks

Characteristics of the disorder

Clinical picture

One of the main symptoms of panic attacks are recurrent episodes of severe anxiety, which occur suddenly and are not associated with specific situations. For this reason, they are impossible to predict. Symptoms may differ widely from case to case, but usually include a number of physical symptoms, which sometimes appear to be life threatening, such as shortness of breath or a feeling of suffocation, feeling faint or dazed, palpitations or tachycardia, trembling, sweating, nausea or abdominal complaints, depersonalization or derealization, numbness or tingling, hot flushes or shivering, thoracic pain or discomfort, fear of dying or fear of losing control.

These attacks typically last for a number of minutes and occur with variable frequency (anything between a few per month and several per day). Although panic attacks usually are not bound to specific situations, some patients report this connection. If this is the case, such situations are anxiously avoided, e.g. taking the bus or being in a crowd.

In the differential diagnosis, panic attacks must be distinguished from physical disorders. Therefore careful physical examination is necessary before a psychogenic cause can be assumed. Panic attacks must also be distinguished from other anxiety disorders and obsessive-compulsive disorder.

Aetiology and pathogenesis

Despite a number of recent studies, the aetiology and pathogenesis of panic attacks remain unclear. However, two sorts of factors appear to play a part.

Genetic factors and predisposition

As opposed to phobic syndromes, there is no evidence suggesting premorbid predisposition for excessive anxiety reaction in patients with panic attacks. The role of genetic factors is thus still speculative. One remarkable fact is that panic attacks respond well to both tricyclic antidepressants and benzodiazepines, which is not the case with monosymptomatic phobias. Thus it seems that panic attacks are etiologically more closely related to generalized anxiety disorder (formerly called anxiety neurosis) than phobias. In some families there seems to be a predisposition for excessively anxious reactions, and it is possible that through this mechanism, genetic factors do play a role.

Psychopathological mechanisms

Patients frequently express their anxiety by means of physical symptoms, which suggests that psychopathological mechanisms may play a part in the aetiology and pathogenesis of panic attacks. This presumes that physical symptoms represent the primary event, with anxious emotions occuring as the secondary event. The repeated association of physical symptoms with a severe panic attack leads to conditioning of the reaction, which with repetition becomes fixed. According to this theory, a feedback mechanism between physical symptoms and the secondary anxiety symptoms result in panic attacks. Thus internal physical symptoms also play a part in the development of panic attacks. This view is supported by more recent studies. Physical symptoms function as 'triggers' for panic attacks and in the course of time, a 'fear of fear' develops with physical symptoms escalating, ultimately causing panic attacks. Palpitations and hyperventilation are the most important physical symptoms causing panic attacks, and the observation that panic attacks or agoraphobia and hyperventilation syndrome overlap, support this theory. Nevertheless, such theories cannot explain the onset or precipitation of the initial attack.

Psychotherapy and guidance

According to current theories, heightened vigilance of physical symptoms may trigger panic attacks. New treatment methods therefore, stress the importance of exposure to physical stimuli (Ollendick et al., 1994). The following approaches have proved successful.

Exposure

This approach was developed primarily for patients with panic attacks but no agoraphobia (Margraf and Schneider, 1989). The disorder must be diagnosed with confidence. On one hand, physical illness should be ruled out, whilst on the other hand, the function of physical symptoms as triggers for anxiety attacks should be meticulously identified. As in all cases, it is important to explain the treatment to the patient in detail. The approach is specific and depends on the physical sensation which precipitates a panic attack. If, for instance, hyperventilation triggers an attack, treatment should concentrate on breathing exercises. If, on the other hand, palpitations are the trigger, this track should be pursued. It is advisable to induce all physical stimuli physiologically, e.g. through intense physical activity. The patient should then compare symptoms during a panic attack and the sensation he has while exercising (Sturm, 1987). Biofeedback methods can be helpful with this technique.

Developing coping strategies

Most patients have already developed some coping strategies for dealing with their panic attacks. These should be identified and frequently serve as a basis for the development of treatment strategies. Therapy may be aided by relaxation training, e.g. autogenic training, progressive relaxation and biofeedback techniques, in order to control heart rate or breathing rate.

Cognitive approaches

Cognitive aspects play an important part in all of the methods mentioned so far. They can normally be used quite often in adolescence but are less applicable in childhood. When using cognitive approaches, it is important to remember the following points.

- Precise instructions should be given to the patient about the approach. This includes information on pathogenesis, which the patient usually finds helpful.
- Reattribution of panic attacks needs to be practised. This involves comparing sensations which occur during a panic attack with those that occur under normal conditions. Precise self-observation plays a major part in this approach. The patient often has to be taught self-observation because he will tend to concentrate only on physical symptoms during a panic attack and only to a limited extent on his reaction to these symptoms.
- Cognitive techniques will help the patient to assess physical and mental symptoms. The patient is taught to see the interaction between irrational anxieties and physical symptoms and is shown how to influence these symptoms, e.g. relaxation techniques or self-instruction. As soon as the patient has experienced this once, the sense of helplessness and incompetence will begin to be lost.

Additional medication

Both tricyclic antidepressants and monoamine oxydase inhibitors are effective as adjuvant therapy. The newer medications no longer cause serious side effects, e.g. an increase in blood pressure with certain foods. Benzodiazepines are also effective, but antidepressants are the preferred treatment because of the risk of addiction. Medication must always be combined with psychotherapy because the risk of recurrence is great after discontinuing medication.

Agoraphobia

Characteristics of the disorder

Clinical picture

The term agoraphobia was formerly used to describe a fear of wide and open places, but its use has now broadened considerably. Today, agoraphobia refers also to a general dread of public places and crowds in many different places. For this reason, the term 'phobia of multiple situations' has been suggested to be more appropriate for this disorder.

It is not difficult to see how this disorder severely interferes with normal life. Patients are often concerned that they will faint on entering an open place, boarding a bus or entering a department store. They usually search out escape routes, e.g. when entering a church or a department store, which may serve to reassure them for a while. The lack of an escape route can trigger symptoms of agoraphobia. Real or anticipated restriction of movement is an important aspect of agoraphobia. It is frequently associated with depressed mood, obsessional symptoms or social phobia. The fact that several anxious symptoms may be associated with one another illustrates how difficult it can be to distinguish between different anxiety disorders.

Agoraphobia usually begins in adolescence. Anxieties are typically related to the adolescent's individual stage of development. Females are more often affected than males.

Aetiology and pathogenesis

It is interesting to compare the role predispositional or genetic factors play compared with psychological and psychosocial factors.

The role of genetic factors remains unclear; however, it has been repeatedly found that anxiety disorders including phobias, depressive disorders and alcoholism occur more frequently in families where one member suffers from agoraphobia (Marks, 1987). Due to the paucity of adoption and twin studies it remains unclear whether these well-founded results point to genetic factors or indicate psychosocial influences within the family.

Psychological and psychosocial factors

It has long been known that agoraphobia may be triggered by traumatic life events. This is not the case with panic attacks. Such events include illness or surgical procedures, but also financial difficulties or conflicts in the partnership or family. Often patients are unable to remember the initial precipitating event. Agoraphobias can be subdivided into two categories (Goldstein and Chambless, 1978). According to this classification, simple agoraphobia is caused by traumatic events which induce a fear of the identical situation that initially triggered the anxiety. Complex agoraphobia, on the other hand, is basically a 'fear of fear', including all ensuing effects. This assumption conforms to the idea that perceptions of physical change are, in fact, internal stimuli which trigger panic attacks. It also emphasizes the close relationship between panic attacks and agoraphobia.

Generally, both disorders (panic attacks and agoraphobia) are rare in childhood. They are more frequent in adolescence and occur most frequently in early adulthood.

Psychotherapy and guidance

Agoraphobia is treated along similar lines as other anxiety disorders. If agoraphobia is combined with panic attacks, methods to treat panic attacks are used and modified to include the symptoms of agoraphobia.

Exposure is by far the most effective method for treating agoraphobia. If possible, this method should be undertaken in vivo. Initially the therapist is present, but in later stages the patient must learn to endure the situation alone. Two methods can be distinguished in treatment:

- stepwise therapy with a gradual extension of the range of action, and
- massed tasks with direct exposure to anxious situations on several consecutive days.

Patients tolerate both of these approaches to varying degrees. Few patients object to therapy in steps, whereas intense exposure leads 25% of patients to discontinue treatment.

Group therapy is reported to be successful. It is important to gather homogeneous groups of patients and motivation for therapy must be high. Group therapy has two main advantages: first, it improves mutual understanding and reduces feelings of loneliness and isolation to which adolescents may be particularly prone; secondly, discussing the disorder with others helps patients to discover new coping strategies, which can then be included in treatment. The feeling of mutual support which develops during group therapy is also helpful in its own right and helps the patient in his treatment programme.

Additional medication

Medication with tricyclic antidepressants and benzodiazepines is also effective in the treatment of agoraphobia. However, if medication alone is used, the risk of recurrence is great. It should therefore never be the only approach to treatment. A combination with other treatment methods is advisable. This advice is based on results from the treatment of adults. There are no comparable studies in children and adolescents.

Course and prognosis

Panic attacks and agoraphobia are rare in childhood. Only 10% of all cases occur before the age of 16 years. Incidence peaks between the age of 20 and 30 years. In most cases symptoms of both disorders first occur suddenly in public, e.g. in church, in public places, in department stores, at school. The course of the disorder varies greatly and often there are phases in which symptoms occur frequently and symptom-free phases. Both disorders, however, have a strong trend towards chronicity if they remain untreated or have persisted for a long time (over 1 year). Spontaneous remissions are known to occur, but chances diminish once the disorder has persisted for a significant length of time.

Marked avoidant behaviour can be one social consequence of both disorders, preventing patients from taking part in the usual activities of members of their peer group. There is a risk of patients developing alcoholism or drug dependency, especially considering that alcohol and medications (most commonly benzodiazepines) are frequently used as 'self-medication' over longer periods of time.

Generalized anxiety disorder (anxiety neurosis)

Characteristics of the disorder

Clinical picture

Free-floating anxiety independent of any specific situation is the main symptom of generalized anxiety disorder. The anxiety does not occur suddenly in short episodes, but persists as an underlying sensation which is frequently associated with a multitude of physical symptoms such as muscle tension, sweating, trembling, constant nervousness, palpitations, dizziness and occasional epigastric discomfort. Patients often express anxiety about the future, e.g. that they or a relative might fall ill or have an accident.

Classification in ICD-10 distinguishes three groups of syndromes:

- apprehension about future misfortunes, poor concentration and occasionally excessive alertness (hypervigilance).
- motor symptoms such as muscle tension, restless fidgeting, tension headaches, trembling and inability to relax, and
- autonomic overactivity such as sweating, tachycardia, tachypnoea, dizziness, dry mouth and lightheadedness.

Cardiovascular or lung disease, depression and other affective disorders, obsessional syndromes, psychoses and physical illness, e.g. thyrotoxicosis, must be ruled out in the differential diagnosis.

Aetiology and pathogenesis

A marked premorbid predisposition for anxiety in both the patient and his family are assumed to facilitate the development of generalized anxiety disorder. Frequently accompanying depression or at least a predisposition to depression is present. Generalized anxiety disorder is very rare in childhood and usually begins in late adolescence. The age at which the disorder most often becomes apparent is between 20 and 30 years. The disorder frequently initially occurs following an episode of depressed mood. Females are more frequently affected than males.

Psychotherapy and guidance

Because the disorder has no specific triggers, treatment aimed at specific situations, e.g. exposure is difficult. Treatment is therefore limited to attempts to generally control anxiety and develop coping strategies. The following measures are possible.

Relaxation training

Autogenic training or progressive relaxation are particularly effective. Autogenic training may be combined with repeated statements out loud of the patient's intentions concerning his exaggerated anxieties.

Incorporation of physical symptoms in treatment

As in the case of panic attacks, physical symptoms should be induced in the treatment of agoraphobia. The patients suffer just as much from their physical symptoms as from anxiety. Anxiety can be reduced by drawing the patient's attention to physical complaints and incorporating these in treatment, e.g. by means of relaxation training. Improvements may also be achieved by asking the patient to compare the physical symptoms during an attack with those which occur with ordinary physical activity, e.g. palpitations, tachycardia, sweating. Biofeedback techniques may help with this because they can help the patient both to relax and also influence the physical symptoms. Biofeedback techniques are particularly effective in those children and adolescents who are extremely tense and do not know how to relax. In addition, these techniques improve assertiveness and help the child to mature. Thus he learns to trust himself, which leads to improved self-esteem.

Additional medication

An antidepressant medication is frequently given, especially as the disorder often follows a depressive episode. Treatment with benzodiazepines has also been shown to be effective. However, they are almost never prescribed in childhood and only rarely in adolecence. They should only be given for short periods of time (never longer than 2 months) because of the risk of addiction.

Medication must never form the only approach to treatment of generalized anxiety disorder. First, patients may attribute improvement of symptoms to the medication alone and no longer make any attempt to develop coping strategies; secondly, recurrence rates after medication has been discontinued are high, particularly if no attempt has been made to develop coping strategies.

Course and prognosis

The course of generalized anxiety disorder is variable. Periods without symptoms alternate with periods during which anxiety is severe. The disorder usually develops during late adolescence or in early adulthood and tends to become chronic. The longer the disorder has persisted, the worse is the prognosis.

REFERENCES

Eisen, A. R., Kearney, C. A. and Schaefer, C. E. (ed.) (1995). *Clinical handbook of anxiety disorders in children and adolescents*. Northvale, NJ: Aronson.

Freud, S. (1909). Analysis of a phobia in a five-year-old boy. In *Standard edition of the works of Sigmund Freud*, vol. 7, pp. 125–243.

Goldstein, A. J. and Chambless, D. L. (1978). A reanalysis of agoraphobia. *Behavior Therapy*, **9**, 47–59.

Hand, I. (1993). Verhaltenstherapie und Kognitive Therapie in der Psychiatrie. In *Psychiatrie der Gegenwart*, ed. K. P. Kisker, H. Lauter, J-E. Meyer, C. Müller and E. Strömgen, pp. 277–306. Berlin: Springer.

Harbauer, H., Lempp, R., Nissen, G. and Strunk, P. (1980). *Lehrbuch der speziellen Kinder- und Jugendpsychiatrie*, 4th edn. Berlin: Springer.

Kammerer, E. and Mattejat, F. (1981). Katamnestische Untersuchungen zur stationären Therapie schwerer Schulphobien. *Zeitschrift für Kinder- und Jugendpsychiatrie*, **9**, 273–87.

Kanfer, F. H., Karoly, P. and Newman, A. (1975). Reduction of children's fear of the dark by competence-related and situational threat-related verbal cues. *Journal of Consulting and Clinical Psychology*, **43**, 251–8.

Kendall, P. C., Howard, B. L. and Epps, J. (1988). The anxious child. Cognitive-behavioural treatment strategies. *Behaviour Modification*, **12**, 281–310.

Lindemann, K. (ed.) (1996). *Handbook of the treatment of anxiety disorders*, 2nd edn. Northvale, NJ: Aronson.

Margraf, J. and Schneider, S. (1989). *Panik. Angstanfälle und ihre Behandlung*. Berlin: Springer.

Marks, I. M. (1987). *Fears, phobias, and rituals. Panic, anxiety and their disorders*. Oxford: Oxford University Press.

Mattejat, F. (1981). Schulphobie. Klinik und Therapie. *Praxis der Kinderpsychologie und Kinderpsychiatrie*, **30**, 292–8.

Minuchin, S. (1974). *Families and family therapy*. London: Tavistock.

Ollendick, T. H., King, N. J. and Yule, W. (ed.) (1994). *International handbook of phobic and anxiety disorders in children and adolescents*. New York: Plenum Press.

Remschmidt, H. (1973). Observations on the role of anxiety in neurotic and psychotic states at an early age. *Journal of Autism and Childhood Schizophrenia*, **3**, 106–14.

Remschmidt, H. (1992). Angstsyndrome und Phobien. In *Psychiatrie der Adoleszenz*, pp. 284–307. Stuttgart: Thieme.

Remschmidt, H. and Mattejat, F. (1990). Treatment of school phobia in children and adolescents in Germany. In *Why children reject school*, ed. C. Chiland, J. G. Young, pp. 123–44. New Haven: Yale University Press.

Seligman, M. E. P. (1970). On the generality of the laws of learning. *Psychological Review*, **77**, 406–18.

Seligman, M. E. P. (1971). Phobias and preparedness. *Behavior Therapy*, **2**, 307–20.

Skynner, A. C. R. (1976). *One flesh, separate persons. Principles of family and marital psychotherapy*. London: Constable.

Sturm, J. (1987). Ein multimodales verhaltensmedizinisches Gruppenkonzept für die Behandlung von Herzphobikern. In *Herzphobie. Klassifikation, Diagnostik und Therapie*, ed., D. O. Nutzinger, D. Pfersman, T. Welan and H. Zapotoczk, pp. 136–44. Stuttgart: Enke.

Wolpe, J. (1958). *Psychotherapy by reciprocal inhibition*. Stanford: Stanford University Press.

World Health Organization (WHO) (1992). *The ICD-10 classification of mental and behavioural disorders: clinical descriptions and diagnostic guidelines*. Geneva: WHO.

16 Obsessive-compulsive disorder

Helmut Remschmidt and Gerhard Niebergall

Clinical picture

Obsessive-compulsive disorders are characterized by persistent obsessional thoughts or compulsive acts. Both phenomena occur repeatedly in a repetitive, stereotypic manner. The patient recognizes these thoughts and acts as senseless, but is unable to resist them. Obsessional thoughts are ideas, beliefs or impulses, which disturb the patient intensely, impairing his freedom to act. Compulsive acts or compulsive rituals are actions that are experienced as alien to the personality but which the patient feels compelled to undertake, so that he is unable to resist them permanently. Obsessive-compulsive symptoms are closely associated with anxiety. If patients refrain, or are prevented, from performing their compulsive ritual, they frequently experience severe anxiety or agitation.

In assessing the clinical picture it is important to bear in mind a number of points (Remschmidt, 1992): the varying severity of symptoms, the fact that symptoms to a great extent are situational, co-morbid symptomatology (most commonly anxiety, depression, sleep disorders, tics and occasionally aggressive impulses), premorbid personality traits, e.g. excessively adaptive behaviour, anxiousness, withdrawal, and the frequent occurence of specific conditional stimuli in up to one-third of all affected children and adolescents. In childhood and adolescence precipitating stimuli should be sought, e.g. sexual experiences, separation, illness of the child or a family member, death of a family member, etc. Obsessive-compulsive disorder may occur as a syndrome in its own right, but also as a constituent of other morbid states, e.g. organic psychiatric syndromes, anxiety disorders, schizophrenia and Gilles de la Tourette syndrome.

In ICD-10, obsessive-compulsive disorders are classified under the headings 'predominantly obsessional thoughts or ruminations' (F42.0), 'predominantly compulsive acts [obsessional rituals]' (F42.1) and 'mixed obsessional thoughts and acts' (F42.2).

Epidemiology, aetiology, pathogenesis

Epidemiology

Epidemiological studies have shown that obsessive-compulsive disorders are rare. In a review of ten studies Knölker (1987) found that incidence rates of patients with morbid obsessive-compulsive symptoms varied between 0.2 and 3.0%. These figures are based on studies in adults. In child and adolescent psychiatric inpatient populations, these figures vary between 0.3% (Flament et al., 1998) and 4.6% (Steinhausen, 1988). In an unselected sample of school children ($n = 1969$) using the Child Behavior Checklist (Achenbach and Edelbrock, 1983), Remschmidt and Walter (1989) found a prevalence of 0.86% for compulsive acts, 4.21% for obsessional anxieties and 14.32% for obsessional thoughts.

Aetiology

There are several factors that appear to play a role in the aetiology and pathogenesis of obsessive-compulsive disorders.

Genetic factors and constitutional influences

Obsessive-compulsive syndromes are observed much more frequently in the parents and siblings of affected children than in the general population.

Organic factors

Brain dysfunction is increasingly recognized as a possible cause of obsessional disorders, particularly fronto-temporal dysfunction and developmental delay (Knölker, 1987). Recently, a number of findings have indicated that dysfunction of basal ganglia may also play a part.

Premorbid personality traits

Children and adolescents who are anxious and depressed, withdrawn and shy, frequently have few social contacts at preschool age and may suffer from anxiety at that time. During prepuberty these children may develop obsessive-compulsive symptoms, frequently precipitated by external events.

Psychopathological factors

Neuropsychiatric theories assume that obsessive-compulsive disorders are associated with depression.

Psychological theories are largely still based upon the dual nature of learning model (Mowrer, 1947), which originally was presumed to explain the onset and

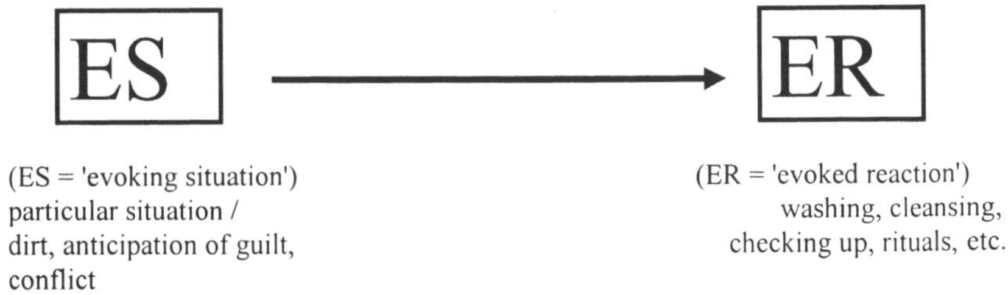

Fig. 16.1. Clinical model of the link between conditional situations and obsessional rituals (Reinecker, 1991).

maintenance of neurotic anxieties. However, it is also relevant to obsessive-compulsive disordes, particularly to compulsive acts. According to this model, stressful conditions provoke a process whereby a previously neutral situation gradually accquires the properties of an unpleasant stimulus (first factor), which is subsequently avoided. The individual learns to avoid these situations by means of certain referential stimuli. Because the individual expects the unpleasant situation to arise despite his attempts at avoidance, acts are performed to prevent the aversive situation from occuring. These preventive acts are reinforced and performed even more frequently (second factor). Because these acts reduce anxiety, they are subjectively experienced as 'successful'. They increasingly become fixed as strategies to neutralize and dispel aversive stimuli and situations. Due to the fact that the acts must be performed each time aversive stimuli are perceived or even imagined, the individual experiences them as 'compulsions', e.g. compulsive washing of hands, although the compulsion is seen as senseless and inappropriate ('I must wash my hands at least three times before meals in order not to contaminate myself with bacteria').

Reinecker (1991) has summarized this link in a simple 'clinical model' (Fig. 16.1).

Pathogenesis

The cause and maintenance of obsessional thoughts can also be explained systematically in terms of Reinecker's 'chain-link model' (Fig. 16.2).

In this 'chain-link model' cognitive components (e.g. subjective 'assessments' or 'estimations') have an important role. In the last few years Mowrer's 'dual nature of learning' model has been modified and cognitive components have been added. Seligman's concept of 'preparedness' has also been influential (Seligman, 1971). This theory suggests that the content of a patient's anxiety can be explained by phobias which developed during the course of evolution (see also Chapter 15). Thus the reactions patients may have when they encounter animals, humans, objects or specific situations that may precipitate

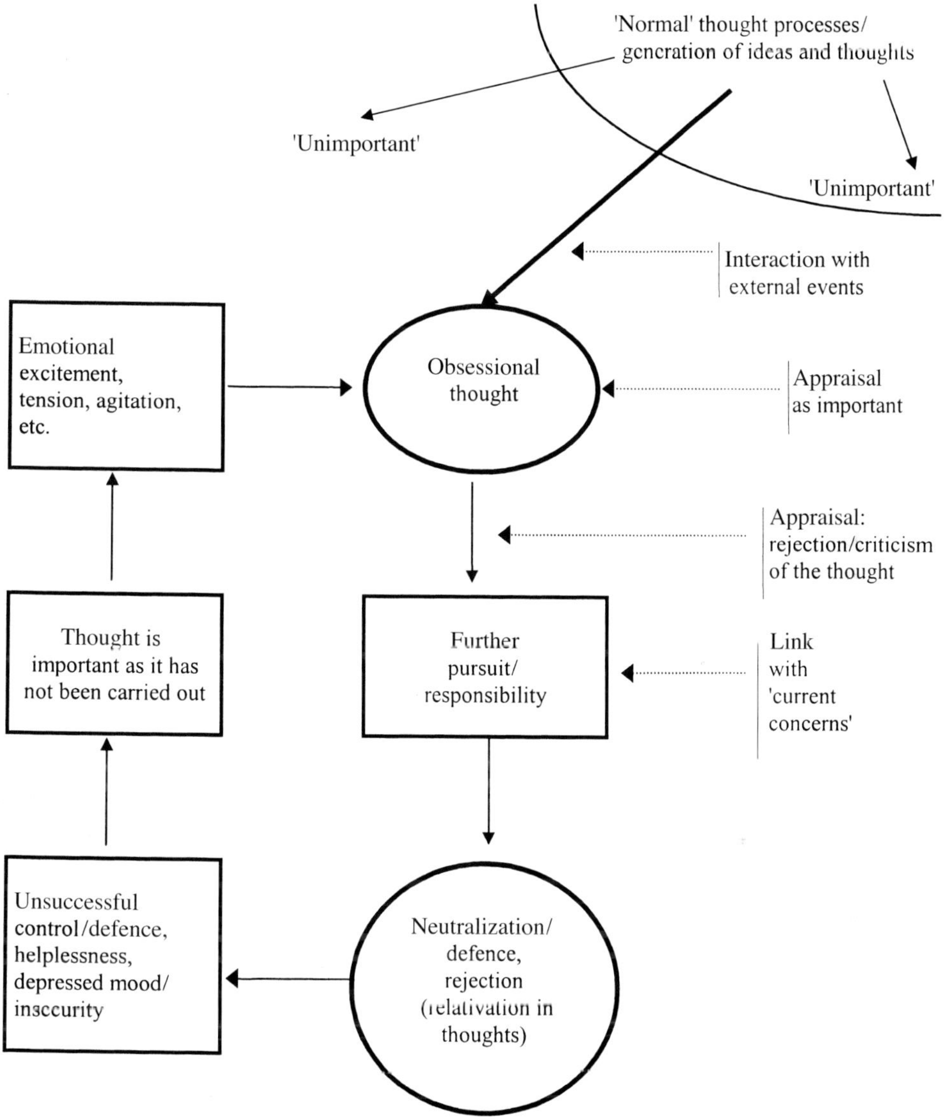

Fig. 16.2. Important elements of a 'chain link model' to explain obsessive-compulsive symptoms (particularly obsessional thoughts) (Reinecker, 1991).

phobias are, in fact, anxiety reduction and avoidance strategies that have spontaneously developed over the course of time. In terms of pathogenesis, a similar mechanism can be proposed for the development of compulsive symptoms as that for phobic anxiety and avoidance reactions. Thus many obsessional rituals, such as avoiding or stepping on lines in the pavement, touching the door knob three times before opening a door, or regularly saying a prayer or magic spell when thinking of a family member's death bring about a subjective reduction in anxiety.

From a psychoanalytic perspective, obsessive-compulsive symptoms are associated with the anal–sadistic phase and early toilet training. According to Freud (1895), instinctual impulses regress in the form of obsessional neurosis. In particular, adolescents with obsessive-compulsive symptoms may experience intrapsychic conflicts when impulses of sexual or aggressive nature intrude upon them. Carrying out respective acts is frequently experienced as forbidden (by the 'superego'). However, impulses continue to intrude (through the 'id') and provoke the experience of anxiety. In this conflict obsessive-compulsive symptoms ensue as a sort of compromise. Symptoms frequently contain parts of the impulses and defence mechanisms at an unconscious level. Regression is one of these defence mechanisms. Regression to a pregenital or 'anal–sadistic' phase may occur if the basis for fixation of libidinous drive has been established in that phase, e.g. by excessive emphasis on toilet training. This results in a predisposition for the development of obsessive-compulsive symptoms (Quint, 1984, 1988).

Treatment methods

Psychoanalytically orientated psychotherapy

Psychoanalytically orientated therapy is still based on the assumption that obsessive-compulsive symptoms represent a defence of the ego. The defence mechanism is that of compromise between drive impulses from the id and restriction by the super ego. In the course of the psychotherapeutic process, which always begins with creating a trusting relationship (Strunk, 1985), the following issues should be addressed:

- the tendency for premorbid personal relationships and emotions to be inhibited,
- the anxiety-reducing function of compulsive acts,
- the frequent association of symptoms with sexual problems,
- the commonly found aggressive component of obsessive-compulsive behaviour,
- the tendency of patients to split interpersonal relationships, representing the internal conflict between the patient's perception and reality,
- the restricted access of patients to their emotional selves.

These variables freqently complicate therapy significantly. Due to their tendency towards inhibition, treatment should incorporate artistic and creative techniques, e.g. drawing or painting, modelling, use of daydream therapy, etc.

In many cases patients can rediscover their emotional world using one of these techniques. Coping with everyday life plays an important part in psychotherapy with adolescents. Adolescents with obsessive-compulsive symptoms frequently develop idiosyncratic mechanisms to deal with their anxiety and obsessions, i.e. improve social adaption and live with less suffering. During the course of therapy, which should gently proceed, the therapist should attempt to understand the function of the coping strategies which the patient has already developed. These strategies may even become an integral part of obsessive-compulsive symptomatology, e.g. in a case of obsessional washing of hands due to fear of bacterial contamination. The therapist should try to understand the function of these coping strategies together with the patient and then proceed to modify them gradually.

Treatment techniques are chosen in each case depending on the age, stage of development, cognitive and emotional capacity of patients and their families. Non-verbal approaches to therapy are more appropriate for children, such as play therapy or other creative methods. They facilitate the trustful relationship which patients undergoing treatment need. These techniques also allow some insight into patients' defence mechanisms. A child with obsessive-compulsive symptoms should perceive the therapeutic situation as supportive and protective. In such a situation the child can experience the acting out of impulses, e.g. aggression without being punished for his behaviour by adults. The child learns to gain insight into the dynamics of drives and can then attempt to express them in a socially acceptable manner.

Verbal techniques are much easier to use with adolescents than with children. A number of factors play an important part in the practice of pychoanalytically orientated psychotherapy: the attitude of the therapist, the manner in which discussion takes place, the subjects spoken about, the precipitation factors relevant to the obsessive-compulsive symptoms and what function they fulfil. It is also important to address the typical problems and conflicts of adolescence in general. The therapist's attitude should clearly demonstrate his willingness to understand and accept the patient's obsessive-compulsive symptoms. This helps the patient to accept his symptoms as a temporary part of his personality, without having to depreciate himself or 'split off' the symptoms. A benevolent attitude, particularly towards seemingly senseless sympoms, helps the adolescent to reveal and discuss all of his obsessional symptoms. Frequently the complexity of symptoms and the extent of their impact on everyday life only becomes apparent at this point. It is appropriate to outline theories about pathogenesis and the function of symptoms to the patient in order to reassure that symptoms are not unique to the patient and that successful outcome is possible with treatment. It may be helpful to point out that some obsessional symptoms may have the function of preventing the exposure of a drive impulse opposing the obsessional symptoms. For example, a patient may deny the wish to dirty himself both literally and figuratively and therefore prevent himself from doing so by means of obsessional washing. Alternatively, aggressive impulses towards family members may be concealed behind exaggerated concern for their well-being, etc. This latter example illustrates the fact that obsessive-compulsive symptoms frequently involve parents and siblings, who often suffer more than the patient. Family-orientated measures are therefore often indicated during certain phases of therapy (see Chapter 12).

Drive-components and other psychodynamic aspects of obsessive-compulsive symptoms should always be addressed very cautiously with the patient, avoiding criticism or depreciation. In adolescents these aspects frequently relate to common challenges associated with development, e.g. sexuality, detachment from parents, attempts to achieve autonomy, demands on performance in school and at work. Special attention should be paid to problems related to autonomy in adolescence. The importance of conflicts concerning autonomy is reflected by fastidious attempts to comply with therapy on the one hand, whilst therapy is essentially boycotted by their obstinate refusal to reveal emotions or block therapy on the other hand, demonstrating their strong desire for autonomy. It should also be mentioned that repressed attempts to achieve autonomy may emerge as aggressive and dissocial behaviour, which may even be directed at the therapist. The psychoanalytic literature unanimously states that such a phase of undirected and unrestrained aggression is a necessary transition stage on the way to personal autonomy and symptom elimination, which must be endured by the therapist (Quint, 1993).

Although a number of theories about obsessional disorders have been put forward and many reports on psychoanalytically orientated treatment of patients with obsessional symptoms have been published, e.g. Benedetti (1978), behavioural methods of therapy have proved superior in treating compulsive behaviour.

Behavioural methods

Behavioural methods of therapy are based on the assumption that obsessional symptoms are conditioned. It should therefore be possible to recondition patients using appropriate techniques. Modern behavioural therapy goes far beyond past methods of behaviour modificaton (March and Mulle, 1998). From today's point of view, these appear much more mechanistic and were applied in a somewhat restricted manner. Previously, treatment was based on the link between 'stimulus' and 'response'. Today treatment is based on a more complex analysis of situations which provoke symptoms and those which sustain them (Hand, 1993).

Aversion therapy

In this method, aversive stimuli are applied when obsessive-compulsive symptoms occur. In the literature there are several reports of the successful treatment of obsessional syndromes by this technique (mostly isolated compulsions). If this manner of treatment is still used, however, it should be used in combination with other methods. Today, it should only be included as part of a comprehensive treatment plan, which should not be predominantly aversive.

Massed practice

With this method, an attempt is made to reduce symptoms by excessive repetition of behaviour. This technique is related to the 'paradox intervention' of Victor Frankl and has been successfully employed to treat compulsive acts and tics (Walton, 1961).

Thought stopping

This technique was introduced by Taylor (1963) and was successfully used in the treatment of obsessional symptoms involving anxiety, i.e. obsessional thoughts, obsessional fears. The patient is asked to verbalize his obsessional thoughts. Subsequently, the therapist interrupts the patient's train of thought by shouting or making a loud and distracting noise. Recent developments in the field of behavioural therapy have shown that the three methods mentioned above are no longer suitable as isolated techniques.

Systematic desensitization

This method is still successfully used today, particularly with compulsive symptoms involving anxiety and in the treatment of phobias. This treatment is based upon learning theory, which emphasises the close link between anxiety and obsessional symptoms. The patient usually finds that obsessional symptoms reduce anxiety. Obsessional symptoms may therefore be regarded as being secondary to anxieties, usually phobias. Hence the treatment should address the primary anxiety rather than secondary obsessional symptoms (Niebergall, 1998).

Flooding

This technique was developed by Meyer (1966) and is based on two principles. In a psychotherapeutic setting the patient is instructed in pertinent aspects of learning theory and the results of treatment using this method are explained. Then the patient is confronted with a situation in which obsessive-compulsive symptoms usually occur. In most cases this results in a severe anxiety attack, which the patient with the help of the therapist must endure. As frequency of exposure to the relevant situation is increased, the intensity of the anxiety is reduced due to absence of negative consequences. The patient experiences having endured a difficult situation. In planning treatment, the therapist tries to evaluate the patient's own coping strategies in order to select those out and utilize those which the patient has previously found useful. Special emphasis is put upon these strategies. This method of therapy is particularly suited for the treatment of children (see the following case report).

Case report

In this case report a combination of therapeutic interventions is demonstrated. The patient was almost 17 and received inpatient treatment over a period of 5 months. The pictures that he drew were of great importance for the successful outcome. Until the age of 15, his development had been unremarkable. His parents had separated when he was $13\frac{1}{2}$ years of age. Shortly afterwards, a vehement conflict took place with his mother, he dyed his hair, began to smoke and took to drinking alcohol. After a short while he developed anxiety that the house was contaminated. He therefore felt unable to touch things, e.g. door knobs. Due to his contamination anxiety he washed his hands frequently (up to 15 times per day). Over the course of time his symptoms worsened both in frequency and in nature. Finally, he would touch objects, e.g. furniture only after having put plastic bags over his hands. Walking around the house he stuck to certain paths and regularly checked he had touched nothing on the way. For a while he was able to control his anxiety by waking his mother in the middle of the night to reassure himself by checking with her whether he had touched certain objects. He was diagnosed as 'obsessive-compulsive disorder, predominantly compulsive acts [obsessional rituals]' (F42.1 in ICD-10). During inpatient treatment, which the patient was eager to begin, cooperation was excellent, he demonstrated good insight and high intelligence (WISC: IQ = 117). Individual psychotherapy was characterized by a combination of psychoanalytically orientated therapy and behavioural methods. During the second session he indicated that he was having difficulties speaking about certain biographical events. As these events seemed to be important for the understanding of his disorder, a non-verbal therapeutic technique was added. The patient was asked to portray the stages in the development of his disorder retrospectively.

Table 16.1. Hierarchy of tasks in behavioural therapy

(i)	Touching own clothing
(ii)	Picking up something from the floor
(iii)	Touching the door to the patient's room
(iv)	Touching the door to the ward
(v)	Touching the toilet door
(vi)	Receiving objects brought from home
(vii)	Touching own shoes
(viii)	Sitting on a chair his mother had just sat on

The order reflects the severity of anxious symptoms (i = easy, viii = very difficult task).

These pictures were discussed with the patient, and helped him to explore important aspects of the anxious and obsessional symptoms.

Towards the end of therapy, the patient was finally able to discuss a sexual conflict – involving an homosexual encounter – with the aid of the pictures. He was obviously relieved to be able to reveal this taboo issue, which was closely associated with feelings of guilt. It was possible to analyse the source of the guilt (parents) and the way in which they were linked to the obsessional symptoms (compulsive washing). Following behaviour therapy, which was undertaken in addition to psychoanalytical therapy, the patient achieved greater mobility. When treatment began, he had been unable to leave the ward. The behavioural method was based on a list of tasks the patient was asked to proceed by. This included objects, places and acts that were in some way relevant to his obsessional symptoms on the ward. Initially the symptoms were severe. Touching a door knob, for instance, led to repetitive washing of hands. The tasks were ranked hierarchically according to their severity, the rank of a task reflecting first perceived difficulty (see Table 16.1). The patient was able to carry out tasks 1 to 3 (touching own clothing, picking up something from the floor, touching the door to the patient's room) after four sessions. However, the fourth task (touching the door to the ward) proved to be much more difficult and was associated with severe anxiety. Anxiety was particularly intense if the patient thought about the fact that he would not be allowed to wash his hands afterwards.

Let us illustrate a practical approach to this method of treatment in more detail. First of all, the patient was asked what anxieties he would experience when touching the door. It turned out to be a fear of contamination by pathogenic bacteria (from the other patients). In a discussion on this subject, he was given 'medical advice' on the true risk of infection. The hope was, that the patient would experience a reduction of his anxiety through desensitization in imagination (Wolpe, 1958), which in fact he did. In the next phase of treatment the patient was permitted to touch the ward door with a glove. The therapist accompanied him whilst performing this step. The patient reported only mild anxiety. But, in order to touch the door with his bare hands, he had to be encouraged much more vigourously. Obviously, the patient was torn in two as to whether he should touch the door or not: he repeatedly approached the door, only to retreat again. Finally, with sustained effort and some persuasion by the therapist, he touched the door for a number of seconds. This task was practised repeatedly (direct confrontation with the anxiety-inducing object and subsequent response prevention). The patient was finally able to touch the door with his bare hands for several minutes, without experiencing associated marked anxiety. However, even at the end of in-patient treatment, the patient still experienced a certain amount of discomfort in carrying out this task. After successfully having completed the other anxiety-inducing tasks on the list, the patient was given positive reinforcement by being permitted to take part in outings and other pleasant activities (in the sense of 'positive reinforcement'). Encouragement by the therapist and nursing staff also had a positive effect on the outcome. After discharge from hospital, therapy was continued in a psychotherapeutic hostel for adolescents. The patient was subsequently able to successfully complete an apprenticeship in carpentry. He re-established contact with his parents and achieved age-appropriate independence. Obsessive-compulsive symptoms had almost ceased. The sexual topic referred to above was taken up in a number of sessions and the patient learnt to cope with this subject.

The behavioural therapy techniques described above are most often used to treat compulsive acts. The techniques available to treat obsessional thoughts are less elaborate. In these cases behavioural therapy should include a combination of thought stopping and desensitization techniques. A number of confrontation techniqes have also been tried.

Finally, it should be mentioned that obsessive-compulsive symptoms in children and adolescents can be so severe that they are refractory to all therapeutic efforts. Such persistent symptoms tend to be obsessional thoughts rather than compulsive acts, e.g. obsessional doubts. Behavioural and mental strategies should be developed which help patients to avoid or circumvent these symptoms. Attempts to influence obsessional symptoms directly are inadvisable. Rather, coping strategies such as cognitive restructuring are developed, which produce subjective relief and adequate social functioning despite ongoing obsessional symptoms.

Medication

Antidepressant drugs have been used for quite some time considering the aetiological and pathogenetic relationship between obsessive-compulsive disorders and depression. Today, clomipramine is the most widely used drug for the treatment of obsessional syndromes. Children under 14 years of age may take 50–75 mg per day, adolescents over the age of 14 may take 75–150 mg per day. In some cases the daily dose will have to exceed this range in order to achieve an effect.

The patients are started on low doses, e.g. 10–25 mg depending on age. The dose is then gradually increased. Medication should not be discontinued prematurely, since reliable assessment of a drug's effectiveness is possible only after 8–10 weeks' time. Existing studies, performed mainly with adults, show that marked improvement can be achieved with clomipramine. Symptoms did not improve in all cases, but patients were able to control their obsessional thoughts and compulsive behaviour more effectively and were more tolerant of remaining symptoms.

The question as to whether the positive effect of clomipramine and other antidepressants on obsessional symptoms is specifically related to antidepressant action is discussed in the literature. Current opinion is not in favour of this theory.

Successful treatments with serotonin reuptake inhibitors have been reported recently. In these studies Fluvoxamine (Price et al., 1987) and Fluoxetine (Turner et al., 1985) were used.

In very severe cases of obsessive-compulsive disorder ('malignant obsessional disorder') treatment has been attempted with neuroleptic drugs, e.g. haloperidol, clozapine. These drugs have proved to be useful. In these cases psychotherapy alone is clearly insufficient for treatment. The use of neuroleptics should be limited to severe cases, whilst antidepressants are indicated for less severe obsessional symptoms.

Course and prognosis

It is generally felt that obsessive-compulsive disorders have a tendency to become chronic. This also seems to be the case in children and adolescents (Wewetzer et al., 1999). In remarking on the course and prognosis of the disorder one must distinguish between two types of obsessive-compulsive disorders in childhood and adolescence:

- temporary obsessional syndromes during early puberty that do not involve all aspects of the adolescent's life have a good prognosis;
- severe obsessional syndromes (obsessional thoughts, compulsive acts, obsessional rituals) that develop in adolescents with primary abnormal personality traits tend towards chronicity.

The possibility of transition from one type to the other will not be addressed here. The number of follow up studies is small. Statements regarding prognosis must therefore be viewed with caution. However, the literature suggests that obsessional syndromes in childhood and adolescence tend to become chronic (Harbauer, 1969; Probst et al., 1979). Follow-up studies have drawn the following conclusions.

- Over a 4–8-year period, obsessional symptoms improve markedly in 60% of all cases; patients show relatively good social integration (Probst et al., 1979; Siefen and Martin, 1984).
- Chronicity with poor social adaptation occurs in 30% of all cases.
- In 10–20% of all cases a severe psychiatric disorder, e.g. schizophrenia develops subsequently to obsessive-compulsive disorder. These rare cases suggest that symptoms may reflect an alternative psychiatric disorder and that obsessional symptoms may be misdiagnosed at an early stage.

Knölker (1987) identified four types of outcome which obsessive-compulsive disorders may have. This study had a follow-up period of $2\frac{1}{4}$ years. The outcomes were characterized by: (i) short episodes and longer difficult courses, without residual symptoms; (ii) development of obsessional neurosis without residual symptoms; (iii) development of obsessional neurosis with residual symptoms or unchanged symptoms requiring further treatment and (iv) syndromes with possible or definite transition to schizophrenia. Of this sample of 49 children and adolescents, 50% were in the first group (those considered recovered), 30% were in the third group and 20% in the fourth group.

Factors associated with good prognosis included: absence of abnormal premorbid personality traits, a short course of the disorder, short time elapsed prior to beginning treatment, absence of additional symptoms, commencement of treatment at an early stage and good compliance with the treatment regimen.

Predictably, the factors indicating a bad prognosis are inverse to those indicating a good one: marked premorbid personality disorder, severe obsessive-compulsive symptoms, an increase in the severity of symptoms, a strong family history of obsessional and anxious disorders and refractory symptoms.

REFERENCES

Achenbach, T. M. and Edelbrock, C. S. (1983). *Manual for the child behavior checklist and revised child behavior profile*. Burlington, VT: University of Vermont.

Benedetti, G. (1978). *Psychodynamik der Zwangsneurose*. Darmstadt: Wissenschaftliche Buchgesellschaft.

Flament, H. M., Whitaker, A., Rapoport, J. et al. (1988). Obsessive-compulsive disorder in adolescents. An epidemiological study. *Journal of the American Academy of Child and Adolescent Psychiatry*, **27**, 764–71.

Freud, S. (1895). Obsessions and phobias, their psychical mechanism and their aetiology. In *Standard edition of the works of Sigmund Freud*, vol. 3, ed. J. Strachey, pp. 25–42. London, Hogarth Press.

Hand, I. (1993). Verhaltenstherapie und Kognitive Therapie in der Psychiatrie. In *Psychiatrie der Gegenwart*, vol. 1, ed. K. P. Kisker, H. Lauter, J-E. Meyer, C. Müller and E. Strömgen, pp. 277–306. Berlin: Springer.

Harbauer, H. (1969). Zur Klinik der Zwangsphänomene beim Kind und Jugendlichen. *Jahrbuch für Jugendpsychiatrie und Grenzgebiete*, **7**, 181–91.

Knölker, U. (1987). *Zwangssyndrome im Kindes- und Jugendalter. Klinische Untersuchung zum Erscheinungsbild, den Entstehungsbedingungen und zum Verlauf.* Göttingen: Vandenhoeck & Ruprecht.

March, J. S. and Mulle, K. (1998). *OCD in children and adolescents. A cognitive-behavioral treatment manual.* New York: Guilford Press.

Meyer, V. (1966). Modification of expectations in cases with obsessional rituals. *Behaviour Research and Therapy*, **4**, 273–80.

Mowrer, O. H. (1947). On the dual nature of learning. A reinterpretation of 'conditioning' and 'problem-solving'. *Harvard Educational Review*, **17**, 102–48.

Niebergall, G. (1998). Psychotherapie bei phobisch-anankastischen Syndromen. *Praxis der Psychotherapie mit Kindern und Jugendlichen*, ed. H. Remschmidt, p. 116–27. Köln: Deutscher Ärzteverlag.

Price, L. H., Charney, D. S., Goodman, W. K. et al. (1987). Treatment of severe obsessive-compulsive disorders with fluvoxamine. *American Journal of Psychiatry*, **144**, 1059–61.

Probst, P., Asam, V. and Otto, K. (1979). Psychosoziale Integration Erwachsener mit initialer Zwangssymptomatik in kindes- und Jugendalter. *Zeitschrift für Kinder- und Jugendpsychiatrie*, **7**, 106–21.

Quint, H. (1984). Der Zwang im Dienst der Selbsterhaltung. *Psyche*, **38**, 717–37.

Quint, H. (1988). *Die Zwangsneurose aus psychoanalytischer Sicht.* Berlin: Springer.

Quint, H. (1993). Psychoanalytische Therapie von zwangsneurotischen Patienten. In *Therapie psychiatrischer Erkrankungen*, ed. H-J. Möller, pp. 528–34. Stuttgart: Enke.

Reinecker, H. (1991). *Zwänge. Diagnose, Theorien und Behandlung.* Bern: Huber.

Remschmidt, H. (1992). *Psychiatrie der Adoleszenz.* Stuttgart: Thieme.

Remschmidt, H. and Walter, R. (1989). *Evaluation kinder- und jugendpsychiatrischer Versorgung Analysen und Ehrbungen in drei hessischen Landkreisen.* Stuttgart: Enke.

Seligman, M. E. P. (1971). Phobias and preparedness. *Behavior Therapy*, **2**, 307–20.

Siefen, R. G. and Martin, M. (1984). Katamnesen bei zwangskranken Kindern und Jugendlichen. In *Psychotherapie mit Kindern, Jugendlichen und Familien*, ed. H. Remschmidt, pp. 112–19. Stuttgart: Enke.

Steinhausen, H-C. (1988). *Psychische Störungen bei Kindern und Jugendlichen.* München: Urban & Schwarzenberg.

Strunk, P. (1985). Zwangssyndrome. In *Kinder- und Jugendpsychiatrie in Klinik und Praxis*, vol. III, ed. H. Remschmidt and M. H. Schmidt, pp. 140–7. Stuttgart: Thieme.

Taylor, J. G. (1963). A behavioural interpretation of obsessive-compulsive neuroses. *Behaviour Research and Therapy*, **1**, 237–44.

Turner, S. M., Jacob, R. G., Beidel, D. C. and Himmelhoch, J. (1984). Fluoxetine treatment of obsessive-compulsive disorder. *Journal of Clinical Pharmacology*, **5**(4), 207–12.

Walton, D. (1961). Experimental psychology and the treatment of the ticquer. *Journal of Child Psychology*, **2**, 148–55.

Wewetzer, C., Jans, T., Bücherl, U. et al. (1999). Zwangsstörungen bei Kindern und Jugendlichen. Daten zum Verlauf. *Verhaltenstherapie und Verhaltensmedizin*, **20**, 421–34.

Wolpe, J. (1958). *Psychotherapy by reciprocal inhibition*. Stanford: Stanford University Press.

17

Depressive syndromes and suicide

Beate Herpertz-Dahlmann

Definition and classification

As recently as 20 years ago, the issue of depressive syndromes in children was controversial. Many psychiatrists felt that children and adolescents lacked the cognitive and emotional capacity to develop depression. At most, the term 'masked depression' was used, where symptoms of some other disorder – usually anxiety or conduct disorder – were thought to reflect underlying low mood. Today, depression is generally recognized as an important psychiatric disorder, frequently occuring in children and adolescents (Beckham and Leber, 1995; Reynolds and Johnston, 1994).

The ICD-10 International Classification of Mental and Behavioural Disorders (WHO, 1992) assumes that the psychopathology of depression in childhood and adulthood is similar. As opposed to ICD-9 (WHO, 1978), aetiology and nosology of depressive syndromes are no longer addressed in ICD-10 (WHO, 1992). This development is based on the clinical findings that both the treatment with antidepressants and the use of specific psychotherapeutic methods are effective in treating 'neurotic' and 'endogenic' depression.

The diagnostic guidelines in ICD-10 distinguish recurrent bipolar affective disorders from unipolar affective disorders. Subclassification is based on the severity of the disorder. Persistent affective disorders are subdivided into cyclothymia and dysthymia. Milder forms of depression are also classified under 'reaction to severe stress' ('brief' and 'prolonged' depressive reaction).

Depressive disorder of conduct is the only form of depression specific to childhood. Recent theories propose that this disorder, classified as 'mixed disorder of conduct and emotions', differs from other depressive disorders in two distinct ways: first, with regard to familial predisposition and secondly, with respect to prognosis.

Recent approaches to the classification of depressive disorders in childhood and adolescence view the disorder as similar to that which occurs in adults. Naturally, however, symptomatology will be influenced by the developmental stage of the child. This aspect of the disorder is increasingly being recognized by research.

Epidemiology

As the definition of depression has become more precise, prevalence data have become more accurate. Prevalence increases markedly from childhood (0.5–2.5%) to adolescence (2–8%) (Harrington, 1994). From puberty onwards, girls are affected more frequently than boys. In a study using the Child Behavior Checklist (Achenbach and Edelbrock, 1983) the item 'depression' was checked in 26% of the 12–17-year-old girls and in 16% of the 12–17-year-old boys (Remschmidt and Walter, 1990).

Aetiology

Genetic and biological causes of depression can only be outlined briefly here. More emphasis is placed on social and psychological theories of the aetiology of depression, as these are particularly relevant for the psychotherapeutic treatment methods discussed later.

Genetic causes

The familial risk for depressive disorders is much higher for bipolar disorders (at least 18%) than for unipolar disorders (at least 7%). Familial risk for depression has also been shown for reactive depressive disorders (about 5%) (Propping, 1989).

Biological causes

The effectiveness of antidepressant medication contributed to the monoamine theory of depression, which assumes that a dysfunction of the brain's monoaminergic system causes depression. Particular importance has been attributed to the noradrenergic system (noradrenalin reuptake inhibitors) and the serotoninergic system (serotonin reuptake inhibitors). Biological indicators include EEG abnormalities during sleep and diminished cortisol suppression after administration of dexamethasone.

Psychosocial factors

Children of depressed parents are usually both gene carriers and an integral part of the parents' environment. This makes it difficult to distinguish gentic and environmental influences. Whereas in non-depressed mothers and their children, there is a correspondence between facial expression and behaviour of the child, infants of depressed mothers showed less positive engagement. Infants of depressed mothers become accustomed to their mother's facial expression and tend not to protest in the way normal children would (Herpertz-Dahlmann and Remschmidt, 1995).

Traumatic life events, e.g. separation of parents, death of a parent frequently precede the development of a depressive disorder. The precipitating event must usually be considered as part of several persistent adversive circumstances, e.g. insufficient emotional support following the death of the mother, child abuse, chronic neglect.

Psychological theories and approaches to treatment

Psychodynamic approaches

Most psychodynamic therories assume that a real or imagined loss leads to the development of depression (Finch and Saylor, 1984). The type of loss and the intrapsychic level, on which coping takes place, is more controversial, and depends upon which theory opinion is based. Depression is considered largely dependent on the development of the ego. As a result, assumptions about the age at which a depression can first occur, are contradictory.

Freud (1917) assumed that depression is principally caused by the introjection of a lost object. The ambivalence formerly directed at the object is now directed at the introjected object, which has become a part of the self. Freud assumed a conflict between ego and superego, whilst Bibring (1953) assumed a conflict between ego and id, explaining the occurence of depression in children of 6 or 7 years old. According to this theory, early traumatization persists at an unconscious level. These children tend to be injured easily and regard every small conflict as an indication of their own helplessness.

The aim of psychodynamic therapy is to allow the patient to recognize the source of the aggressive impulses directed at the self. The patient should make the attempt to integrate these impulses and learn to improve his self-esteem in the therapeutic relationship. As in adults, therapy with adolescents is based on conversation, whilst play therapy is more appropriate for the treatment of children.

Behavioural and cognitive methods

In Lewinson's behavioural approach (Lewinson et al., 1976), reinforcement plays a major part in depression. According to this theory, depression is caused by an individual's inability to experience reinforcement by his own environment. Therapy is aimed at increasing the patient's activity and improving social interaction. Kashani et al. (1981) support the theory that a lack of social competence and communication skills contribute to the development of depression in childhood.

Cognitive theories include the idea of 'learned helplessness' (Seligman, 1975) and the idea of 'cognitive distortion' (Beck et al., 1979). Both have gained considerable credence over the course of time.

According to Seligman's theory, the depressed individual experiences success or failure as entirely independent of his own influence and behaviour, resulting in a feeling of great helplessness. This causes a negative attitude with respect to future events. Depressed individuals constantly expect detrimental events to occur, which they perceive as being outside their range of control. The theory of learned helplessness implies that a depressed individual tends to attribute all failures to his own behaviour ('personalization'), focuses on details of a situation while ignoring other aspects that are equally important ('selective abstraction'), draws negative conclusions on the basis of insufficient evidence ('arbitrary inference') and draws general conclusions from single incidents ('overgeneralization').

Beck et al. (1979) described his method of cognitive behaviour therapy as an active, directive, time-limited and structured psychotherapeutic method, based on the assumption that an individual's emotions and behaviour are determined by the way in which the individual shapes his environment. This method has gained great importance in the treatment of adults and has been evaluated in detail. Encouraging attempts have been made to apply this technique also to children and adolescents (Dudley, 1997; Wilkes et al., 1994). The technique is described in greater detail in Chapter 7.

Beck's theory of depression is based on three assumptions, which explain the development and maintenance of depressive symptoms (Beck et al., 1979).

(i) The patient has depreciative thoughts about himself (negative self-appraisal).
(ii) He is only able to see failures, disadvantages and disappointments in his interaction with the environment (negative perspective).
(iii) He assumes that failure and frustration will continue perpetually (negative expectations).

Depressed individuals typically make these basic assumptions. Thus, both past and present events are interpreted to a negative perspective, which cannot be countered by rational argument. Depressive thought patterns thereby prevent the planning of constructive and optimistic actions.

These dysfunctional beliefs, in addition to negative self-esteem, negative interaction with the environment and negative expectations, have been shown to be present in depressed children and adolescents (Kovacs and Beck, 1977; Kazdin et al., 1983).

Case report

This case report is intended to illustrate the typical logical mistakes and distorted information processing which depressed adolescents have, in this case a 16-year-old girl. The case serves to illustrate the use of cognitive treatment methods, which Wilkes and Rush (1988) have adapted for use with adolescents.

The patient presented to an ENT-hospital requesting a cosmetic operation for her nose because she felt it was ugly and disfiguring. The doctors were unable to perceive any abnormality and refused the operation. The patient subsequently withdrew from all social activities and isolated herself. If she had to go to town, she would cover her nose with her hand. She avoided entering shops and public places. In the family she was apathetic, neglected her appearance and wore only black clothes. She was admitted for inpatient child and adolescent treatment because of depressed mood and attempted suicide.

Several distorted cognitions described by Beck et al. (1979) became apparent during the first interview.

Arbitrary inference

'After I took the tablets to kill myself, I vomited. My mother thought I had an upset stomach and didn't notice how I really felt. A mother who loves her child notices something like that. Therefore, she doesn't care about me.'

Personalization

'Yesterday my father was in a bad mood. He was probably in that mood because he couldn't bear looking at my ugly face.'

Minimization

'I won the sports event, but anyone could have done that with a little bit of practice.'

Maximization

'My nose is too big. Therefore, I cannot accept other parts of my body either.'

Over-generalization

'When I came back to school after the holidays, a fellow pupil ignored me. That proved that no one in school likes me.'

Dichotomous thinking

'Either one has a nice nose and looks attractive, or one is ugly and looks unattractive.'

Cognitive therapy concentrates on changing things in the 'here and now' and does not make attempts to uncover any conflicts of early childhood. The therapist plays an empathic and active role by asking questions. By asking questions he avoids imposing his opinion on the patient. Allowing the patient to consider the pros and cons of his opinions ultimately helps the patient to (i) recognize, (ii) examine and (iii) alter his fixed cognitions and become more realistic in his ways of thinking.

The patient (P.) talks to her therapist (Th.) about a weekend spent at home:

P.: 'When I went to the fair, everybody looked at me because of my big nose.'

Th.: 'How do you know they were looking at your nose? Did you ask someone?'

P.: 'I didn't ask anyone. But lots of young people came and asked why I had been away for so long.'

Th.: 'Did they perhaps look at you because they hadn't seen you for such a long time?'

P.: 'Um. They wanted to know if I would like to do something together with them next weekend.'

Th.: 'Would you invite someone whom you don't like and who you think is ugly?'

P.: 'No, I don't think I would. Maybe they do like something in me after all.'

These kinds of thoughts are typical for the depressed patient. By analysing such thoughts, the therapist may elucidate the patient's dysfunctional assumptions. In this example, the patient is convinced that her esteem and success depend entirely on her appearance. In the course of therapy, many patients learn to pursue similar internal dialogues in situations which cause anxiety.

At the end of each session the patient is given a task as 'homework'. The tasks should increase in difficulty from session to session, but should not be too difficult for the patient to fulfil. The patient should be permitted to experience some success in order to improve self-esteem and motivation to continue therapy.

In this case the patient participated in outings into town, during which she was not permitted to cover her nose. Later on, shopping trips and visits to a youth club were added to her list of tasks. The patient was asked to write down her impressions and experiences and discuss them during therapy.

At the end of treatment, the patient had still not learnt to accept the appearance of her nose. However, she was increasingly able to overcome her tendency to withdraw and her anxiety of being rejected. She found new friends, participated in age-appropriate activities and coped well with re-integration in school. The relationship towards her mother had changed during therapy, so that she was finally able to discuss some problems together with her mother.

Emotional training

Cognitive behaviour therapy may include several approaches, including emotional training. Children and adolescents should be allowed to explore their own emotional world and have the opportunity to experience the way other individuals feel, e.g. the wide spectrum of emotions including happiness, indifference, sadness, disconsolation. In therapy, identifying expressions or gestures, e.g. in illustrations may help the child discover his emotional world (Stark et al., 1991).

Self-control methods

An attempt to change depressive cognitions can be made by means of self-observation, self-appraisal and self-reinforcement (Rehm, 1977).

Self-observation helps to identify stressors and negative thoughts in everyday life and allows the child to recognize the effects of therapy. In self-appraisal training, children are taught to see themselves in a more realistic and optimistic perspective. They are also taught to perceive the good sides of themselves and recognize positive development. Children learn to reward themselves by self-reinforcement for developing constructive coping strategies (Stark et al., 1991).

Activating the patient

In most cases of depression in childhood or adolescence, it is helpful to make a timetable for all activities or outings the child is required to participate in. A healthy level of activity is incompatible with several symptoms of depression: the tendency to withdraw, a passive attitude and reduced motivation. This activation can help the child to understand the association of positive experiences and improved mood.

Social skills training

Social skills training should include both verbal and non-verbal skills, e.g. eye contact, facial expression, which are important for expressing and perceiving both positive and negative emotions. It usually includes instruction, modelling and practice of appropriate social behaviour, with feedback from the therapist. The child should learn to think about a problem first, develop coping strategies and consider the consequences of actions before proceeding to act.

Problems in the course of therapy

There are several commonly encountered problems when treating children and adolescents. Cognitive behaviour therapy requires that patients play an important part in promoting treatment. However, depressed patients are often passive and have a tendency to say very little in therapy. Therefore, a child or adolescent may find it difficult even to carry on a conversation. The hopelessness and anhedonia typical for depression may cause children or adolescents to doubt that therapy will improve their situation ('There's no point to it all'). Due to his depression, activities intended as positive reinforcement may not be perceived as such. Problems with concentration and difficulty in making decisions may also impair the therapeutic progress.

In treating depressed children and adolescents, the therapist should give the utmost attention to maximizing compliance, including demonstrating professional commitment and providing pleasant surroundings. Role playing, storytelling and looking at pictures are more helpful than words alone to help the patient to participate in therapy. Therapeutic interventions and advice should not be vague or general, but should fit the child's and the family's individual circumstances. The family should be included regularly in the treatment of adolescents. This ensures that all persons involved in treatment relate to the patient in a similar understanding manner and do not submit the patient to undue stress.

Evaluation studies

Whilst the effectiveness of cognitive behaviour therapy has been evaluated in a large number of studies in adults, there are few studies on this type of therapy in children and adolescents.

Reynolds and Coats (1986), with a sample of 30 children and adolescents, compared the effect of cognitive behaviour therapy or relaxation training using patients on a waiting list as a control group. Both methods of treatment were applied twice a week for a total of 5 weeks. Compared to the patients on the waiting list, both treatment groups experienced a significant reduction of depressive symptoms which persisted for at least 5 weeks after the end of therapy.

Stark et al. (1987) studied 29 depressed school children 9–12 years old, who participated either in a self-control programme or in behavioural training of problem-solving skills. The self-control programme included self-observation, self-appraisal and modulation of attributions. Behavioural training of problem-solving skills emphasized emotional training (see above), self-observation during pleasant situations, planning of activities and acquisition of social skills. Both groups showed a significant reduction of depressive symptoms compared to the group on waiting lists. Improvement was particularly marked in the self-control group.

Stark et al. (1991) performed a further study in 24 children treated either with cognitive behaviour therapy or traditional supportive therapy. The children met in groups of four with two therapists to a group. Treatment consisted of 24–26 sessions held over $3\frac{1}{2}$ months, with additional family sessions once a month. After treatment, both groups showed improvement, which was significantly more marked in the group with cognitive behaviour therapy. This difference was no longer detectable 7 months after termination of therapy. The authors attribute this to the fact that the treatment goups were incomplete at the time of follow-up. Long-term outcome of cognitive behaviour therapy in childhood and adolescence has not yet been conclusively evaluated. However, a recent meta-analysis based on seven studies in clinically diagnosed depressed adolescents demonstrated that cognitive behaviour therapy is significantly superior to the comparison interventions (Harrington et al., 1998).

Suicidal behaviour

Definition

Attempted suicide implies the occurrence of an action with the intention of putting an end to one's life. In completed suicide, this intention is actually achieved.

Suicide and attempted suicide may occur in a various psychiatric conditions. Therefore, there is no single diagnostic category in ICD-10 (nor in other classification systems) in which to classify suicide. However, in the case of emotionally unstable personality disorder (borderline type), suicidal behaviour is explicitly mentioned as a typical symptom.

In differential diagnosis, one must distinguish between suicidal behaviour and acts of self-harm.

Epidemiology

The prevalence of completed suicide in childhood (age 5–14 years) is 0.5–1.0 per 100 000 individuals of this age group. Prevalence increases in adolescence and early adulthood (age 15–24 years) and thereafter reaches a prevalence of 12–16 per 100 000.

The rate of attempted suicide is more difficult to determine because of a large probable number of unknown cases. In children it is assumed to be about 1% and in adolescents 2–9% (Shaffer and Piacentini, 1994; Pfeffer, 1991).

In Western cultures, the rate of completed suicide is higher in males, whereas the rate of attempted suicide is higher in females. This difference does not apply to all cultures. This may be explained by the fact that males tend to use harsher suicide methods (firearms, hanging) than females (intoxication, jumping from great height), which are more likely to cause death (Shaffer and Piacentini, 1994).

Aetiology

The families of individuals who complete suicide frequently have an increased familial risk of suicide. Neurochemical studies suggest that abnormalities of serotonin metabolism in the brain may be involved in patients with suicide. Imitation and 'contagion' also play a part. After the suicide of prominent individuals, suicide rates particularly in adolescents increase for about 1–2 weeks. Televised dramatizations of suicide have a similar effect on suicide rates (Gould et al., 1988).

Psychiatric disorders are an important cause of suicide. About 15% of individuals with mood disorders, 10% of those with schizophrenia and 2–4% of those with chronic alcoholism commit suicide. Drug addiction is also associated with a high suicide rate. Previous suicide attempts increase the risk of completed suicide. Rates of completed suicide in male adolescents who had already attempted suicide, were 100 per 100 000. The suicide rate for depressed adolescents is 270 per 100 000 and for the normal population it is only 4 per 100 000 (Gould et al., 1990).

Triggering events

In cases of suicidal behaviour in adolescents, preceding crises can usually be identified, e.g. fear of punishment after commiting a crime, rejection, problems with school, drugs or alcohol, end of a relationship, etc. The most frequent cause of attempted suicide appears to be conflicts in the family (Remschmidt, 1992).

Family environment

There are frequently problems in the families of patients who perform suicidal acts. Findings include an above average rate of psychiatric disorders and a style of upbringing with frequent punishment, disinterest or lack of understanding. Many adolescents who attempt suicide feel that their parents make excessive demands on them. There is a significant association of suicide and child abuse in families. This issue should be addressed in therapy.

Assessment of risk

The physician or psychotherapist is frequently confronted with the question as to the risk of suicide in a particular individual, i.e. they have to decide in individual cases whether or not treatment in an inpatient facility is necessary. If a patient has presented for assessment, the appropriateness of inpatient treatment should be discussed with a senior child and adolescent psychiatrist, particularly if compulsory admission is being considered.

The following criteria have proved helpful in identifying an increased risk for suicide:

- active suicide ideas, rejection of alternatives and precise plans for committing suicide;
- presence of depression or another psychiatric disorder;
- previous suicide attempts; the risk of completed suicide seems to be highest during the year after a suicide attempt;
- previous suicide attempts using methods other than overdosing;
- the patient is a relative or close friend of someone, who has also made an attempt at suicide;
- social isolation;
- discord between the adolescent and his environment; violence in the family or impending divorce of parents;
- stressful events outside the family, e.g. failure in school, conflicts due to anti-social behaviour, drug or alcohol abuse;
- the patient's wish to be admitted to hospital.

Treatment

The steps to be taken in cases of attempted suicide or suicidal threats are detailed in Table 17.1.

Acute phase and initial treatment

If suicide has already been attempted, an intervention should be made as early as possible, ideally at the site of the incident. After the adolescent's 'return to life', both the adolescent and the parents will be in an emotionally charged state, which can be used to facilitate therapeutic steps (Remschmidt, 1992). This time should be used to obtain information on motives and the background facts of the suicide attempt. The first steps to building a trusting relationship with the patient should be made. The therapist's attention and concern may help to counteract the patient's typically depressive view that he is worthless and without hope.

During inpatient psychotherapy, an attempt should be made together with the patient to develop ideas other than thoughts of suicide. Strategies for coping with difficult situations should be developed. This approach is similar to the cognitive behavioural treatment of depression. The therapist should encourage the adolescent to discuss those thoughts and emotions which caused the suicide attempt. It is helpful to develop a written plan of how to cope with situations in which ideas of suicide recur frequently. It should contain several alternative strategies and should always be accessible to the patient.

Table 17.1. Steps to be taken in the case of attempted suicide or suicidal threats

Acute phase 1 (inpatient treatment)	Acute phase 2 (inpatient treatment)	Recovery phase (inpatient treatment)	Remission phase (outpatient treatment)
Intensive care unit	Psychiatric/ psychotherapeutic ward	Psychiatric/ psychotherapeutic ward	Clinic, private practice
Treatment of physical complications	Observation and care by nursing staff	Extended range of action, e.g. leaving the ward in company of other patients	Observation at home by persons close to the patient
Consultation of psychiatric/ psychotherapeutic liaison services for assessment of motives for suicide	Regular individual conversations to assess conflicts triggering attempted suicide; development of coping strategies	Continued individual therapy sessions, development of a suicide prevention plan	Frequent sessions with the therapist, possibly supported by telephone calls
	Integration of the patient in groups, e.g. group psychotherapy, occupational therapy	Continued group therapy	
Initial approach to the family	Decision about the type and frequency of sessions with the family, e.g. counselling, family therapy, etc.	More frequent sessions with parents; family sessions to prepare for discharge	Continued sessions with parents or family sessions ; addressing new stressful situations or conflicts
		Steps to change environmental factors, e.g. inform other persons close to the patient	Help with social re-integration, e.g. informing the school
Goal: acute medical care, assessment of remaining suicide risk, building a trusting relationship, 'diagnosis' of familial background	Goal: to prevent self-injurious impulses, intensify the relationship with the therapist, reduce social isolation, discuss the familial conflicts leading to attempted suicide	Goal: to stabilize the therapeutic relationship; change conditions leading to attempted suicide; prepare social re-integration	Goal: prevention of any further suicide attempts; activation of 'co-therapists'

In addition to individual therapy, group therapy with patients of the same age group is recommended. This approach facilitates social integration and activity. The patient may otherwise continue to be isolated, and thus remain at higher risk for further suicide attempts.

Outpatient treatment

It must be ensured that the patient has adequate support by persons close to him after discharge. Apart from outpatient treatment, the patient must be carefully observed in his own environment. Frequently ideas of suicide recur after discharge. A contract should be made with the patient, in which he agrees to refrain from attempting suicide for a defined length of time. The higher the risk of suicide, the shorter the length of time should be. The contract should be signed by both the patient and the therapist. This helps to demonstrate to the patient that he is being taken seriously. Regular telephone conversations are recommended in the interval between sessions. During these telephone conversations, the patient is asked to briefly report on his present situation. The telephone calls should take place punctually at regular times. They serve to structure the jeopardized adolescent's time between sessions. The patient should be instructed to call the therapist immediately if suicidal impulses occur. Every session should include the making of a new appointment at a fixed date and time. Follow-up should not be terminated too soon, because the risk of recurrence in adolescents is fairly high (see below).

Participation of the family and the social environment

After an initial phase of 'family diagnostics', the form and intensity of further collaboration must be decided upon, e.g. whether parents desire advice or wish to participate in family therapy etc. Certain topics must be discussed with parents, such as offended feelings, attributions of guilt or possible discord in the family, which may have precipitated the suicide attempt.

If possible, other individuals close to the patient, e.g. teachers or persons also involved in upbringing should be included in the treatment, provided they can help the patient deal with any conflicts which arise. Confronting the patient with the individuals held responsible for the suicide attempt may be helpful, but should always aim to be constructive. No promises should be made which cannot be kept.

As in the treatment of depressed children and adolescents, the therapist will have to use all of his talent and creativity in therapy in order to impart a feeling of security, competency and self-assurance. This feeling will help the patient to develop alternative problem solutions in difficult situations in the future.

Prognosis

There are very few studies that compare psychotherapeutic methods of treating children and adolescents after attempted suicide. Cognitive behavioural methods of treating children, adolescents and their families have been shown to be encouraging (Rotheram-Borus et al., 1994).

The risk of recurrence is very high: up to 50% of adolescents who attempted suicide make further attempts; 4–10% of these are fatal. Therefore, preventive measures are very important.

REFERENCES

Achenbach, T. M. and Edelbrock, C. S. (1983). *Manual for the child behavior checklist and revised child behavior profile*. Burlington: Queen City Printers.

Beck, A. T., Rush, A. J., Shaw, B. F. and Emery, G. (1979). *Cognitive therapy of depression*. New York: Guilford.

Beckham, E. E. and Leber, W. R. (ed.) (1995). *Handbook of depression*, 2nd edn. New York: Guilford Press.

Bibring, E. (1953). The mechanism of depression. In *Affective disorders*, ed. P. Greenacre, pp. 13–48. New York: International Universities Press.

Dudley, C. D. (1997). *Treating depressed children. A therapeutic manual of cognitive behavioral interventions*. Oakland, CA: New Harbinger Publications.

Finch, A. J. and Saylor, C. F. (1984). An overview of child depression. *Progress in Pediatric Psychology*, pp. 201–38.

Freud, S. (1917). Mourning and melancholia. In *Standard edition of the works of Sigmund Freud*, vol. 14, ed. J. Strachey, pp. 243–58. London: Hogarth Press.

Gould, M. S., Shaffer, D. and Kleinmann, M. (1988). The impact of suicide in television movies. Replication and commentary. *Suicide and Life-Threatening Behavior*, **18**, 90–9.

Gould, M. S., Shaffer, D. and Davies, M. (1990). Truncated pathways from childhood. Attrition in follow-up studies due to death. In *Straight and devious pathways from childhood to adulthood*, ed. L. Robins and M. Rutter, pp. 3–10. Cambridge: Cambridge University Press.

Harrington, R. (1994). Affective disorders. In *Child and adolescent psychiatry. Modern approaches*, ed. M. Rutter, E. Taylor and L. Hersov, pp. 330–50. Oxford: Blackwell Scientific.

Harrington, R., Wood, A. and Verduyn, C. (1998). Clinically depressed adolescents. In *Cognitive-behaviour therapy for children and adolescents and families*, ed. P. Graham, pp. 156–93. Cambridge: Cambridge University Press.

Herpertz-Dahlmann, B. and Remschmidt, H. (1995). Entwicklungsabweichungen infolge von Störungen der Kind-Umwelt-Interaktionen im Säuglingsalter. *Kindheit und Entwicklung*, **11**, 15–24.

Kashani, J. H., Husain, A., Shekim, W. O., Hodges, K., Cytryn, L. and McKnew, D. H. (1981). Current perspectives on childhood depression. An overview. *American Journal of Psychiatry*, **138**, 143–52.

Kazdin, A. E., French, N. H., Unis, A. S. and Esveldt-Dawson, K. (1983). Assessment of childhood depression. Correspondence of child and parent ratings. *Journal of the American Academy of Child and Adolescent Psychiatry*, **22**, 157–64.

Kovacs, M. and Beck, A. T. (1977). An empirical–clinical approach toward a definition of childhood depression. In *Depression in childhood. Diagnosis, treatment and conceptual models*, ed. J. G. Schulterbrandt and A. Raskin, pp. 1–25. New York.

Lewinson, P. M., Biglan, A. and Ziess, A. M. (1976). Behavioral treatment of depression. In *The behavioral management of anxiety, depression and pain*, ed. P. O. Davidson, pp. 91–146. New York: Brunner and Mazel.

Pfeffer, C. R. (1991). Suicide and suicidality. In *Textbook of child and adolescent psychiatry*, ed., J. M. Wiener, pp. 507–14. Washington, DC: American Psychiatric Press.

Propping, P. (1989). *Psychiatrische Genetik*. Berlin: Springer.

Rehm, L. P. (1977). A self-control model of depression. *Behavior Therapy*, **8**, 787–804.

Remschmidt, H. (1992). *Psychiatrie der Adoleszenz*. Stuttgart: Thieme.

Remschmidt, H. and Walter, R. (1990). *Psychische Auffälligkeiten bei Schulkindern*. Göttingen: Hogrefe.

Reynolds, W. M. and Coats, K. I. (1986). A comparison of cognitive-behavioural therapy and relaxation-training for the treatment of depression in adolescents. *Journal of Consulting and Clinical Psychology*, **54**, 653–60.

Reynolds, W. M. and Johnston, H. F. (ed.) (1994). *Handbook of depression in children and adolescents*. New York: Plenum Press.

Rotheram-Borus, M. J., Piacentini, J., Miller, S., Graae, F. and Castro-Blanco, D. (1994). Brief cognitive-behavioral treatment for adolescent suicide attempters and their families. *Journal of the American Academy of Child and Adolescent Psychiatry*, 4, 508–17.

Seligman, M. E .P. (1975). *Helplessness. On depression, development, and death*. San Francisco: Freeman.

Shaffer, D. and Piacentini, J. (1994). Suicide and attempted suicide. In *Child and adolescent psychiatry. Modern approaches*, ed. M. Rutter, E. Taylor and L. Hersov, pp. 407–24. Oxford: Blackwell Scientific.

Stark, K. D., Reynolds, W. M. and Kaslow, N. J. (1987). A comparison of the relative efficacy of self control therapy and a behavioral problem solving therapy for depression in children. *Journal of Abnormal Child Psychology*, **15**, 91–113.

Stark, K. D., Rouse, L. W. and Livingston, R. (1991). Treatment of depression during childhood and adolescence. Cognitive-behavioral procedures for the individual and family. In *Child and adolescent therapy cognitive-behavioural procedures*, ed. P. C. Kendall, pp. 165–206. New York: Guilford Press.

Wilkes, T. C. and Rush, A. J. (1988). Adaptions of cognitive therapy for depressed adolescents. *American Journal of the Academy of Child and Adolescent Psychiatry*, **27**, 381–6.

Wilkes, T. C., Belsher, G., Rush, A. J. and Frank, E. (1994). *Cognitive therapy for depressed adolescents*. New York: Guilford Press.

World Health Organization (WHO) (1978). *Mental disorders. Glossary and guide to their classification in accordance with the ninth revision of the classification of diseases*. Geneva: WHO.

World Health Organization (WHO) (1992). *The ICD-10 classification of mental and behavioural disorders. Clinical descriptions and diagnostic guidelines*. Geneva: WHO.

18 Dissociative [conversion] disorders

Helmut Remschmidt

General considerations, definition and classification

The term 'conversion' (Freud, 1894) was originally used to describe the process whereby psychic energy contained in an instinctual wish is transformed – or 'converted' – into physical symptoms. Conversion symptoms are thus a symbolic representation of repressed instinctual wishes. Psychic equilibrium is restored at the price of a mismatch between the severity of symptoms and the indifferent attitude of the affected individual towards the symptoms ('belle indifference'). Conversion symptoms are closely related to hysteria. However, in recent years the term hysteria has not only been used in the psychoanalytic sense, but increasingly in a phenomenological and descriptive sense. In the 1920s, hysterical symptom neurosis (conversion) was distinguished from hysterical character (hysterical character neurosis). However, this classification is not precise and allows only a rough distiction, because conversion symptoms also occur frequently in hysterical personalities.

Classification

In the last few years, attempts have been made to distinguish between the disparate symptoms associated with the term hysteria. In ICD-10 the term 'hysteria' is avoided 'in view of its many and varied meanings' (WHO, 1992). Instead, three different categories associated with the concept are described:

(i) dissociative [conversion] disorders (F44), e.g. dissociative amnesia, dissociative stupor, dissociative convulsions;

(ii) somatoform disorders (F45), e.g. somatization disorder, hypochondriacal disorder, somatoform autonomic dysfunction, persistent somatoform pain disorder;

(iii) histrionic personality disorder (F60.4), which is simalar to the classic 'hysterical personality'.

In the following section only those conversion symptoms or hysterical disorders relevant to childhood and adolescence are discussed. Individual symptom profiles are discussed separately. However, because aetiology and treatment are similar, despite the symptoms, these are discussed together.

Dissociative convulsions

Characteristics of the disorder

Dissociative convulsions are the most common manifestation of hysteria in childhood and adolescence, followed by dissociative loss of movement and dissociative trance (Blanz et al., 1987). However, it is important to bear in mind that additional epileptic seizures occur in about 10% of patients with dissociative convulsions. The most important characteristics of dissociative convulsions are:

- they may begin either suddenly or gradually;
- they usually occur in the presence of other persons;
- their duration is usually longer than epileptic seizures;
- they are often triggered by an unusual occurrence or stressful situation;
- they include bizarre and uncoordinated acts which usually differ from the typical movements of epileptic seizures;
- there are usually no neurological or electrophysiological signs, e.g. Babinski's sign, EEG abnormalities, tongue biting, passing urine, deep sleep after a seizure;
- injuries only rarely occur during dissociative convulsions.

Although the characteristics listed above are typical, differential diagnosis can still pose problems. Dissociative convulsions must not only be distinguished from epilepsy, but also from other neurological disorders, syncope, hyperventilation tetany, hypoglycaemic disturbance of conciousness, personality disorders, schizophrenia and movement disorders, e.g. tics, dystonia, myoclonus.

Dissociative loss of movement

Characteristics of the disorder

In this disorder, there is a loss or interference with complex movements like walking, standing or other intentional movements. Extent and type of impairment frequently does not correspond with any true neurologic condition, but rather resembles a lay person's concept of physical disorder. Muscle tone may vary depending on posture. When changing posture, muscle groups may be used which the patient was apparently unable to use shortly before. Supportive posturing may be observed. During attempts to stand up, the bending of knees can frequently be observed. Patients who fall over, rarely suffer injury.

Occasionally 'paralysis' with total loss of movement occurs.

The following psychopathological abnormalities may be found.

- Symptoms appear to be intentional and seem to be connected with the precipitating situation in some way.
- Symptoms frequently appear to be demonstrative.
- The severity of symptoms often contrasts remarkably with the patient's indifference or indolence ('belle indifference').
- The patient is unaware of the aim of his/her symptoms, whilst their underlying motive may be apparent to outside observers.

Differential diagnosis

There is a wide spectrum of different symptoms that may be associated with dissociative loss of movement (pain syndromes, sensory loss, stupor, etc.). Differentiating this from neurological disorders is often difficult. Co-morbidity with additional neurological disorder is common and therefore careful neurological examination and investigation is appropriate. In the past there has been great concern over missing physical disorders, with up to 20% of patients with conversion disorders later developing physical disorders which explain symptoms. With appropriate investigation, this now appears less common.

Hysterical personality disorder

Characteristics of the disorder

In this disorder, emotions tend to be shallow and unstable. Emotions largely depend on the response by others and are easily hurt. Behaviour is often theatrical and is to a great extent determined by the patient's wish for acknowledgement and attention. Patients tend to be very suggestible, easily affected by others or influenced by particular circumstances. In ICD-10 and DSM-IV (APA, 1994) these symptoms and ways of behaviour are classified under 'histrionic personality disorder'.

This personality disorder is mentioned here for completeness, because it is one of the manifestations of hysteria. However, in this condition hysteria is not characterized by physical or specific mental symptoms, but pervades the entire personality.

Diagnosis and differential diagnosis of hysterical manifestations

Diagnosis is based on a detailed history, a negative neurological examination (including additional diagnostic procedures) to look for inconsistencies

Table 18.1. Differential diagnosis of psychophysiological (psychosomatic) reactions and (hysterical) conversion symptoms

Psychophysiological (psychosomatic) reactions	Conversion reactions
(i) Areas supplied by the autonomic nervous system are affected	(i) Areas supplied by motor nervous system are affected
(ii) Symptoms do not reduce anxiety	(ii) Symptoms reduce anxiety
(iii) Symptoms do not have symbolic meaning	(iii) Symptoms have symbolic meaning and express a conflict
(iv) Injury of tissue may be life-threatening	(iv) No injury of tissue (atrophy at most), never life-threatening

Modified after Alexander (1943).

indicating hysteria, a detailed psychiatric interview and a psychological examination using standardized tests. Cognitive abilities, emotional state and the individual's personality should be assessed. Special attention should be paid to a possible connection between symptoms and specific precipitating situations (Remschmidt, 1992).

In differential diagnosis, the following disorders need to be distinguished from symptoms of hysteria or conversion.

(i) Psychosomatic disorders: several important aspects of differential diagnosis were summarized by Alexander (1943); they are shown in Table 18.1.

(ii) Paralysis and dissociative loss of movement should be distinguished from other psychogenic disorders of movement. Conversion symptoms may be distinguished from epileptic seizures by means of EEG. They should also be distinguished from tics, hyperventilation tetany, hypoglycaemic disturbance of consciousness and movement disorders, e.g. tics, dystonia, myoclonus.

(iii) Schizophrenia: particularly in adolescence, schizophrenia may present with apparently 'hysterical' symptoms. Often, distinction between the two is possible after a time of observation.

Aetiology and pathogenesis

A large number of theories relating to the aetiology and pathogenesis of hysterical symptoms have been put forward. However, none of them has been able to explain the disorder conclusively and without contradiction and they are therefore not discussed here. However, a number of individual propositions have been postulated, and these are discussed in detail below.

Genetic predisposition

Hysterical syndromes, especially conversion syndromes, occur more frequently in some families. This fact may be interpreted in two ways: as a result of genetic predisposition or due to a familial tradition of specific symptoms. Environmental factors are known to play a part in the aetiology of neurotic manifestations, to which hysterical symptoms belong. However, genetic factors are also increasingly recognized to be important (Schepank, 1974).

Personality structure

Personality structure is a factor which influences predisposition.

Models in the family or neighbourhood

Several studies have shown, that about 60% of patients with hysterical symptoms (especially conversion syndromes and dissociative convulsions) had models in their family environment or in their immediate surroundings. Patients 'imitated' the symptoms of these models. However, the process occurs unconsciously and must not be confused with intentional imitation or conscious simulation.

Conflicts and excessive demands

Biographical analysis of symptomatology often reveals that hysterical symptoms frequently occur in conflicts or situations in which excessive demands are made on patients. Symptoms frequently have some symbolic meaning. However, psychoanalytical theory, according to which symptoms are caused by repressed instinctual impulses of oedipal or incestual nature, cannot be supported empirically, as symbolic motives cannot always be uncovered.

Past illness determining the 'choice of symptoms'

An illness in someone's medical history may contribute towards the subsequent pattern of symptoms, e.g. an accident with ensuing paralysis may lead to dissociative paralysis later on in life. Again, it is important to recognize that this occurs unconsciously.

Primary and secondary gain

Hysterical symptoms lead both to primary gain, where the internal conflict is resolved, and to secondary gain from the assumption of the sick role, where the patient is relieved from normal responsibility and receives increased care and attention.

Promotion of symptoms through organic disorder

Brain injury may facilitate the occurrence of dissociative symptoms. This is demonstrated by the frequent co-morbidity with epilepsy.

Berblinger (1960) proposed several components in the pathogenesis of conversion symptoms, including inactivation of organ systems, e.g. in the case of paralysis or sensory loss, increased autonomy of the psyche, e.g. in dissociative convulsions and excessive motor activity, and reduced functional autonomy of the psyche, e.g. trance, amnesia. However, these basic mechanisms serve only to describe symptomatology and do not contribute to aetiological theories.

Psychotherapy and guidance

Treatment aims to eradicate the precipitating conflict and enable the child to cope better in future with potentially stressful situations (Silberg, 1996). Treatment usually includes changing the patient's home situation. Frequently, specific practical methods are used to treat the symptoms, e.g. in dissociative loss of movement, physiotherapy may be used. An appropriate explanation should be offered, for example, that the patient has 'forgotten' how to walk due to the disorder and must now relearn the skill lost.

The patient is usually treated individually in small steps. Group therapy may serve to satisfy the patient's wish for attention and dominance and may therefore aggravate symptoms at the start of treatment.

If the family is involved in the development, precipitation or maintenance of symptoms in any way, they should also be included in therapy. Usually, conflicts and excessive demands are closely associated with the family or the surroundings. However, changing the home situation is not easy. Often, as the therapist, one has to be satisfied with small changes, which relieve the patient from the immediate threat of further conflicts.

If additional disorders are present, e.g. epileptic seizures, treatment should follow the same principles. However, medication is naturally an important adjuvant to treatment.

The most important general principles of treatment are as follows.

(i) After identifying the conflict (or trigger), it is important to impart (or develop) alternative coping strategies by means of behavioural therapy and cognitive methods.

(ii) Practise coping strategies in appropriate situations. This approach should always begin with individual sessions.

(iii) If necessary, suggestive techniques should be used. It has been known that hysterical patients are generally very suggestible. Hysterical symptoms may, for instance, be produced by suggestion, which may in turn be used to treat hysterical symptoms, e.g. hypnosis, direct suggestive influence. The exclusive use of suggestive techniques is not recommended, but it may be useful at the beginning of treatment.

(iv) The family and the social environment should wherever possible be included, although how this is undertaken depends on the individual circumstances. The aim of restructuring is to modify external conditions, in order that the patient no longer obtains inappropriate reinforcement.

(v) A combination of medication and psychotherapy is required in the presence of additional physical conditions, e.g. epilepsy.

(vi) The symbolic content of symptoms should be discussed only as a second or third step of therapy. Usually the patient is unaware that symptoms may have symbolic meaning. If this aspect is addressed too early in therapy, the patient is at risk of feeling guilty or humiliated. However, if he/she shows some insight into his/her personality and into ways of reacting, the patient may recognize the final aim of the symptoms in the course of treatment (usually lasting several weeks). Eventually the patient may even perceive the symbolic content of his/her symptoms.

Two factors are essential for successful therapy: account should be taken of the patient's precarious condition. The therapist should be very careful not to make rash interpretations of the patient's symptoms. It is important rather to impart coping strategies, to enable the patient to cope without recourse to hysterical symptoms.

It is difficult to describe specific steps of treatment in a generally applicable way. The biographical context of symptoms and the aim of therapeutic interventions can best be rendered in an individual case report.

Case report

A 16-year-old patient, Cornelia, was admitted to a paediatric hospital for suspected meningitis. The family physician had found a slightly stiff neck and the patient complained of a severe headache, loss of strength in both legs and allowed her left leg to hang. Subsequent 'paralysis' of both legs occurred and the patient was unable to leave her bed. Her mother (working as a social worker after a career break) spent hours in the hospital at her daughter's bedside. The patient seemed remarkably unconcerned in the face of the severe symptoms and sometimes even lay in bed smiling. Both the internal medical and the neurological examinations were unremarkable and did not reveal features to account for the patient's condition. A child and adolescent psychiatrist was consulted, who diagnosed a conversion syndrome. He was able to convince the mother of the necessity of psychiatric treatment. The patient was then admitted for inpatient treatment on a child and adolescent psychiatric ward. There she was treated for 6 weeks. Treatment included physiotherapy, individual psychotherapy and family therapy. The patient was subsequently discharged entirely without symptoms.

The detailed family history, and conversations with the family, revealed that the patient was a highly motivated sportswoman, who had won several prizes. She had been anxious about an approaching competition. Family communication was severely disturbed. The father (an out-of-work alcoholic) refused to speak with the other family members and communicated by writing only. His position was entirely outside the family system. The patient's younger sister seemed to suffer least from the situation. During family therapy it was possible to persuade the family to resume speaking with one another. They were able to speak together about everyday topics, but also about interpersonal difficulties. After discharge, the father went on holiday with both children. This was considered a good indication of the vast improvement in the atmosphere within the family. The patient's symptomatology was understood as a cry for help in a seemingly hopeless situation and as an unconscious avoidance reaction to problems which the patient perceived as unsolvable. Follow-up 1 year after discharge showed that the effects of therapy were lasting.

This example highlights several important aspects associated with hysterical and dissociative disorders.

(i) The difficult diagnostic task of distinguishing between neurological and psychiatric symptoms, which may occur simultaneously.
(ii) The developmental psychological perspective on symptoms in childhood and adolescence. As a result of the various physical and mental changes taking place at this time, conversion symptoms tend to occur more frequently and in unusual ways.
(iii) The importance of predisposing factors in the family, in this case alcoholism of the patient's father.
(iv) The inclusion of the family in diagnosis and treatment. Considerable experience with families is required. Knowledge about family interaction and the influence of one family member's symptomatology on the family structure is necessary.
(v) The combination of various therapy techniques and their integration in a treatment plan, in which several individuals play a major role.

Course and prognosis

Conversion symptoms which only occur once are usually easy to treat. Therapy is difficult if symptoms have persisted for a long time and if they have caused a large amount of secondary gain. The following conditions can make therapy much more difficult:

- a chronic disorder (with a duration of more than 2–3 years);
- additional medical conditions, e.g. epileptic seizures with dissociative convulsions;
- severe mental sequelae of a medical condition, e.g. brain injury or dementia;
- insufficient guidance of the child or adolescent by those individuals caring for him;
- mental retardation or an undifferentiated personality structure;
- an extremely hysterical personality structure.

REFERENCES

Alexander, F. (1943). Fundamental concepts of psychosomatic research. *Psychosomatic Medicine*, **5**, 205–10.

American Psychiatric Association (APA) (1994). *Diagnostic and statistical manual of mental disorders*, 4th edn (DSM-IV). Washington, DC: APA.

Berblinger, K. (1960). Hysterical crisis and the question of hysterical character. *Psychosomatics*, **1**, 270–9.

Blanz, B., Lehmkuhl, B., Lehmkuhl, G., Lehmkuhl, U. and Braun-Scharm, H. (1987). Hysterische Neurosen im Kindes- und Jugendalter. *Zeitschrift für Kinder- und Jugendpsychiatrie*, **15**, 97–111.

Freud, S. (1894). The neuro-psychoses of defence. In *Standard edition of the works of Sigmund Freud*, vol. 3, ed. J. Strachey, pp. 43–61. London, Hogarth Press.

Remschmidt, H. (1992). Hysterie und Konversionssyndrome. In *Psychiatrie der Adoleszenz*, ed. H. Remschmidt, pp. 327–41. Stuttgart: Thieme.

Schepank, H. (1974). *Erb- und Umweltfaktoren bei Neurosen. Tiefenpsychologische Untersuchungen an 50 Zwillingspaaren*. Berlin: Springer.

Silberg, J. L. (ed.) (1996). *The dissociative child. Diagnosis, treatment, and management*. Lutherville, MD: Sidran Press.

World Health Organization (WHO) (1992). *The ICD-10 classification of mental and behavioural disorders. Clinical descriptions and diagnostic guidelines*. Geneva: WHO.

19

Disorders of sexual development and sexual behaviour

Matthias Martin and Helmut Remschmidt

Characteristics of the disorders and classification

In assessing sexual abnormalities in childhood and adolescence, four aspects should be observed:

- specific phase-related aspects of biological development,
- timing and contents of sexual education and the development of gender specific behaviour,
- the present abnormal situation, including possible 'triggers',
- the psychosexual situation, including mental or physical disorders and the assessment for premature or protracted sexual development.

Normal variants of sexual behaviour

Masturbation

Definition

Intentional self-arousal by manual stimulation of the genitals with the aim of achieving sexual gratification is called masturbation (synonym: onanism). Masturbation is a common expression of human sexuality and is a normal phenomenon in the course of adolescence. However, excessive masturbation may require treatment. For retarded children, excessive masturbation may be a way of achieving substitute gratification and may require treatment if it is performed excessively and without regard for other individuals.

Under adverse conditions, masturbation may be associated with psychiatric symptoms in adolescence, e.g. by inappropriate sexual education, excessively religious upbringing (where masturbation is considered 'sinful'), etc. The adolescent may experience feelings of guilt, which encourage the development of hypochondriasis with physical symptoms. Even paranoid symptoms may subsequently develop. Feelings of guilt are often accompanied by concern about the possibility of being sexually deviant. These adolescents tend to be inhibited in their contacts with peers. The combination of these two aspects may lead the adolescent to believe that he is sexually deviant and incapable of maintaining a normal sexual relationship, thus exacerbating his withdrawal.

Case report

A 6-year-old girl was referred with the following symptoms: she had been about 4 years old when her parents separated. Following this, she withdrew from almost all social contacts and showed oppositional behaviour towards her mother, who was the primary care-giver. Her mother reported that her daughter had masturbated excessively ever since her parents' separation. She frequently withdrew, crossed her legs and stimulated herself by sliding back and forth on the edge of a chair. She would not respond when spoken to.

Symptoms improved following outpatient treatment. However, after commencing school, symptoms became increasingly severe, particularly at school, such that day-hospital treatment was required. Treatment focused on the following aspects:

- advising the mother how to relate with her daughter in a more structured manner;
- individual psychotherapy of the patient, which revealed a loyalty conflict towards her father;
- occupational therapy;
- school attendance in order to improve the patient's attitude regarding achievement at school.

Symptoms disappeared during treatment and the relationship between mother and child improved. A follow-up examination no longer revealed any symptoms of the disorder ('emotional disorder with difficulties in relations').

Therapy

Masturbation should be regarded as a widespread act in a temporary developmental phase. It usually does not require any specific treatment. However, when interviewing adolescents with psychiatric problems, sexual topics should always brought up at some point. The therapist should have an idea of how the patient achieves sexual gratification, how this topic is dealt with in the family and which sexual fantasies are relevant for the patient. The way a patient copes with sexuality may be discussed in individual psychotherapy. During sessions, the following issues should be covered:

- educating the patient on age-appropriate sexuality,
- reassuring the patient with regard to those sequelae of masturbation that he is afraid may occur,
- discussing the the patient's individual situation and his (sexual) fantasies,
- encouraging adolescents who are withdrawn and have problems establishing

social contacts to approach members of the other sex (possibly in a group setting directed by a social worker).

Homosexuality

In ICD-9 (WHO, 1978), homosexuality was classified in a separate category. This category no longer exists in ICD-10 (WHO, 1992). Homosexuality may now be classified with 'psychological and behavioural disorders associated with sexual development and orientation' (F66). However, sexual orientation alone is not regarded as a disorder in ICD-10.

Sexual maturation disorder

Affected individuals suffer from uncertainty regarding their gender identity or sexual orientation, causing anxiety or depression. This disorder usually occurs in adolescents, who are uncertain whether their sexual orientation is homosexual, heterosexual or bisexual. The disorder may also occur in individuals who become uncertain about their sexual orientation after a long duration of apparently stable sexual orientation, or individuals who discover their sexual orientation has changed, sometimes after relationships have lasted for many years.

Egodystonic sexual orientation

Gender identity or sexual preference is unequivocal, but the affected individual wishes this were not so, because of the mental or behavioural stress involved. Affected individuals occasionally request treatment. However, as mentioned above, sexual orientation alone is not regarded as a disorder in ICD-10. The following conditions should be distinguished:

(i) homosexuality as a temporary developmental phase,
(ii) pseudohomosexual behaviour,
(iii) fixed homosexuality (homosexual orientation).

Homosexual behaviour is fairly common during puberty. It may indicate insecurity concerning the aim of drives or an insufficiently developed gender identity. Homosexual behaviour may also occur in adolescents around the ages 16–18 years, who experience a peak of instinctual impulses, but lack the opportunity to satisfy drives in a heterosexual partnership ('homosexuality by necessity'). Finally, victimization may occur, for example, in prisons, where homosexual activity is enforced upon other adolescents. Homosexual acts or disorders of sexual development and orientation are fairly common reasons for psychotherapy.

The term 'pseudohomosexual behaviour' (Bräutigam, 1979) is used to describe homosexual behaviour in the absence of homosexual preference, e.g. working as a male prostitute. In this case, psychotherapy in a strict sense is not indicated, because the problem often involves a wider picture of deprivation, delinquency and drug abuse.

According to current opinion, there is no indication for the psychotherapy of fixed homosexuality (homosexual orientation), except in cases of egodystonic sexual orientation. This implies that the affected individual intends to change his sexual orientation.

Case report

An adolescent was admitted for inpatient treatment after attempted suicide. The suicide attempt was apparently triggered following interrogation by the police. The patient was accused of not helping a friend of his, who had attempted suicide the night before. The patient reported that his own suicide attempt had not been a sudden and irrational act, but that he had been contemplating suicide for quite some time. He gave as his reason the fact that a relationship with a homosexual friend 3 years older than himself had come to an end. The patient subsequently felt hopeless regarding his future as a homosexual in a small town.

During therapy the patient's main problem became clear: he had feelings of intense inadequacy and felt victimized by others, in particular, by some of his homosexual friends, who would occasionally take advantage of him, subsequently abandoning him. The patient required hospital treatment for his emotional disturbance and protracted depressive reaction. After discharge he successfully attended a boarding school.

Therapy

Individual psychotherapy is useful in adolescents with temporary homosexual behaviour. Therapy should then focus on helping the adolescent to overcome his identity crisis and integrate his psychosexuality with his personality. It is also then important, in addition, to educate the parents who should not aggravate the situation by laying blame on the adolescent.

It has been claimed that approximately 35% of homosexuals would like to change their sexual preference (Giese, 1967). However, the attempt to change sexual preference raises a number of ethical problems and has led to this practice being criticized for the following reasons (Bancroft, 1983).

(i) Every attempt to change sexual preference reinforces negative public attitude towards homosexuality.

(ii) Individuals, who express the desire to change their sexual preference, do so because of social pressure and not by their free will.

(iii) Treatment of homosexuals to change their preference is undesirable. Treatment is unnatural, because it is aimed at changing homosexuals' natural preference for members of their own sex.

Individual psychotherapy may be conducted on the basis of psychoanalytically orientated theories or behavioural theories. Long-term psychoanalytical treatment is successful in 19% of cases at most. In homosexual men, treatment usually focuses on conflicts associated with excessively close attachment to the mother on one hand and on the father's disinterest on the other.

Older behavioural approaches to treatment relied upon aversion techniques, which were intended to suppress homosexual reactions. Today, these techniques are no longer considered helpful. Later, several conditioning techniques were introduced to reinforce positive responses to heterosexual stimuli (Bancroft, 1974). Therapy to change sexual preference has two facets: first, switching patients' fantasies and secondly, changing actual behaviour towards a potential heterosexual partner. Fantasies are influenced by 'fantasy shaping', during which homosexual masturbatory fantasies are supplemented by heterosexual fantasies, which in time, should generalize (Bancroft, 1972). Masters and Johnson (1979) reported successful treatment by means of a heterosexual partner. This approach resembles the treatment of heterosexual couples with sexual dysfunction.

Advising the majority of homosexuals who accept their sexual preference is an important task of psychotherapeutic guidance. It is important to identify specific problems and associated emotions, which frequently involve:

- feelings of guilt due to homosexual preference and difficulty accepting the way affection is expressed between homosexuals;
- difficulties in approaching members of the same sex and maintaining intimate relationships;
- sexual problems within the homosexual relationships;
- problems in dealing with the social stigmatization of homosexuals in society (Bancroft, 1983).

Gender identity disorder

Gender identity disorder of childhood

As defined in ICD-10 (F64.2), this disorder most frequently occurs during early childhood (and always well before puberty). The disorder is characterized by the intense and persistent wish to be (or insistence that one is) of the other sex. The child rejects his own sex and is constantly preoccupied with the clothes or behaviour of the other sex. No desire for sex change is expressed, and the disorder cannot be diagnosed after reaching puberty.

The aetiology remains unclear; however, several factors also relevant in therapy have been proposed to be relevant (Green, 1975, 1994). In addition to a genetic predisposition, specific styles of upbringing are thought to play a role. In boys, an excessively strong bond with the mother, fixation with an immature, childish role and discouragement of gender appropriate behaviour, e.g. aggressive play in boys are also said to be contributory. The lack of a same sex role model, e.g. friends of the same sex is also said to be important.

Therapy

Therapy is only indicated if the adolescent expresses a desire to acquire a sexual identity corresponding to his biological sex. If the adolescent has no motivation for change, therapy is inappropriate. Instead, treatment may be limited to offering the adolescent advice about the nature of the disorder. Further steps include helping the patient work through the consequences of his condition, discussing sexual desires and fantasies and helping the adolescent integrate with his peer group. Depression, social isolation and the development of neurotic traits are common. The parents should be offered the opportunity to participate in treatment. They should be informed about the nature of the disorder and should learn to accept the adolescent's desire to receive no treatment to alter the situation. This is best achieved in family sessions, in which unanswered questions may be discussed openly by both sides. In some cases, gender identity disorder develops to true transsexualism. In this case, the patient usually requests sex realignment surgery. Prognosis is much better in cases when the patient wishes to attain a sexual identity that corresponds to his biological sex. In these cases, the rate of secondary psychiatric disorders occurring is much lower than in cases of true transsexualism (Remschmidt, 1992).

Transsexualism

In ICD-10, transsexualism (F64.0) is defined as 'a desire to live and be accepted as a member of the opposite sex, usually accompanied by a sense of discomfort with, or inappropriateness of, one's anatomic sex and a wish to have hormonal treatment and surgery to make one's body as congruent as possible with the preferred sex' (WHO, 1992).

Diagnostic guidelines

Transsexual identity must have been present persistently for at least 2 years. It must not be a symptom of another mental disorder, e.g. schizophrenia, and must not be associated with any other intersex, genetic or sex chromosome abnormality.

Transsexualism occurs more frequently in women than in men (about 3 to 2). The fixation with an opposite gender role can frequently be traced back to early childhood. Adolescents who dress in clothes of the opposite sex are often encountered in child and adolescent psychiatric clinics. Several theories have been put forward to explain the aetiology of the disorder.

Prenatal neuroendocrine imprinting of gender identity

According to this theory, androgens affect the hypothalamus of the developing female fetus and cause imprinting of opposite gender identity, leading to transsexualism in girls. Lack of androgens in the developing male fetus causes transexualism in boys (Dörner, 1972).

Abnormal central nervous control of sexuality

According to this theory, transsexuals may have a functional abnormality of the temporal lobe (Kockott and Nusselt, 1976).

Familial factors

Several factors have been considered relevant for male transexualism, including absent parental role model, disturbed gender role in the patient's father, a symbiotic mother–son relationship and a style of upbringing contrary to the child's gender.

Genetic factors

A genetic influence in transsexualism is suspected because of the above average rate of transexuality in some families (Sigusch et al., 1979).

Therapy

Earlier attempts to treat transexualism by means of psychotherapy aimed at switching gender identity to that of the biological sex have now been abandoned. However, adolescents do require psychotherapeutic guidance and support. Whilst sex realignment surgery is not performed on adolescents, they need not only to learn to live with continuing conflicts, which may cause additional psychiatric complications, e.g. attempted suicide, neurotic traits, but also to begin the process of adjusting for any future surgery.

In Germany, a number of requirements must be met before a patient undergoes sex realignment surgery.

(i) Psychosexual development should be completed. Sex realignment surgery should not be performed before the patient is 19 years old.

(ii) The patient needs to have lived with his or her intended gender identity for at least 1 or 2 years. Hormone therapy should be used during this time. This condition is made in order that the patient has become familiar with his or her new gender role before permanent surgery is contemplated. A further issue is the relinquishment of an unequivocal sex within a future relationship.
(iii) Usually the patient has to be a German citzizen or at least live in Germany for sex change to be contemplated.
(iv) The patient should be carefully examined and investigated. Postoperative care and support should be ensured. Both assessment prior to surgery and follow-up should include individuals close to the patient.
(v) At least two physicians with expert experience in the field should agree before referral for realignment surgery.
(vi) Sex realignment is contraindicated where transexualism is caused by schizophrenia or organic brain damage because of the risk of complications postsurgery.
(vii) If a psychiatric indication for sex realignment is approved, but medical reasons preclude an operation, e.g. age, physical illness, the patient should at least be granted the opportunity to change his or her civil status.

Follow-up studies have shown that results of this treatment method are much less encouraging than was initially expected. In many cases today, psychotherapeutic approaches are preferred, i.e. behavioural therapy techniques.

Disorders of sexual preference (paraphilias)

Disorders of sexual preference are classified in ICD-10 together under F65: fetishism (F65.0), fetishistic transvestism (F65.1), exhibitionism (F65.2), voyeurism (F65.3), paedophilia (F65.4), sadomasochism (F65.5) and multiple disorders of sexual preference (F65.6).

Disorders of sexual preference (paraphilias, sexual deviations) require psychotherapy in some, but by no means in all cases. In these disorders, several approaches to therapy are possible (Kockott, 1993): counselling, physical treatment, psychoanalytically orientated psychotherapy, behavioural therapy and treatment methods not bound to any particular school of therapy ('multidimensional approach'). Counselling should fulfil several different functions.

- Simply listening taking the patient's problems seriously often brings about relief.
- Along with a frank discussion regarding the wide range of normal sexual experiences, the issue as to whether or not the patient's own behaviour is abnormal, should be addressed early on.

- It should be clarified who wants behavioural change (the patient himself, his partner, or his or her parents).
- Counselling should involve the patient's partner or parents in order to help them better understand the patient's sexual deviance.
- The parents and the partner should be asked to consider whether the sexual deviance is acceptable to them (at least to some extent).
- Counselling should also serve to discuss therapeutic options with the patient.

Therapy

Psychotherapy may be indicated if, as a result of his deviance, the patient is suffering, e.g. if the deviant behaviour increases and becomes more disturbing to the patient, or if he or she feels uneasy about being increasingly compelled to perform certain acts. Psychotherapy may also be indicated if other individuals are suffering from the patient's behaviour (Kockott, 1993). In some cases, therapy is ruled by order of court, which does not necessarily reduce the chances of successful treatment (Schorsch et al., 1985).

Psychoanalytically orientated psychotherapy was at first not used as a first-line treatment of deviations. Schorsch et al. (1985) have shown that it is possible to motivate patients and to successfully undertake therapy.

Aversion treatment was the first behavioural therapy technique used in treating sexual deviations. However, the exclusive use of aversion techniques is regarded today as unethical. Cases were reported, in which patients suffered a 'post-therapeutic vacuum', which led to depression, due to the fact that deviant behaviour was abated without any increase in heterosexual behaviour (Kockott, 1993). Current behavioural approaches combine self-control methods with 'orgasmic reconditioning' (modifying masturbatory fantasies and reducing deviant fantasies). Several behavioural approaches should be combined to compile a treatment plan. Treatment should not be aimed at the deviancy alone and should also address any other problems (self-confidence, attachment anxiety, social difficulties).

Exhibitionism

In ICD-10, exhibitionism is defined as 'a recurrent or persistent tendency to expose the genitalia to strangers (usually of the opposite sex) or to people in public places, without inviting or intending closer contact. There is usually, but not invariably, sexual arousal at the time of the exposure and the act is commonly followed by masturbation. This tendency may be manifest only at times of emotional stress or crises, interspersed with longer periods without such overt behaviour.' The diagnostic guidelines add: 'most exhibitionists find their urges difficult to control and ego-alien.'

Exhibitionism is fairly commonly encountered in child and adolescent psychiatric clinics. Those adolescents who are referred for assessment, usually have withdrawn personalities, are inhibited and have problems with heterosexual contacts. They tend to be shy and bashful. In addition to feelings of physical inadequacy they often experience feelings of general low self-esteem and appear to be retarded in their psychosexual development. Patients frequently come from families which avoid discussing sexual topics or demonstrate an attitude generally opposed to sexuality.

Therapy

Many adolescents with exhibitionism are subjected to treatment by order of court, i.e. treatment is involuntary. Therefore, initially motivation for therapy should be a major goal. Exhibitionism being a petty offence ('disorderly conduct'), treatment is usually undertaken in an outpatient setting. Contrary to general opinion, it is possible in most cases to motivate adolescents for therapy, build trusting relationships and lead them to understand that they may benefit from treatment.

During treatment, the following points should be remembered: the affected adolescents usually have inadequate knowledge about sexuality and often have great difficulties discussing the topic. These adolescents require information on sexual matters and age-appropriate sexual behaviour. Therapy must address the adolescent's entire personality and development such as the common feelings of severe inadequacy, social inhibition and lack of self-confidence. Finally, therapy should also address the adolescent's social situation and improve his social behaviour towards members of the opposite sex. This may be achieved by self-assertion training and guidance by social workers in peer group settings. Prognosis is fairly good if therapy succeeds in reducing the patient's social inhibitions and improving his social behaviour. Additional counselling of the parents may be helpful in order to alter their behaviour and help them to support the patient in his psychosexual development.

Treatment of adolescent sexual delinquency

About one-quarter of all cases of rape are committed by adolescents and young adults. Sexual delinquency in adolescence is a fairly common problem with a variety of different causes. The background of each individual case must be carefully analysed.

Directive and behavioural methods of psychotherapy are the preferred approaches to treatment of sexual delinquency (Bancroft, 1983). Treatment should be aimed at any specific underlying causes and should be focused on the problems of the individual patient. The following common issues should be taken into account:

- difficulties in establishing sexually gratifying relationships;
- difficulties in establishing relationships of any kind;
- issues of self-confidence, inadequate assertiveness and narrow repertoire of pleasurable activities;
- inadequate sexual arousal following 'normal' sexual stimuli;
- problems in self-control and inappropriate sexual arousal following deviant sexual stimuli.

In behavioural therapy, one should distinguish between methods that focus on a specific symptom and those which address a variety of symptoms. Symptom-specific methods (Schorsch et al., 1985) include aversion therapy, in which the occurrence of sexual arousal following deviant stimuli results in the application of an aversive stimulus. Covert sensitization is another symptom-specific method, in which the patient is asked to imagine a situation which stimulates him to perform sexually deviant acts. Adverse thoughts incompatible with sexual arousal are induced simultaneously and arousal is thus reduced by means of extinction. Biofeedback methods may also be used to control sexual arousal following deviant stimuli.

A positive and constructive approach to therapy is important, i.e. the attempt to help the patient discover and reinforce new and appropriate behaviours, instead of merely extinguishing old and undesirable behaviours. Social skills training and assertiveness training in individual or group psychotherapy settings will help the patient to establish relationships more easily. Behaviours can be analysed using video recordings and the therapist may offer feedback by commenting on behaviour and suggesting modifications. Novel appropriate behaviours may be modelled and practised repeatedly (Bancroft, 1983).

Methods addressing a variety of symptoms include both conditioning sexual arousal following 'normal' stimuli and systematic desensitization, combined with social competency training. In a study undertaken by Schorsch et al. (1985) in sexual delinquents treated with behavioural therapy and counselling, about one-half of the 86 patients were successfully treated with outpatient psychotherapy. Psychotherapy was performed by a psychotherapist who did not have special qualifications for treating sexual delinquents. Good results may be achieved by a multi-dimensional approach, i.e. combining behaviour therapy and psychodynamic elements.

REFERENCES

Bancroft, J. H. J. (1972). The relationship between gender identity and sexual behaviour. Some clinical aspects. In *Gender differences. Their ontogeny and significance*, ed. C. Ounsted and D. C. Taylor. Edinburgh: Churchill Livingstone.

Bancroft, J. H. J. (1974). *Deviant sexual behaviour. Modification and assessment.* Oxford: Clarendon Press.

Bancroft, J. H. J. (1983). *Human sexuality and its problems.* Edinburgh: Churchill Livingstone.

Bräutigam, W. (1979). *Sexualmedizin im Grundriss. Eine Einführung in Klinik, Theorie und Therapie der sexuellen Konflikte und Störungen*, 2nd edn., Stuttgart: Thieme.

Dörner, G. (1972). *Sexualhormonabhängige Gehirndifferenzierung und Sexualität.* Vienna: Springer.

Giese, H. (1967). *Die sexuelle Perversion.* Frankfurt: Akademische Verlagsgesellschaft.

Green, R. (1975). Atypical sex role behavior during childhood. In *Comprehensive textbook of psychiatry*, 2nd edn, vol. II, ed. A. M. Freedman, H. I. Kaplan and B. J. Sadock., pp. 1408–14. Baltimore: Williams & Wilkins.

Green, R. (1994). Atypical psychosexual development. In *Child and adolescent psychiatry. Modern approaches*, ed. M. Rutter, E. Taylor and L. Hersov, pp. 749–58. Oxford: Blackwell.

Kockott, G. (1993). Therapie von Sexualstörungen. In *Therapie psychiatrischer Erkrankungen*, ed. H-J. Möller. Stuttgart: Enke.

Kockott, G. and Nusselt, L. (1976). Zur Frage der cerebralen Dysfunktion bei der Transsexualität. *Nervenarzt*, **47**, 310–18.

Martin, M. and Dauner, I. (1985). Störungen der Sexualentwicklung und des Sexualverhaltens. In *Kinder- und Jugendpsychiatrie in Klinik und Praxis*, vol. III, ed. H. Remschmidt and M. H. Schmidt, pp. 299–322. Stuttgart: Thieme.

Masters, W. H. and Johnson, V. E. (1979). *Homosexuality in perspective.* Boston: Little Brown.

Remschmidt, H. (1992). *Psychiatrie der Adoleszenz.* Stuttgart: Thieme.

Schorsch, E., Galedary, G., Haag, A., Hauch, M. and Lohse, H. (1985). *Perversion als Straftat. Dynamik und Psychotherapie.* Berlin: Springer.

Sigusch, V., Meyenburg, B. and Reiche, R. (1979). Transsexualität. In *Sexualität und Medizin*, ed. V. Sigusch. Köln: Kiepenheuer & Witsch.

World Health Organization (WHO) (1978). *Mental disorders. Glossary and guide to their classification in accordance with the ninth revision of the classification of diseases.* Geneva: WHO.

World Health Organization (WHO) (1992). *The ICD-10 classification of mental and behavioural disorders. Clinical descriptions and diagnostic guidelines.* Geneva: WHO.

20

Substance abuse and addiction

Andreas Warnke

The management of children and adolescents with substance abuse or addiction is a common field for child and adolescent psychiatrists (Washton, 1996). More than 150 000 children and adolescents in Germany are involved with substance abuse or addiction. The estimated total number of individuals with alcohol addiction in Germany is between 1.5 and 2.5 million. Additionally, 200 000–500 000 individuals are addicted to medication and 100 000–120 000 to illicit drugs. The fact that individuals with substance abuse or addiction constitute the largest group of patients undergoing psychiatric treatment facilities highlights the enormous challenge to child and adolescent psychiatry in terms of preventive work. More than 700 000 children live with an alcohol-dependent parent. The risk of these children also becoming alcohol dependent is high. The percentage of those children and adolescents between 14 and 18 years old, associated with drug-related crimes, e.g. registered as suspects by the police, has ranged between 8% and 25% during the last 25 years. Psychiatric disorders due to substance abuse or addiction frequently require child and adolescent psychiatric treatment. It is likely that a high percentage of affected children and adolescents already had another disorder before the beginning of substance abuse or addiction. In many cases of substance abuse or addiction, co-morbidity is sufficiently severe that social work and psychological assistance alone are insufficient. Substance abuse and addiction, including co-morbid psychiatric disorders, require prevention, psychiatric treatment and rehabilitation, areas in which child and adolescent psychiatry services bear a significant responsibility.

The disorders associated with psychoactive substance abuse and addiction are complicated. They are influenced by pathogenetic and maintaining factors, by the addictive properties of the substance abused and the way it influences the individual development of the affected child or adolescent. Individual coping strategies and environmental factors also play a part in the disorder.

The following section addresses the most important psychotherapeutic methods and approaches for children and adolescents with substance abuse or addiction.

Definition and classification

With respect to treatment, it is useful to distinguish between acute intoxication, harmful use and dependence syndromes using ICD-10 (WHO, 1992) to define the disorders. Acute intoxication (F1x.0) is a temporary state after administration of psychoactive substances and involves a disturbance of physical, mental and behavioural functions and responses. Harmful use (F1x.1) refers to health disturbances caused by psychoactive substances, e.g. hepatitis or a depressive episode. Dependence syndrome (F1x.2) is characterized by a compelling desire to consume psychoactive substances, difficulties in controlling the substance-taking behaviour in terms of its onset, termination or levels of use, with the aim of preventing withdrawal symptoms. Addiction is characterized by evidence of tolerance, narrowing of the personal repertoire of patterns of psychoactive substance use, e.g. consuming substances in inappropriate situations, progressive neglect of alternative sources of pleasure or interests and persistent substance abuse in spite of harmful physical, mental and social consequences (WHO, 1992, 1996). Psychological addiction and the wish to continue drug abuse in order to achieve gratification or relief from discomfort is the basis of all dependence syndromes. Physical addiction is characterized by withdrawal symptoms. Some substances may cause physical addiction, e.g. morphine derivates and barbiturates, whereas others do not, e.g. amphetamines and cocaine. The characteristics of the substance determine whether or not medication needs to be considered as part of the treatment plan.

Symptoms and diagnosis

Physical, mental and social symptoms, as well as co-morbid psychopathology, differ between individuals. They must be diagnosed in order that an appropriate treatment plan can be drawn up.

Physical symptoms

Physical symptomatology tends to be non-specific and to a great extent depends on the psychoactive substance consumed. Some of the many symptoms are briefly mentioned here:

Delirium may occur following abuse of barbiturates or alcohol: the first stage (prodromal state) consists of sleep disturbance, sweating, morning trembling, morning vomiting, organic seizures; in the second stage (full delirium), disturbance of consciousness and orientation, delusions, hallucinations and autonomic nervous system abnormalities occur, including hyperthermia, hypotension and, more seriously, cardiac and pulmonary complications.

Barbiturate intoxication causes nystagmus, myosis, ataxia, disturbance or loss of consciousness, central respiratory depression, circulatory failure, cerebral seizures.

Cannabis abuse causes mydriasis, muscle aches, sweats and shivers, rhinorrhoea, loss of appetite (anorexia); during withdrawal: goose-skin, tear secretion and diarrhoea.

Cocaine abuse causes loss of appetite and weight loss (cachexia), psychosis, chronic inflammation of nasal mucosa, deprivation with organic psychosyndrome.

Opiate intoxication causes myosis, central respiratory depression, pulmonary oedema, cerebral oedema, pressure paralysis, cerebral seizures, skin disorders, cutaneous abscesses, phlebitis, immunological abnormalities, amenorrhoea, impotence.

Abuse of volatile solvents causes symptoms of organic psychosyndrome, general cerebral atrophy, adrenal disorder.

Amphetamine intoxication causes mydriasis, facial redness, dry mouth, tachycardia, arrhythmia, high blood pressure, headache, trembling, loss of appetite (anorexia), nausea and vomiting, tinnitus.

Mental and social symptoms

The disorder is diagnosed by means of taking a careful history from the patient and where possible also from an informant. Mental status examination, physical examination, laboratory tests and psychological questionnaires are also necessary. A positive screening test for drugs may prove consumption, but not addiction. It may help in distinguishing acute intoxication from other psychiatric disorders, such as acute schizophrenia.

The history may reveal hints suggesting drug abuse, such as a sharp drop in school achievement or performance at work, a change in personality, declining personal reliability and general disinterest. Further signs of drug abuse include deterioration in conduct, conflicts with the aquaintances or neighbours, withdrawal from family and friends and increasingly close association with the drug scene. The occurrence of motor vehicle accidents and criminal offences should lead to drug abuse being queried. The doctor should always be aware that psychiatric symptoms and/or personality traits may be the consequence of drug abuse, e.g. agitation, nervousness, paranoia, hallucinations, depersonalization, derealization and suicidal behaviour.

The possibility of a primary psychiatric disorder or unsolved conflict should always be borne in mind, such as poor socialization, personality disorder, specific developmental disorder (particularly dyslexia or spelling disorder), hyperkinetic disorder, depression or psychosis. Even young drug users may have experienced physical or sexual abuse at home or by other drug users, which has an impact on self-esteem. It is important to enquire about drug abuse by parents and other care-givers as well as the influence of peers. Frequently there is a strong attachment to the family, despite the fact that affected adolescents often show oppositional behaviour and say that they do not wish to return home.

A developmental perspective is important for assessing the influence drug abuse and addiction has had on the individual's premorbid physical and psychological development. Drug abuse is fairly rare before the age of 14 years and becomes more frequent towards the age of 18 years. The problems of drug abuse affect developmental issues such as mental and physical maturation, coping in school, vocational choice, social detachment from the family, sexuality and finding a partner. It is normal in adolescence to question values, seek to escape from the usual environment and acquire new interests and goals.

Treatment should be aimed at all of the above mentioned problems associated with drug abuse and addiction. Therapy should therefore address:

(i) the detrimental effects of the substance itself,
(ii) withdrawal symptoms,
(iii) psychological addiction, and
(iv) the primary cause or conflicts associated with the disorder.

Treatment should take into account the physical, mental and social aspects of drug abuse and addiction.

Therapy

General principles of treatment

The aims of treatment largely determine the phases of treatment:

(i) contact phase
(ii) withdrawal (if required)
(iii) rehabilitation treatment
(iv) follow-up phase.

About 90% of all patients undertaking rehabilitation treatment for alcoholism experience a relapse. A significant number, however, are able to maintain abstinent after two or three further attempts at treatment. This demonstrates that treatment is not usually a straightforward procedure, but may often involve continued therapeutic and rehabilitative efforts for several years (Table 20.1).

The contact phase includes all measures taken to motivate the patient for a course of treatment lasting weeks to several years. The patient should be supported in accepting the diagnosis and treatment opportunities should be explained. The young patient and his family should be motivated to reattempt treatment, despite previous failures. The short-term, medium-term and long-term aims of treatment should be discussed. Supportive therapy sessions should be held frequently and mental and physical complaints treated promptly.

Motivation involves improving insight into the necessity of changing the present situation ('I can't continue like this'), realizing one's helplessness ('I can't cope by myself'), accepting help ('I will allow others to help me'), admitting to substance abuse or addiction ('I am addicted'), accepting abstinence as an aim ('I must never drink alcohol again') and accepting the necessity of changing one's lifestyle ('I have to change my life if I don't want to relapse') (Feuerlein, 1995).

Quite frequently it is intoxication with a pychotropic substance which leads to treatment being sought. Counselling the patient and the family is required in every case, as emotional disturbance, behavioural disorder and poor coping skills must be expected.

Counselling should concentrate on education of the patient and – if possible – the family and other care-givers on the substance abused and the signs and risks of continued abuse. Intoxication with suicidal intent must be ruled out. In some cases, counselling may address an underlying psychiatric disorder (depression, anxiety disorder, bulimia), a present conflict (familial discord, disappointed love affair, etc.) or excessive demands made on the adolescent (failure in school or at work). The aims of the contact phase should be pursued further, particularly establishing the importance of rehabilitation treatment after withdrawal.

Acute complications of substance abuse require specific measures. Cutaneous abscesses or septicaemia may require medical treatment, whereas severe agitation, aggressive behaviour, delirium or acute suicidal behaviour may require crisis intervention on a psychiatric ward.

In cases of withdrawal symptoms in newborn infants from drug-dependent mothers, advising the parents is essential. First, appropriate medical treatment of the child must be ensured. It must be determined to what degree the

Table 20.1. Treatment network for patients with addiction

Therapy phase	Outpatient facilities	Partial hospitalization	Inpatient facilities	Other facilities
Contact phase	Primary care physician Psychologist Child guidance centre Psychiatric clinic Specialized clinic Drug addiction counselling services Public Health Office	Day-patient treatment Night-patient treatment	General hospital Psychiatric hospital	School Workplace Self-help group Family Other relatives Youth Welfare Office Penal institution
Detoxification	Primary care physician Psychiatric clinic (Specialized clinic)		General hospital Psychiatric hospital Special hospital for addiction	Penal institution
Supportive treatment	Specialized clinic Psychiatric clinic (Primary care physician)	Day-patient treatment Night-patient treatment	Special hospital for addiction Psychiatric hospital General hospital	
Follow-up phase	Primary care physician Psychologist Psychiatric clinic Public Health Office	Day-patient treatment Night-patient treatment Temporary residential facility	Residential facility Residential groups	School Workplace Self-help group Family Other relatives Youth Welfare Office Penal institution

From Feuerlein (1995).

drug-dependent mother will be able to provide adequate care for the child, and what kind of support she is likely to require from youth welfare services. The mother should be encouraged to undergo treatment. In cases of teenage mothers, it is important to consider to what extent their relatives or guardians will be able to help with the care of the infant. About one-third of drug-dependent mothers continue to abuse drugs and thus put the well-being of their child at risk. The question of putting the child up for adoption at an early point or transferring the child's care and custody to someone else may have to be addressed.

Psychotherapy during withdrawal and detoxification

Detoxification is the phase during which the physical effects of withdrawal and other problems associated with drug abuse, e.g. weight loss, eczema, abscesses, parasites are treated. Withdrawal may be attempted in an outpatient setting, however, in many cases it is necessary to admit the patient to hospital. The risk of relapse is especially great after withdrawal from certain substances, because patients may not be able to resist consumption. Frequently outpatient treatment is not possible due to family or social conflicts, social isolation or close ties to the drug scene.

Psychotherapy during withdrawal in hospital should be performed by an experienced therapist, who should see the patient on a daily basis if possible. Individual psychotherapy should be supplemented by counselling the relatives. If necessary, the Youth Welfare Office and the school or educational facility should also be involved. It is important to ensure abstinence during inpatient treatment. This involves regular urine screening tests for drugs as well as restriction of visits and correspondence by friends. Patients should be encouraged to participate in group activities and the inpatient treatment programme as soon as possible.

It is important to inform patients in detail about their disorder and to motivate them to continue treatment, usually in the form of rehabilitation after a withdrawal phase. A further important issue is to explain the ward rules, especially to adolescents, very clearly. Eventually patients should be introduced to self-help groups.

The initial interview should not focus on just taking a detailed history of drug consumption, but should concentrate on listening to all of the adolescent's present problems. The therapeutic relationship should serve to focus on the patient's subjective cares and difficulties, his fears and expectations. Attempting to coerce the adolescent or making rash remarks about drug abuse can easily provoke resistance. The aim is to discuss the adolescent's individual situation and discover exactly what part drug abuse plays in his life. Contracts may serve to structure the course by means of specific tasks. One should ensure that the patient fulfils the tasks he is assigned to. The therapist should aim to be impartial and avoid the impression that he is acting on the parents' behalf. The rules of the treatment programme should be explained carefully to both the patient and the parents.

Rehabilitation

Rehabilitation is indicated if there is a risk of developmental disturbance and the adolescent is unable to stay abstinent. Rehabilitation may be undertaken in a variety of different settings: as an outpatient, as a day-patient or as an inpatient for either short-term (4–8 weeks), medium-term (2–6 months) or long-term (> 6 months) treatment.

Outpatient treatment is relatively economical and may allow the adolescent to remain in his usual environment, which includes maintaining social contacts and continuing at school or at work. The patient must be willing and able to remain abstinent, keep outpatient appointments, commit himself to the rules of the treatment plan and pursue the normal activities of daily life, e.g. regular attendance at school or work, stable accommodation and adequate family support.

A family situation which facilitates drug abuse, ongoing court cases, imprisonment, or severe physical, mental or social disorders preclude outpatient rehabilitation. The drop-out rate of outpatient rehabilitation is quite high (up to 50%). Duration of treatment is usually about 1 year, with 1–2 sessions per week. Therapy of drug-dependent adolescents is usually performed by means of individual psychotherapy. It may be necessary to restrict treatment to 'supporting' the patient, who may be unable to discontinue drug abuse. In these cases the therapist should limit himself to counselling the patient in crises and should then refer him for withdrawal treatment.

Inpatient treatment is necessary if outpatient treatment cannot be undertaken, either because the patient is unable to comply or because appropriate facilities are unavailable. This may be the case if an adolescent is unable to keep appointments, if his environment facilitates continued drug abuse (sometimes requiring removal of the patient from his environment) or if frequent relapses after outpatient treatment make admission to hospital advisable. If the family is to be included in therapy, a local treatment facility will be required. When choosing an appropriate facility for rehabilitation, one should consider the presence of co-morbid psychiatric disorders which also require treatment (eating disorder, psychosis, hyperkinetic syndrome, specific developmental disorder, mental retardation). If possible, treatment should take place in a hospital specializing in the problems of adolescents. Rehabilitation treatment should last for about 6 months. Treatment of short or medium duration (6–8 weeks) may be offered by ordinary child and adolescent psychiatric inpatient units, but ideally longer-term rehabilitation should follow.

Rehabilitation treatment, which should immediately follow withdrawal, attempts to achieve continued abstinence and regaining mental and physical health. It is also ideally aimed at social reintegration and returning the adolescent to school or work. For a chance of success, the adolescent should develop a feeling of responsibility, have the capacity for realistic self-appraisal and have resources for adequate coping with a variety of problems. In practice, a number of compromises must be made, relapses must be managed and, over the course of several years, ways and means to achieve goals must be developed with the patient. If addiction has progressed so far that the adolescent is indifferent about sequelae of the disorder, or if there is risk of self-harm, the patient may have to be admitted for compulsory treatment.

If there is a waiting list for admission to an inpatient unit and withdrawal symptoms are expected, regular consultations and physical and occupational therapy can be performed in order to support the patient until admission and distract him from withdrawal symptoms to some extent. Treatment with psychopharmacological medication such as neuroleptics, e.g. thioridazine, chlorprothixene or antidepressants has proved useful for interim periods. In addition to individual psychotherapy, group therapy taking place once or twice a week is a good method for supporting outpatient rehabilitation.

The formal structure and substance of psychotherapy

The principles of treatment discussed here represent basic components of treatment. Whether or not they are used in individual cases depends on the situation, the addictive behaviour of the patient and the treatment facilities available. Only inpatient treatment will be discussed here. Psychotherapy must always be viewed as part of a larger context of physical, occupational, vocational and social treatment methods. Psychotherapy has a structure (in terms of time and place), a particular method and specific contents or topics.

As in situational therapy, the daily life of adolescents treated for addiction should be structured in terms of time, place and type of activity. Treatment should provide a supportive 'framework', in which the patient can develop and try out alternative coping strategies, which will enable him to live in abstinence.

The inpatient environment has an important therapeutic function. By admission to a ward, a number of external stimuli associated with the consumption of psychotropic substances are eliminated. Because psychotropic substances are unavailable in hospital, conflicts, e.g. with other patients cannot lead to drug consumption. In this way, stimulus–response cycles are interrupted and inappropriate coping strategies are prevented. Contacts with the drug scene are cut off and restriction of visits, inspection of patient's rooms and urine screening-tests for drugs help to ensure drug-free wards and the abstinence of patients. Any breach of rules should lead to sanctions or denial of privileges. The inpatient unit should be a place for 'health education', where the harmful effects of drugs and alcohol are clearly explained, where stimulants such as cigarettes as well as medication are used in a disciplined way and where a regular lifestyle is pursued, consisting of alternating periods of meaningful tasks and periods of leisure.

Strict ward rules help adolescents to acquire ways to cope with the demands of daily life. Ward rules should be made clear to the patient and nursing staff should ensure that rules are respected. Patients should get up with other patients at a similar time in the morning, take their meals together and participate in the usual ward activities. At the beginning of treatment, restrictions are usually necessary. The patient should not normally leave the ward and visitors are inspected in order to prevent them from bringing psychoactive substances onto the unit. It is important for patients to help with household work, meet basic hygiene requirements and avoid neglect. The inpatient community represents a social environment, in which patients find support and can practise dealing with daily life. Patients have to learn to deal with peers, engage in meaningful leisure activities and manage daily tasks.

Most patients find practising social and communication skills much easier in an environment with their peers. It is important for them to practise living in a social environment as they frequently have severe social difficulties which often lead to social isolation. Difficulties, which occur amongst the community of the unit, provide opportunities for learning appropriate ways of solving conflicts. Group therapy sessions or communicative groups may help in achieving this goal. Initial privilege restrictions are gradually lifted, so that adolescents may be allowed outside the unit accompanied by nursing staff. Eventually, patients may be allowed to go on outings in the company of other patients and finally leave the hospital premises alone. In this way patients can re-attain the social privileges previously denied to them because of the high risk of relapse.

A patient's willingness to learn and achieve something meaningful should be supported by a structured treatment programme. Initially, the patient is required to participate in recreational activities, e.g. sports, later there is participation in occupational therapy, with the opportunity of exercising capabilities and improve concentration and fine motor skills. Occupational therapy may also help the individual to participate in activities useful for spending leisure time in a sensible way, e.g. cooking, painting. School attendance should be re-assumed during hospital treatment, perhaps as individual instruction at first. Eventually, external school attendance may be attempted.

Vocational therapy puts greater demands on adolescents than occupational therapy alone. Vocational therapy is more appropriate for adolescents who normally work and may help them maintain interest in their work. Im some cases patients may be able to attend a vocational training facility outside the hospital and go to work there regularly.

Exercises such as self-assertiveness training or improvement of self-esteem may help to facilitate personality development. Someone with a mature personality is more likely to develop specific coping mechanisms for dealing with conflicts. Inpatient treatment can be structured by combining individual psychotherapy and activities with group psychotherapy and activities.

Psychotherapeutic methods and content

Psychoanalytically orientated psychotherapy, behavioural approaches, counselling and family therapy are frequently combined in a pragmatic approach to treatment.

Sessions should include educating the patient about psychoactive substances, their effects and the risks involved. Individual psychotherapy concentrates on the adolescent's individual situation and is intended to help the patient to remain abstinent and solve current problems. During interviews the tasks of daily life, such as planning the day, organizing leisure time and searching for work or housing may be discussed. Defining small steps gives the therapist the opportunity of reinforcing improvements. Abstinence should be positively rewarded by the therapist, whilst relapses or breaches of ward rules should have negative consequences.

In individual psychotherapy, additional mental disturbances such as anxiety or depression should also be addressed. If the patient is concerned about failing to fulfil demanding tasks or is anxious about failure in social situations, desensitization techniques may be appropriate. Some patients may find writing a diary helpful as a form of 'dialogue'. This may better enable the patient to cope with phases of social isolation on the ward, social helplessness, boredom and insufficient opportunity for communicating with others. With the patient's consent, the diary may serve as the basis for conversation during psychotherapy sessions. The therapist should remember to go beyond narrow intervention techniques and support the patient in dealing with his social situation outside the ward and coping with tasks in school or at work and in his family environment.

Group psychotherapy can be a great help in addressing these problems. Role play, self-assertiveness training and dealing with social situations can all be practised in a group setting as may desensitization techniques. During role play, different situations can be acted out with other patients, for instance, how one might react when insulted or hurt in a social situation, and how to deal with being invited to have a drink or on approach by a drug dealer.

The group is able to support an individual during a motivational crisis, on the other hand, it can point out an individual's problematic behaviour and propose means of correcting it. Dealing with disappointments is often a time of high risk, and group support and role play can be helpful. Creative methods (completing a fairytale or story, drawing about a given theme) may be used to introduce certain topics, particularly when dealing with sensitive issues.

Cooperation with families is important from the start, provided the family is supportive and does not promote substance abuse. A degree of cooperation should be sought even if treatment is aimed at removing an adolescent from a home environment in which substance abuse is tolerated or facilitated.

The therapist should aim to be impartial. Some families fail to realize that the adolescent is at risk for addiction and requires treatment. This may be the case when a parent is drug or alcohol dependent or where child abuse has occurred. Parents may fear that their reputation or the family's whole existence is put at risk if they give their consent for treatment.

Family sessions are aimed at informing parents about drug addiction, psychoactive substances, signs and symptoms of the disorder, about which they are often insufficiently informed. Cooperation with the family should serve to improve their ability to manage conflicts and offer guidance and support. Facilitating factors in the family should be identified and modified.

Contact should also be made with the school, the employer, local drug addiction counselling services, self-help groups and residential groups, in order to keep them fully informed, as they are likely to play an important role in follow-up. It should be established early on whether the patient can continue to attend school or resume work after discharge, in order that plans drawn up do not later fall through.

The demands made on the therapist and nursing staff who work with patients dependent on psychoactive substances are great. On the one hand, they will experience successful treatment, but see failures, discontinuation of treatment and relapses are also to be expected. The therapist, who is frequently initially idealized by the patient as 'the only trustworthy and helpful person' (in contrast to parents, the Youth Welfare Office, the police, etc.), may suddenly find himself the victim of deliberate deceit by the patient. There is a risk of the therapist reacting unduly harshly to the patient for this breach, and it is important not to give up to despondency and punishment at this time. On the other hand, untoward goodwill and excessive indulgence can be equally unhelpful. After all, it is the addiction which leads to ignorance restrictions, breaching of rules, telling of lies, hatching of intrigues and disappointment of the trust put in the patient. Those treating the patient run the risk reacting in a confused, split and inconsistent way and they may lose their motivation for treatment. Instead of treating the disorder, they may turn against the adolescent, eventually rejecting him.

For this reason, multidisciplinary discussions, Balint-group type sessions and personal supervision are essential. The patient's situation should be reconsidered at regular intervals, reassessing his needs and resources and considering alternative treatment options. Attempts made to deceive therapists or nursing staff should be interpreted as inappropriate coping mechanisms and addressed as such with the patient. Alternative behavioural strategies should be developed with the patient so that he can experience success, thus reinforcing the behaviour. The adolescent should be encouraged to define his own therapeutic goals, accept and pursue them. He should also be helped to find replacements for external and internal stimuli, which usually precipitate drug consumption, e.g. visiting a discotheque, experiencing anxiety or depression by seeking less risky alternative activities. If the patient succeeds in reaching short-term goals, the therapist will be motivated to continue the difficult task of making greater therapeutic gains.

Follow-up treatment

Rehabilitation is succeeded by follow-up treatment, in which the patient should play a much more active part. The risk of relapse is greatest in the 6–12 months after treatment. Follow-up appointments should be made at short intervals and should help adolescents to improve their coping skills, provide the opportunity to discuss transitional problems and develop ways of solving them. The adolescent should be continuously encouraged and praised for his effort.

Follow-up may also serve to reduce the risk of relapse by means of regular screening tests for drugs. Important risk factors associated with relapse should be identified, e.g. mood disorder, depression, anxiety, social conflicts, an environment conducive to drug abuse and discussed with the patient. Problems of debt, pressure at school, vocational training and finding work must be addressed. In some places there are schools and vocational training facilities specializing in adolescents with drug or alcohol abuse.

Supportive groups are an important part of follow-up treatment. Groups may be conducted by professionals (drug addiction counselling services) or can be held as self-help groups (Alcoholics Anonymous, Narcotics Anonymous). In some places, the parents of adolescents with alcohol or drug addiction have formed parent support groups. Particularly in larger cities, appropriate residential homes or groups are available, in which adolescents can continue a social integration programme after discharge from an inpatient unit.

Evaluation

Studies on treatment of alcoholism indicate a high risk of patients discontinuing treatment, both in outpatient and inpatient settings. Relapse rates are high, particularly during the first year after inpatient treatment. A prospective multicenter study in Germany (Küfner et al., 1988) showed that about 53% of patients were abstinent 18 months after treatment and 46% were abstinent after 4 years of treatment. Patients who underwent detoxification more than once remained abstinent in 39% of cases (which is a surprisingly high rate). These results emphasize the fact that multiple treatments do improve outcome.

Even when taking into account a spontaneous remission rate of somewhat less than 20% in the long run, the rates for abstinence, controlled drinking or marked reduction of consumption are likely to improve further over time. Abstinence rates after treatment for drug addiction are between 23% and 43% (Ladewig, 1987). Success rates are lower if patients discontinue treatment or if they refuse further treatment after detoxification.

Case report

A 17-year-old female patient was referred by a drug addiction counselling service. She requested admission to a child and adolescent inpatient unit out of her own initiative and against the explicit wish of her parents. Her paternal grandfather had been an alcoholic who committed suicide by hanging. Her father also abused alcohol heavily. Three years prior to admission, the patient had been treated in a child and adolescent psychiatric unit for anorexia nervosa, marked hysterical personality traits and infantile behaviour (interest in infant's toys, desire to be in a play pen, fear of the dark). At that time the patient was admitted because of suspected physical abuse by her father. The patient was discharged upon her parents' wish and against medical advice. Thereafter, the patient completed secondary school and domestic science school with good results and commenced an apprenticeship as a shop assistant.

Asked about alcohol and drug abuse, the patient revealed that her mother had given her beer when she was just 4 years old so that she would sleep better. From the age of 7 years she occasionally consumed beer, wine and spirits. At the age of 16 years, she was already consuming alcohol regularly, beginning in the morning. Shortly before admission she was used to consuming up to six cans of beer before work and carbonated lemonade mixed with spirits during work. Her school referred her to a drug addiction counselling service, whilst her parents denied their daughter's alcohol abuse. Both parents denied knowing anything about their daughter's alcohol problem, but the mother admitted to having searched her daughter's handbag for bottles. The patient defended her use of alcohol as a 'medicine' in order to 'self-medicate' herself for depressed mood, fear of failure but also finally to alleviate withdrawal symptoms. She declared that alcohol had no longer helped 'as medicine' during the weeks before admission.

During withdrawal she had sufferd trembling, stomach cramps, agitation, anxiety and depression almost to the point of suicide. During the initial interview the patient denied hallucinations and declared a wish for abstinence.

Additional complaints included a fear of failing at work and in trade school, difficulties in going to sleep or staying asleep and frequent nightmares. She also had severe bulimia. She was socially isolated and was also withdrawn within the family, also due to her fear of being physically abused by her father. Occasionally, she had experienced depressed moods and had thoughts of suicide.

Therapy and course

Immediatly after admission to hospital the patient discontinued alcohol consumption. However, on the third day of her hospital stay she was discovered behind a shower curtain, secretly drinking a small bottle of cognac that she had hidden under her mattress in order to be able to avoid withdrawal symptoms. She had severe withdrawal symptoms: trembling, shivering, acrocyanosis, tachycardia, agitation, anxiety, nausea, stomach cramps, loss of appetite and an extreme craving for alcohol. She was subsequently treated with clomethiazole for 5 days.

Initially, she received individual psychotherapy and attended group therapy every day. Physical therapy was added soon to improve her physical self-esteem and activity. All other activities were restricted to the ward. Contact with parents was restricted to 1 hour per week in accordance with the patient's wish. She expressed feelings of hate towards her parents and was afraid they might take her out of hospital, in which case she threatened to commit suicide. During family therapy sessions severe discord ensued between the patient and her parents, which had a negative effect on her mood for several days. For this reason family sessions were discontinued. Both parents, especially the mother, denied their daughter's addiction.

Instead, the parents complained that the patient was immoral and ungrateful towards her mother. It was difficult to persuade the parents to allow their daughter to remain in the child and adolescent psychiatric unit. The patient refused to return home and threatened to commit suicide if she was made to return to the family.

Individual psychotherapy sessions soon concentrated on the patient's daily diary entries. Her aggressive and sadistic impulses were discussed, which were ususally directed at persons close to her. During psychotherapy, a trusting relationship ensued and the patient eventually 'admitted' to hearing two 'spirits' converse in her head. The patient said that she also conversed with the spirits and that they advised her. They had forbidden her to speak about them. These symptoms were viewed as an alcohol-induced hallucinosis.

In the course of therapy, topics such as her anorexic symptoms, anxiety, social phobia, guilt and low self-esteem were also discussed. The patient was eventually able to leave the premises accompanied by other patients and nursing staff. Later, she went on outings with other patients only and was finally able to go out alone without relapse. However, due to the fact that psychological addiction persisted, the patient was at considerable risk for relapse in situations which she perceived as particularly demanding throughout the 2 months of inpatient treatment.

The patient's social behaviour vastly improved in the course of weeks, in spite of her great reluctance on admission. She remained friends with another patient for months after discharge. This caused marked improvement of self-esteem and thus had a positive effect on her mood.

A treatment plan was agreed upon at the time of discharge. It combined two steps: first, the patient was referred to an an adult psychiatric inpatient unit, it being felt that she should engage with an adult facility prior to discharge from hospital. Secondly, the patient agreed to move into a residential facility for women, where therapy was to continue after discharge. Her employer had agreed to allow her to complete her apprenticeship as a saleswoman. The patient approached the drug addiction counselling services. There, she made friends with a former patient who had also maintained abstinence, and was able to receive ongoing informal support.

Follow-up

Due to intervention of her parents, the patient was unfortunately not referred from the adult psychiatric unit directly to the residential facility, and in the family environment, she suffered an immediate relapse. After 3 months the patient again approached the drug addiction counselling services and attended weekly counselling sessions. With the aid of the drug addiction counselling services, the patient was able to obtain funding for a place in the residential facility to which she had intended to move into after discharge. The patient continued the first year of her apprenticeship.

However, before being able to move into the residential facility, the patient suffered a further relapse including delirious symptoms and required hospitalization for several weeks.

After finally moving into the residential facility, the patient was able to remain abstinent and repeated the first year of her apprenticeship successfuly. Marked bulimia, phases of depressed mood without hallucinations and thoughts of suicide were still present after the end of the follow-up period. She had cut off contact with her family, had a boyfriend who also lived in the residential facility and she had also made other appropriate social contacts.

REFERENCES

Feuerlein, W. (1995). Definition, Diagnose, Entstehung und Akutbehandlung der Alkoholkrankheit. In *Handbuch Alkohol, Alkoholismus, alkoholbedingte Organschäden*, ed. H. K. Seitz, C. S. Lieber and U. A. Simanowski, pp. 1–20. Leipzig: Barth.

Küfner, H., Feuerlein, W. and Huber, M. (1988). Die stationäre Behandlung von Alkoholabhängigen. Ergebnisse der 4 Jahreskatamnesen, mögliche Konsequenzen für Indikationsstellung und Behandlung. *Suchtgefahren*, **34**, 157–271.

Ladewig, D. (1987). Katamnesen bei Opiatabhängigkeiten. In *Langzeitverläufe bei Suchtkrankheiten*, ed. D. Kleiner, pp. 55–69. Berlin: Springer.

Washton, A. M. (1996). *Psychotherapy and substance abuse. A practitioner's handbook*. New York: Guilford Press.

World Health Organization (WHO) (1992). *The ICD-10 classification of mental and behavioural disorders. Clinical descriptions and diagnostic guidelines*. Geneva: WHO.

World Health Organization (WHO) (1996). *Multiaxial classification of child psychiatric disorders. The ICD-10 classification of mental and behavioural disorders in children and adolescents*. Geneva: WHO.

21 Eating disorders

Matthias Martin

Anorexia nervosa

Characteristics of the disorder

The diagnostic guidelines for anorexia nervosa in ICD-10 (WHO, 1992) include the following features: marked weight loss to at least 15% below expected weight or a Quetelet's Body Mass Index (BMI) of 17.5 (BMI = body weight in kg/[height in m]^2). The weight loss is self-induced predominantly by avoiding highly caloric food. Additional symptoms include: self-induced vomiting, self-induced purging, excessive physical exercise and the use of appetite depressants and/or diuretics (Brownell and Fairburn, 1995).

The patient has a distortion of body image with the persistent, intrusive and overvalued idea of being 'too fat' or being 'flabby'. Endocrine abnormalities involving the hypothalamic–pituitary–gonadal axis are also present. If the disorder begins prepubertally, development during this period, including growth, is disturbed (Szmukler et al., 1995).

Progressive cachexia is associated with a number of physical changes, which are described in Table 21.1.

Extreme cachexia is associated with neuropsychological disturbances, including poor concentration, mental fatigue and repetitive and obsessional thoughts, which usually concern food and eating. Cranial computed tomography has demonstrated that pseudoatrophy of the brain may occur at this stage, with enlargement of the sulci and the longitudinal cerebral fissure, and in a few cases, even enlargement of the ventricles. Psychological tests usually reveal disturbed concentration, and prolonged reaction times, reduced ability to perceive visual figures, deficient visual–motor coordination and reduced visual memory. These deficits are relevant in psychotherapy, demonstrating the importance of not making excessive cognitive or emotional demands on patients at the beginning of therapy (Remschmidt and Herpertz-Dahlmann, 1988a).

Table 21.1. Physical changes in patients with anorexia or bulimia nervosa

Physical examination	Dry and scaly skin (A*) Lanuginous hair (A) Acrocyanosis, cutis marmorata (A) Hair loss Swelling of salivary glands Marked caries (B*) Calloused skin on the backs of the hands (due to repeated manual induction of vomiting) Insufficient growth
Laboratory findings	Pathological blood cell count (leucopenia, anaemia and thrombocytopenia Fluid and electrolyte disturbance Elevated transaminases, amylase, creatinine, urea Changes in lipid metabolism Reduced albumin and other plasma proteins
Endocrinology	Disturbance of the hypothalamic–pituitary–adrenal, thyroid and gonadal axes Elevated growth hormone
Other	Abnormal cranial CT scan (pseudoatrophy of the brain) Oesophagitis EKG-abnormalities Complications due to misuse of laxatives, e.g. osteomalacia, malabsorption syndrome, severe constipation, osteoarthropathy Osteoporosis

*Symptoms applicable to anorexia only are indicated by (A), those applicable to bulimia only are indicated by (B).

Psychological findings

Whereas physical findings in patients are usually similar, psychological findings tend to be variable. Despite this, several psychopathological symptoms are characteristically present: loss of control over food intake, persistent denial of the disorder and distortion of body image, which in most cases relates to the size and shape of the abdomen, buttocks and thighs (see Figs. 21.1 and 21.2).

In the course of the disorder patients often lose their sense of hunger and satiety. Low self-esteem is almost always present. As the disorder progresses and patients continue to lose weight, they also lose their interests, social contacts and increasingly become depressed. Frequently elaborate eating

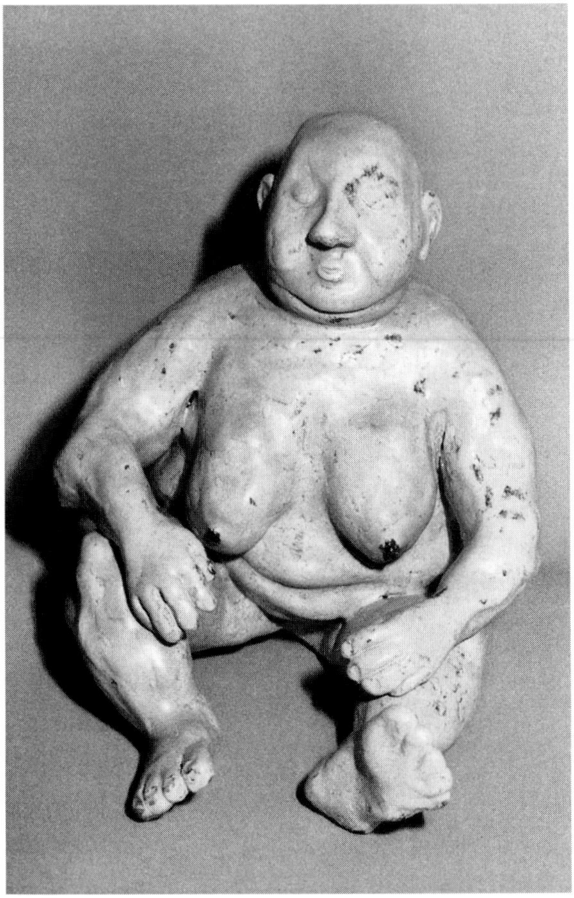

Figs. 21.1 and 21.2. Models made by a patient with anorexia nervosa to illustrate body image disturbance. The patient is anxious about being either too fat or too thin. She said: 'I don't like either.'

rituals develop together with obsessive thoughts involving food and calories. These psychopathological findings depend to some extent on body weight and some, especially depression, may disappear once the patient approaches normal body weight (Table 21.2).

In approaching therapy, it is important to distinguish between anorexic patients who only restrict food intake and those who have occasional bulimic episodes ('bulimanorexia'). Dietary treatment usually begins with a restriction of sweet, highly caloric and carbohydrate-rich foods. In the course of the disorder some patients lose control over their diet. These patients may subsequently experience an intractable urge to over-eat, followed by self-induced vomiting or excessive purging by means of excessive laxative use (Fig. 21.3).

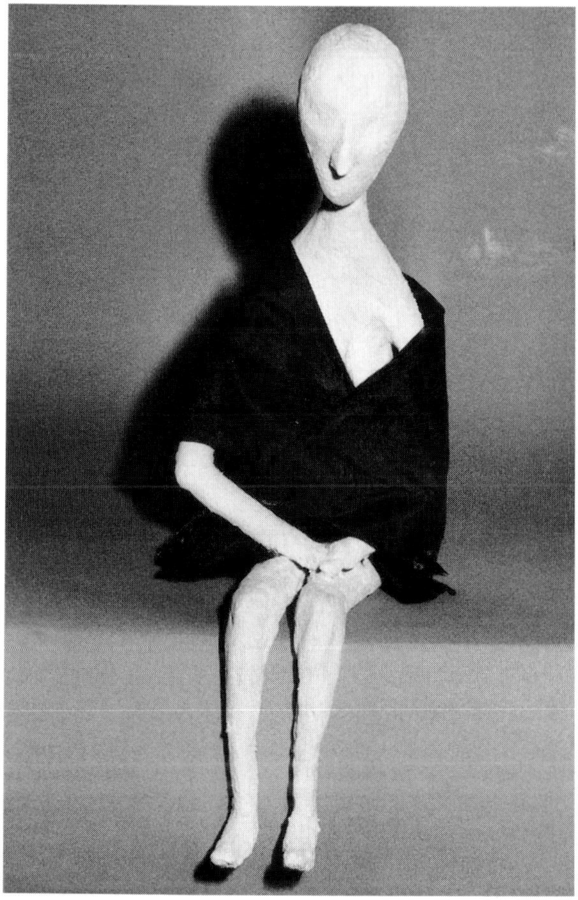

Fig. 21.2. (See caption of Fig. 21.1).

Aetiology

Eating disorders are today said to be caused by several factors, including biological, cultural, familial and psychological ones. Some of these factors are also held responsible for the increasing incidence of eating disorders in our society.

Biological factors may include a genetic predisposition or biological changes during adolescence, triggering eating disorders at that age (Remschmidt, 1992). Monozygotic twins have a concordance rate of 50%, whereas in dizygotic twins the risk is less than 10%. In addition, relatives of patients with an eating disorder have an eightfold risk of also being affected.

It has been suggested that the many physical changes taking place during puberty contribute to the biological risk of the disorder. Interaction between physical and mental factors are also presumed to play a role, particularly in

Table 21.2. Psychological and psychopathological findings in anorexia nervosa

Loss of control over 'diet'
Denial of the disorder
Body image disturbance
Loss of the sense of hunger and satiety, also occasionally the loss of other emotions
Low self-esteem
Loss of interests
Loss of social contacts
Depressed mood
Eating rituals and obsessional thoughts, particularly concerning food and eating
Reduced libido
High achievers

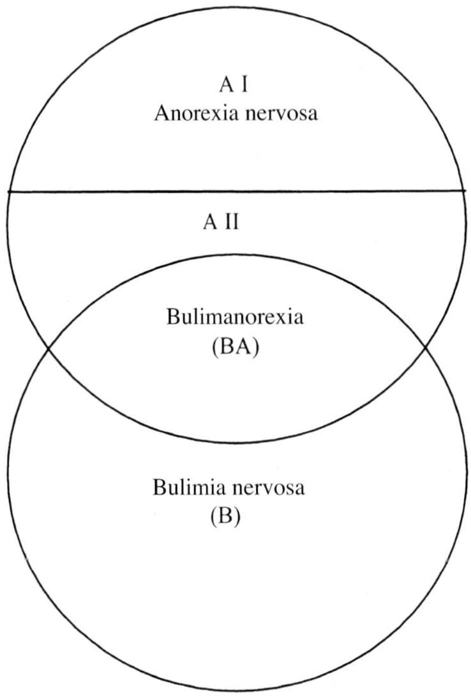

Fig. 21.3. Association of anorexia nervosa with bulimia nervosa (Remschmidt and Herpertz-Dahlmann, 1988).

terms of coping psychologically with the physical changes occurring. The adolescent is confronted with his or her growth and maturation, particularly psychosexual, at the same time as increasing autonomy and detachment from the family (Remschmidt, 1992). Social pressure towards being thin has increased since the 1950s, when being thin became increasingly associated with success and attractiveness. Thus social and cultural factors contribute to the aetiology of eating disorders.

Almost no other psychosomatic or neurotic disorder in adolescence is, to such a great extent, associated with the typical problems of this developmental phase: problems of identity, conflicts with authority and autonomy, disturbance of psychosexual development and problems of gender role. A commonly encountered interpretation of anorexia nervosa is that of 'solving problems by losing weight'. The physical signs of sexual development are made to disappear, thus enabling the patient to 'remain a child' and avoid the demands of appropriate psychosexual development. Problems with autonomy and authority are transferred to the 'battlefield' of food intake. However, problems with autonomy and identity are ubiquitous in adolescence, and they cannot alone account for the pathogenesis of anorexia nervosa. Minuchin et al. (1978) extended the psychopathology to include families. They used the term 'psychosomatic families' to describe patterns of interaction typical for families with an anorexic patient: emotional overinvolvement, overprotective behaviour, rigidity, avoidance of conflicts and inappropriate approaches to problem-solving within the family. These findings have, at best, only been partially confirmed by others (Kog et al., 1987). Others have suggested an ideology over several generations of renunciation, sacrifice and selflessness (Stierlin and Weber, 1987). The unanswered issue in these family studies is whether the behavioural patterns described were present before the beginning of the disorder or were secondary. Family interaction seems to be disturbed in more families with an anorexic patient than in normal families, whilst families with a bulimic patient are even more severely disturbed than those with anorexia (Humphrey, 1988). The risk factors for eating disorders are summarized in Table 21.3.

Therapy

General considerations

The most important aim of any approach to the treatment of anorexia is to restore a 'healthy' body weight (Garner and Garfinkel, 1997). This implies a weight, at which the most important symptoms of this psychosomatic disorder, i.e. those caused by the disturbance of the hypothalamic–pituitary–gonadal axis, are no longer present. In this respect osteomalacia – due to low estrogen

Table 21.3. Risk factors for eating disorders

Age (around puberty)
Female sex
High pressure towards thinness (models, athletes)
High achievers, e.g. medical students
Inability to perceive one's emotional state
Family conflicts and excessively close bonds
Very early puberty
Twins
Insulin-dependent diabetes mellitus

levels – may be a good indicator. The target weight may be estimated by several different methods. Whereas the Broca Index is no longer widely used in the assessment of eating disorders, the body mass index (BMI) has gained increasing importance in this respect. In calculating target weight, it is important to allow for the patients' age. It has been suggested that the 25th BMI-percentile is an appropriate target weight (Hebebrand et al., 1996). Age-adjusted BMI-percentiles may be used for this purpose (Fig. 21.4). A clear agreement should be made with the patient concerning the course of treatment, because subsequent weight gain is frequently associated with conflicts and quarrels with the therapist and nursing staff. The BMI-percentiles may be useful in explaining to the patient how and why a particular target weight was determined.

Continuous weight gain over a reasonable period of time (about 0.5 kg per week) is essential for other therapeutic efforts to succeed. Many symptoms – including several of the severe psychopathological symptoms – disappear once the patient has regained normal body weight, e.g. depressive mood, obsessional thoughts concerning food and eating, reduced social contacts. However, this is not the case in all patients. Specific treatment is therefore essential if symptoms persist.

The decision as to whether admission to hospital is required or whether outpatient treatment is sufficient, largely depends upon the patient's body weight. With very low body weight the patient has usually completely lost control over the disorder and only inpatient treatment is likely to be successful.

For treatment of anorexia nervosa on an outpatient basis, the patient must be highly motivated and should have a supportive family background. Usually, outpatient treatment is successful only if the disorder is of recent onset. It is essential to agree upon regular assessment of body weight and the patient

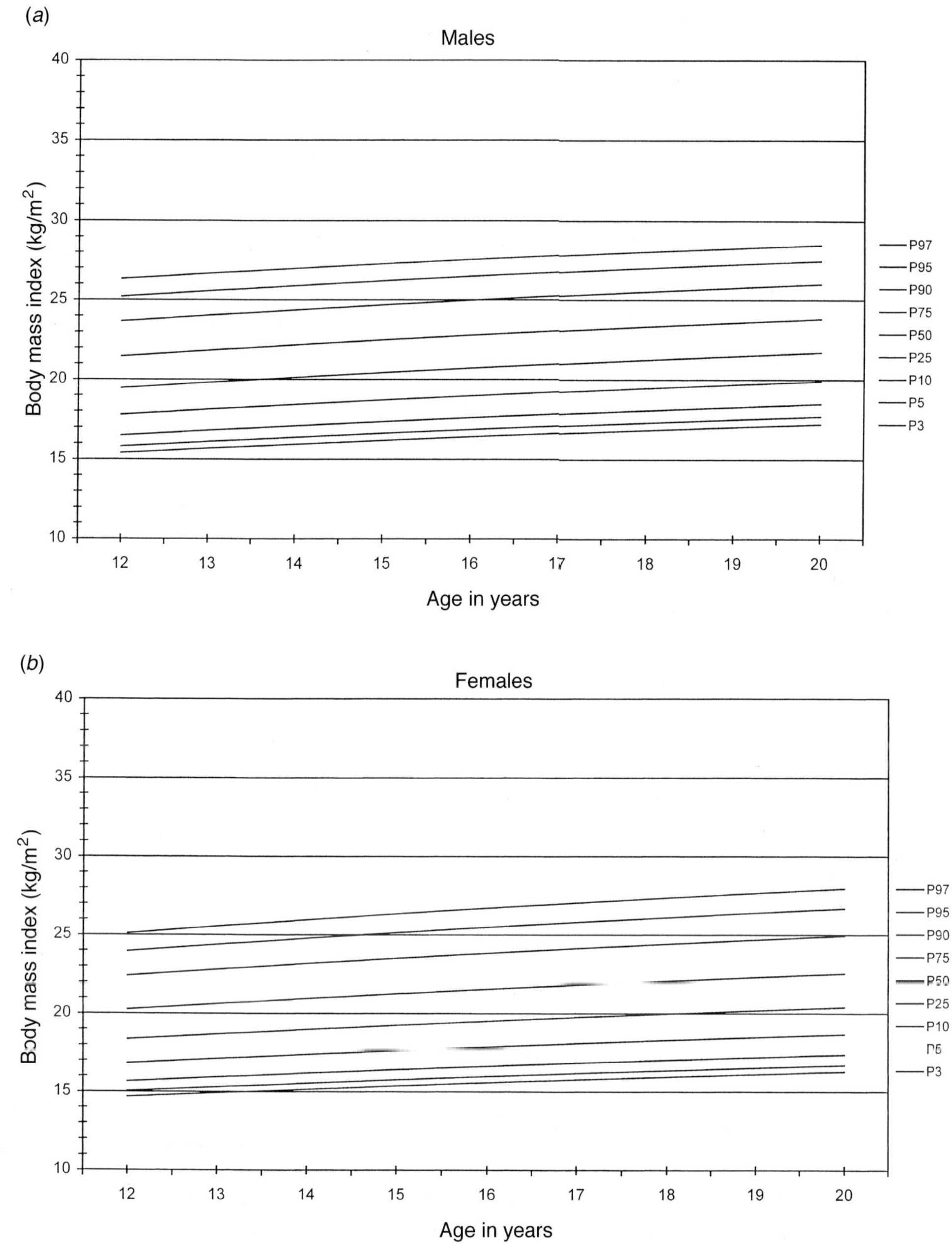

Fig. 21.4. Age-adjusted BMI-percentiles (Hebebrand et al., 1996).

should be willing to continuously gain weight (about 0.5 kg per week). The patient should also agree to continue treatment in hospital if weight gain is insufficient. Treatment of anorexia nervosa without regular assessment of body weight must be regarded as malpractice.

Case vignette

The following case vignette of a patient we assessed, serves as an example of how things may go wrong with inappropriate therapy techniques. This female patient with anorexia nervosa underwent psychoanalytically orientated family therapy. In the course of treatment, only family therapy sessions and no individual therapy sessions had been held. The therapist did not assess the patient's body weight. During the course of therapy, the patient continued to lose weight and was eventually so weak that her father was forced to carry her to therapy sessions. Eventually, her father noticed her increasing dyspnea. After admission to an intensive care unit, pericardial effusion was diagnosed, requiring immediate surgical treatment.

Several therapy methods are usually combined in the treatment of anorexia in an inpatient setting, because a disorder as complex as anorexia nervosa rarely responds to one treatment method alone. Attempts to see the disorder as unifactorial or to treat it by a single method alone are inappropriate. A combination of symptom-orientated behavioural approaches (in order to influence eating behaviour), psychodynamic approaches and family therapy are appropriate in treatment. In outpatient settings individual therapy may be combined with family therapy, whereas in hospital a combination of individual therapy, group therapy, counselling of parents and family therapy should be used, accompanied by compulsory ward activities, occupational therapy and physiotherapy aimed at influencing the disturbance of body image.

In some cases of anorexia nervosa with persistent and severe depression, antidepressant medication may additionally be required.

Specific approaches to therapy

The specific therapeutic approaches discussed below are primarily intended for an inpatient setting and hence are aimed at severely disturbed patients. However, in modified form these approaches may be used in an outpatient or day-hospital setting (Garner and Garfinkel, 1997).

The different phases of inpatient treatment are listed in Table 21.4. Therapy may be divided into four phases, followed by follow-up after discharge. The first essential phase of therapy is to improve food intake and raise body weight; during the second and third phases individual psychotherapy is emphasized,

Table 21.4. Phases of inpatient treatment of anorexia nervosa

Phase 1: Increase in body weight
Tube feeding required in some cases
Exclusion of the family required in some cases
Phase 2: External control of food intake
Ready-to-eat meals
Increasing involvement of the family
Frequent individual psychotherapy
Phase 3: Self-control of food intake
Family therapy
Continued individual psychotherapy
Phase 4: Family therapy
Increasing participation in the activities of daily life
Preparation for discharge
Phase 5: Follow-up on an outpatient basis and continued family therapy

From Remschmidt and Herpertz-Dahlmann (1988a).

whereas during the fourth phase the family is increasingly included in treatment.

Steps to improve weight and food intake

Despite the fact that patients with anorexia are often 'experts' at counting calories, they usually have distorted assumptions about the composition and content of different foods. Thus many anorexic patients keep up the notion that fat and carbohydrates should be eliminated from meals as far as possible. Advising patients about the necessity of a well-balanced and healthy diet is therefore an essential part of initial treatment. Accommodations may be made for a patient's intense dislike of certain foods. Some patients may be used to a vegetarian diet, which should be respected. However, the larger volume of food that must be consumed may present a problem.

In an inpatient setting the patient's eating behaviour may be observed for 1–3 days in order to assess the extent of the problem. However, in the case of extremely emaciated patients, tube feeding may be necessary immediately following admission. At this stage, patients frequently experience tube feeding as a relief.

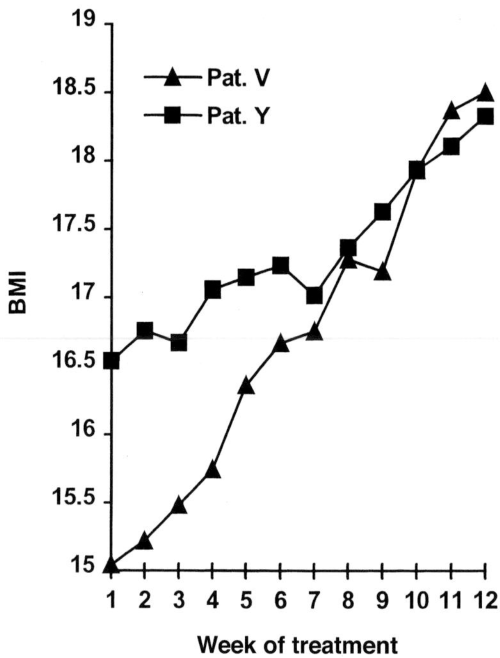

Fig. 21.5. Weight gain of two female patients (V and Y) compared, shown as an increase of the Body Mass Index (BMI).

Case vignette

A 16-year-old female patient with a weight of 36 kg on admission and a height of 178 cm reported that she had been unable to sleep during the past few weeks before admission. She suffered insomnia because of obsessional thoughts concerning the question of whether she should eat one or half an apple and one or half a tablespoon of yoghurt the next day (as a daily ration). Tube feeding was started immediately, and her obsessional thoughts and insomnia disappeared with increasing body weight

Weight gain should be continuous but not too rapid (see Fig. 21.5). Too steep an increase in body weight may impair prognosis because patients find it more difficult to accept and sustain their weight (Remschmidt et al., 1990). Fig. 21.5 shows the weight gain of two female patients over a course of 12 weeks. Patient V shows a faster rate of weight gain than patient Y. Follow-up 3 months after discharge showed that patient Y had sustained her weight, whereas patient V had relapsed with severe weight loss. These observations (Remschmidt et al., 1990) suggest that optimal rate of weight gain is relevant to prognosis and should therfore be one important aim of treatment.

Most patients initially require controlled food intake, i.e. scheduled meals with determined caloric content, fixed meal times and time limited duration. Detailed meal schedules may be helpful (see Table 21.5).

A total of six meals per day are served to ensure that individual servings need not be too large. Small meals tend to be better tolerated by patients. The total number of calories required per day will depend on the weight on admission. This will need to be reviewed and increased as weight increases and normal activities are resumed.

Methods using positive reinforcement to increase weight have proved helpful during this initial phase. This may be aimed at either weight gain or eating behaviour. In practice, focusing on weight gain has proved more helpful. Reinforcing weight gain has the advantage that patients maintain the responsibility and autonomy when eating, conflicts with parents or nursing staff about eating behaviour are avoided and the criterion for reinforcement, i.e. weight gain can be determined precisely (Steinhausen, 1993). In effect, a behavioural contract with the patient is set up (see Table 21.6). Through achieving projected goals, i.e. progressive weight gain the patient is granted increasingly more privileges, which reinforce weight gain.

During treatment there is a constant risk of deception by the patient. Common methods of manipulating weight are drinking water or binging prior to weighings, which may then trigger bulimic episodes.

Towards the end of treatment, reinforcement should be gradually discontinued. Treatment should aim to support the patient in attaining more and more self-control over her eating behaviour. Once the desired behaviour change has developed in an inpatient setting, it is necessary to take steps to generalize this to the home setting and ensure that weight gain continues. This can be achieved by gradually lengthening periods of home leave for the patient, prior to discharge.

Apart from this behavioural approach, inpatient psychotherapy is restricted in the first phase of treatment to providing empathy and support. Problems and conflicts should not be directly addressed at this point as many patients are unable to properly engage in psychotherapy because of the cognitive impairment resulting from malnutrition and cachexia.

Psychotherapy

Individual psychotherapy should be undertaken in addition to behavioural methods. A wide spectrum of different methods are described in the literature, ranging from psychoanalytically orientated psychotherapy, behavioural and cognitive therapy to approaches based on feminist principles.

Table 21.5. Example for a meal schedule: 2400 kcal/day

	Protein	kcal
1. Breakfast:		
75 g wholegrain roll	3.60	120
20 g butter	1.40	155
25 g jam/marmalade	0.20	64
or 25 g honey	0.10	76
or 30 g chocolate spread	1.50	165
40 g cottage cheese	6.30	58
2. Snack (10: 00 am):		
150 g high-fibre yoghurt	6.10	147
or 150 g fresh fruit	0.45	82
or 150 g cottage cheese with fruit	7.90	185
3. Lunch		
120 g meat	24.20	191
10 g fat	0.04	76
150 g vegetables	3.70	42
10 g fat	0.04	76
or 1 serving of salad	0.90	20
30 g sour cream	0.80	38
100 g wholegrain noodles	3.90	117
or 100 g wholegrain rice	2.10	111
or 100 g potatoes	2.00	87
or 100 g mashed potatoes	5.90	162
3a. Dessert		
150 g fresh fruit	0.45	82
or 150 g high-fibre yoghurt	6.10	147
or 150 g pudding	4.10	150
or 1 serving of icecream	4.00	205
4. Tea (2: 30 pm)		
50 g wholegrain bread	3.60	120
10 g butter	0.70	78
25 g jam	0.20	64
50 g cottage cheese (2% fat)	6.30	58
or 1 piece of cake	8.00	200
5. Supper		
75 g wholegrain bread	5.20	180

Table 21.5. (*cont.*)

	Protein	kcal
20 g butter	1.40	155
30 g cheese (45% fat)	7.50	120
30 g sausage	3.70	110
150 g salad or fresh fruit	0.90	20
6. Late meal		
150 g high-fibre yoghurt	6.10	147
or 325 g muesli	10.60	445
Total	84.33	2371

Thursdays and Sundays 1 egg/1 piece of cake or 2 snack bars.

Table 21.6. Behavioural contract with patient Y

Current weight	37.3 kg	Short walks in a small group, activities on the ward
	38.5 kg	Occupational therapy
	39.5 kg	Attendance at hospital school
	40.5 kg	Unrestricted visits by the family
	41.5 kg	Walks in a larger group, physical therapy
	42.0 kg	Unsupervised meal, e.g. tea
	42.5 kg	Unrestricted visiting hours
	43.0 kg	Unsupervised meal, e.g. snack
	43.5 kg	Group activities outside the ward
	44.0 kg	Unsupervised meal, e.g. late meal
	44.5 kg	All meals gradually unsupervised (as agreed)
	45.5 kg	Outings with other patients unaccompanied by nursing staff
	46.5 kg	Weekend visits at home (one day at first, eventually two days)
Target weight	48.0 kg	Unaccompanied outings and temporary discharge for a few days

Psychodynamic approaches are recommended particularly for older adolescents, during which current concerns may be discussed in the light of the patient's biography, family background and developmental phase. Therapy frequently revolves around issues such as low self-esteem, feelings of inadequacy, self-depreciation and a desire for harmony, accompanied by the inablity to express conflicts within the family. A further common problem is the tendency of the patient to value achievement-orientated activities over other social or recreational activities. Further tendencies include the inability to view interpersonal relations as other than competitive, a perfectionist attitude, anxiety in sexual topics and insecurity in the female role. Feelings of ineffectiveness, powerlessness and inadequacy lead to a situation in which personal autonomy can be expressed only by rigorous control over the body.

Psychodynamic therapy aims to help the patient understand the aetiology of the disorder, analyse the role which morbid attitudes play and develop new patterns of thinking and acting. It should be borne in mind that the ability to be retrospective is still limited in adolescence. Therapy should therefore focus mainly on current concerns rather than attempts to reinterpret the past. Treatment should address current problems and develop appropriate ways of coping with future developmental demands.

Cognitive approaches to therapy

Frequently severe dysfunctional thoughts and attitudes develop in the course of anorexia nervosa, which tend to be persistent and difficult to correct. Therapy needs to address these thoughts and attitudes. Cognitive therapy has been shown to be useful in treating chronic cases of anorexia nervosa, and is also useful as a method of brief psychotherapy.

Dysfunctional attitudes towards the body, weight and nutrition may be treated with cognitive methods. They are also appropriate for treating low self-esteem, feelings of inadequacy and distortion of self-perception (Steinhausen, 1993).

Behavioural theory views the symptoms of anorexia as being reinforced by cognitive mechanisms: weight reduction by restricting food intake is in fact cognitive reinforcement of the behaviour because the patient experiences competency, autonomy and self-control. Asking the patient 'What remains, if you give up fasting?' touches the central point of this problem. Cognitive therapy also addresses the patient's severely disturbed self-esteem. Usually patients have a large number of negative attitudes concerning themselves, their emotions, self-appraisal and the assessment of their own abilities. These symptoms may be treated by cognitive therapy, first devised for the treatment of depression (Beck, 1976).

Using cognitive therapy, the anorexic patient learns to improve the perception of her thoughts and emotions, she recognizes the connection between dysfunctional thoughts, emotions and inapproppriate behaviours. She can then be more realistic in the evaluation of her attitudes, reinterpreting them more appropriately and eventually modify the basis of her initial assumptions (Steinhausen, 1993).

Example

Many patients with anorexia say: 'Everyone thinks that thin people are more attractive and competent.' This 'hypothesis' is discussed during therapy.

- Do other people really believe that thin people are more interesting?
- Is this relationship really proportional (the thinner people are, the more attractive they seem)?
- Does this apply to everyone, or only to a subgroup, who follow every fashion trend?
- Do most people instantly think of thinness when using the words 'interesting', 'attractive' or 'competent'?

A dialogue incorporating these points can lead to a discussion of culturally determined ideals concerning body image, ideals of being thin, the feminine role, the purpose of physical attraction, etc.

Family therapy

Family and environmental interventions are usually included in the treatment of anorexia nervosa. However, the disorder can not be viewed as a symptom of dysfunctional family interaction alone (Vandereycken, 1987; Kog and Vandereycken, 1985). Individual psychotherapy should be meshed with family therapy sessions, both in terms of time and content. An overview of this approach is shown in Table 21.7.

In addition to individual diagnostic procedures, family assessment should be undertaken before commencing therapy (see Chapter 12). Parents should be educated about the disorder and the therapeutic steps which are planned (Table 21.7). Family therapy has two main aims: first, to structure the course of therapy and to help to improve interactions within the family. Secondly, to focus on specific relationships within the family and address family conflicts, e.g. between the patient and her parents. At this stage, some topics from individual psychotherapy sessions may be introduced into family therapy. In this way, individual and family therapy are complementary parts of treatment as a whole.

During follow-up, therapy should continue on an outpatient basis, focusing alternately on individual and family problems. One session of individual psychotherapy per week should be undertaken, supplemented by one family therapy session per month. However, very few controlled studies exist empirically showing the efficacy of family therapy in anorexia nervosa. Russell et al. (1992) found that familiy therapy is particularly effective in younger, more acutely ill patients. However, family therapy as the sole treatment should be

Table 21.7. Example of the course of treatment in a case of anorexia nervosa (both in- and outpatient therapy)

Therapy phase	Duration	Individual psychotherapy	Family therapy
Assessment	1st week	Initial assessment ⇩	Initial assessment ⇩
First phase of inpatient therapy	3 weeks	Tube feeding, medical care, antidepressant medication ⇩	Informing and counselling parents (2 sessions with parents) ⇩
Second phase of inpatient therapy	2 months	Behavioural therapy aimed at eating behaviour (daily); individual psychotherapy (2 sessions per week); group therapy (2 hours per week), additional physical therapy (2 sessions per week) ⇩	Counselling and instructing parents (2 sessions per week) ⇩
Third phase of inpatient therapy	2 months	Self-controlled behavioural therapy to improve eating behaviour (daily); nutritional education (total of 2 hours); individual psychotherapy (2 sessions per week); group therapy (2 hours per week); social competency and generalization training; weekend visits home; school attendance at school outside the hospital ⇩	Family therapy: structuring the course of therapy and advising parents (aim of improving family interaction); 1 session every 2 weeks ⇩ Family therapy: addressing family conflicts between the patient and her parents; 1 session every 2 weeks ⇩
Outpatient follow-up	7 months	Weight check every week by the family physician Individual psychotherapy; 1 session per week	Family therapy: addressing family conflicts between the patient and her parents; 1 session per month

reserved for a highly selected group of young patients whose disorder is of short duration. In addition, a high degree of cooperation from the parents is required and the family must not be severely disturbed (Hall, 1987).

Including the family must be considered an essential part of the treatment of anorexia nervosa, even if the main emphasis of treatment is individual work. The family-orientated approach to the treatment of anorexia includes counselling, improving personal interaction and resolving conflicts within the family.

Prognosis and evaluation of treatment

The criteria suggested by Morgan and Russell (1975) are helpful for determining the outcome of therapy: good outcome comprises regained weight (± 15% of normal weight) and regular menstruation, fair outcome is reflected by marked fluctuation in weight and irregular menstruation, whereas in poor outcome body weight remains below 85% of normal weight and amenorrhoea is present. Data from follow-up studies (Herzog et al., 1992; Remschmidt et al., 1988) show that 40% of patients can be classified as good outcome, 30% as fair and 30% as poor. With longer follow-up intervals, success rates for all patients with anorexia are about 60–70% (Herpertz-Dahlmann and Remschmidt, 1994).

It is generally agreed that most patients benefit from a multimodal approach to treatment. However, there is insufficient data to prove the effectiveness of every component of treatment programmes (Steinhausen, 1994). The effectivity of operant behavioural therapy has been best evaluated (Bemis, 1987). In a controlled study, Crisp et al. (1991) compared three groups comprising inpatient treatment, outpatient treatment with individual and family therapy, and outpatient group therapy. All three treatment programmes additionally utilized behavioural therapy aimed at increasing weight and improving eating behaviour. All three approaches to treatment were reported to be equally effective in terms of target weight, regular menstruation and psychosexual development. These results also applied to the follow-up 1 year later.

Russell et al. (1992) reviewed the results of three studies which looked at the effect of family therapy on patients with anorexia nervosa, and concluded that family therapy was effective in early onset anorexia when the disorder has not progressed to a chronic state. Persistent improvement was confirmed after a follow-up period of 5 years. Continued supervision of eating behaviour by the parents was reported to be the key to successful treatment.

Bulimia nervosa

ICD-10 defines bulimia nervosa (F50.2) as 'repeated bouts of overeating and an excessive preoccupation with the control of body weight, leading the patient to adopt extreme measures so as to mitigate the fattening effects of ingested food.' The following criteria should be met to make the diagnosis (WHO, 1992).

(i) Persistent preoccupation with eating and irresistible craving for food; the patient succumbs to episodes of overeating in which large amounts of food are consumed in very short periods of time.

(ii) The patient attempts to counteract the fattening effects of food by one or more of the following: self-induced vomiting, purgative abuse, alternating periods of starvation, use of medications such as appetite suppressants, thyroid preparations or diuretics.

(iii) The psychopathology consists of a morbid dread of fatness; the patient sets herself sharply defined weight thershold, well below the premorbid weight that constitutes the optimum or healthy weight in the opinion of the physician.

(iv) There is often, but not always, a history of an earlier episode of anorexia nervosa, the interval between the two disorders ranging from a few months to several years. This earlier episode may have been fully expressed, or may have assumed a minor cryptic form with a moderate loss of weight and/or a transient phase of amenorrhoea.

Characteristics of the disorder

Epidemiology

All epidemiological studies support the current opinion that anorexic and bulimic behaviour has increased in civilized countries of the western world. However, the increase in bulimia nervosa is more difficult to prove than the increase in anorexia. Bulimia nervosa was only described as a disorder in its own right in the late 1970s (Russell, 1979). In 1980, bulimia nervosa was included as a diagnostic category in DSM-III (APA, 1980).

Many patients with bulimia manage to keep their symptoms secret to a large extent for long periods of time. This means that many cases remain undetected (Remschmidt and Herpertz-Dahlmann, 1989). In a study by Paul et al. (1984) the majority of patients were between 20 and 30 years old, 16% were younger and 22% were older. In the majority of cases the disorder began between 14 and 20 years of age. Incidence peaked at 18 years of age. The population prevalence of bulimia in women between the ages of 18 and 35, is 2–4% using DSM-III criteria (Fichter, 1984).

Symptoms

The main symptoms are bulimic episodes, characterized by an irresistible craving for food followed by episodes of overeating and frequently self-induced vomiting. Between bulimic episodes, patients usually keep to a strict diet.

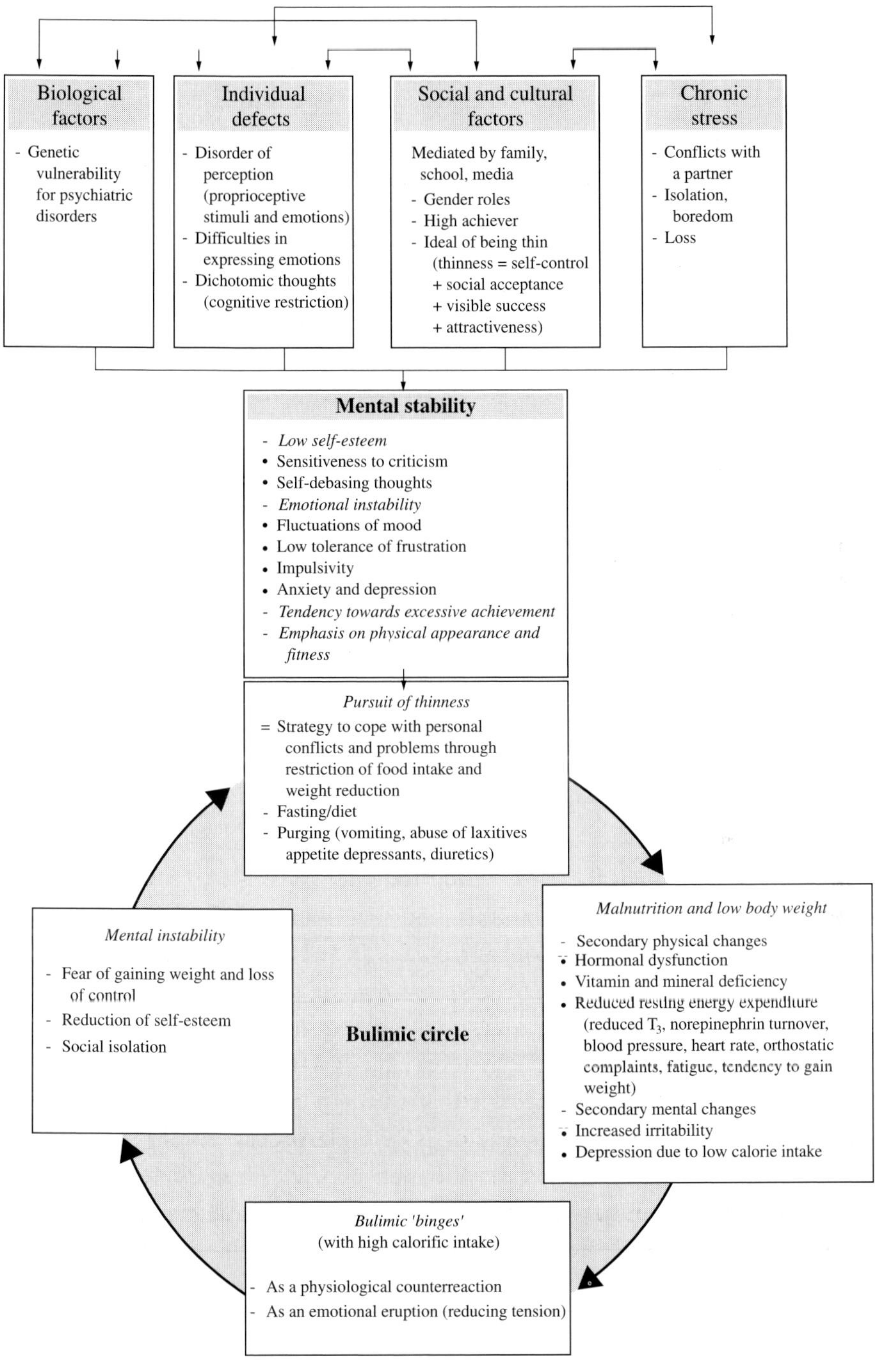

Fig. 21.6. Model for the aetiology and maintenance of bulimic eating disorders (Fichter, 1989a).

Certain foods are avoided, only to be consumed in great amounts during a bulimic episode. Body weight – which is usually insufficient – is rigorously controlled. Some patients have marked depression and become increasingly socially isolated as the disorder progresses. In some cases addictive behaviour (alcohol, medication, drugs) may additionally complicate the disorder. As in anorexia, body image is usually disturbed (Remschmidt and Herpertz-Dahlmann, 1988b).

Aetiology

In order to comprehend the various contributing factors in the aetiology and maintenance of bulimia, long term mulifactorial analyses are necessary. An overview of factors precipitating and sustaining the disorder is shown in Fig. 21.6. These factors determine the nature of therapy used in treatment.

Social and cultural influences, e.g. female role; ideal of being thin, individual psychological and psychopathological factors, e.g. affective disorders; impulse disorders, genetic factors and physiological effects of disturbed eating behaviour (biological factors), family influences and the developmental demands of late adolescence all contribute to the aetiology of bulimia nervosa. Family problems, e.g. separation of parents, excessive demands at school, increasing environmental demands or denied autonomy during adolescence or psychiatric disorder of a parent may trigger bulimia. Bulimia frequently occurs if an individual's personal and social development has been disrupted (Herpertz-Dahlmann, 1991)

The many aetiological factors acting together have led to several different approaches to treatment of bulimia nervosa (Vanderlinden et al., 1992). If bulimia is viewed as the symptom of an underlying affective disorder, an approach similar to treating depression may seem appropriate; if it is regarded as a symptom of impulse disorder, an approach similar to treating addiction may be considered helpful; if it is seen as a reaction which is continuously negatively reinforced, an approach to treatment resembling that of anxiety disorder will seem appropriate; if it is considered the result of disturbed cognition, congnitive treatment may be preferred; if it is regarded as a dissociative symptom, an approach to treatment aimed at dissociative disorder will seem promising; if it is seen as a symptom of a type of socialization process forced upon women, an approach to therapy based on feminist principles may seem appropriate.

Treatment

It is inappropriate simply to apply methods of treating anorexia to the treat-

Table 21.8. Assessment of bulimia nervosa

History, current complaints
Physical examination
Assessment for additional psychiatric disorders
Assessment of eating behaviour
Nutritional diary
Comparing past and present eating habits
Discussion of attitudes concerning eating
Patient's subjective target weight
Body perception
Functional analysis of eating behaviour and other behaviours
Identifying triggers and sustaining conditions
situational conditions
patient's reactions (emotions, thoughts, behaviours)
results of reactions (positive, negative, short term, long term)
Connection with daily life, the family and social environment
Diary of nutritional and emotional matters in order to recognize functional connections between emotions and eating behaviour
Assessment for further deficits or resources
Introspection
Emotional perception
Social perception
Thoughts and attributions
Self-efficacy
Emotional expression
Ability to communicate
Ability to resolve conflicts

ment of bulimia. Several different approaches to treating bulimia have been suggested (Garner and Garfinkel, 1997); however, no single approach has proved to be superior. The modes of treatment tried include behavioural therapy, cognitive behaviour therapy, several types of group therapy including self-help groups, psychoanalytically orientated therapy, hypnosis and multimodal approaches. Treatment approaches should always be chosen after appropriate assessment. There are two aims to treatment, first, restoring normal eating behaviour, secondly, addressing the patient's individual problems.

Table 21.8 shows essential steps in assessing eating behaviour. It is important to include initial assessment, functional analysis of eating behaviour, individual perceptions and possible deficits in assessing the disorder. Individual resources

Table 21.9. Psychotherapeutic steps to encourage normal eating behaviour

Information about the disorder
Explaining the nature of the disorder
Keeping a diary
Sharing experiences in a group setting
Nutritional education
Energy and nutrient requirements
Set point theory of body weight
Supporting an 'antidiet' attitude
Normal weight fluctuations
Stimulus control
Control of precipitating conditions
Buying food, preparing meals, storing provisions
Reaction control
Gradual reduction of binges, vomiting and laxative abuse
Reaction prevention if necessary
Scheduled meals with regular meal times and balanced nutrition
Normal eating behaviour (serving size, speed, chewing, tasting, swallowing)
Perception of hunger and satiety
Progressive self-control
Self-observation, keeping a diary
Eating in a group
Eating 'forbidden' kinds of food
Pleasure perception training
Relaxation training
Reducing dysfunctional attitudes towards physical appearance and weight ('I am only liked if I am thin')
Improving self- and body perception
Video feedback, group feedback
Relapse prevention

which may help the patient to cope better with the disorder also need to be considered. Most patients are not well informed about the disorder, its sequelae nor the various treatment options. From the assessment phase on, patients need to be informed about healthy eating behaviour and the possible complications of bulimia (Brownell and Fairburn, 1995). Patients also need to be informed about the good prospects for improvement, the duration and scope of treatment and the opportunities for self-help or self-help group attendance.

Table 21.10. Psychotherapeutic steps to improve psychosocial competency

Indentify conflicts, e.g. in the family, in a partnership, at work
Early recognition of stressful situations
Perception of emotions in oneself and others
Expression of emotions
Reduction of dysfunctional thoughts and attitudes ('all-or-none', catastrophic thoughts, depressive point of view)
Perception of one's positive sides
Reduction of irrational anxieties
Social competency training
Self-assertiveness training
Develop strategies to cope with conflicts
Communication training, e.g. listening, speaking, paying compliments
Methods
Cognitive restructuring
Role play and group sessions
Family and partner therapy

Issues related with food must be discussed openly, directly and in detail with the patient. Patients' feelings of guilt or shame should be taken into account during conversations. Dysfunctional thoughts, e.g. that regular meals inevitably cause weight gain need to be challenged. The connection between dieting and bulimic binges should be explained. Frequently, the ability to perceive the normal internal stimuli of hunger and satiety and eat accordingly has been lost (Szmukler et al., 1995).

After the eating behaviour has been assessed, an individual treatment plan is developed, aim at improving eating behaviour. Important points to remember are shown in Table 21.9. The patient needs to learn the following ways of behaviour in order to normalize eating behaviour: all meals should be consumed at regular times, including snacks. Nutrition should be varied and should avoid special diet products. Patients should avoid drinking large amounts of fluid, as this may induce a false feeling of satiety and may facilitate vomiting (Herpertz-Dahlmann, 1991). Consuming meals together with other patients may by helpful. It is important to ensure that meals are eaten neither too hastily nor too slowly (Fichter, 1989a).

A further requirement is to identify those factors which trigger and sustain the disorder. Encouraging the patient to keep a journal may help to explore both eating behaviour and the factors which precipitate binges and purging.

Table 21.11. Indication for inpatient treatment of bulimia nervosa

Impaired general health
Unsuccessful outpatient treatment
Lack of opportunity for outpatient treatment
Severe eating disorder
Day-to-day lifestyle prevents alteration of eating patterns
Conflicts in the family or with a partner
Additional addiction to medication, alcohol or drugs
Additional psychiatric disorders
Extreme social isolation
Suicide risk
Multisymptomatic bulimia nervosa

From Fichter (1989b) and Vanderlinden et al. (1992).

Therapy may serve to develop alternative behaviour patterns and encourage behavioural change.

In addition to treatment aimed at changing behaviour, psychotherapy sessions addressing emotional and psychosocial problems should also be undertaken (Table 21.10).

Depending on the emphasis of treatment, several different approaches may be used: counselling, behavioural therapy or cognitive behaviour therapy. Cognitive behaviour therapy is particularly suitable for the treatment of dysfunctional and irrational thoughts, attitudes and values (see Chapter 7). When discussing dysfunctional thoughts, convictions and values, certain attitudes are frequently encountered, e.g. 'Only if I am thin, will I be successful and feel accepted. If I am fat, I will be totally useless, unsuccessful and lonely' (Fichter, 1989b). The aim of cognitive therapy is to challenge these irrational convictions and values, which constantly impair the patients' self-esteem, and replace them with more realistic and healthy attitudes. Patients' self-esteem and self-acceptance should be distinguished in the patient's mind from physical appearance.

If these undertakings do not bring about marked improvement within 3 months, at least in terms of how often binges occur, then referral for inpatient treatment should be considered (Table 21.11).

Inpatient treatment has the advantage of interrupting the bulimic circle (Fig. 21.6) in order that the patient has the opportunity to try out new behaviour. An inpatient setting also permits several therapy methods from different theoretical backgrounds to be combined, e.g. behavioural therapy, physical therapy, counselling, psychoanalytically orientated therapy.

The family should always be included in the treatment of children and adolescents. Parents frequently have strong guilty feelings towards the patient, which may sometimes be expressed as rejection of therapeutic measures. Such feelings should be addressed at an early stage (Herpertz-Dahlmann, 1991). Discussing important emotional aspects in therapy sessions reduces tension between family members.

Prognosis and evaluation of treatment

Vanderlinden et al. (1992) described the following good prognostic indicators: rapid response to treatment and the absence of personality disorder, addiction and self-inflicted injury, no previous anorexic phase and a negative psychiatric family history. High self-esteem and a positive attitude towards one's body improved prognosis. However, about 20% of the patients in their study either failed to respond or responded only poorly to treatment.

Nutzinger and de Zwaan (1989) analysed 20 studies looking at behavioural therapy of bulimia nervosa. Most treatment programmes consisted of a combination of different behavioural therapy techniques. After treatment about 40% of all patients no longer binged, 30% experienced a marked reduction of binges to about one-half of the number prior to treatment, and 30% failed to show any significant improvement. The studies illustrate the importance of improving eating behaviour and preventing relapses.

Waadt et al. (1992) reported similar findings. They found that behavioural therapy methods were used most frequently (self-observation, self-control, cognitive restructuring, self-assertiveness training, stimulus control). On average, 38% of all patient were reported to be without symptoms at the end of treatment, and 42% had not binged during the follow-up interval of 8-months on average. Unfortunately, follow-up studies of bulimia nervosa have not been as long as those of anorexia nervosa.

REFERENCES

American Psychiatric Association (APA) (1980). *Diagnostic and statistical manual of mental disorders*, 3rd edn (DSM-III). Washington, DC: APA.

Beck, A. T. (1976). *Cognitive therapy and the emotional disorders*. New York: International Universities Press.

Bemis, K. M. (1987). The present status of operant conditioning for the treatment of anorexia nervosa. *Behavior Modification*, **11**, 432–63.

Brownell, K. D. and Fairburn, C. G. (ed.) (1995). *Eating disorders and obesity. A comprehensive handbook*. New York: Guilford Press.

Crisp, A. H., Norton, K., Gowers, S. et al. (1991). A controlled study of the effect of therapies aimed at adolescent and family psychopathology in anorexia nervosa. *British Journal of Psychiatry*, **159**, 325–33.

Fichter, M. M. (1984). Epidemiologie der Anorexia nervosa und Bulimia. *Aktuelle Ernährungsmedizin*, **9**, 8.

Fichter, M. M. (1989*a*). Bulimia nervosa und bulimisches Verhalten. In *Bulimia nervosa. Grundlagen und Behandlung*, ed. M. M. Fichter, pp. 1–10. Stuttgart: Enke.

Fichter, M. M. (1989*b*). Psychologische Therapien bei Bulimia. In *Bulimia nervosa. Grundlagen und Behandlung*, ed. M. M. Fichter, pp. 230–47. Stuttgart: Enke.

Garner, D. M. and Garfinkel, P. E. (ed.) (1997). *Handbook of treatment for eating disorders*, 2nd edn. New York: Guilford Press.

Hall, A. (1987). The place of family therapy in the treatment of anorexia nervosa. *Australian and New Zealand Journal of Psychiatry*, **21**, 568–74.

Hebebrand, J., Himmelmann, G. W., Heseker, H., Schäfer, H. and Remschmidt, H. (1996). Use of percentiles for the body mass index in anorexia nervosa. Diagnositic, epidemiological, and therapeutic considerations. *International Journal of Eating Disorders*, **19**(4), 359–69.

Herpertz-Dahlmann, B. (1991). Die Bulimie der jungen Mädchen. *Zeitschrift für Allgemeinmedizin*, **67**, 325–33.

Herpertz-Dahlmann, B. and Remschmidt, H. (1994). Anorexia und Bulimia nervosa im Jugendalter. *Deutsches Ärzteblatt*, **91**, 1210–18.

Herzog, W., Rathner, G. and Vandereycken, W. (1992). Long-term course of anorexia nervosa. A review of the literature. In *The course of eating disorders*, ed. W. Herzog, H-C. Deter and W. Vandereycken, pp. 15–29. Berlin: Springer.

Humphrey, L. L. (1988). Relationships within subtypes of anorexic, bulimic and normal families. *Journal of the American Academy of Child and Adolescent Psychiatry*, **27**, 544–51.

Kog, E., and Vandereycken, W. (1985). Family characteristics of anorexia nervosa and bulimia. A review of the research literature. *Clinical Psychology Review*, **5**, 159–80.

Kog, E., Vertommen, H. and Vandereycken, W. (1987). Minuchin's psychosomatic family model revised. A concept-validation study using a multitrait-multimethod approach. *Family Process*, **26**, 235–53.

Minuchin, S., Rosman, B. L. and Baker, L. (1978). *Psychosomatic families. Anorexia nervosa in context*. Cambridge, M. A.: Harvard University Press.

Morgan, H. G. and Russell, G. F. M. (1975). Value of family background and clinical features as predictors of long-term outcome in anorexia nervosa. Four-year follow-up study of 41 patients. *Psychological Medicine*, **5**, 355–71.

Nutzinger, D. O. and de Zwaan, M. (1989). Verhaltenstherapie bei Bulimia. Rückblick und Ausblick anhand der bisherigen Forschung. In *Bulimia nervosa. Grundlagen und Behandlung*, ed. M. M. Fichter, pp. 248–61. Stuttgart: Enke.

Paul, T. H., Brand-Jacobi, J. and Pudel, V. (1984). Bulimia nervosa. Ergebnisse einer Untersuchung an 500 Patientinnen. *Münchner Medizinische Wochenschrift*, **126**, 614.

Remschmidt, H. (1992). Anorexia nervosa. In *Psychiatrie der Adoleszenz*, ed., H. Remschmidt, pp. 434–9. Stuttgart: Thieme.

Remschmidt, H. and Herpertz-Dahlmann, B. (1988a). Anorexia nervosa im Jugendalter. *Monatsschrift Kinderheilkunde*, **136**, 718–23.

Remschmidt, H. and Herpertz-Dahlmann, B. (1988b). Bulimia nervosa im Jugendalter. *Monatsschrift Kinderheilkunde*, **136**, 712–17.

Remschmidt, H. and Herpertz-Dahlmann, B. (1989). Bulimia und Bulimarexie im Jugendalter. In *Bulimia nervosa. Grundlagen und Behandlung*, ed. M. M. Fichter, pp. 62–75. Stuttgart: Enke.

Remschmidt, H., Wienand, F. and Wewetzer, C. (1988). Der Langzeitverlauf der Anorexia nervosa. *Monatsschrift Kinderheilkunde*, **136**, 726–31.

Remschmidt, H., Schmidt, M. H. and Gutenbrunner, C. (1990). Prediction of long-term outcome in anorectic patients from longitudinal weight measurements during inpatient treatment. A cross-validation study. In *Anorexia nervosa. Child and youth psychiatry. European perspectives*, vol. 1, ed. H. Remschmidt and M. H. Schmidt, pp. 150–67. Toronto: Hogrefe & Huber.

Russell, G. F. M. (1979). Bulimia nervosa. An ominous variant of anorexia nervosa. *Psychological Medicine*, **9**, 429–48.

Russell, G. F. M., Dare, C., Eisler I. and LeGrange, P. D. F. (1992). Controlled trials of family treatments in anorexia nervosa. In *Psychobiology and treatment of anorexia nervosa and bulimia nervosa*, ed., K. Halmi, pp. 237–61. Washington, DC: American Psychiatric Press.

Steinhausen, H-C. (1993). Anorexia und Bulimia nervosa. In *Handbuch Verhaltenstherapie und Verhaltensmedizin bei Kindern und Jugendlichen*, ed. H-C. Steinhausen and M. von Aster, pp. 383–40. Weinheim: Psychologie Verlags-Union.

Steinhausen, H-C. (1994). Anorexia and bulimia nervosa. In *Child and adolescent psychiatry. Modern approaches*, 3rd edn, ed. M. Rutter, E. Taylor and L. Hersov, pp. 425–40. Oxford: Blackwell Scientific.

Stierlin, H. and Weber, G. (1987). Anorexia nervosa. Family dynamics and family therapy. In *Handbook of eating disorders*, vol. I, ed. P. J. V. Beumont, G. D. Burrows and R. C. Casper, pp. 319–47. Amsterdam: Elsevier Science.

Szmukler, G. I., Dare, C. and Treasure, J. (ed.) (1995). *Handbook of eating disorders. Theory, treatment and research*. Chichester: Wiley.

Vandereycken, W. (1987). The constructive family approach to eating disorders. Critical remarks on the use of family therapy in anorexia nervosa and bulimia. *International Journal of Eating Disorders*, **6**, 455–68.

Vanderlinden, J., Norré, J., Vandereycken, W. and Meermann, R. (1992). *Die Behandlung der Bulimia nervosa*. Stuttgart: Schattauer.

Waadt, S., Laessle, R. G. and Pirke, K. M. (1992). *Bulimie. Ursachen und Therapie*. Berlin: Springer.

World Health Organization (WHO) (1992). *The ICD-10 classification of mental and behavioural disorders. Clinical descriptions and diagnostic guidelines*. Geneva: WHO.

22 Psychotherapy in chronic physical disorders

Ingeborg Jochmus

Introduction

During the past few years, the number of children requiring treatment for a chronic paediatric illness has continually increased. Prevelance rates of 5–12% have been reported (Roghmann, 1981). Chronic physical illness may last for years, or go on for a whole lifetime and influence or dictate the daily life of affected children and their parents to varying degrees. Usually, there is no curative treatment, but ongoing observation and management may be required (Ryan et al., 1998).

The clinical picture may be stable, relapsing or remitting, or progressive and may be complicated by life-threatening acute episodes (McMahon et al., 1998). Frequently life expectancy is reduced, and some chronic physical disorders are associated with pain (McGrath and Goodman, 1998; Allen and Mathews, 1998). Sequelae may include physical disability or handicap, and in some cases progressive mental handicap. Acute psychological crises are a common feature of these disorders.

Compared to children and adolescents with psychiatric disorders, those with a physical illness have entirely different characteristics and needs. About two-thirds have no psychopathological findings prior to the onset of their illness. A psychologist or child and adolescent psychiatrist is usually consulted in order to help the patient maintain as much quality of life as is possible with the illness. Treatment is aimed at giving support, facilitating self-help and imparting crisis intervention (Wehmeier, 2000).

Parents and patients are free to decide whether they wish to see a therapist in addition to the physicians treating their physical illness. This may be proposed at the onset of inpatient treatment or perhaps during an outpatient appointment. Establishing a trusting relationship will enable the therapist to identify children with premorbid psychopathology and to identify high-risk families.

Many oncology and nephrology units have psychosocial professionals working on the team. They should be included in the care of the patient from the beginning, in order to observe, listen and assess the patient's mental condition and the family's general situation. The information may then be used to develop appropriate coping strategies. If they are only consulted in a crisis, there may be suspicion and mistrust.

Cooperation within multiprofessional teams should take place in an atmosphere of tolerance, mutual understanding and clarity, which implies good and clear communication. This facilitates a better understanding of patients' and parents' behaviour and eases the burden of looking after these difficult patients.

Studies looking at the types and frequencies of mental disorder encountered in chronic physical illness are few, and most are based on relatively small samples. Remschmidt and Walter (1990) found a prevalence of 12.7% of psychiatric disorders amongst children and adolescents in the general population in Germany. Patients with a chronic illness are generally considered at much greater risk. Using the Child Behavior Check List (Achenbach and Edelbrock, 1983), Hürter (1990) found 33% of 101 chronically ill children to have a psychiatric disorder. Broken down by illness, psychiatric disorder was found in 20% of diabetic children, 30% of oncological patients, 42% of acutely ill children, 44% of children with impaired movement and 50% of patients with cystic fibrosis. However, there is a paucity of longitudinal studies looking at the relevance of physical symptoms for psychiatric disturbance and it is not clear whether disturbances tend to be temporary or persistent.

Studies on individual strategies of coping with physical illness and on concepts of illness are few and far between. However, clinical experience suggests that younger children frequently feel guilty, whereas children between 7 and 10 years begin to understand the concept of external aetiology of illness, and expect treatment to make them well again or link treatment with improvement. Children of this age usually understand that something physical is not in order. However, despite this, children often suffer severe emotional distress, anxiety and dispair, which leads to feelings of guilt and a tendency to regress. As these children may find it difficult to express their feelings verbally, non-verbal communication techniques, e.g. drawing, modelling, play, music may be helpful in establishing a relationship and supporting the child emotionally. Psychological instability, negative expectations and anxiety regarding the future may complicate the cause of any therapy and in these cases counselling (individually or in a group) is often additionally necessary.

Many physically ill adolescents are taciturn, withdrawn and tend towards depression and anxiety. They often do not share their problems spontaneously and do not express their concept of illness or their concerns about it. Denial and minimalization are often used as defence mechanisms in order to make life easier. However, some adolescents act out their feelings in an aggressive manner, which may disrupt treatment and lead them to refuse further therapy.

In order to be able to offer appropriate psychiatric support to such patients, baseline information regarding the patient's psychological make-up and family communication is needed. However, empirical findings are few. Schmitt (1991) combined standardized methods and individual assessment of adolescents with cystic fibrosis (CF). Both the patients with CF and the comparison group of patients with Crohn's disease and hemophilia expressed very similar thoughts and plans, implying that the outlook, goals and coping strategies of patients with chronic physical illnesses are similar (Schmitt, 1991).

There is also a paucity of studies evaluating the results of psychotherapy in chronic physical illness. However, clinical experience and published case reports suggest that treatment may be effective, e.g. behavioural therapy to treat phobia of syringes, compliance therapy, reinforcing self-competency, improvement of self-esteem, modelling in group therapy sessions, special education etc.

In this chapter several physical disorders are discussed which often become chronic during childhood or adolescence. Special emphasis is given to the psychiatric management of such patients, their families and other care-givers, e.g. hospital, school, peers. The approaches to psychotherapy described elsewhere in this book may also be helpful. In many cases continuous support of the families is also required, sometimes for several years. This kind of management usually comprises general psychological support rather than treatment of specific problems or conflicts. The aims of this approach have been summarized by Steinhausen (1996) and are shown in Table 22.1.

Specific chronic illnesses

Insulin-dependent diabetes mellitus (IDDM)

Epidemiology

IDDM is a chronic disorder affecting carbohydrate, protein and fat metabolism. Genetic factors and cytotoxic effects are thought to cause dysfunction of the insular cells of the pancreas. The inadequate secretion of insulin results in hyperglycemia, causing serious short-term and long-term complications. Prevalence is reported to be 1 in 1000 children under 17 years. The age of onset is usually 4–12 years. In Germany about 1500 new cases are diagnosed every year.

Table 22.1. Aims of general psychological support of children with a chronic illness

Responsibility of the parents
Developing an appropriate approach to upbringing by:
• emotional attention
• appropriate guidance and control
• supporting social integration
• supporting appropriate physical exercise
Responsibility of physicians or psychologists
Providing information
Advising the family and others regarding:
• medical issues
• psychological and educational issues
• reducing fear of diagnostic and therapeutic procedures by appropriate preparation and instruction
Psychotherapy
• individual sessions
• group sessions
• parent groups and parent training
• partner therapy
• behavioural therapy
• family therapy

From Steinhausen (1996).

Clinical picture, treatment and course

The severity of the disorder depends on the extent of the hypoinsulinemia. The predominant symptoms are polydipsia, polyuria, hyperglycemia, glucosuria and weight loss. In severe cases, ketoacidosis may occur (diabetic coma). Lifelong substitution of insulin is required at regular intervals (3–5 times per day). Meals should be fairly regular (6–7 per day) and not too large. Regular physical excercise is advisable.

Treatment is difficult in children and adolescents and optimal control may be difficult to achieve (Burger et al., 1991). Unfortunately, long-term complications such as nephropathy, retinopathy or neuropathy are common. Severe symptoms often occur after a course of 15–20 years and life expectancy tends to be reduced.

A high degree of cooperation is demanded of patients and their parents (usually mothers in particular), who may eventually become experts in managing the disorder. Assessment of blood glucose levels by the patient requires careful and detailed instruction. Children can learn to inject insulin on their own when they are about 8 years old.

Psychological management

About 80–90% of the mothers react with shock when the diagnosis has been confirmed. They often then dedicate themselves to learning about the disorder and acquainting themselves of the basics of treatment (Jochmus, 1971). It is important that the affected children have someone close, who is able to explain the situation to them and support them. The treatment of diabetes involves many restrictions and is difficult for children to understand, especially as they do not feel ill and fail to realize the seriousness of the disorder with its consequent grave complications. The reason for treatment should be explained patiently in an age-appropriate manner. The common psychological difficulties that children with diabetes have should also be addressed to try to improve compliance. Patients up to the age of 12 years old often tend to consume food between meals, 'forget' to measure their blood glucose and attempt to keep their disorder a secret, and this tendency should be addressed. An atmosphere of understanding and support may help the patient to reduce feelings of anger and aggression, facilitating behavioural change and improving compliance.

Counselling of parents in order to help them better understand their child's behaviour is also important. Group sessions may provide the parents with additional support. Psychological problems in diabetes differ according to age (Hürter, 1981). It is therefore advisable to constitute groups of parents with diabetic children of a similar age, so that they can meet others in a similar situation, sharing their anxieties and concerns. Parents need to learn to accept their child's disorder and avoid a reproachful attitude towards the child. They should also avoid getting involved in power struggles with the child. Threatening the child with the long-term risks invariably increases the child's resistance. When severe family conflicts occur, brief family therapy may be indicated. The role of any siblings should always be addressed.

Crises during puberty, a time when adolescents normally detach from home and gradually take up increasing responsibility, should also be addressed in individual or group sessions. The realization that one is different, that one will be ill throughout life and any anxieties concerning the future (work, partners, etc.) may contribute to feelings of resignation, thoughts of suicide or rebellious acts. Individual sessions are often preferable in such situatons. However, group sessions may also help diabetic adolescents to realize that others are in a very similar situation, thus relieving them of their social isolation. In cases of severe emotional or behavioural disturbance or increasing conflicts with a parent, individual psychotherapy may be indicated.

Chronic renal disease

Epidemiology

Chronic renal failure frequently initially goes unrecognized. In children the cause of chronic renal failure is usually genetic or congenital renal disease. The duration of the preterminal stage varies, the age peak in this stage of progressive renal failure is between 11 and 15 years (Koch, 1990). In Germany about 40–60 new cases are diagnosed each year.

Clinical picture, treatment and course

At the stage of uremia, with increasing metabolic acidosis, affected children complain of fatigue and headache and suffer from loss of appetite, weight gain, anaemia, polyuria and occasionally bed wetting. Eventually, electrolyte imbalance, hypertension and oligouria occur, making haemodialysis and/or renal transplantation necessary for survival. Affected children are generally faced with a difficult day-to-day life.

The necessity of an arteriovenous shunt being fashioned indicates progression of the illness and impending dialysis. Canulation is painful and causes anxiety, particularly initially. Dialysis takes 4–5 hours and physical symptoms often occur during the procedure. In addition to dialysis 2–3 times per week, patients must adhere to a strict diet, restrict their fluid intake and take an average of 16 tablets per day. All of these measures cause considerable problems to most children. Additional complications include retarded physical growth, anaemia, osteopathy, retarded puberty and sexual development. The fact that only 50% of children undergoing dialysis survive to the age of 10 years (Schärer, 1988) illustrates the severity of the disorder. In some cases, continuous ambulatory peritoneal dialysis (CAPD) is an alternative to haemodialysis.

Dialysis is usually considered temporary until renal transplatation can be undertaken. However, any delays in physical growth are not made up for. Transplantation requires lifelong treatment with immunosuppressant medication, which usually has unpleasant side effects. Parents and the patient have to live with the constant risk of graft rejection, which would require the patient to resume dialysis. Fortunately, 65% of all transplanted kidneys continue to function normally after 5 years. Patients who have undergone unsuccessful transplantation and are resubjected to dialysis are at an increased risk of emotional disturbance.

Psychological management

Patients need the support of their family to cope with their illness, the extensive medical treatment and the serious prognosis. The patient's dependency on medical technology will change the routine of the whole family. A particularly close relationship may develop between mother and patient, sometimes causing siblings to feel neglected. The therapist should be included in patient care well before the terminal stage in order to offer help and support. By developing coping strategies, parents are helped to deal with their child's illness, some learn to accept the situation whilst others find comfort from distracting themselves. Some parents report positive psychological changes as a result of their child's illness (Jochmus and Tieben-Heribert, 1981).

The therapist needs to be an empathic and understanding advisor in a situation which is new and threatening to the patient. It is important to offer support, because many children experience severe anxiety once dialysis is commenced and need specialist attention. School lessons and occupational therapy during dialysis may help to distract the patients and help them to develop new interests.

Patients commonly experience anxiety regarding the future, which often remains unclear. They tend to lose contact with peers and are faced with having to live through the death of fellow patients. They are confronted with the fact that they may never be able to work. In the 1970s, psychosocial teams were set up in many nephrology departments and continue to tackle the ever-changing issues in the field of rehabilitation.

A system-orientated care programme has been developed by Stein (1985) to support individual patients and to counsel the family, school and hospital 'systems'. In this programme, family therapy was given in only a small number of cases due to the complications of dialysis, and travel to the centre. Psychological preparation was offered prior to transplantation and procedures. Continual assessment and integration with other professionals enabled behavioural change in the patient to be recognized early and addressed immediately by the therapist.

Psychosocial teams need to be familiar with the family's resources in order to utilize strengths within the family. Autonomy should be encouraged, as it reduces feelings of dependency and anxiety.

Admission for inpatient psychotherapy may be required if there is a risk of graft rejection or if the patient has severe compliance difficulties. Individual psychotherapy may be required in cases of persistent depression.

Children with cancer

Epidemiology and assessment

Cancer in children most commonly comprises haematologic malignancies, neoplasias of embryonal tissue and sarcomas (malignant tumours of muscle, connective tissue or bone). In Germany about 1200 new cases are diagnosed every year. Children usually present with general symptoms, and when indicated, diagnostic procedures are performed, e.g. blood count, bone marrow biopsy, chest X-ray, CT-scan.

The diagnosis of cancer is always associated with ideas of suffering and death. The diagnosis is therefore often shocking for both patient and parents, generally causing severe distress. Parents may entertain the hope of a diagnostic error. As treatment usually has to commence immediately after the diagnosis is confirmed, those involved have little time to deal with the new situation. The revelation of the diagnosis is usually possible from the age of 5 years onwards, although frequently parents want the help of a doctor to raise the issue of diagnosis and treatment with the patient. All discussions should be conducted in an open and trusting atmosphere. For as long as possible, hope should be conveyed that treatment can be successful. The psychiatrist or psychologist working on the team should be included in discussions right from the start if possible, or at least from an early stage.

Clinical picture, treatment and prognosis

If chemotherapy or radiotherapy is required, the mother is usually asked to stay with the child in hospital. Chemotherapy may take up to 10 weeks. Despite their mother's presence, most children feel homesick during their stay in hospital. In disorders such as acute lymphoblastic leukaemia (ALL), preventive radiotherapy to the brain and spinal chord may be required for between one-quarter and one-third of children. In some departments patients are discharged after 10–12 days and treatment is continued on an outpatient basis with two to three appointments per week lasting several hours. Back home, children must be isolated to some extent from their friends in order to prevent infection. Thus patients need more support from their family, especially their mother. The side effects of chemotherapy (nausea, vomiting, loss of hair) can be very stressful for both child and parents. The treatment of solid tumours may require additional procedures, such as radiotherapy or surgery. Children with ALL must usually undergo outpatient treatment for 2 years, and the disease is only considered cured if the patient remains free of recurrence for 5–6 years. Today, about 70% of all cases of ALL and more than 50% of all malignant tumour cases are curable. Cancer has changed from an acute and usually fatal illness to a chronic disease with uncertain prognosis. The risk of recurrence remains 2–3% (Gutjahr, 1993), and this risk continues for several years, constantly present for both patients and their families. Follow-up is often associated with much concern and waiting for the results of medical assessment may reactivate anxieties which had previously been overcome. Dealing with a recurrence is especially demanding of patients and their families.

Psychological management

This is especially appropriate during the first 2 years of the illness, in cases of recurrence and in cases of terminal illness. When a child is diagnosed with a life-threatening illness, the whole family is faced with the crisis. During this unstable phase, counselling the family is an important task for the psychotherapist. The physicians will remain the primary point of contact for families, but the psychotherapist should aim to identify the family's resources for coping with crises. This may require several sessions to help families develop appropriate coping strategies.

In the acute phase, the therapist should attempt to convey an attitude of personal availability, genuineness and empathy (Schmitt, 1983). After dealing with the first shock, parents usually feel intense grief and frequently develop guilty feelings whilst searching for the cause of the illness. Children can only cooperate if they perceive that their parents are willing to accompany them in accepting the disease. However, initially patients may be withdrawn, taciturn and express a dislike of anything that is associated with treatment, which is usually perceived as threatening. Behaviour tends to be influenced by the child's experience of physical weakness, helplessness and vulnerability. Having to undergo amputation of a limb is a cause of extreme emotional stress, involving as it does, a major loss of physical self-determination. Such matters need to be addressed early on, in order to allow the patient to express his opinion and work through the feelings associated with subsequent loss of autonomy.

There is a paucity of empirical data on the psychosocial problems that families with chronically ill children have to face. However, Knispel et al. (1985) have studied the psychosocial support offered to families of pediatric patients with malignancy. They found that children with cancer and their families do not usually require any specific psychotherapy, but do need general support. Caring for a child with cancer is very stressful and may be almost too much to bear in some cases. Some degree of decompensation has to be considered 'normal' considering the extreme circumstances. Self-help groups may be of particular importance to parents in dealing with their anxieties and fears.

There is also a paucity of follow-up studies looking at the quality of life of children with cancer, perhaps understandably in view of the sensitivities included. Petermann et al. (1992) have followed up 18 former patients with bone malignancies. The individuals were 15–25 years old and were seen on average of 4 years after discharge. All individuals were physically handicapped to some extent. The interviews were analysed to draw out common features. The main problem for most individuals was accepting their altered body image. They were also concerned about the future, feeling restricted regarding their occupational options. Some also reported positive effects of the illness, 78% said that they now were much more aware and conscious of their options in life.

A long-term follow-up study from the United States (Kaplan, 1982) was less optimistic, showing that families do not always manage to accept the illness. Parental divorce is more common and some children have difficulties, developing anxiety disorders and psychosomatic symptoms, e.g. enuresis, encopresis. The issue of whether behavioural disorders resolve if the cancer is cured, remains controversial (Ritter, 1991).

Haemophilia

Epidemilogy and aetiology

Haemophilia is a rare, X-linked recessive condition, in which the blood-clotting factor VIII (haemophilia A) or IX (haemophilia B) is reduced, causing excessive bleeding. The disorder affects males only. The severity of the condition depends on the extent to which the clotting factor is reduced in the blood. Haemophilia A is ten times as common as haemophilia B, with incidences of 1 to 10 000 and 1 to 20 000, respectively.

Clinical picture, treatment and course

The condition is usually recognized in the second year of life, when the child becomes more mobile. Extensive tissue haemorrhages, haematomas and haemarthroses occur. Haemarthroses usually first occur in the ankle joints. From the age of about 4 years onwards, elbow and knee joints are more frequently involved. Intracranial bleeding is rare.

During the past 25 years, clotting factor concentrates have become widely available to treat the condition. Treatment at home in close cooperation with a haematology department has improved life expectancy and quality of life dramatically. Physicians may treat when necessity arises or administer the required clotting factor on a regular basis (two to three times per week) until the end of the growth period (Pollmann, 1991). Thereafter, the factor is administered as necessary.

The clear benefit felt after injection, helps patients' motivation considerably.

Parents can be taught how to administer intravenous injections, and from the age of 12 years onwards, patients can often undertake this themselves. Today, contractures and physical diability can be avoided by careful treatment.

The steady improvement in the quality of life of haemophiliacs was thwarted by the onset of HIV infections through infected blood clotting factors in the 1980s. Today, about 50% of haemophiliacs are HIV-positive and a number have died of AIDS. Since 1985, blood from donors has been tested for HIV.

Many patients with haemophilia report that emotional stress influences the frequency and duration of the bleeding (Kipnowski and Kipnowski, 1979). Older children and adolescents with severe haemophilia or HIV infection also appear to recognize the negative influence of stress on haemophilia (Hamel, 1994).

Psychological management

Many haemophiliacs adopt a stoic attitude and repress aspects of the condition which threaten their self-esteem, e.g. physical handicap, risk of HIV infection, sexual problems. Individuals seek a high degree of self-control and responsibility with regard to their life and treatment. They often lead an outwardly normal life and tend not to show signs of resignation or hopelessness. This attitude appears to be independent of the degree of physical handicap or their HIV status (Hamel, 1994).

However, clinical experience reveals that adolescents may indeed react with anxiety in crises and occasionally discontinue treatment when HIV infection supervenes. Disturbed relationships within the family may also lead parents to refuse treatment, a situation which requires intensive psychotherapeutic intervention (Friedrich, 1985). Haemophiliacs and their families may benefit from the opportunity of discussing these issues openly, which is often possible in self-help groups.

HIV infection is a particularly sensitive issue, which many parents find difficult to discuss with their children. The therapist can help to prepare such conversations and devise lines along which conversation can take place, although this should not distract from the importance of the child's emotional reaction.

Cystic fibrosis (CF)

Epidemiology and aetiology

Cystic fibrosis (also called mucoviscidosis) is the most common congenital metabolic disorder in caucasians. It is inherited as an autosomal recessive and occurs in about 1 in 2000 births. About two thirds of all patients survive to adult age if they are managed at specialist centres. Today, average life expectancy is 25 years, whereas in former times 80–90% of children born with the condition died during the first 2 years of life.

In 1989, the CF-gene was identified on chromosome 7, and about 200 different mutations have been discovered. As a result of a mutation, the secretions of all exocrine glands are abnormally viscid, obstructing the gland ducts. The most commonly involved organs are the gut, pancreas and lungs, resulting in intestinal obstruction and chronic lung and pancreatic disease. The proteinacious secretions are an ideal substrate for bacterial infection, particularly in the lungs, and antibiotic treatment (sometimes also prophylactically) is commonly required. Pulmonary involvement and right ventricular function determine the course of the illness and influence survival.

Diagnosis is confirmed by a sweat test, which determines the electrolyte concentration in the sweat. There is no reliable neonatal screening test for the condition. Prenatal diagnosis should be considered in high-risk families only.

Clinical picture, treatment and prognosis

The severity of the condition varies and the course is not uniform. Symptoms such as diarrhoea and failure to thrive are usually first noticed in infancy. Intestinal obstruction due to meconium ileus occurs in about 10% of all cases. Pulmonary symptoms usually become manifest only after the age of 6 months.

Ideally, medical treatment should commence in infancy. This comprises a high-calorie diet and the administration of fat-soluble vitamins (A, D, E, K) and pancreatic enzymes. Prevention of pulmonary involvement is attempted by a number of measures including the administration of broad-spectrum antibiotics, oral expectorants, and regular chest physiotherapy. From 4–6 years, children may learn methods of postural drainage.

Complications such as diabetes mellitus, biliary cirrhosis, oesophageal bleeding, haemoptysis and pneumothorax may occur, especially in severe and late disease stages. Male patients are usually infertile, whereas for females pregnancy involves great risks.

The terminal stage of CF is associated with bouts of severe dyspnoea and extreme anxiety. In some cases transplantation of heart and lungs is undertaken and whilst this prolongs survival it is not curative and continuous immunosuppressive medication is required.

Psychological management

Soon after the birth of their child, parents are faced with a devastating diagnosis, which results in severe emotional stress. In this situation 65% of parents have been found to be willing to accept psychological support (Jedlicka-Köhler and Götz, 1989). Self-help groups provide a useful opportunity to help parents cope with the problems associated with diagnosis and treatment.

There is little data on the behaviour of younger patients with CF. However, there appears to be a risk of overprotection and parents may convey their anxieties and depression unconsciously. This risk should be addressed by the team managing the patient. Unfortunately, there are relatively few therapists working in teams treating children with CF. An open style of communication in the family and access to fellow sufferers is often the most useful way to help the family cope with the illness. Psychiatric support should not be considered essential in all cases, and many families adapt well to the situation.

Emotional crises in patients with CF usually occur during adolescence, when stigmata, e.g. retarded physical growth, low weight, sexual immaturity, coughing, flatulence may lead to feelings of low self-esteem and depression. Adolescents also come to realize that their life expectancy is relatively short. Individual counselling and support are appropriate in order to help adolescents to come to terms with these issues and improve their self-competency.

Patients with CF are often described as taciturn and withdrawn, with minimalization and denial said to be common defence mechanisms (Boyle et al., 1976; Bywater, 1981), enabling patients to better adapt to the circumstances of daily life. The therapist should respect such defence mechanisms and the patient should be encouraged to direct the areas of discussion, thus indicating his limits. Client-centred counselling is an appropriate technique in the treatment of patients with CF.

In an empirical study, Schmitt (1991) analysed the outcome of patients in a variety of standardized and client-centred methods as well as group psychotherapy. He found that patients tended to emphasize learning to cope with the illness and make the best out of their albeit short life. They tended, on the other hand, to avoid mentioning existential anxieties, worries and self-defeative thoughts. This stoic attitude is all the more remarkable, given the poor prognosis in CF both in terms of morbidity and mortality.

Cardiac disease

Epidemiology

About 0.8% of all newborns have a congenital cardiac disorder, which is usually initially managed in a pediatric cardiology unit. Over 90% of all congenital cardiac abnormalities can be treated by surgery. Since the introduction of modern surgical techniques, the mortality associated with cardiac surgery during the first year of life has fallen from 85% to 10% today (Stoermer, 1990).

At least 80% of children in need of surgery have a better quality of life post-surgery. Nevertheless, physical fitness is usually reduced, and these children must be considered chronically ill, although about 80% of patients do survive to adult age. In the last few years, cardiac transplantation has been increasingly performed in children. Whilst this represents a good opportunity for the affected child, it remains associated with many risks and may lead to additional morbidity.

Clinical picture, treatment and prognosis

In about half of all cases the diagnosis is made in the first year of life. In addition to cyanosis, several rather uncharacteristic symptoms may also be present: failure to thrive, psychomotor retardation, general weakness, dyspnoea or compromised circulation. Affected children may be withdrawn, and mothers may notice that their child is somehow 'different'. Children frequently commence school later than usual and puberty is also delayed in comparison to healthy children. However, some children show no signs of abnormality before school age.

Assessment of the cardiac disorder requires admission to hospital to perform cardiac catheterization and angiography. When indicated, the optimal age for surgery must be agreed upon. The diagnosis of congenital heart disease may cause severe emotional disturbance in the parents. The heart symbolizes life and they dwell for many years on the idea of losing their child. Parents' coping style depends to a great extent on their personality structure, but also on the extent of the child's heart disease. Low social class also appears to be a risk factor. Parents tend towards overindulgence and overprotection, and they may feel alone with their distress (Kahlert, 1985). Support and counselling by a family therapist should always be considered.

Some publications refer to 'child-psychiatric disorder' or 'behavioural disturbance' in these children. A wide range of symptoms has been described such as nail-biting, thumb-sucking, restlessness, eating disorders, tics, aggression and attention-seeking behaviour. Symptoms such as these tend to increase after surgery, whereas anxiety is usually reduced. However, excessive pampering post-surgery may impair patients' ability to adapt to the normal social environment, despite their good physical health.

Adolescents frequently feel at a social disadvantage because of restrictions made on sports and other social activities at school. They may also express anxiety concerning physical stigmata (scars, cyanosis), limited occupational options and fears of recurrence or worsening of their condition, including death. These anxieties may persist, even after successful surgery (Ratzmann et al., 1991). Some adolescents with severe heart disease may attempt to compensate by striving for academic excellence at school (Kahlert, 1985).

Psychological management

The paediatrician will remain the main source of support for both the patient and the parents over the years of treatment. During this time, parents may go through a number of crises and experience feelings of great anxiety regarding the child's future. Families may require psychological help in order to cope with issues which arise within the family and with the patient's individual development. If the style of upbringing appears to be causing problems, this must be addressed and parents offered feedback and alternative solutions. Discussions between professionals and the family should be held in an open and trusting atmosphere. As a result of this the patient will learn to ask questions and discuss problems openly with physicians, parents and peers. Over time, the patient will require increasingly detailed information about his condition and the prognosis. Anxieties concerning the future are frequently repressed, but may come out, particularly in threatening situations. When raised, such anxieties should be addressed, and time should be offered to the patient to discuss these issues as fully as he feels is necessary (Jänsch and Tröndle, 1982).

Epilepsy

Epidemiology and aetiology

Chronic recurrent seizures are due to disturbed cerebral function, associated with abnormal synchronized action of groups of neurons. Epilepsy is a common chronic disorder which arises as a result of genetic factors, trauma, inflamation, tumour, etc., but may also be idiopathic. A combination of several factors may also cause epilepsy. The incidence in children under 16 years old is approximately 1–2%. As seizures tend to first occur at the age of 1–4 years, paediatricians and neuropaediatricians usually manage these children, but child and adolescent psychiatrists often become involved later, especially if learning difficulties or secondary behavioural disorders occur.

Clinical picture, treatment and prognosis

Seizures must be fully assessed in order to make an accurate diagnosis which informs treatment. The classification of seizures is complex, and whether the type and frequency of seizures predicts behavioural symptoms is still debated. However, it is clear that children with epilepsy suffer more frequently from behavioural problems than those without epilepsy (Rutter, 1977). There is no specific or typical behavioural disorder associated with epilepsy, however, learning difficulties are often present. Remschmidt (1973) found that children with epilepsy tend to have reduced gross and fine motor skills, visuomotor coordination, and verbal expression, and may show stereotypical behaviour.

Some seizures (infantile spasms, grand mal seizures, absences) are commonly associated with mental retardation. Whilst IQ is below average in some cases, others may have normal intelligence. The association between epilepsy and IQ may be difficult to establish. Problems may be apparent prior to the first fit, or developmental retardation and the loss of mental, motor and social functions may be accompanied by an increasing frequency of fits. Sixty to seventy per cent of patients respond well to treatment with anticonvulsive medication, with no further seizures. A further 15–20% at least improve on medication.

In the assessment of children with epilepsy, it is important to consider organic, mental and social factors, all of which may contribute to the pathogenesis of the disorder. The behavioural side effects of anticonvulsive medications must also be taken into account (Blank, 1989). The occurrence of seizures in public may cause stigmatization and rejection of the patient by his peers. In such situations, support by family members is especially important in order to avoid subsequent behavioural problems. Conflicts within the family may also have a detrimental effect on the child's behaviour. Regular medical examinations (EEGs), medication, and restrictions in life style, sports and play may all cause problems for the child.

The patient may be assigned to a special role in the family system, especially if the parents see epilepsy as a stigmatization. They may make special demands of the child to assuage their disappointment. Under such excessive pressure school achievement may decline, and, as a result, secondary psychological reactions such as conduct disorder and emotional outbursts may occur. Personality structure will depend on a number of factors, but as a result of additional pressures a tendency towards immaturity may persist longer than in other children.

Psychological management

The physician has the task of helping parents to accept the diagnosis of epilepsy. After appropriate investigation, any additional problems such as learning or behavioural problems should be discussed with the parents, and ways to facilitate healthy development sought. It is important to consider both the child's strengths and weaknesses. If parents are allowed to dwell on unrealistic expectations, this may further disadvantage the child, impeding any progress he is capable of. Parents should be warned of this danger and psychotherapeutic intervention may be required in some cases.

Patients with epilepsy may feel hopeless and become depressed, especially when they become able to recognize the differences between themselves and their siblings or peers. They need to be helped to achieve a more positive attitude and should be granted extra time if this will help them to catch up in certain areas. Adolescents are in particular need of their parents' help to enable appropriate detachment from home. They should be offered help in making vocational choices and finding realistic occupational opportunities.

Bronchial asthma

Clinical picture, epidemiology and aetiology

Bronchial asthma is an obstructive pulmonary disorder causing dyspnoea due to constriction of the large and small airways. Asthmatic attacks may be life threatening. Asthma is the most common chronic illness in childhood and adolescence, with a prevalence of 2–4%. A large proportion of cases (30–40%) first occur during adolescence. Asthmatic attacks are characterized by dyspnoea due to bronchial spasms, prolonged expiratory phase, increased secretion of abnormally viscous mucus and occasional bronchial oedema. It is considered a typical 'psychosomatic' disorder, as psychological factors often play a role in triggering or maintaining attacks. The course of the illness is very variable, many patients have no symptoms between attacks, but some develop a tendency to chronicity and progression. The relationship of physical and emotional factors in asthma remains a controversial area.

In ICD-10 (WHO, 1992), asthma may be classified as purely psychological or as behavioural factors associated with asthma (F54). The latter category should be used to record the presence of psychological or behavioural influences thought to have played a major part in the manifestation of physical disorders classified elsewhere in ICD-10. The diagnosis F54 should be combined with an organic diagnosis, in this case asthma (J45).

Today, bronchial asthma is considered an illness of multifactorial aetiology. Genetic vulnerability, hyperreactive bronchi and precipitating stresses such as infection, immunological factors or emotional stress are all considered relevant in its development. Both individual psychological make-up and the family situation seem to influence pathogenesis. Whilst not actually causing the condition, they contribute to triggering and sustaining the illness. Older theories of a specific personality defect or a pathologic relationship between mother and child no longer have credence. Factors thought to be involved in the aetiology of bronchial asthma are shown in Fig. 22.1.

Psychotherapy and psychological management

In addition to medication, which is usually required, individual psychotherapy,

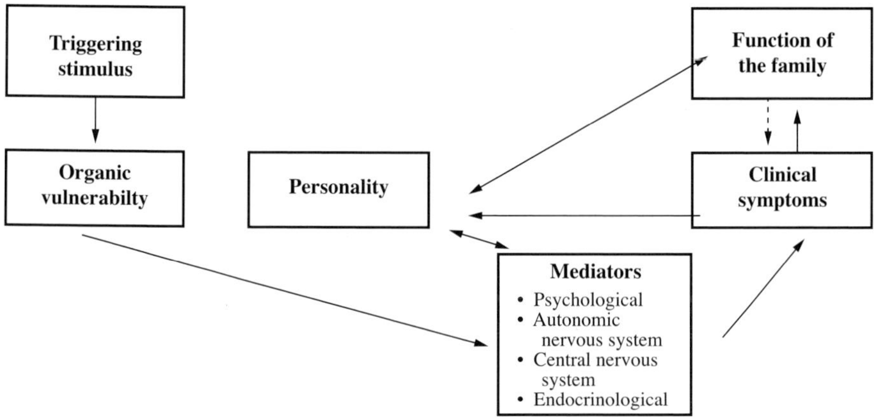

Fig. 22.1. The aetiology of bronchial asthma (Steinhausen, 1996).

family therapy or group therapy may be helpful in the management of the asthmatic child. Psychotherapy aims to support medical treatment and help the patient to pursue a healthy lifestyle. Through education and explanation, the therapist may be able to improve compliance with medication, which is of paramount importance, as well as helping patients avoid precipitating factors.

Almost all approaches to psychotherapy have been attempted to treat bronchial asthma. The following methods have been shown to be effective:

- attempts to reduce the occurrence of asthmatic attacks by behavioural therapy techniques, e.g. systematic desensitization or conditioning;
- relaxation training such as progressive relaxation or autogenic training;
- individual psychotherapy (client centred or psychodynamic) if assessment shows that important individual conflicts are present. Conflicts are often related to the family, the school or the situation at work;
- problem-centred family therapy if disagreements are present, if the family avoids conflict or if there are unhealthy alliances within the family. In some cases it can be helpful to point out that asthmatic attacks may be symptomatic of family conflicts and that symptoms may indicate a dysfunctional family system;
- group psychotherapy may help to reduce the sense of social isolation which is often present. It is an opportunity for developing coping strategies and comparing individual strategies with others.

In addition to these general principles, behavioural therapy programmes are available. Based on a functional behavioural analysis of asthmatic attacks, these programmes aim to identify frequent and infrequent behaviours and assess their relevance. Behavioural goals are identified and strategies to attain these goals are developed. Behavioural goals may be set on any of several planes:

- physiological parameters, e.g. expiratory volume, breathing rate, etc.,
- self-observational symptoms, e.g. anxiety, irritability, fatigue, dyspnoea, etc.,
- objective behaviour, e.g. asthmatic attacks, rate of consultation, etc.

After detailed functional analysis, intervention aimed at the goal is planned. Additional techniques may also be useful, e.g. relaxation training, biofeedback, systematic desensitization, cognitive control strategies. Relaxation training and biofeedback techniques are most appropriate in anxiety and tension, whereas cognitive control strategies are more helpful for treating patients who either ignore or exaggerate their symptoms, and try to help patients to improve their appraisal of symptoms.

Course

In 25% of cases, bronchial asthma becomes chronic, despite a combination of medication and psychotherapeutic treatment, although it is only severe in under half of these. In childhood asthma has a stable course in 30% of cases, remission occurs in 20% provided allergens are avoided, whereas 20% go on to suffer additional allergic symptoms (Steinhausen, 1996). Mortality is about 1%. Prognosis is good if symptoms only occur with infection. Frequent asthmatic attacks, additional eczema and significant behavioural problems are associated with a poorer outcome.

REFERENCES

Achenbach, T. M. and Edelbrock, C. (1983). *Manual for the child behavior checklist and revised behavior profile*. Burlington, VT: University of Vermont.

Allen, K. D. and Mathews, J. R. (1998). Behavior management of chronic pain in children. In *Handbook of child behavior therapy*, ed. T. S. Watson and F. M. Gresham. New York: Plenum Press.

Blank, R. (1989). Psychopathologie und Leistungsverhalten unter Antikonvulsiva bei Kindern und Jugendlichen. *Zeitschrift für Kinder-und Jugendpsychiatrie*, **17**, 140–9.

Boyle, I. R., di Sant'Agnese, P. A., Sack, S., Millican, F. and Kulczycki, L. L. (1976). Emotional adjustment of adolescents and young adults with cystic fibrosis. *The Journal of Pediatrics*, **88**, 318–26.

Burger, W., Weber, B., Enders, I. and Hartmann, R. (1991). Therapie des Diabetes mellitus im Kinder- und Jugendalter. *Monatsschrift Kinderheilkunde*, **139**, 62–8.

Bywater, M. (1981). Adolescents with cystic fibrosis. Psychosocial adjustment. *Archives of Disease in Childhood*, **56**, 538–43.

Friedrich, H. (1985). Chronisch kranke Kinder und ihre Familien. *Praxis der Kinderpsychologie und Kinderpsychiatrie*, **34**, 296–302.

Gutjahr, P. (1993). Sekundärmalignome nach Krebserkrankungen bei Kindern. *Deutsches Ärzteblatt*, **90**, 1032–7.

Hamel, A. (1994). *Selbsterleben bei chronischer Erkrankung am Beispiel hämophiler Jugendlicher und junger Erwachsener*. Doctoral Dissertation, University of Münster.

Hürter, A. (1990). Psychische und soziale Belastungen und der Wunsch nach professioneller Hilfe bei verschiedenen chronischen Erkrankungen. In *Krankheitsverarbeitung bei Kindern und Jugendlichen*, ed. I. Seiffge-Krenke. Berlin: Springer.

Hürter, H. (1981). Kinder und Jugendliche mit Diabetes und ihre Familien, Erfahrungen aus Gruppendiskussionen mit diabetischen Kindern, Jugendlichen und ihren Eltern. In *Chronisch kranke Kinder und Jugendliche in der Familie*, ed. M. C. Angermeyer and O. Döhner. Stuttgart: Enke.

Jänsch, G. and Tröndle, C. (1982). Psychologische Untersuchungen an herzkranken Kindern vor und nach der Herzoperation. *Sozialpädiatrie*, **4**, 506–11.

Jedlicka-Köhler, I. and Götz, M. (1989). Reaktionen von Patienten und Familien mit cystischer Fibrose auf psychologische Betreuung. *Monatsschrift Kinderheilkunde*, **137**, 75–9.

Jochmus, I. (1971). *Die psychische Entwicklung diabetischer Kinder und Jugendlicher*. Stuttgart: Enke.

Jochmus, I. and Tieben-Heibert, A. (1981). Belastungen der Familie durch chronisch niereninsuffiziente Kinder und Möglichkeiten ihrer Bewältigung. In *Chronisch kranke Kinder und Jugendliche in der Familie*, ed. M. C. Angermeyer and O. Döhner. Stuttgart: Enke.

Kahlert, G. (1985). *Jugendliche mit schweren Herzkrankheiten*. Doctoral Dissertation, University of Münster.

Kaplan, D. M. (1982). Intervention strategies for families. In *Psychological aspects of cancer*, ed. J. Cohen, J. W. Cullen and L. R. Martin, pp. 221–33. New York: Raven Press.

Kipnowski, A. and Kipnowski, H. J. (1979). Psychosomatische Aspekte bei genetisch determinierter Krankheit. Eine Untersuchung an erwachsenen Hämophilen. *Psychotherapie, Psychosomatik, Medizinische Psychologie*, **29**, 178–83.

Knispel, J., Thiel, R. and Wallis, H. (1985). Bereiche psychosozialer Betreuung krebskranker Kinder und ihrer Familien. Auswertung eines ganzheitlichen Versorgungsmodells. *Klinische Pädiatrie*, **197**, 183–8.

Koch, U. (1990). *Abschlussbericht 'Chronische Niereninsuffizienz, Mukoviscidose und Krebserkrankungen im Kindes und Jugendalter'. Krankheitsübergreifende Evaluation der Modellprogramme des Bundesministeriums für Arbeit und Sozialordnung (BMA)*. Freiburg.

McGrath, P. J. and Goodman, J. (1998). Pain in childhood. In *Cognitive-behaviour therapy for children and families*, ed. P. J. Graham. New York: Cambridge University Press.

McMahon, C. M., Lambros, K. M. and Sylva, J. A. (1998). Chronic illness in childhood. A hypothesis-testing approach. In *Handbook of child behavior therapy*, ed. T. S. Watson and F. M. Gresham. New York: Plenum Press.

Petermann, F., Dobmeyer, A., Noeker, C. and Bode, U. (1992). Psychosoziale Situation krebskranker Jugendlicher, *TW Pädiatrie*, **5**, 238–43.

Pollmann, H. (1991). Die Gelenkblutung hämophiler Kinder und Jugendlicher. Substitutionsbehandlung bei Bedarf im Vergleich zur Dauerbehandlung. *Ellipse*, **26**, 370–5.

Ratzmann, U., Schneider, P. and Richter, H. (1991). *How do children and their parents cope with congenital heart disease?* Report on the conference of the Association of European Paediatric Cardiologists, Hannover (Germany), ed. H. C. Kallfelz.

Remschmidt, H. (1973). Testpsychologische und experimentelle Untersuchungen zur Psychopathologie der Epilepsien. In *Psychische Störungen bei Epilepsie*, ed. H. Penin, pp. 135–56. Stuttgart: Schattauer.

Remschmidt, H. and Walter, R. (1990). Psychische Auffälligkeiten bei Schulkindern. *Zeitschrift für Kinder- und Jugendpsychiatrie*, **18**, 121–32.

Ritter, J. (1991). Psychische Störungen nach onkologischen Erkrankungen im Kindesalter. Möglichkeiten ihrer Behandlung und Prävention. *Sozialpädiatrie in Praxis und Klinik*, **13**, 18–22.

Roghmann, K. J. (1981). Die Familie als Patient. Zum Wandel des Krankheitsbegriffs der Pädiatrie chronisch kranker Kinder. In *Chronisch kranke Kinder und Jugendliche in der Familie*, ed. M. C. Angermeyer and O. Dörner. Stuttgart: Enke.

Rutter, M. (1977). Brain damage syndromes in childhood. Concepts and findings. *Journal of Child Psychology and Psychiatry and Allied Disciplines*, **18**, 1–21.

Ryan, R. M, Sundheim, S. T. P. V. and Voeller, K. K. S. (1998). Medical diseases. In *Textbook of pediatric neuropsychiatry*, ed. C. E. Coffey and R. A. Brumback, pp. 1223–72. Washington, DC: American Psychiatric Press.

Schärer, K. (1988). Dialyseverfahren und Indikation zur Nierentransplantation im Kindesalter. *Monatsschrift Kinderheilkunde*, **136**, 307–12.

Schmitt, G. M. (1983). *Die psychologische Betreuung des krebskranken Kindes*. Göttingen: Vandenhoeck & Ruprecht.

Schmitt, G. M. (1991). *Cystische Fibrose*. Göttingen: Hogrefe.

Stein, L. (1985). Systemorientierte Betreuung chronisch nierenkrannker Kinder und ihrer Familien. *Zeitschrift für personenzentrierte Psychologie und Psychotherapie*, **4**, 39–52.

Steinhausen, H-C. (1996). Psychische Störungen bei Kindern und Jugendlichen. München: Urban & Schwarzenberg.

Stoermer, J. (1990). Entwicklung der Kinderkardiologie. *Der Kinderarzt*, **21**, 930–5.

Wehmeier, P. M. (2000). Psychische Störungen bei chronischen Erkrankungen und Behinderungen. In *Kinder- und Jugendpsychiatrie. Eine praktische Einführung*, 3rd edn, ed. H. Remschmidt, pp. 313–21. Stuttgart: Thieme.

World Health Organization (1992). *The ICD-10 classification of mental and behavioural disorders. Clinical descriptions and diagnostic guidelines*. Geneva: WHO.

23

Enuresis and faecal soiling

Kurt Quaschner and Fritz Mattejat

Enuresis (the involuntary passing of urine during sleep) and faecal soiling (encopresis) are common conditions in childhood and a frequent reason for consultation of child and adolescent psychiatrists. Enuresis is much more common than faecal soiling. The apparent simplicity of the symptoms may suggest that treatment should also be quick and simple; however, unfortunately this is often not the case. Several different theories of aetiology and numerous approaches to treatment have been suggested. Defining the disorders has proved challenging in terms of defining age criteria and distinguishing clinical subtypes.

The disorders are discussed separately, both for aetiological reasons and in terms of treatment.

Enuresis

Clinical picture

Essential data on enuresis (definition, classification, prevalence, aetiology, prognosis) are summarized in Table 23.1.

Approaches to treatment

A large number of different approaches to treatment have been suggested (Mellon and Houts, 1995; Friman and Jones, 1998). Some are based on a single aetiological theory, implying that a particular method of treatment should be used in treating every case, e.g. exclusive use of a night alarm or play therapy as the only technique. Such narrow approaches are now considered rather outdated. Today, combinations of several different techniques are thought to be most effective.

Different treatment techniques may be used simultaneously or in sequence. The sequential approach is more common and is based on a succession of 'easy' steps, usually avoiding any drastic measures, followed by a succession of

Table 23.1. Clinical profile of enuresis

Definition and classification

In ICD-10 enuresis (F98.0) is defined in the following way: 'A disorder characterized by involuntary voiding of urine, by day and/or night, which is abnormal in relation to the individual's mental age and which is not a consequence of a lack of bladder control due to any neurological disorder, to epileptic attacks, or to any structural abnormality of the urinary tract. The enuresis may have been present from birth, i.e. an abnormal extension of the normal infantile incontinence or it may have arisen following a period of acquired bladder control. The later onset (or secondary) variety usually begins about the age of 5 to 7 years.' The diagnostic guidelines add: 'There is no clear-cut demarcation between an enuresis disorder and the normal variations in the age of acquisition of bladder control. However, enuresis would not ordinarily be diagnosed in a child under the age of 5 years or with a mental age under 4 years.'

Prevalence

Due to the application of different diagnostic criteria, it is difficult to exactly determine incidence and prevalence rates. About 15–29% of 5 year olds, 10% of 10 year olds and 2% of 12–14-year-old children are affected. Enuresis is about twice as common in boys as in girls.

Aetiology

Three main aetiological theories have been proposed:

(i) a disturbed learning process
(ii) a medical/genetic condition
(iii) sign of emotional disturbance

Prognosis

The proportion of individuals with enuresis decreases in the course of adolescence. In the general adult population about 1–2% continue to suffer from the condition.

From WHO (1992), Liebert and Fischel (1990), Walker et al. (1989).

'difficult' steps, involving more invasive techniques. This approach has been shown to be helpful (Schmidt and Esser, 1981). The simultaneous approach to treatment involves using several techniques at the same time, e.g. dry bed training (Azrin et al., 1974).

The approach to treatment discussed here is problem centred and interactional, using behavioural methods to treat symptoms. Treatment must be based on the findings of a thorough assessment and should be flexible and avoid dogmatic restrictions. In the past, enuresis has often been inadequately assessed and current trends are towards a more thorough work-up of enuresis, which results in better treatment plans (Grosse, 1991, 1993). In some cases, medication may be required in addition to psychotherapeutic methods.

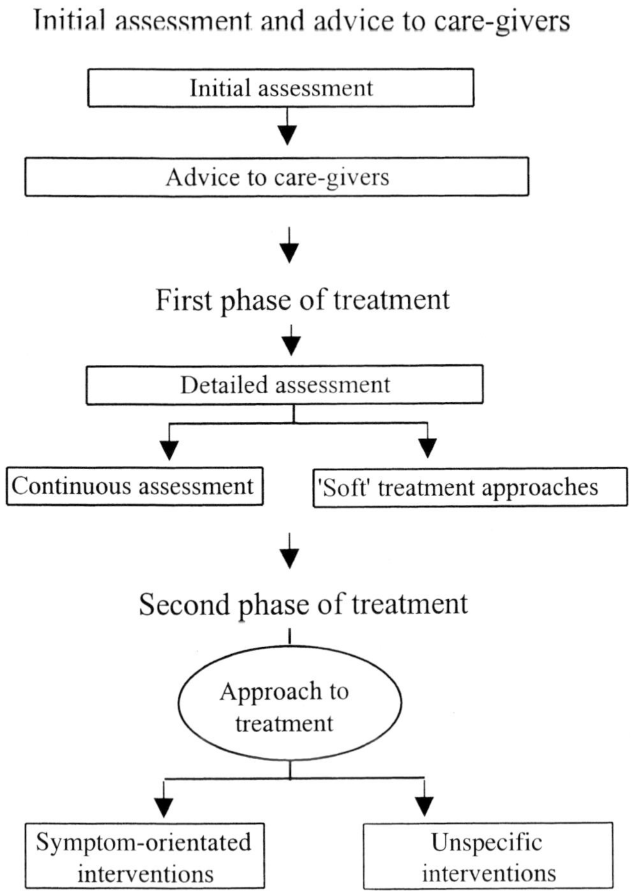

Fig. 23.1. The approach to treating enuresis.

The technique chosen depends not only on symptomatology, but also on the patient's psychosocial context. To some extent, the choice of technique also depends on the degree of cooperation possible from both patient and family. The technique must take into account both family interaction and interaction between family members and the therapist (Mattejat and Quaschner, 1985; Quaschner and Mattejat, 1989). The approach to treating enuresis is summarized in Fig. 23.1.

Treatment techniques

Initial assessment and offering advice to care-givers

Initial assessment

When assessing enuresis, the possibility of co-morbidity must be borne in mind. In the case of co-morbidity, one should be pragmatic with regard to which condition is more serious and which problem should be addressed first. A management plan must then be drawn up addressing the relevant symptoms to be treated and the order of the therapeutic steps to be undertaken. Pertinent questions, such as whether treatment can be recommended at all, should also be addressed early on, e.g. should one treat a 4-year-old child with enuresis?.

Advising care-givers

During the initial assessment phase, parents or other care-givers should be offered advice and information. This should include details of treatment, e.g. the setting, frequency of appointments, duration of therapy, emphasis on cooperation, distribution of responsibility as well as the condition itself, e.g. aetiology and maintaining factors, information on toilet training, regarding toilet training as a learning process which may be disturbed, possible connections between physical symptoms and mental state.

First phase of treatment

The first steps of treatment naturally aim to improve the condition; however, they must go hand in hand with an ongoing assessment process with the aim of recording symptoms in detail.

Detailed assessment

If in the process of initial assessment the enuresis is declared a target symptom, detailed assessment of the disorder should be undertaken. The choice of treatment is based on the results of this assessment. A semistructured interview may be helpful and in some cases questionnaires may provide additional help (Grosse, 1991). A proforma for such a questionnaire is shown in Table 23.2, and it should include general psychological symptoms as well as inquiring about symptoms relevant for a functional behavioural analysis. The list of topics may be extended to include additional aspects which are relevant if a particular treatment approach is being considered.

In addition to the presenting symptoms, the developmental history and physical findings, it is essential to enquire about any specific situations which seem to trigger symptoms or any life events which seem to relate to onset. It is also important to ask about previous attempts at treatment and how the family

Table 23.2. Initial assessment: topics suitable for a questionnaire

Presenting symptoms	Symptoms depend on	Development of symptoms
Day/night enuresis Primary/secondary Frequency (week/night/day) Amount (variation?)	A specific situation (location, time) The general life situation	Variations in frequency Duration of the longest dry phase Occurrence of dry and wet phases Toilet training Physical assessment

Previous attempts at treatment	Coping strategies of the parents and the patient
Medication Homeopathic treatment Night alarm Advice to parents symptom orientated non-symptom orientated Non-symptom orientated treatment of the child Health resort Other treatment	Waking up the child Fluid restriction (allowing child to drink less) Reinforcement (promises, rewards) Specific punishment Non-specific punishment/expressing displeasure Baby nappies (diapers) Rubber sheet Making child change own bed/wash bedclothes Other attempts

Patient's environment
Socioeconomic status Family members Living and sleeping conditions (toilet) Situation at school or in kindergarten Social contacts Interests, preoccupations Stressful events in the course of the patient's development Family interaction

has coped with symptoms so far. Reviewing coping mechanisms may help the therapist to discover the family's own aetiological view of the condition and will also help to assess the family's motivation for treatment and their willingness to cooperate. It is also important to inquire about the patient's environment, i.e. general living conditions and obtain information more directly related to the symptoms: where does the child sleep? Where is the toilet located?

If physical assessment was omitted in the initial stage, this must be undertaken by someone familiar with paediatrics before pychotherapy is commenced.

Ongoing assessment

Despite detailed initial assessment, assessment should be continued throughout the course of treatment. This allows feedback to be given which may in itself have a therapeutic effect. The recording of data may be restricted to determining the frequency of the enuresis, but may also be more elaborate.

Involving the patient or the parents in the recording of symptoms on a chart can be a great help. Initially, symptoms are simply observed in order to establish a baseline. It may be helpful to fill in a weekly schedule in order to reinforce behaviour, e.g. allowing the patient to draw a sun on those days he remains dry at night. However, this reinforcement technique is often used indiscriminately and must be accompanied by appropriate advice and encouragement.

When recording symptoms, both the type and frequency of symptoms should be noted. If possible, any triggers and the consequences should also be recorded. The chart should subsequently be discussed together with both the patient and parents in order to help them to identify relevant factors and improve their coping strategies. The manner in which a family deals with this task may help the therapist to assess the family's degree of cooperation ('compliance') or any reluctances regarding treatment ('resistance'). In some cases the patient may 'forget' to fill in the form or his mother may take over the task for him. As well as permitting insight into the family mechanisms, this task may also allow the therapist to assess the patient's own capacity and power within the family.

'Soft' treatment approaches

Diagnostic undertakings always have therapeutic relevance because they may influence symptoms. Thus whereas the procedures discussed above are primarily aimed at establishing a diagnostic baseline, they also represent the first 'soft' steps of treatment. It is proposed to the family and patient that they refrain from doing anything which might influence symptoms, so that the therapist can obtain an optimal baseline. This implies not restricting fluid intake, not waking the child at night, not admonishing the child or refering to the symptoms in a debasing manner. The only permissible measure is a rubber sheet in the patient's bed.

Paradoxically, this (self-)observation period may result in a brief reduction of symptoms, and in some cases symptoms may disappear entirely. It is well described that close observation may attenuate a behaviour, but in addition the task of (self-)observation may be considered a type of 'symptom prescription' or 'paradoxical intervention'. Patients and families experience the acceptance or even request to show symptoms as a great relief, in some cases improving symptoms.

Second phase of treatment

In the second phase, treatment is more specifically focused. Hypotheses regarding any aetiological or maintaining factors and about appropriate specific therapy should be based on the findings from the assessment phase. Thus, there are no predetermined preferred therapies; rather, an individual approach to treatment is devised. The most common techniques used are the well-known methods of behavioural therapy, e.g. self-observation, conditioning techniques, night alarm. These are usually helpful; however, they should never form the sole treatment. It is just as important to consider the individual context, in which symptoms occur, the relationship between the patient and the therapist, communication within the family, etc.

Techniques

Typically, the therapist suggests an approach and explains the technique to the patient and parents. Discussion should include information about the therapist's hypotheses on the aetiology of symptoms and maintaining factors as well as a rationale for the choice of a treatment method. Account should be taken of the family's understanding of the condition and accomodations made if necessary, i.e. the family should trust in the proposed approach to treatment.

The treatment plan is discussed in detail with the patient and his family and any adaptions suggested are considered. During this phase any difference of opinion should be confronted as this may lead to discontinuation of treatment unless they can be resolved, e.g. if a child refuses a night alarm due to a previous demoralizing experience despite the fact that the therapist sees it as the treatment of choice.

Such extreme differences in opinion are rare and usually it is possible to agree on a treatment method. The most important criteria for the choice of specific treatment techniques are summarized in Table 23.3.

Table 23.3. Criteria for the indication of techniques

Criteria for the choice of specific treatment techniques	
Symptoms	Type of enuresis and clinical condition
Patient: age / developmental status / capacity for self-control	Degree of suffering Intelligence Capacity for self-control
Cooperation of the family	Degree to which it is considerd a problem Ability to cooperate, e.g. intelligence, social status Willingness to cooperate
Treatment experience	Previous attempts at treatment
Additional problems / additional symptoms	. . . in the patient . . . in the family . . . in the patient's environment ('external conditions')

Table 23.4. Operant conditioning schedule (summary)

Operant conditioning schedule	
Indication	Appropriate as an additional or supportive measure in the treatment of all types of enuresis
Technique	(i) Determine the target behaviour (ii) Select the reinforcement (together with the patient) (iii) Define the contingencies, e.g. accumulative way of counting (iv) Written record ('contract' or 'schedule') (v) Practical details ('Who is responsible for what?')
Problems	Duration of therapy 'Wrong' selection of reinforcements Incorporation of reinforcements into interactional problems

Symptom-orientated techniques

The techniques discussed below are classified according to the aims of treatment or clinical condition. They are summarized in Tables 23.4 to 23.8.

Operant techniques

Indication

Operant techniques usually make use of a reinforcement schedule. This technique is helpful as a single method to treat mild enuresis. The technique can

Table 23.5. Enuresis alarm (summary)

	Enuresis alarm
Indication	Frequent night enuresis (habitualized symptom), i.e. primary night enuresis and some cases of secondary night enuresis
Technique	Explain and demonstrate the device Define the exact order of treatment steps Address all questions and concerns in detail Discontinue treatment gradually rather than abruptly
Problems	Motivational difficulties Negative expectations due to unsuccessful previous treatments Discouraging external conditions, e.g. residential situation, different night nurses, etc. Patient unable to cope with treatment without aid High relapse rate (up to 40%)

Table 23.6. Retention control (summary)

	Retention control training (various methods of retaining or interrupting micturation)
Indication	All types of enuresis (advantage: patient 'contributes' to treatment)
Technique	(Increased fluid intake) More or less systematic practice of retention, e.g. gradual increase in difficulty (Exact recording of steps if necessary)
Problems	Motivation must be high, particularly if the technique is complex or in other ways demanding

also be combined very conveniently with other methods, in which case it serves as additional support. Thus reinforcement schedules have a very broad spectrum of indications, including secondary night enuresis, day enuresis and as an additional measure in combination with a night alarm to treat primary night enuresis.

Technique

Techniques based on reinforcement are commonly used in behavioural therapy and have been shown to be effective. Use of the technique has been

Table 23.7. Medication for enuresis (summary)

	Medication for enuresis
Indication	To achieve initial improvement (in cases of severe enuresis) To help the patient cope with stressful situations, e.g. school outings To support other treatment methods, e.g. night alarm
Problems	Extremely high relapse rate after discontinuing medication (90–100%)

Table 23.8. Interactional treatment (summary)

	Interactional treatment (= steps taken to better cope with symptoms)
Indication	Day enuresis Secondary night enuresis Primary night enuresis
Technique	Refrain from negative comments, e.g. criticizing the patient, blaming, reprimanding or well-meant 'reminding') Give patient responsibility for ammending the sequelae of symptoms, e.g. changing clothes or bedclothes Change setting if necessary, e.g. separating patient and parents Toilet training in day enuresis, e.g. toilet schedule, etc.
Problems	Other symptoms may require treatment first Interactional problems may be more severe than expected and may include symptoms other than enuresis

explained in more detail elsewhere, so that only the specific application in the treatment of enuresis is discussed here. Determining the target behaviour in enuresis is fairly straightforward, because the symptom is defined quite precisely. Initially, days or nights without symptoms ('dry' days or nights) are an appropriate aim, however, in some cases it may be necessary to project a less demanding goal, e.g. half a 'dry' day or night, in order to enable the patient to have a successful experience, making the use of reinforcement possible.

It is important to discuss the choice of reinforcements together with the patient and the family. It may be helpful to use an 'accumulative' way of counting symptoms to define contingency criteria, e.g. the patient is required to 'collect' a certain number of 'dry' days in order to obtain the reward, regardless of whether days with enuresis have occurred in the meantime. If the time during which the patient is required to be without symptoms is too long, frustration may result, e.g. if the patient is required to stay dry for 1 week, but only manages to do so for 6 days. Frustration leads to a decrease in motivation and can be avoided by using the approach discussed above.

Keeping a precise record of the reinforcement schedule and defining the responsibilities of every individual involved in a written contract may help adherence to the schedule. However, in some families agreement may be achieved verbally. The reinforcement schedule should be used for a predetermined duration. Naturally, the option of continuing or modifying the schedule may be discussed with the patient and the family, perhaps with the ultimate aim of gradually discontinuing the schedule.

Problems

Insufficient motivation for treatment or a lack of concern regarding the symptoms preclude the use of reinforcement techniques. It is important to remember that motivation declines if the treatment lasts too long without success, even if patients were enthusiastic initially. Depending on the success, it may be appropriate to extend treatment, restrict or modify it, or even terminate it.

Problems may arise in choosing appropriate reinforcements, particularly if the therapist discusses the choice only with the parents. It is very important to include the patient in discussing the reinforcements. Additional problems may occur if reinforcements are somehow incorporated into current interactional problems between the patient and his parents and no longer serve the intended purpose.

Night alarm

Several different night alarm devices are available for use in children and adolescents (Stegat, 1978).

Indication

In a study by Quaschner and Mattejat (1989), they found that about a quarter of the patients had previously used a night alarm for treatment of enuresis without success. This demonstrates the importance of selecting and educating patients appropriately when using this treatment method. In their study, they found patients and parents had had inadequate instructions initially and insufficient support during treatment. In addition, many patients have been prescribed the device indisciminately. When prescribed in cases with appropriate indications and used properly, it is a very effective and safe treatment.

The method is particularly useful when enuresis is frequent, e.g. occurring almost every night. In primary night enuresis, this is usually the case, as the symptom is, to a great extent, habitualized.

Using a night alarm is also appropriate if symptoms are extremely frequent in secondary enuresis. However, apart from having become a habit, additional factors play a role in secondary enuresis, and the use of a night alarm should be considered carefully.

If enuresis is infrequent or variable, the chances of treatment being successful with a night alarm are low.

Technique

Using a night alarm is not as straightforward as it may seem. Instruction in its use is essential and families should never be simply given the device, as this may lead to misunderstandings and inappropriate use. Before treatment is commenced, the way the device works should be explained and demonstrated to all involved. The therapist should explain the steps in treatment. It may be helpful to practise using the device. The therapist should answer any questions and address any doubts, concerns or anxieties regarding the use of the device. Only following this process can treatment be initiated.

Ongoing assessment is usually required, and this should be done in person and never simply by letter or telephone. Frequent appointments with the family should be made, with telephone back-up if necessary between appointments if the family are concerned.

Termination of treatment should be gradual rather than abrupt, preferably after the patient has attained a particular therapeutic goal, e.g. 2 weeks without enuresis. The end of treatment should always be discussed with the patient and the parents beforehand. The technique of gradually discontinuing the night alarm should be explained to them, e.g. using the device only every second or third night. After having discontinued using the device with relief of symptoms, a few follow-up appointments should be offered over increasing time intervals.

An example of the course of treatment with a night alarm is shown in Fig. 23.2. The patient was a 6-year 8-month-old girl with primary night enuresis. The figure shows the frequency of symptoms, the number of times the alarm was activated and the number of times she got up at night of her own accord.

Problems

Several specific problems may occur in the course of treatment with a night alarm. First, if the child is unable to cope as a result of his age or developmental level, a parent may have to help him, e.g. switching off the alarm, waking up the child, sending him to the toilet, changing the wet pyjamas, setting the

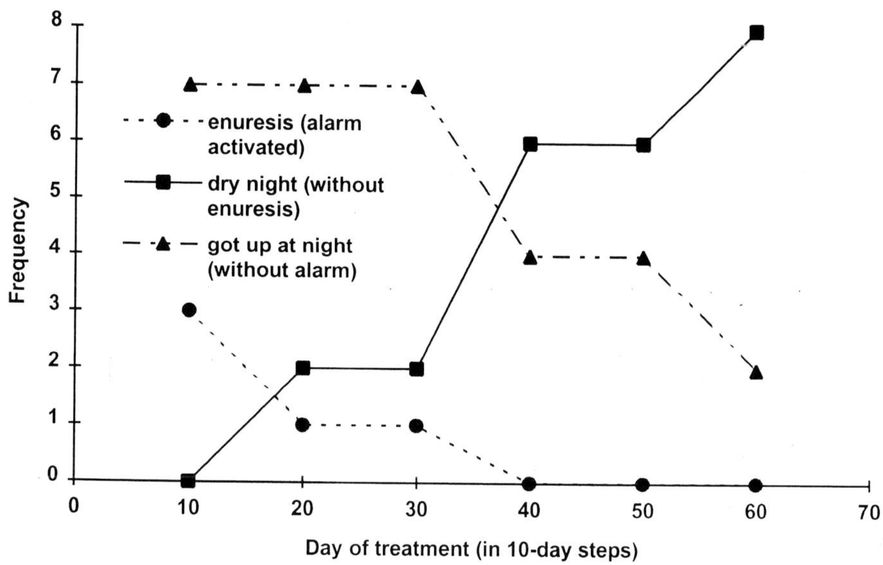

Fig. 23.2. The course of treatment of a patient with enuresis using a night alarm.

device for renewed use. Secondly, it may sometimes be difficult or even impossible to use the device if the patient sleeps in the same room as his siblings. Finally, problems may arise as a result of difficult housing conditions, e.g. the toilet is too far away, it is located on another floor, the child is afraid of going to the toilet in the dark, etc.

Negative experiences with alarms used in the past frequently cause problems over the course of treatment and these can be exceptionally difficult to overcome. In some cases patients have used a night alarm for extended periods of time (up to 1 year), although, in our experience, the further use of alarms may be successful in some cases. However, the indication should be clear and the course of treatment should be planned particularly carefully. The therapist should be aware of the great difficulty in motivating such patients and additional motivational therapy may be neccessary prior to restarting the treatment to optimize compliance.

Retention control training

Several different approaches to retention control training are available. Common techniques include deferring or interrupting micturition with the aim of eventually increasing the functional bladder capacity (FBC) and improving the patient's perception of the urge to micturate.

Indication
Retention control training is a technique which may be used for treating all types of enuresis. Although the effectiveness of retenion control training is limited (Fielding, 1980; Geffken et al., 1986), it can be used as a supplement to other techniques, allowing the patient and the family to make some contribution to treatment, thus encouraging cooperation.

Technique
Retention control training is usually combined with increased fluid intake. As soon as the patient perceives the urge to micturate, he is instructed to retain the urine for as long as possible or – depending on the technique used – to interrupt micturation repeatedly. These steps are repeated as often as possible and are precisely recorded, e.g. the duration of retention or the number of times micturation was interrupted. Programmes such as these may either be applied on special 'training days' or integrated into the patient's daily schedule.

Problems
Retention control training requires very good cooperation, although this varies depending on the particular technique used. It should only be attempted where a high degree of motivation of both patient and family is present.

Medication
The use of medication is widespread in the treatment of enuresis; however, the disadvantage is that in an extremely large proportion of cases, symptoms recur after discontinuation of the medication. This type of treatment should therefore be restricted to the small number of cases in which it is truly indicated. Medication may be helpful in supporting other types of treatment, such as the night alarm, particularly if symptoms do not improve with one method alone. Medication may be the treatment of choice in severe cases of enuresis in order to provide an initial success and prepare the way for other methods, thus improving motivation. Temporary medication may be useful in specific stressful situations, e.g. on a school outing.

Although several different medications have been used in the treatment of enuresis, e.g. synthetic diuretics, sympathomimetic stimulants, anticholinergics, tricyclic antidepressants have been shown to be most effective (Remschmidt, 1993).

Combination of approaches
Several approaches to treatment are described in the literature, which combine two or more of the techniques explained above. The more well known

methods include the 'Dry Bed Training' (Azrin et al., 1974) and the 'Full Spectrum Home Training' (Houts and Liebert, 1984; Houts et al., 1983). These methods tend to be rather elaborate, which may cause problems during treatment. In the literature, a dropout rate of 60% is reported for the Full Spectrum Home Training (Liebert and Fischel, 1990). Nevertheless, a combination of the methods above may be very useful, although they should not be applied in a stereotypical fashion, but adapted to suit the requirements of the individual.

Interactional treatment

Indication

Enuretic symptoms should always be considered in their interactional and familial context, regardless of which 'approach' or 'technique' the therapist favours. The context in which enuresis occurs affects resistance, compliance and cooperation to a great extent.

Technique

The therapist should allow the patient to take a considerable amount of responsibility in his treatment, regardless of the techniques or interventions which are planned. The patient's age and developmental stage must be taken into account. It happens all too frequently that adults (parents or therapist) take an active role, whilst the patient is assigned to a more passive role. This may lead to the patient showing avoidance, resistance or refusal.

For instance, expecting the child to change his bedclothes after wetting the bed may be a useful means to emphasize the child's own responsibility. However, it is essential that the child does not perceive the task as a punishment, but rather as a sign of responsibility. This is often not the case, leading to disagreements and tension in the family, such that family interaction gradually deteriorates and symptoms remain static.

It is thus important to address not only motivation, but also the family relationship and interactions. Patterns of interaction and disagreements may be sustaining symptoms and this issue should be raised. Treatment must be specific and tailored to each individual case. The examples discussed below should not be regarded as standardized approaches, but are intended to illustrate the range of possibilies of influencing family interaction.

Parents should refrain from reprimanding, blaming or criticizing the patient and avoid constantly 'reminding' the child, even when it is done in a well-meaning way, e.g. suggesting the child tries harder, sending him to the toilet frequently, advising him to drink less, questioning his motivation, etc.

Changing the therapeutic setting may lead to marked improvement of symptoms, e.g. asking a patient who has always come to appointments accompanied by his mother, to come to the next appointment alone. The patient should decide himself whether he wants to take part in school outings or spend the night at a friend's home.

In summary, interactional treatment encompasses all steps conductive to reducing the patient's feelings of guilt, shame and low self-esteem.

Problems

Therapeutic steps when treating enuresis may prove to be insufficient if other problems or symptoms turn out to be more severe than expected. In this case treatment should shift focus and concentrate on these problems initially.

Non-symptom-specific approaches

Psychiatric screening prior to treatment ensures that enuresis should indeed be the main focus of treatment. In the course of therapy, however, the necessity for non-symptom-specific treatment may arise and these problems and symptoms need to be addressed. This occurs in both secondary enuresis and day time enuresis. The most common additional problems include:

- excessive dependency, inadequate responsibility, low self-esteem;
- fear of failure, e.g. regarding the success of treatment, fear of excessive demands, e.g. sibling rivalry;
- additional psychological symptoms which may become apparent during treatment and which may become more important than the initial enuretic symptoms.

Faecal soiling (encopresis)

Clinical picture

Table 23.9 summarizes the definition, classification, prevalence, aetiology, and prognosis of faecal soiling.

Approaches to treatment

The treatment of faecal soiling has not been addressed in such detail in the literature as enuresis. This reflects the fact that faecal soiling is much rarer, that the clinical picture is more variable and that treatment is more difficult.

Approaches to treating faecal soiling are therefore more varied than those used in the treatment of enuresis (Mellon and Houts, 1995; Friman and Jones, 1998). However, using a similar approach seems appropriate, and has, in our experience, produced satisfactory results. Treatment usually begins with assess-

Table 23.9. Clinical profile of encopresis

Definition and classification

In ICD-10 non-organic encopresis (F98.1) is defined in the following way: 'Repeated voluntary or involuntary passage of faeces, usually of normal or near-normal consistency, in places not appropriate for that purpose in the individual's own sociocultural setting. The condition may represent an abnormal continuation of normal infantile incontinence, it may involve a loss of continence following the acquisition of bowel control, or it may involve the deliberate deposition of faeces in inappropriate places in spite of normal physiological bowel control.'

The diagnostic guidelines include the following additional points:

(i) Encopresis can be the result of inadequate toilet-training;
(ii) It can reflect a psychologically determined disorder in which there is normal physiological control over defecation, but for some reason, a reluctance, resistance or failure to conform to social norms in defecating in acceptable places;
(iii) It may stem from physiological retention, involving impaction of faeces, with secondary overflow and deposition of faeces in inappropriate places. In some cases the encopresis may be accompanied by smearing of faeces over the body or over the external environment.

Prevalence

Depending on the definition of the disorder, the literature indicates prevalence rates of 0.3–8.0%. The condition is four to five times more common in boys than in girls. About 50–60% of patients experienced a loss of continence following the acquisition of bowel control, i.e. secondary encopresis. In almost 100% of patients the symptoms occurred only in the daytime.

Aetiology

Two main aetiological theories have been proposed:

(i) Faecal soiling as the result of an emotional disturbance
(ii) Faecal soiling as the result of a disturbed learning process

Prognosis

The number of cases of faecal soiling in a sample decreases with increasing age of the individuals. Faecal soiling is rare after the age of seven years. Rutter et al. (1970) found the presence of faecal soiling among 10–12 year olds to be only 0.3–1.3%.

From WHO (1992), Liebert and Fischel (1990), Walker et al. (1989).

ment, with special emphasis on a medical assessment. Once any relevant medical conditions have been ruled out, additional symptoms should be assessed and treatment planned. Finally, a symptom-specific assessment of the faecal soiling is performed, including questions about present symptoms, associations with external or internal stimuli, a history of the development of symptoms, previous treatment attempts, family and social environment, etc.

In this phase it is paricularly important to assess the patient's and the family's motivation for treatment and their willingness and ability to cooperate with the therapist. The patient and the family should be aware that treatment is elaborate and takes time.

A combination of treatment techniques are discussed below. Medical treatment and behavioural techniques are generally important components of any treatment programme.

Techniques

The techniques discussed below are usually applied roughly in the order in which they are described here (Liebert and Fischel, 1990).

Achieving regular and normal defecation

A majority of patients retain faeces, resulting in severe constipation. Thus it is important to clear the bowel and encourage regular and pain-free defecation by appropriate use of laxatives. In some cases an enema or microenema may be required to clear the bowel. The use of laxatives may be required over an extended period of time.

During this initial phase, the patient and the parents should be informed of the treatment options and educated about normal bowel function and the physiology of defecation.

Recording symptoms

It is important to record symptoms as treatment proceeds. Two target behaviours should be noted: first, the frequency of inappropriate defecation and the conditions under which it occurs, and secondly, appropriate toilet-seeking behaviour.

Toilet training

The aim of toilet training is to achieve regular defecation and establish appropriate bowel control. Usually a fixed schedule with two to four predetermined times per day for visiting the toilet are agreed upon. These times may be coordinated with meal times, the administration of laxatives or other regular daily activities. Toilet training may have to be assigned to the patient as a task, depending on the patient's age, developmental stage and general motivation. Some patients may initially require help or support, e.g. help in cleaning themselves after defecation. Later in treatment, they then learn how to cope with the task on their own.

Training hygiene and cleanliness
Faecal soiling may indicate an inadequate appreciation or skills in hygiene and cleanliness. Therefore, in addition to toilet training it may be necessary to educate the patient about what to do when he has soiled himself. This may include helping him change his clothes, depositing the soiled clothes in an appropriate place, cleaning himself, etc. The patient may also require help in other areas of hygiene, e.g. washing himself and changing clothes regularly, regardless of whether they are soiled.

Operant techniques
Operant techniques are quite effective in the treatment of faecal soiling, particularly the systematic use of positive reinforcement of appropriate target behaviour. This technique, incorporating a written reinforcement schedule, is an essential part of many faecal soiling treatment programmes. It must be emphasized that depositing faeces in the appropriate place is the target behaviour to be reinforced, particularly in patients with faecal retention and constipation. Merely reinforcing the absence of soiling may cause patients to retain faeces, thus aggravating constipation and leading to overflow soiling.

Family-orientated approaches
The family should be included in treatment, particularly as symptoms always affect family interaction in some way. Treatment may be aimed at developing strategies to cope with symptoms or may focus on the expectations the parents have towards the patient or towards treatment. Working with parents is essential in order to sustain motivation and cooperation, both of which are important for successful treatment.

Conclusions

Good cooperation between the therapist and the family is essential for successful treatment, and is a requirement for the effective application of all treatment techniques. Without sufficient cooperation, all attempts at treating faecal soiling are compromised.

Treatment should be discontinued gradually rather than abruptly. The family should be offered the opportunity to return for assessment or treatment immediately, should symptoms reccur. Making follow-up appointments may help to dispel any anxieties which may occur upon termination of treatment and help to convey a feeling of support and trust.

REFERENCES

Azrin, N. H., Sneed, T. J. and Fox, R. M. (1974). Dry bed training. Rapid elimination of childhood enuresis. *Behaviour Research and Therapy*, **12**, 147–56.

Fielding, D. (1980). The response of day and night wetting children and children who wet only at night to retention control training and the enuresis alarm. *Behaviour Research and Therapy*, **18**, 305–17.

Friman, P. C. and Jones, K. M. (1998). Elimination disorders in children. In *Handbook of child behavior therapy*, ed. T. S. Watson and F. M. Gresham. New York: Plenum Press.

Geffken, G., Johnson, S. B. and Walker, D. (1986). Behavioural interventions for childhood nocturnal enuresis. The differential effect of of bladder capacity on treatment progress and outcome. *Health Psychology*, **5**, 261–72.

Grosse, S. (1991). *Bettnässen*. Weinheim: Psychologie Verlags Union.

Grosse, S. (1993). Enuresis. In *Handbuch Verhaltenstherapie und Verhaltensmedizin bei Kindern und Jugendlichen*, ed. H-C. Steinhausen and M. von Aster, pp. 433–60. Weinheim: Psychologie Verlags Union.

Houts, A. C. and Liebert, R. M. (1984). *Bedwetting*. Springfield, IL: Charles C. Thomas.

Houts, A. C., Liebert, R. M. and Padawer, W. (1983). A delivery system for the treatment of primary enuresis. *Journal of Abnormal Child Psychology*, **11**, 513–20.

Liebert, R. M. and Fischel, J. E. (1990). The elimination disorders. In *Handbook of developmental Psychopathology*, ed. M. Lewis and S. M. Miller, pp. 421–9. New York: Plenum Press.

Mattejat, F. and Quaschner, K. (1985). Zur ambulanten Behandlung von Enuretikern. *Zeitschrift für Kinder- und Jugendpsychiatrie*, **13**, 212–29.

Mellon, M. W. and Houts, A. C. (1995). Elimination disorders. In *Handbook of child behavior therapy in the psychiatric setting*, ed. R. T. Ammerman and M. Hersen. New York: Wiley.

Quaschner, K. and Mattejat, F. (1989). Kooperation und Behandlungsabbruch. Eine Untersuchung zum Verlauf von Therapien bei Kindern mit Enuresis. *Zeitschrift für Kinder- und Jugendpsychiatrie*, **17**, 119–24.

Remschmidt, H. (1993). Reaktive, alterstypische und neurotische Störungen. In *Lehrbuch der Kinderheilkunde*, ed. F. J. Schulte and J. Sprange, pp. 795–806. Stuttgart: Gustav Fischer.

Rutter, M., Tizard, J. and Whitmore, K. (1970). *Education, health and behaviour*. London: Longman.

Schmidt, N. J. and Esser, G. (1981). Einflüsse auf die Effizienz der verhaltenstherapeutischen Behandlung der Enuresis. *Zeitschrift für Kinder- und Jugendpsychiatrie*, **9**, 217–32.

Stegat, H. (1978). Enuresis. In *Handbuch der Psychologie. Klinische Psychologie*, ed. L. J. Pongratz, pp. 2626–65. Göttingen: Hogrefe.

Walker, C. E., Kenning, M. and Faust-Campanile, J. (1989). Enuresis and encopresis. In *Treatment of childhood disorders*, ed. E. J. Mash and R. A. Barkley, pp. 423–48. New York: Guilford Press.

World Health Organization (WHO) (1992). *The ICD-10 classification of mental and behavioural disorders. Clinical descriptions and diagnostic guidelines*. Geneva: WHO.

24 Dyslexia and dyscalculia

Andreas Warnke and Gerhard Niebergall

Introduction

Dyslexia (also known as specific reading and spelling disorder) and dyscalculia (also known as specific disorder of arithmetical skills) influence performance at school to a great extent. Dyslexia usually leads to conflicts not only at school but also at home. Many additional psychological symptoms may occur, resulting sometimes in serious psychiatric disorders (Esser, 1990).

The many psychiatric and behavioural sequelae of dyslexia are generally of a 'neurotic' nature. Thus, symptoms arise as a result of conflicts between the desire to achieve at school, and the difficulty in fulfilling this expectation. Eventually, the child is unable to cope with the excessive demands and constant failure, and there is a resultant loss of self-esteem. Thus a vicious circle is established (Fig. 24.1), usually involving the school, parents and the peer group.

The conflicts I to IV in Fig. 24.1 directly affect the child. The child is less involved in conflict V, unless other children side with the dyslexic child in opposition to the school. Secondary symptoms are usually similar regardless of whether the child suffers from dyslexia or dyscalculia. Thus, the approach to treatment must be broad: after assessment and diagnosis, patients should be treated with a specific treatment programme aimed at their specific problem (reading, writing, arithmetic skills), but, in addition, individual psychotherapy may be required for any accompanying mental or behavioural symptoms (Skinner, 1998). Parents or families should be included in treatment, and in order to optimize results treatment programmes should be coordinated with the school.

Treatment of dyscalculia differs to some extent from the treatment of dyslexia in several points. However, many aspects of treatment apply to both disorders (Maughan and Yule, 1994). Here, the general management is discussed first and the specific issues relating to each disorder are then considered.

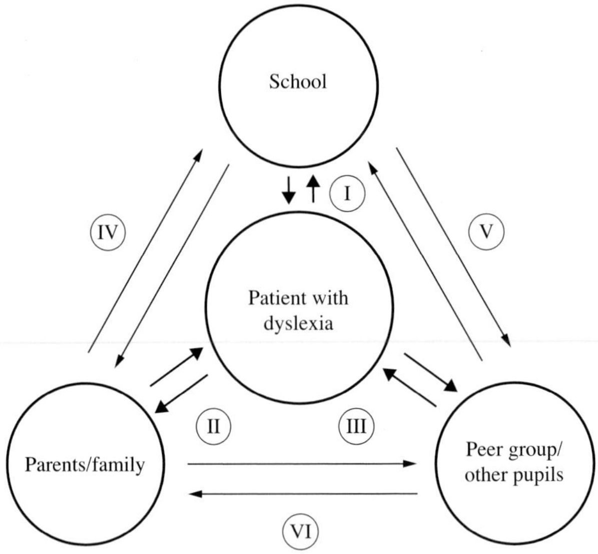

Fig. 24.1. Vicious circle involving the patient, school, parents and the peer group (I–IV = areas of conflict).

Characteristics of the disorders, definitions, classification and assessment

Dyslexia

Dyslexia is a specific impairment in the development of reading and spelling skills. Symptoms include impaired reading out loud, word recognition and reading comprehension. During reading out loud or writing, letters or words are frequently omitted, switched around or substituted. Both recognition of individual letters and the synthesis of a word from these letters is impaired (Weinschenk, 1965). Primary associated symptoms are quite common, including specific developmental disorders of language ('phonological awareness'), arithmetic skills, and motor function. Probably up to 10% of children with dyslexia have a visual information processing impairment. Psychopathological abnormalities often occur as secondary associated symptoms; these include:

- learning difficulties and low achievement at school (usually due to lack of motivation, although in rare cases excessive efforts at school may cause problems);
- emotional problems (anxiety, depression, fear of failure at school, school refusal);
- hyperactive symptoms (restlessness, fidgeting, attention deficit);
- psychosomatic complaints (headache, abdominal pain, nausea associated with demanding situations at school);

- conduct disorder (difficulties with discipline at school, aggression, social isolation, disagreements about homework, antisocial behaviour). In some cases, severe interactional difficulties between child and parents may occur (Warnke, 2000).

Considering the variety of secondary symptoms that may be associated with dyslexia or dyscalculia, all children who present to a child and adolescent psychiatric practice or clinic for conduct disorder should be assessed for specific learning disorders, i.e. reading, spelling, arithmetic skills.

In ICD-10 (WHO, 1992), dyslexia and dyscalculia are classified as 'specific developmental disorders of scholastic skills'. Both disorders are not considered to be the result of inadequate opportunity to learn, low intelligence or brain damage, but are considered to develop fairly early in life, becoming apparent at school age. In order to make the diagnosis, there must be a 'clinically significant degree of impairment in the specified scholastic skill'. This may be judged on the basis of severity as defined in scholastic terms, i.e. a degree that may be expected to occur in less than 3% of school children. The prevalence of dyslexia among school children is 2–8% and about 1% of the general population are thought to have severe dyslexia.

ICD-10 distinguishes between specific reading (F81.0) and spelling (F81.1) disorders. In specific reading disorder, 'reading comprehension skill, reading word recognition, oral reading skill, and performance of tasks requiring reading may be all affected. Spelling difficulties are frequently associated with specific reading disorder and often remain into adolescence even after some progress in reading has been made.'

In specific spelling disorder, 'the main feature [. . .] is a specific and significant impairment in the development of spelling skills in the absence of a history of specific reading disorder, which is not solely accounted for by low mental age, visual acuity problems, or inadequate schooling. The ability to spell orally and to write out words correctly are both affected.'

The ability to process visual and auditory information is typically disturbed in dyslexic children (Schulte-Körne et al., 1999). They have difficulties in transforming visual information into phonemes (reading) and, verbal information into script by means of visually controlled motor acts (writing).

Considering the complex nature of scholastic skills, the aetiology of disorder is very likely to be multifactorial. Several factors are presumed to be relevant in the aetiology of dyslexia: a genetic predisposition for dyslexia and minor abnormalities in brain development before and after birth appear to contribute to the condition (Warnke, 1999).

Table 24.1. Assessment of the primary symptoms of dyslexia

Assessment of the primary symptoms of dyslexia
(i) Dictation of numbers (usually normal)
(ii) Dictation of letters (usually normal)
(iii) Copying words and sentences (usually normal)
(iv) Reading numerals (usually normal)
(v) Reading letters (usually normal)
(vi) Reading sentences (slow, disrupted, incorrect)
(vii) Reading phonetically (usually normal)
(viii) Writing words (incorrect, disturbed)
Also:
History (patient, family)
Physical examination (senses, neurological assessment, additional investigations)
Assessment of general intelligence, e.g. WISC
Specific reading and spelling tests

From Niebergall, 1987.

Assessment of dyslexia

The clinical assessment of dyslexia is summarized in Table 24.1. An assessment should be made of the child's ability to write the letters of the alphabet, a short sentence, and a text dictation. In addition, the child should be asked to read numbers consisting of several digits as well as letters, words and sentences. When dyslexia is suspected, an age-appropriate standardized reading and/or spelling test should be administered.

Physical examination is essential to rule out any physical illness, particularly disorders of the senses or the central nervous system. An intelligence test should be undertaken to detect significant differences between the IQ and spelling test results. A significant difference suggests dyslexia. Dyslexia can only be diagnosed with confidence if the IQ is within the normal range and the spelling test results are below 85–90% of the normal control group. However, this operationally defined approach to diagnosing dyslexia is controversial (Warnke, 1990, 1999).

Dyscalculia

This disorder (also known as specific arithmetic retardation) may occur as a specific developmental disorder, with primary impairment of arithmetic skills, or as a result of brain damage, causing secondary loss of arithmetic skills. Arithmetic skills may also be impaired by congenital or acquired mental retardation, or as a result of psychogenic stress. Here, we will focus only on the specific developmental disorder.

In ICD-10 (WHO, 1992) specific disorder of arithmetical skills (dyscalculia) is defined thus: 'This disorder involves a specific impairment in arithmetical skills, which is not solely explicable on the basis of general mental retardation or of grossly inadequate schooling. The deficit concerns mastery of basic computational skills of addition, subtraction, multiplication, and division (rather than the more abstract mathematical skills involved in algebra, trigonometry, geometry, or calculus). [. . .] The child's arithmetical performance should be significantly below the level expected on the basis of his or her age, general intelligence, and school placement, and is best assessed by means of an individually administered, standardized test of arithmetic.'

Most individuals who are familiar with solving arithmetic problems are unaware that learning arithmetic is a 'qualitative learning process'. This process can be broken down into six steps (Weinschenk, 1975).

(i) The words for the numerals used must be understood and used in the right order.
(ii) The numerals must be understood to refer to specific amounts; specific amounts must be associated with the corresponding numerals.
(iii) Illustrations of objects eventually replace the actual objects.
(iv) Abstract concepts gradually replace the concept of actual objects, e.g. the concept of three apples is replaced by three dots or marks to represent the number '3'.
(v) The first few numerals of the number sequence are learnt.
(vi) The ability to imagine a number, rather than perceive it, must be acquired.

In dyscalculia, it is particularly step (vi) which is impaired. Epidemiological studies have shown that about 2% of children attending primary school have symptoms of primary dyscalculia (Remschmidt et al., 1990).

The curriculum for the first year of primary school usually includes teaching children basic arithmetic skills (addition, subtraction) within a numerical range of 1 to 20. During the second year, the numerical range is extended to 100 and multiplication and division are introduced. During the third year, the numerical range is extended to 1000 and methods of written arithmetic are taught. In the fourth year of primary school, the numerical range is extended beyond 1 million. Primary school teachers have observed that children approach the task of arithmetic in different ways and develop a surprisingly wide range of strategies to solve arithmetic problems. When doing decimal arithmetic, children generally tend to have difficulties changing to the next unit of ten, e.g. from tens to hundreds, etc.

Assessment of dyscalculia

School children with dyscalculia can frequently be identified by the great discrepancy between their arithmetic skills in comparison to all other subjects at school. These children tend to develop similar secondary symptoms as children with dyslexia, which affect mental and physical well-being and may involve conduct disorder. To make the diagnosis of dyscalculia, an assessment of intelligence and a standardized arithmetic skills test are required.

In our experience it has been useful to follow the six steps described above (see also Geary, 1994; Miles and Miles, 1992). Arithmetic tasks involving addition, subtraction, multiplication and division within the numerical range of 1 to 100 help to further assess the child's skills. Just a few questions are sufficient to assess which of the six steps the child has not yet attained. Children with dyscalculia usually do not have an abstract idea of what a numeral signifies. Thus they often require fingers or other objects to help them count out an answer as they have not yet learnt how to perform calculations by abstract means. The diagnosis can usually be made with confidence at the end of the second year of primary school. A qualitative analysis of the child's arithmetic skills is helpful for planning future treatment.

Treatment

General principles

The treatment of dyslexia and dyscalculia involves several aspects:

- offering advice to the patient, parents and teachers;
- individual instruction;
- psychotherapy of associated emotional and/or behavioural disturbance;
- parent training when appropriate;
- helping with the financial aspect of treatment, which may require involving school authorities, health insurance, social services etc.

Treatment focusing directly on the child includes psychotherapy, a motivational phase prior to individual instruction, individual instruction in reading and spelling (or arithmetic) and associated skills, e.g. concentration, visual–motor coordination, language comprehension, teaching the child to cope with the diagnosis of a learning disorder, and treatment of any secondary symptoms.

It may be helpful to begin instruction in an individual setting and then attempt to transfer improvement to a school situation. In addition to individual treatment, parents and the school need to be included, particularly if secondary symptoms are present.

It is advisable to commence treatment by explaining the diagnosis of dyslexia or dyscalculia and the consequences the diagnosis has for the child. At this stage, parents tend to express misconceptions, make accusations, or feel guilty, whereas the patient on the other hand usually has low self-esteem. The sessions should therefore focus initially on the recent stress which the family has gone through, and only later proceed to address the patient's scholastic goals and vocational plans. Any uncertainty or conflicts associated with these topics need to be discussed openly with the patient and the family. An analysis of daily life activities may help to identify areas in which the patient and the family particularly require support, and these provide a useful focus for initial therapy.

It is important to stress the fact that the learning disorder is neither a result of the child's laziness or stupidity nor a sign of failings in either the child's upbringing or education. Clearly stating that the disorder is not the child's fault usually eases stress considerably. The child may be told:

> You have dyslexia (or dyscalculia). No one knows why you of all people have this disorder. Just like some people are good at music and others are not, or some people have good eyesight and others wear glasses, you have more difficulties than others learning to read and write (or learning arithmetic). It's not your fault, and you are certainly clever enough to improve your achievement. However, you will need more time than the others, you will have to be patient, work hard and accept the extra help which you will get from your parents, teachers and other professionals.

It may be helpful to focus on three main areas when offering support to the family:

(i) Resolution or help with family conflicts, which occur as a result of the child's learning difficulties. In cases of severe disorder, the relationship between the parents and the child may be quite tense and both the child and the parents (particularly the mother) may become depressed.

(ii) Offering advice to parents on how best to help their child with homework. Supervising the homework of a child with dyslexia or dyscalculia is a difficult and demanding educational task. Unfortunately, the child's efforts are frequently accompanied by undue pressure and criticism, frequently resulting in tearful outbursts or arguments. Homework, which has taken many hours of toil, may be rewarded with comments from teachers, such as 'needs to take more care with homework'. These conflicts are almost ubiquitous in these learning disorders (Warnke, 1987; Warnke, 2000). Many parents, however, after appropriate advice and support are able to help the child and address any associated emotional issues. On the other hand, severe disturbance of the parent–child relationship may occur despite great efforts by the parents, and in these cases, it may be more appropriate for the therapist to discourage parents from directly supervising their child's homework. The likelihood of parental help being successful depends on the parents having patience in dealing with the child and sufficient time for supervising homework.

(iii) The therapist should encourage cooperation between the family and the school in order to facilitate specific measures to help the child cope with the learning disorder. Parents need to be able to work together with the school in a constructive way and coordinate supportive measures as well as accepting help such as educational aids or individual instruction where this is appropriate.
In many cases of severe dyslexia (or dyscalculia) the support offered by schools or special educational agencies proves to be inadequate, as instruction has been given in a group setting. Individual instruction is frequently required, and in severe refractive cases it may be necessary for the child to attend a school either boarding or day, specializing in instructing children with learning disorders.

Psychotherapy

Patients with a learning disorder may have a broad spectrum of mental symptoms and behavioural abnormalities. During assessment and treatment, one frequently encounters low self-esteem. Self-esteem is an important aspect of personality development, which young children are usually unaware of. Thus, addressing self-esteem is an important task of psychotherapy. The attempt to understand the child and his situation usually helps to establish an empathic relationship. It is important to express sympathy for the stressful experiences the child has been through as a result of his learning disorder and any resulting loss of self-esteem. For example, the child might be told: 'I would expect you to feel rather stupid getting bad marks in school all the time. But I know that you are not really stupid. It's understandable that you're sad after being made fun of and scolded again by your parents. In your place I would probably feel that way. I would also become angry and upset if I felt so hard done by . . .' Such statements help the patient to understand the (compensatory) connection between the primary disorder and the secondary sequelae. It is important to convey hope and give a realistic prognosis for the course, provided that specific individual instruction in reading and spelling (or arithmetic) is undertaken. In this way, the child can learn to distinguish between the way he is assessed at school and his own way of assessing the true effort that is put into his achievements. Self-esteem should also be addressed independent of school achievement, as children may generalize negative experiences made at school and consider themselves a 'failure' in all respects. However, the basic necessity of having to learn to read and spell (or do arithmetic) correctly should not be questioned.

Appropriate self-esteem is best recovered by giving the child the opportunity to make (objective) achievements, thus allowing him to experience (subjective) success. These aspects are the keystones of treatment and of individual instruction. Patients must be encouraged to accept the challenge of learning to read and spell or do arithmetic. Successful learning, positive appraisal and further encouragement help to improve self-esteem and facilitate the development of a normal personality.

Disappointments and anxieties will be common during the many years of treatment. These typically involve school, examination situations, family life and other interpersonal relationships. The use of behavioural therapy programmes developed for anxiety disorders may prove helpful (see Chapter 15) and the patient may improve his strategies for coping with stressful situations in group therapy and using role play (see Chapter 11). The emotional and social difficulties of patients with learning disorders are likely to be due to several symptoms (a 'syndrome') rather than one symptom alone. This syndrome includes both the primary and secondary symptoms, which continually feed back to one another. This complex interaction makes the use of several different treatment techniques most appropriate.

Because of the nature of the disorder, cooperation with the parents and the school is essential. Parents are usually only too willing to cooperate, and work together with teachers from the special school in the hospital is usually straightforward. However, cooperating with schools outside the hospital and coordinating school attendance for inpatients sometimes causes problems. Psychiatrists, psychologists and teachers all have different views of what 'learning disorders' are. They may entertain different concepts of aetiology and approaches to treatment. It is essential to agree upon one approach to treatment in and out of school, in order not to further burden the patient.

Individual instruction for dyslexia

There is no single correct method of treating dyslexia, but despite the broad spectrum of treatment techniques, several basic guidelines may help in choosing an appropriate treatment approach.

- Treatment should begin as early as possible and should continue in addition to normal school attendance. Individual instruction is usually more helpful than group instruction. The formal setting in which individual instruction takes place (the work place, keeping appointments, punctuality) helps to improve the patient's attitude towards achievement. Treatment time should be utilized fully for improving reading and spelling skills and is best undertaken following a schedule. Most children with dyslexia are eager to improve their reading and spelling skills and are likely to be disappointed if individual instruction does not focus on these skills.

- Reading and spelling skill can only be acquired by means of intensive practice.
- Excessive demands, for example, the principle of 'zero tolerance', should not be made of dyslexic children. Progress will largely depend on the child's individual ability and age. Thus, individual instruction should focus initially on aspects of 'phonological awareness', on analysing words and identifying phonemes, synthesizing phonemes to make up words, progressing from two-letter syllables to multi-letter syllables, analysing and correcting individual errors, progressing to reading and writing whole sentences. Comprehension skills of both words and texts should be covered alongside each step and the child should also be taught the specific rules of spelling including exceptions to rules.
- The use of systematic treatment programmes with proven efficacy has been suggested (Kossow, 1975). Many such programmes emphasize the importance of a phonetic approach to language and suggest analysing phonemes, associating phonemes with letters and considering words as a sequence of phonemes. This approach addresses the primary deficit dyslexic children have, namely difficulty in 'phonological awareness' (Klicpera and Gasteiger-Klicpera, 1995). Such treatment programmes begin with teaching phonemes and letters and proceed to teach reading and spelling whole words.
- A broad spectrum of educational material is available for dyslexic children, both commercially or through educational services. The material is generally appropriate for use in individual instruction sessions and may include games with letters and words which are helpful for helping children to relax during treatment sessions and maintaining their motivation.
- Computer programs to help improve reading and spelling skills are available. They can be very useful for increasing motivation; however, they cannot entirely replace individual instruction and should therefore only be used in conjunction with personal reading and spelling instruction.
- The principles of the teaching of reading and writing outlined here do not differ to any significant degree from those used in schools. However, in school children with dyslexia, it is particularly important to respect the individual's speed of learning.
- If dyslexia is associated with additional developmental weaknesses such as language or motor skills, visual–motor coordination, attention or auditory discrimination, these need to be addressed in addition to the dyslexia. However, help in these alone will not improve reading and spelling skills. A specific effect on the dyslexia is only likely when the additional weaknesses are in some way connected with reading and spelling, e.g. verbal articulation, attention

training, and are addressed in conjunction with reading and spelling. Thus the combined functional treatment of fine motor skills (neat handwriting), verbal skills (articulation), language skills (grammar, vocabulary), auditory discrimination, visual and auditory memory, and attention usually improves dyslexia only if reading and spelling skills are also included in the treatment programme.

Individual instruction for dyscalculia

There is a paucity of systematic publications on the treatment of dyscalculia (Grissemann and Weber, 1990; Grissemann, 1996). However, the basic approach to treating the disorder is similar to that of dyslexia and can be considered in several phases:

- psychotherapy and motivational phase,
- cooperation with the parents and the school,
- individual instruction, and
- transfer of skills to the school setting.

Before starting treatment, it is advisable to determine which of the six previously mentioned steps the child is capable of. Children with normal general intelligence but with dyscalculia are usually unable to perform simple calculations on an abstract plane without the aid of actual objects.

To what extent is it then possible to teach the patient to perform abstract calculations? Treatment requires that the patient has at least some idea of amounts and is able to associate defined amounts with the appropriate numerals, using actual objects for help if necessary, e.g. fingers within the numerical range of 1 to 10. Through techniques using extensive practice, children can usually improve their conceptual ability (Weinschenk, 1975).

However, dyscalculia does not necessarily imply total inability in understanding the concept of amounts and numerals. The disorder varies in severity, and most patients have some basic skills. Normal school lessons are often unable to improve on these skills, and secondary symptoms may develop, ultimately resulting in severe emotional or behavioural disturbance (Weinschenk, 1975).

In order to avoid excessive demands, children should first learn to feel entirely comfortable with addition and subtraction within a numerical range of 1 to 10, eventually without having to use their fingers. The child should then learn strategies with which he may perform calculations on an abstract plane, without having to refer to actual objects. One method is to use small rods to represent numbers. The child is asked to do a simple calculation using the rods. In the next step, the child is asked to close his eyes and imagine a given number of rods and the changes which occur when one or two are removed or added.

This approach encourages a learning experience, through which the child may eventually be able to change from calculation using actual objects to calculation based on the concept of numerals. As arithmetic skills improve, the numerical range can be extended. This method emphasizes the visual sense, but it may be combined with other sensations such as touch or sound, in order to use different sensory stimuli to convey the sense of numbers.

Children with dyscalculia frequently have difficulties in changing to the next unit of ten as the numerical range is extended, e.g. from tens to hundreds. The approach to explaining the phenomenon of an additional place before the decimal is similar each time. It may be helpful to use money (small change and bank notes) to explain the concept of decimal places. An understanding of quantitative ratios may be conveyed by using a ruler or measuring tape. Multiplication and division can thus be explained in a comprehensible way, and the teacher may then gradually move on to explain more abstract calculations (see Geary, 1994).

In most cases of learning disorder, children require systematic treatment and individual instruction, sometimes for several years. A broad spectrum of educational material is available for children with dyscalculia. However, improvement may be difficult and is usually achieved only by means of learning essential arithmetic rules by heart. It is nevertheless helpful to ask the children to verbalize their arithmetic strategies and thoughts in order to correct mistakes immediately. In some cases role play, e.g. 'shopping' may help to improve the child's motivation.

Treating psychogenic disturbance of arithmetical skills

Psychogenic disturbance of arithmetical skills usually requires a different approach to treatment. This disorder develops as a result of fear of failure, e.g. in an examination, experience of failure or by a particularly difficult relationship between a child and the mathematics teacher. When inferior performance is a result of low general intelligence, however, specific treatment of the disturbance of arithmetical skills is unlikely to lead to significant improvement.

Case report

A 16-year-old boy with poor arithmetic skills was presented. He was in his ninth year of school. His performance in mathematics and other science subjects had declined rapidly. Eventually, the boy had been unable to solve even simple tasks in the four fundamental operations of arithmetic. General intelligence was above average (IQ = 122). The assessment of the 'disturbance' revealed that the boy had been victimized by the mathematics and physics teacher in front of the entire class, causing the boy great shame and embarassment. The boy developed a marked fear of failure in school, which generalized and gradually involved other subjects at school.

We advised the parents to seek help from the headmaster of the school, who responded positively to the request to assign the boy to another class. With the support of the new teacher his performance improved rapidly. Several months later his achievements in mathematics had greatly improved.

Evaluation

The prognosis of dyslexia is rather poor: follow-up studies show that, if no intensive and specific treatment is undertaken, dyslexia continues throughout adolescence and into adulthood (Esser, 1990; Strehlow et al., 1992). Children with dyslexia are at increased risk of psychiatric disorder, because it generally impairs social integration and school performance. About 30% of children (Rutter et al., 1976) and about 50% of adolescents with dyslexia (Korhonen, 1984) have a conduct disorder. A high proportion of delinquent adolescents are dyslexic (Weinschenk, 1965; Esser, 1990; Esser and Schmidt, 1994). In long-term follow-up studies, dyslexia has been shown to be extremely persistent (Klicpera and Gasteiger-Klicpera, 1995). However, with intensive treatment, reading and spelling skills may improve markedly (Gäbe, 1990; Kossow, 1975).

The effectiveness of intensive individual instruction has been shown in a study in 44 children with an average of 80 individual sessions per child over an average time of 2 years (Warnke and Niebergall, 1997). Several conclusions were drawn from the results of the study.

- Problems in the family are likely to impair treatment progress.
- Children from an adverse social background tend to discontinue treatment.
- Certain personality traits, e.g. obsessional personality may impair the child's progress despite high general intelligence.
- Some individuals show normal personality development, despite little improvement of primary symptoms.
- Some individuals improve their reading and spelling skills, but continue to have social and behavioural difficulties.
- Systematic individual instruction, including the teaching of orthographic rules, tends to improve dyslexia.
- Treating dyslexia usually causes significant improvement in most cases, however, it is time-consuming and requires much patience from everyone involved.

The psychological and social development of children and adolescents with dyslexia is at risk if no specific treatment is undertaken. A considerable number of adults with dyslexia continue to suffer as a result of the condition: several individuals reported that they continued to experience severe examination anxiety many years after leaving school as a result of the traumatization which they had suffered at school.

There is a paucity of studies assessing the efficacy of treating dyscalculia. Experience shows that treatment is quite demanding and a great motivation is required to achieve improvement. It is likely that younger children (first or second year of elementary school) make faster progress than older children. In younger childern the disorder appears to be due to a great extent to inadequate specific development, whilst in older children the disorder appears to be a result of predisposition. In either case, educational measures and specific individual instruction is indicated for several years. All those involved need to be advised on matters concerning school and vocational choice.

REFERENCES

Esser, G. (1990). *Bedeutung und langfristiger Verlauf umschriebener Entwicklungsstörungen*. Heidelberg: University of Heidelberg.

Esser, G. and Schmidt, M. H. (1994). Children with specific reading retardation. Early determinants and long-term outcome. *Acta Paedopsychiatrica,* **56**, 229–37.

Gäbe, I. (1990). *Schwere Legasthenie. Einzelbehandlung bei Kindern und Jugendlichen*. Freiburg: Lambertus.

Geary, D. C. (1994). *Children's mathematical development*. Washington DC: American Psychological Association.

Grissemann, H. and Weber, A. (1990). *Grundlagen und Praxis der Dyskalkulietherapie*. Bern: Huber.

Grissemann, H. (1996). *Dyskalkulie heute*. Bern: Huber.

Klicpera, C. and Gasteiger-Klicpera, C. (1995). *Psychologie der Lese- und Schreibschwierigkeiten*. Weinheim: Beltz.

Korhonen, T. (1984). A follow-up study of Finnish children with specific learning disabilities. *Acta Paedopsychiatrica*, **50**, 255–63.

Kossow, H-J. (1975). *Zur Therapie der Lese-Rechtschreibschwäche*. Berlin: VEB Deutscher Verlag der Wissenschaften.

Maughan, B. and Yule, W. (1994). Reading and other learning disabilities. In *Child and adolescent psychiatry. Modern approaches*, 3rd edn, ed. M. Rutter, E. Taylor and L. Hersov, pp. 647–65. Oxford: Blackwell Science.

Miles, T. R. and Miles, E. (1992). *Dyslexia and mathematics*. London: Routledge.

Niebergall, G. (1987). Diagnostische Aspekte der Legasthenie. *Monatsschrift für Kinderheilkunde*, **135**, 297–302.

Remschmidt, H., Walter, R., Kampert, K. and Hennighausen, K. (1990). Evaluation der Versorgung psychisch auffälliger und kranker Kinder und Jugendlicher in drei Landkreisen. *Ner-*

venarzt, **61**, 34–45.

Rutter, M., Tizard, J., Yule, P., Graham, P. and Whitmore, K. (1976). Research report. Isle of Wight studies, 1964-1974. *Psychological Medicine*, **6**, 313–32.

Schulte-Körne, G., Deimel, W., Bartling J. and Remschmidt, H. (1999). The role of phonological awareness, speech perception, and auditory temporal processing for dyslexia. *European Child and Adolescent Psychiatry*, **8**, 28–34.

Skinner, C. H. (1998). Preventing academic skills deficits. In *Handbook of child behavior therapy*, ed. T. S. Watson and F. M. Gresham. New York: Plenum Press.

Strehlow, U., Kluge, R., Möller, H. and Haffner, J. (1992). Der langfristige Verlauf der Legasthenie über die Schulzeit hinaus. Katamnesen aus einer Kinderpsychiatrischen Ambulanz. *Zeitschrift für Kinder- und Jugendpsychiatrie*, **20**, 254–63.

Warnke, A. (1987). Behandlung der Legasthenie im Kindesalter. *Monatsschrift der Kinderheilkunde*, **135**, 302–6.

Warnke, A. (1990). *Legasthenie und Hirnfunktion*. Bern: Huber.

Warnke, A. (1999). Reading and spelling disorders: clinical features and causes. *European Child and Adolescent Psychiatry*, **8**, 28–34.

Warnke, A. (2000). Umschriebene Entwicklungsstörungen (Teilleistungsstörungen). In *Kinder- und Jugendpsychiatrie. Eine praktische Einführung*, ed. H. Remschmidt, pp. 131–43. Stuttgart: Thieme.

Warnke, A. and Niebergall, G. (1997). Legasthenie und Rechenstörungen. In *Psychotherapie im Kindes- und Jugendalter*, ed. H. Remschmidt, pp. 322–34. Stuttgart: Thieme.

Weinschenk, C. (1965). *Die erbliche Lese-Rechtschreibschwäche und ihre sozial-psychiatrischen Auswirkungen*. Bern: Huber.

Weinschenk, C. (1975). *Rechenstörungen*. Bern: Huber.

World Health Organization (WHO) (1992). *The ICD-10 classification of mental and behavioural disorders. Clinical descriptions and diagnostic guidelines*. Geneva: WHO.

25 Stuttering

Gerhard Niebergall and Helmut Remschmidt

Introduction and characteristics of the disorder

Stuttering is a disturbance of the fluency of speech, usually occuring during communicational speech (Böhme, 1977). Symptoms may be classified as clonic, tonic or tonoclonic. In clonic stuttering, the fluency of speech is interrupted by frequent repetitions (sounds, syllables, words), whereas in tonic stuttering, speech is interrupted by a prolongation of sounds, especially the initial sound of a word or the first sound of a new sentence.

In ICD-10 stuttering (F98.5) is defined as being 'characterized by frequent repetition and prolongation of sounds or syllables or words, or by frequent hesitations or pauses, that disrupt the rhythmic flow of speech' (WHO, 1992).

If the disorder persists, many children and adolescents develop additional symptoms, e.g. ocular movements resembling tics, grimacing, unintentional tongue movements which make speech difficult, tongue-clicking, grunting noises and shaking movements of the head and extremities.

Pathological stuttering must be distinguished from 'developmental' or 'physiological' stuttering, which may occur in many children 2–4 years old in the course of normal speech development ('developmental dysfluency'). However, pathological stuttering usually evolves from this stage of development, so that prevention and treatment are important if symptoms occur at this stage. If symptoms indicate that stuttering may be developing, parents should always be advised about the treatment options (Miltenberger and Woods, 1998).

Regardless of whether stuttering is regarded as the result of a neurotic tendency or is itself the onset of a neurosis, many children who stutter develop secondary psychiatric symptoms. These symptoms are usually the result of damaged self-esteem, e.g. in kindergarten or at school. Symptoms may seriously affect social contacts, and the child often finds himself in a vicious circle.

Several factors are presumed to be responsible for the pathogenesis and maintenance of early childhood stuttering (Bishop, 1994). There is some

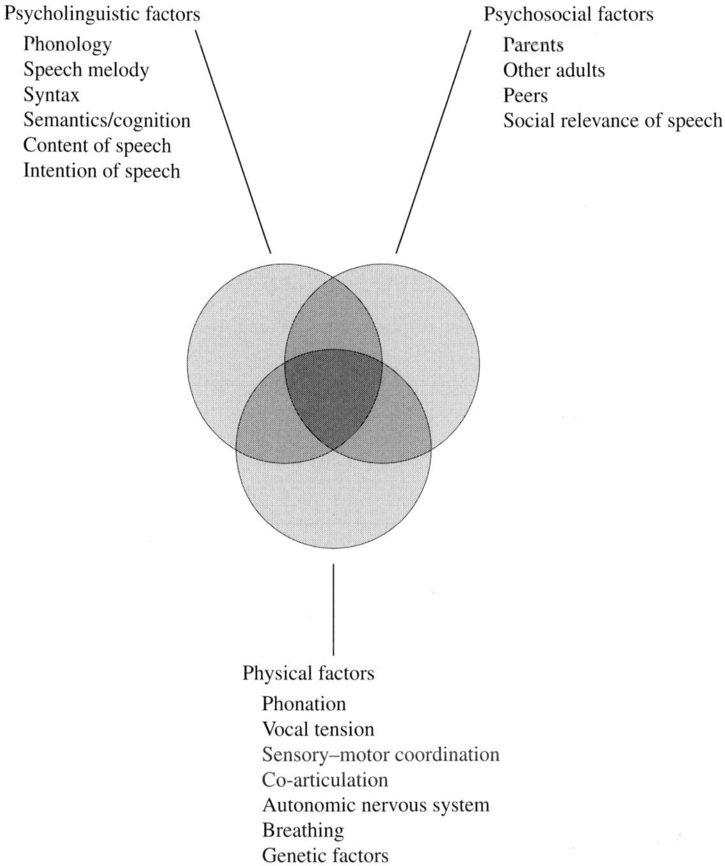

Fig. 25.1. Multifactorial model of the pathogenesis and maintenance of stuttering in early childhood (modified after Myers and Wall, 1982).

evidence that psycholinguistic, psychosocial and physical factors together contribute to the disorder (Myers and Wall, 1982) (Fig. 25.1).

The appropriate treatment depends on the interaction of the relevant factors causing the disorder. It is advisable to pursue treatment according to a multimodal treatment plan, which may include several different therapeutic techniques. There is a broad spectrum of techniques available to treat stuttering, all of which appear to be equally effective. However, recently several distinct therapeutic trends have evolved: psychoanalytically orientated therapy, operant conditioning techniques and desensitization are now less favoured and, in their place, treatment methods which influence speech directly, e.g. by reducing the frequency of suttering or extending periods of stutter-free speech, are used increasingly. Previously, treatment methods targeted at speech skills were thought to be contraindicated because of the presumed risk of the stuttering becoming worse. However, successful treatment of this type has now been reported for preschool children. It is also advisable to counsel parents in addition to treatment of the child (Schulze and Johannsen, 1986).

Approaches to treatment

In the following section, several different approaches to the treatment of stuttering will be discussed as well as the problems surrounding generalization on any gains achieved and the current state of the evaluation of these techniques.

The general therapeutic setting

Theoretical and practical considerations

Empathy is thought to lead to a trusting relationship, allowing patients to relax and approach treatment with sufficient motivation.

Aims of treatment

To create therapeutic rapport.

Practical approach

Empathy and understanding should be conveyed to the patient with regard to the causes, context and the implications of the patient's symptoms. In particular, the therapist must recognize the significance of personal disadvantages such as teasing and loss of self-esteem. The aims of treatment and the prognosis should be discussed openly, with the parents when this is appropriate.

Speech training

Theoretical and practical considerations

A number of factors are thought to influence the speech of the individual. Individual symptoms are regarded as the target behaviour and by reducing these, secondary general improvement is also likely to occur.

Aims of treatment

Reducing suttering and accompanying symptoms.

Practical approach

The patient learns to speak with (a) a sonorous voice, (b) soft consonants, (c) reduced speed. Modified speech patterns, e.g. singing, whispering, stretching vowels, and rhythmic speaking using a metronome are utilized, and the patient stops speaking if stuttering symptoms or accompanying symptoms occur. The different situations in which the patient has to speak are practised, such as reading out loud, talking, asking and answering questions, speaking in the presence of others; role play, e.g. situations at school, in the family, in the presence of persons with authority. Low demands are made initially, and more demanding tasks are introduced gradually. Other techniques used include: self-observation training, practice of incompatible activities, e.g. deep respiration, muscle and larynx relaxation, prior preparation of what is to be spoken, the use of pauses between units of speech, rhythmic speaking, imagining situations which usually induce stuttering. Audiovisual support in assessment and treatment may be very helpful.

Behavioural techniques

These techniques include: systematic desensitization, anxiety coping strategies, operant techniques, emotional and cognitive restructuring, assertiveness training (role play).

Theoretical and practical considerations

Stuttering is considered to be a learnt behaviour. Both individual, e.g. experience of anxiety and environmental factors are responsible for the pathogenesis and maintenance of suttering. Modification of these factors can result in a reduction of symptoms.

Aims of treatment

Modifying the conditions which determine symptoms. Reducing stuttering and accompanying symptoms.

Practical approach

In systematic desensitization, a hierarchy of anxieties is established, the patient is then exposed to anxious stimuli which enhance stuttering, whilst practising relaxation techniques with the aim of reducing the anxiety. Strategies for coping with anxiety include imagining anxious (phobic) situations, such as having to speak with others such that the patient experiences the emotions beforehand. However, elimination of all anxieties will rarely be achieved. Operant techniques, in combination with emotional and cognitive restructuring and counselling of care-givers can have a positive influence on the manner in which patients experience anxiety and hence on their stuttering.

Psychodynamic approaches

This may take the form of psychoanalytically orientated individual psychotherapy or play therapy.

Theoretical and practical considerations

Stuttering is considered to be a symptom caused by the patient's unsolved unconcious psychic conflicts. According to theorists such as Adler, stuttering is associated with unconscious intentions and secondary benefit (source of power). Making the conflicts accessible to conscious thought should thus result in a resolution of symptoms.

Aims of treatment

Modifying the patient's personality structure or solving unconscious conflicts. The patient is asked to consider the function of stuttering as a source of power and consider unsolved conflicts originating in early childhood.

Practical approach

Treatment is undertaken by means of play and/or conversations. The transference and countertransference which occur in this setting are used, in addition to cathartic experiences, interpretation of unconscious material and analysis of defence mechanisms (in particular, those including symptoms). Influencing symptoms directly is not the primary aim of treatment and in play therapy, for example, the direction of therapy is determined by the child.

Play therapy

Theoretical and practical considerations

Play therapy is a sensitive and successful treatment option in children with many different psychiatric (or developmental) disorders. If a child feels insecure and has difficulties in social interaction due to stuttering, play therapy, although somewhat unspecific, may improve the stuttering symptoms.

Aims of treatment

Improving general psychosocial development, addressing conflicts, influencing stuttering symptoms more or less directly.

Practical approach

In addition to supporting the child's development, play therapy can help in improving stuttering symptoms by including specific elements of speech train-

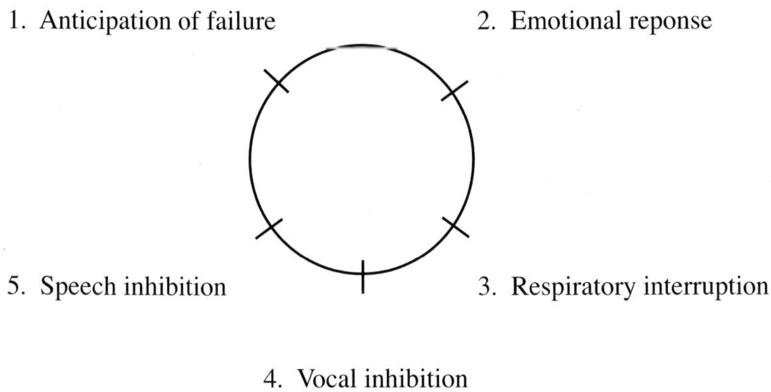

Fig. 25.2. Psychosomatic inhibitory circle in stuttering (Orthmann and Scholz, 1983).

ing, e.g. role playing. It has been shown that the symptoms of children who stutter improve when playing the role of a parent, friend or teacher. The strong emotions that frequently occur during play therapy may help children to speak without stuttering for a short while (many individuals who stutter are able to speak fluently when they are angry). The experience of being able to speak without stuttering is a great relief for the affected individual, who may gradually change his view on the prospect of symptom relief. Patients may feel more able to control their speech and do not therefore feel entirely at the mercy of their stuttering.

Relaxation training and respiratory exercises

Theoretical and practical considerations

Stuttering is associated with excessive 'tension' of muscles during speech and interruption of regular respiration (Fig. 25.2). The inhibitory psychosomatic cycle (Fernau Horn, 1973) presumably plays a role in stuttering:

- anticipation of failure,
- emotional response,
- respiratory interruption,
- vocal inhibition, and
- speech inhibition.

Aims of treatment

Physical relaxation and speaking during controlled expiration both contribute to fluent speech. Therapy should facilitate an excitatory psychosomatic cycle (Fernau-Horn, 1973), which counteracts the inhibitory cycle described above:

- relaxation and confidence,
- inspiration and expiration,
- sequence of vocalizations,
- sequence of speech and
- self-perception.

Practical approach

Training in techniques such as relaxation training may be helpful. Children taught such techniques can induce a state of relaxation which is antagonistic to the physical tension associated with stuttering. This also contributes to disrupting the vicious circle. The patient is taught how to speak during controlled expiration, because inspiration while speaking can disrupt fluent speech. Autosuggestive thoughts such as 'I can speak easily and fluently' may also be helpful. Such exercises to improve the fluency may be combined with other techniques, although considerable patience is required for successful treatment.

Family therapy

Theoretical and practical considerations

According to earlier learning theories, inappropriate reactions of parents, particularly in the developmental dysfluency phase, contributed to a worsening of the child's stuttering. If parents anxiously anticipate the stuttering and constantly make corrections in this labile phase, children may become insecure and develop a speech disorder. Such emotionally charged verbal interaction may contribute to a disturbance of speech fluency.

Aims of treatment

Changing interactional patterns in the family in order to enable the patient to speak fluently.

Practical approach

In family therapy the therapist analyses the communication within the family. Video recordings may be helpful in uncovering interactional patterns. The therapist can feed this information back to the family, demonstrating how familial interaction inhibits the child's impulse to speak. In the course of treatment, the family are encouraged to modify their interaction so as to give the child more attention, allow him to speak without interrupting and refrain from constantly correcting him. It is important to address the guilty feelings the parents frequently have, to support them and help family members to use the resources which are available to them. This may involve modifying the child's role as a 'scapegoat' if he has been assigned this role by other family members due to his stuttering. A change in the parents' attitude towards the stuttering child can be brought about by explaining to them the difficulties of speech development and making them aware of their disappointment in the child. Other aspects of the family therapy which also apply in the treatment of stuttering are identical to those explained elsewhere (see Chapter 12).

Counselling

Theoretical and practical considerations

Counselling sessions, in addition to therapy, advise and reassure care-givers and patients, which helps to contribute to the improvement of symptoms.

Aims of treatment

Explaining the findings and their relevance to all involved.

Practical approach

Issues such as pathogenesis, likely cause of the disorder, treatment options, prognosis, associated physical and mental symptoms, and familial patterns of interaction are addressed. Parents frequently ask whether any change in their behaviour can improve their child's stuttering. Although this is difficult to answer specifically, it is generally helpful for the parents of suttering children to listen patiently and refrain from correcting the children whilst they are speaking. Parents who feel unsure of how to react, may benefit from trying to ignore symptoms completely. It is absolutely inappropriate to punish the child in any way. If there is any indication that one or both parents have a history of stuttering or continue to stutter, this issue should be addressed in counselling sessions. The parents' suffering tends to be interwoven with the children's suffering and these parents frequently express special concern as to the future development of the child. It is therefore advisable to inform parents and other care-givers about the good outcome after treating the secondary symptoms of stuttering, even if in about 30% of all cases the stuttering itself does not improve. It is also helpful to discuss with teachers the influence which their attitudes and behaviours (and those of the other school children) have on the stuttering. Children who stutter usually feel anxious when they are asked to speak at school. Teachers can help to dispel such anxieties by encouraging the child and protecting him where necessary from the reaction of other children. The connection between stuttering and the reaction of other children can be more easily explained in terms of learning theory rather than by means of psychoanalytical theory and can also be more easily accepted for use during school lessons. Counselling sessions may help to stabilize the improvements achieved in the course of individual therapy.

Medication

Although medication has no specific effects on stuttering, in clearly defined situations and in combination with other therapies, some patients may benefit from medication (neuroleptics, tranquilizers, antidepressants). If the therapy techniques described above are unsuccessful, medication may help to bring about some improvement, particularly in stressful situations, e.g. oral examinations. Any medication given should be fully evaluated before being prescribed for a longer period.

Transfer and generalization of successful treatment steps

Frequently, the stuttering improves during treatment, only to recur in everyday situations. It is therefore necessary to generalize achievements made in therapeutic sessions to situations at school, at work, in the family or with friends. To facilitate this, the individual therapy setting may be extended to include a third person, e.g. another patient, a nurse, a parent, friend or teacher, such that the patient is confronted with a more realistic situation. During this phase of treatment it is helpful to discuss some of the experiences the patient has had with stuttering. The patient thus has the opportunity to consider new ways of approaching stressful situations previously associated with recurrent stuttering. Where situational anxiety plays a role, techniques for coping with this should be taught. The patient and the therapist together can develop strategies for anticipating and dealing with negative comments such as 'you still can't speak properly', in order to prevent the patient from suffering further loss of self-esteem. Some patients devolp a motto such as 'stuttering has nothing to do with my self-esteem', with which they are able protect themselves from insult. Patients must be aware that stuttering symptoms can fluctuate in an unpredictable manner and do not necessarily occur in certain situations. The therapist should encourage the patient to continue to work towards improvement without conveying unrealistic hopes. Therapy should be discontinued gradually, increasing the interval between sessions. The sessions become an opportunity to discuss the patient's experience with speaking in ordinary situations, and if required, certain techniques may be reinforced.

Evaluation

The treatment of stuttering is often demanding and may need to continue for several years. Previously it was thought that therapy was only of benefit in or prior to puberty, however, today, some adults are treated successfully for stuttering. Regardless of whether the stuttering itself improves, secondary psychological symptoms certainly merit psychotherapy.

Evaluation studies suggest that about one-third of the patients improve markedly, one-third improve slightly, and one-third do not improve. More recent studies have shown that outcomes differ, depending on which particular sample is studied (Remschmidt and Niebergall, 1981). There is some evidence that early treatment of stuttering improves outcome (Schulze and Johannsen, 1986). These findings refute the theory that stuttering may be worsened by very early treatment of developmental dysfluency.

Many children who stutter have an additional speech disorder, e.g. dyslalia, dysgrammatism, cluttering (Remschmidt and Niebergall, 1981). The treatment of patients should therefore take place in conjunction with other professionals. Whereas a speech therapist may treat a voice disorder, a child and adolescent psychiatrist is more appropriate for treating stuttering.

REFERENCES

Bishop, D. V. M. (1994). Development disorder of speech and language. In *Child and adolescent psychiatry. Modern approaches*, 3rd edn, ed. M. Rutter, E. Taylor and L. Hersov, pp. 546–68. Oxford: Blackwell Science.

Böhme, G. (1977). *Das Stotter-Syndrom*. Bern: Huber.

Fernau-Horn, H. (1973). *Die Sprechneurosen*. Stuttgart: Hippokrates.

Miltenberger, R. G. and Woods, D. W. (1998). Speech dysfluencies. In *Handbook of child behavior therapy*, ed. T. S. Watson and F. M. Gresham. New York: Plenum Press.

Myers, F. L. and Wall, M. J. (1982). Toward an integrated approach to early childhood stuttering. *Journal of Fluency Disorders*, 7, 47–52.

Orthmann, W. and Scholz, H-J. (1983). *Stottern*. Berlin: Marhold.

Remschmidt, H. and Niebergall, G. (1981). Störungen des Sprechens und der Sprache. In *Neuropsychologie des Kindesalters*, ed. H. Remschmidt and M. H. Schmidt, pp. 248–79. Stuttgart: Enke.

Schulze, H. and Johannsen, H. S. (1986). *Stottern bei Kindern im Vorschulalter*. Ulm: University of Ulm.

World Health Organization (WHO) (1992). *The ICD-10 classification of mental and behavioural disorders. Clinical descriptions and diagnostic guidelines*. Geneva: WHO.

26 Hyperkinetic disorders

Kurt Quaschner

Introduction

The terminology used to describe disorders involving attention deficit and overactivity varies, depending on the classification system used. Previously, many children with attention deficit and overactivity would have been classified as having 'minimal cerebral dysfunction' (MCD). Today, the most common diagnosis in use is 'attention deficit and hyperactivity' (ADHD) or 'hyperkinetic conduct disorder'. The characteristics of 'disturbance of activity and attention' as defined in ICD-10 (WHO, 1992) are summarized in Table 26.1.

Assessment and treatment planning

In a child with hyperkinetic disorder, several difficulties become apparent. Whilst the cardinal symptoms are clear, symptoms are often heterogeneous and there is a broad spectrum of additional symptoms. Associated symptoms may be more or less severe, but should not be regarded as unimportant. Frequently, they merit just as much attention as the cardinal symptoms, and treatment may need to focus more on them than the cardinal symptoms.

A further difficulty in assessment is that symptoms may be to some degree situation specific. The behaviour of the child in the clinic, in which the child is seen alone in a structured manner may be remarkably different, resulting in diagnostic error. But, even in a familiar setting, such as the classroom, the child's behaviour may vary considerably depending on the degree of structure and the demands made on the child.

Both chronological age and developmental level must be taken into account when assessing behaviour. The degree of motor activity and associated symptomatology may vary considerably depending on the child's age and developmental status. For instance, the behaviour which in a 3-year-old child would be described as 'lively' would certainly be regarded as inappropriate and perhaps abnormal in a 6-year-old child.

Finally, it is important to determine the parental expectations in order to define what may be considered by them as 'normal' or 'well-adapted' behaviour. Parents' expectations regarding their child's behaviour are usually determined by such norms. They therefore, tend to feel guilty or inadequate if their child develops hyperkinetic symptoms. This reaction will be influenced by the belief that their child is behaving in an 'improper' manner and the therapist needs to bear in mind what effect this must be having in the assessment of hyperkinetic behaviour.

Assessment and diagnostic instruments

Because of such difficulties, assessement needs to be comprehensive and detailed, taking into account all symptoms. It should include standardized tests; however, these should be complemented by observations in several situations by different individuals.

A wide range of rating scales have been developed to reliably assess hyperkinetic behaviour. Prior to using such instruments psychiatric assessment including the history, physical examination, and psychological assessment with a special focus on the hyperkinetic disorder should be undertaken. This should gather information on the role the hyperkinetic behaviour plays in the child's psychopathology as a whole (Schmidt et al., 1991), as well as identifying factors which may later prove relevant for treatment at a later point, e.g. general intelligence.

Specific assessment should include the follwing aspects or dimensions (summarized in Table 26.2).

Instruments

Structured clinical interviews have been developed, which may be used to supplement taking a history. Such interviews tend, however, to be inconvenient in clinical settings, and their use is generally restricted to research purposes.

The same applies to rating scales assessing behaviour by direct observation, which also tend to be inconvenient and impractical. An individually tailored assessment, using a small number of clear criteria in selected relevant situations in the child's daily life may be more appropriate and effective. For instance, the teacher may be asked to record the number of times a child shows certain behaviours (interrupting lessons, starting quarrels, not sitting down, etc.). The importance of 'subjective' parameters such as these has been emphasized in the literature (Eisert, 1993).

Table 26.1. Characteristics of disturbance of activity and attention

Definition and classification

In the ICD-10, the hyperkinetic disorders are subdivided under the category F90. The following characteristics are listed (WHO, 1992):

1. Early onset.
2. A combination of overactive, poorly modulated behaviour with marked inattention and lack of persistent task involvement.
3. Pervasiveness over situations and persistence over time.

The diagnostic guidelines include impaired attention and overactivity as cardinal features. 'Impaired attention is manifested by prematurely breaking off from tasks and leaving activities unfinished. The children change frequently from one activity to another, seemingly losing interest in one task because they become diverted to another. [. . .] Overactivity implies excessive restlessness, especially in situations requiring relative calm. It may, depending upon the situation, involve the child running and jumping around, getting up from a seat when he or she is expected to remain seated, excessive talkativeness and noisiness, or fidgeting and wriggling. [. . .] This behavioural feature is most evident in structured, organized situations that require a high degree of behavioural self-control' (WHO, 1992).

Several associated features may help to sustain the disorder, although they are not sufficient for the diagnosis: 'Disinhibition in social relationships, recklessness in situations involving some danger, and impulsive flouting of social rules [. . .] Learning disorders and motor clumsiness occur with undue frequency [. . .] Symptoms of conduct disorder are neither exclusion nor inclusion criteria for the main diagnosis, but their presence or absence constitutes the basis for the main subdivision of the the disorder' (WHO, 1992). When the overall criteria for hyperkinetic disorder are met, the code should be F90.0, whereas the code should be F90.1 when features of both hyperactivity and conduct disorder are present and the hyperactivity is pervasive and severe.

Prevalence

Prevalence rates of about 3% of children in elementary school are reported in the literature. Boys are more frequently affected than girls. Whilst clinical samples usually include six to nine times more boys than girls, epidemiological studies have shown only three times more boys than girls (Minde, 1985; Barkley, 1989).

Aetiology

Although many aetiological factors have been considered, genetic factors (predisposition) seem to play a decisive role. However, the severity of the disorder, associated symptoms and the course seem to be influenced to a great extent by environmental factors (Barkley, 1989).

Prognosis and course

Although some children may be regarded as abnormally hyperkinetic in their behaviour from the time of birth, most children first show abnormal hyperkinetic behaviour when they are 3–4 years old. The increasingly hyperkinetic behaviour may be tolerated by some parents during

Table 26.1. *(cont.)*

preschool age, but during kindergarten the behaviour usually begins to cause major problems, especially in terms of social contact and interaction. Problems usually increase after transition to school and gradually include other aspects of the child's life. Thus learning difficulties may result in addition to the interactional problems, puting school progress at serious risk, especially when symptoms continue to have negative effects.

Previously it was thought that children would simply 'grow out' of the hyperkinetic symptoms during puberty. However, today it is known that slightly more than three quarters of patients continue to have difficulties at school, during vocational training, in the family and in general social settings. This development usually continues into adulthood. About 60% of young adult patients continue to show hyperkinetic symptoms. In particular, those patients with low intelligence, low socioeconomic status and high aggressive potential are at a greater risk of sustaining the disorder. Impaired social contact with peers, emotional instability and psychopathology of the parents are additional disadvantages for patients. The proportion of hyperkinetic individuals among substance abusers and delinquents is higher than among peers without hyperkinetic symptoms (Minde, 1985; Barkley, 1989; WHO, 1992).

Table 26.2. Aspects relevant for assessment

Instruments
Clinical interviews
Observation of behaviour
Questionnaires
Rating scales
Laboratory parameters
Rater
Therapist
Parents
Teachers, care-givers
Patient
Situation
Structured vs. open situation
Type of interaction, e.g. individual vs. group, child vs. adult, male vs. female
Demands made, e.g. at school, during homework, during tests

Rating scales, on the other hand, are often helpful for recording symptoms objectively. They are not associated with much inconvenience and are easily repeatable to assess symptoms over time. Rating scales have been shown to be helpful in practice, although their theoretical objectivity, validity and reliability have been questioned.

It is possible to distinguish between non-specific questionnaires, such as the Child Behavior Checklist (CBCL) (Achenbach and Edelbrock, 1983, 1987), which aims to assess general psychopathology, and specific rating scales, such as the Conners' scale (Conners, 1973), which deals with specific symptoms.

The term laboratory parameters is used to summarize several objective tests, which have been developed to assess the cardinal symptoms of hyperkinetic behaviour in a research setting.

Attention/concentration

The 'Continuous Performance Test' (CPT) (Rosvold et al., 1956) is commonly used to assess the span of continuous attention. However, the validity of this test in assessing situations in everyday life is limited.

Impulsivity

The 'Matching Familiar Figures Test' (MFFT) (Kagan, 1966) is a well-established test to assess impulsivity in children. The child is presented with a figure and asked to choose the matching figure from a series. Other tests of impulsivity are available; however, scores do not correlate well, which may indicate that the tests are measuring different aspects of impulsivity.

Motor behaviour

Devices which register several different types of movement have been used to measure the physical activity of hyperkinetic children. However, there are no norms available for such devices, and these devices do not take into account the situation, making assessment of situational hyperactive behaviour difficult.

Raters

Standardized tests are usually available in several versions in order to allow for the skills and competencies of different raters, who may view hyperactivity from different perspectives. The raters catered for include mental health professionals, parents, other care-givers, teachers or child-minders. Some older patients may also be capable of assessing their own behaviour and filling in rating scales on their own. This type of self-rating can be a valuable source of information for those treating the patient.

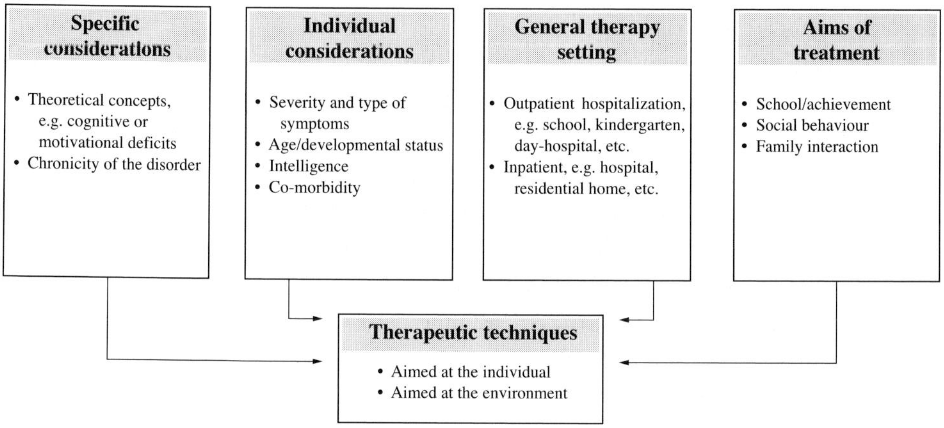

Fig. 26.1. Treatment: indications and planning.

Situations

Raters generally observe the patient's behaviour in a specific environment, e.g. at school, at home, within the family context. Their observations alone are therefore restricted to certain situations. However, to achieve a full picture during assessment, it is important to use more than one observer and vary the situations in which the patient is observed.

In assessing the nature of a particular situation, the degree of external structure is of pivotal importance. The term 'structure' refers to the demands, expectations, rules and limits within which the child has to operate. Fluctuations in hyperkinetic behaviour are remakably sensitive to the degree of structure in any situation.

Another important variable is the degree of 'content' in any situation, for example the child's interactional behaviour. It may be helpful to consider how the child interacts with individuals compared to the whole group, how the child interacts with children as opposed to adults, and whether behaviour differs with regard to sex both in child/child and child/adult interactions. Behaviour in situations in which some effort is expected of the child should also be assessed.

Treatment-indications and planning

The relevant criteria in deciding the appropriate approach to treatment and treatment steps are summarized in Fig. 26.1. The information obtained during assessment, theoretical concepts and practical considerations, all play an important role in this planning phase.

Specific considerations

Which technique a therapist chooses to treat a condition will usually depend on his professional and theoretical background. The therapist who considers hyperkinetic behaviour to result from cognitive deficits will emphasize this aspect in treatment. If, on the other hand, he considers the central problem to be a motivational one, treatment will focus on this issue.

Regardless of this, it is important to remember the fact that hyperkinetic syndrome is a chronic disorder, which will not respond to any 'quick fix', but will require a long course of treatment, which in some cases may take several years (Hinshaw and Erhardt, 1991).

Individual conditions

The overall severity of the condition comprising severity and the nature of symptoms will determine the approach to treatment. Other factors which will influence the therapeutic options include: age and developmental status, which will determine to what extent the patient can participate actively in therapy, intellectual ability, which influences both therapy and the generalization or transfer of any progress made into ordinary situations, and co-morbidity. Hyperkinetic symptoms are frequently associated with conduct disorders; however, learning disorders and emotional disturbances must also be considered during treatment.

General therapy setting

The setting, in which treatment is undertaken, is to a great extent, determined by the severity of hyperkinetic symptoms and the situational conditions of the behaviour. Usually, outpatient treatment is sufficient; however, additional help from the school or kindergarten may be required.

In some cases, partial hospitalization (day-hospital treatment) or inpatient treatment is necessary. Severe hyperkinetic behaviour with serious interactional problems may even require care in a residential home or foster family. In such cases, the potentially negative effects of separating the child from his parents and family must be considered very carefully.

Aims of treatment

It is inappropriate to focus only on a narrow selection of specific symptoms during treatment. Specific symptoms are usually related to one another in some way and frequently involve a particular aspect of the patient's life, e.g. the school or the family. Often, school presents the greatest problem for hyperkinetic patients, whilst the situation at home may be tolerable. In this case, issues relevant to 'school' or 'achievement' should take priority in therapy.

As hyperkinetic disorders tend to be persistent, aims of treatment may vary during the course and should periodically be reviewed. It may be appropriate to shift the focus to the family, difficulties at school, or interactional problems with peers.

Treatment

The treatment of hyperkinetic behaviour is complex and multidimensional, and it should be emphasized to all involved that there is no single approach to treatment (Barkley, 1998). Treatment techniques, often from several theoretical backgrounds, are combined in the course of psychotherapy, thus enabling the therapist to adapt to the patient's particular needs (Munden and Arcelus, 1999).

Techniques directed at the individual can be distinguished from those aimed at the environment, i.e. interactions with the patient and the daily living situation (Quaschner, 1990).

Individual techniques

Behavioural techniques

Operant techniques

Behavioural techniques based on operant conditioning have always formed part of the treatment of hyperkinetic behaviour (Barkley, 1998). They are useful for establishing schedules and programmes, drawing up rules and guidelines for general behaviour and involving parents in treatment. When used systematically, they are one of the most effective methods of influencing and regulating behaviour.

It is often important initially to modify the child's perception of himself. No child is entirely chaotic, and even extremely hyperactive children spend some time in quiet play or perform tasks which they have been assigned to, even if these periods tend to be dishearteningly short. Such periods should be acknowledged and regarded as opportunities for encouraging and establishing further behaviour of this type.

Using this technique, the desired behaviour needs to be reinforced, i.e. rewarded. To be effective, such reinforcements or rewards must be perceived as attractive and desirable from the child's perspective. Initially, these are usually material objects, which may progress to a form of token economy, where tokens given to the child are later exchanged for a predefined reward.

Hyperkinetic children tend not to notice their behaviour and fail to recognize the way it effects others. Rewards which are unclear or given after an extended interval are not helpful. Children require immediate, clear and unequivocal feedback on their behaviour (Taylor, 1986).

One of the most effective reinforcement techniques is rewarding the child with increased attention, i.e. social reinforcement, by means of praise, encouragement or activities together. Withdrawing social reinforcement may also be used therapeutically when the child shows problematic behaviour, a technique often known as time out (Barkley, 1989). This can be particularly useful with aggressive behaviour or tantrums. These often escalate easily and are difficult to interrupt verbally, and removing the child from the situation and withdrawing all attention may be the only way to interrupt events.

Response cost is another technique of withdrawing reinforcement. At the start of a therapy session the child is given a number of tokens, which are withdrawn if he breaks predetermined rules. The tokens left at the end of the session may then be exchanged for a reward or 'saved' for later date.

A further principle common in operant techniques is a stepwise or gradual approach. The treatment goal is achieved after a sequence of successive steps. It is unrealistic and counter-therapeutic to construct a complex system of positive expectations if the child cannot fulfil them, and parents or care-givers should receive help in deciding which steps should be taken first. It is not helpful to address the largest and most difficult problem first. Rather, progress is first made with smaller tasks and subsequently more difficult tasks can be addressed. Therapeutic efforts should initially focus on one area, and as therapy progresses other areas can be incorporated into treatment (Taylor, 1986).

Barkley (1990) has proposed a set of general guidelines for treating hyperkinetic children. These are summarized in Table 26.3. This type of 'contingency programme' uses the principles of operant conditioning to establish a reinforcement schedule, according to which the child is then rewarded. This type of programme may involve giving delayed rewards, an approach which makes considerable demands on the child's intellectual ability. When using such treatment programmes, the therapist should not only consider the child's own role, but also the role of other individuals who interact with the child. Contingency programmes may be particularly useful as a 'standard' or 'point of reference', helping the nursing staff of an institution (hospital, residential home) to deal better with difficult behaviour.

Cognitive behavioural techniques

Whilst operant behavioural therapy techniques rely strongly on external control, cognitive behaviour therapy techniques aim to improve patients' self-

Table 26.3. Guidelines for dealing with the behaviour of hyperkinetic children

(i) Rules and instructions provided to ADHD children must be clear, brief, and often delivered through more visible and external modes of presentation than is required for the management of normal children.
(ii) Consequences used to manage the behaviour of ADHD children must be delivered more swiftly and immediately than is needed for normal children.
(iii) Consequences must be delivered more frequently, not just more immediately, to ADHD children in view of their motivational deficits.
(iv) The consequences used with ADHD children must be often of a higher magnitude, or more powerful, than those needed to manage the behaviour of normal children.
(v) Appropriate and often richer incentives or motivational parameters must be provided within a setting or task to reinforce appropriate behaviour before punishment can be implemented.
(vi) Those reinforcers or rewards that are employed must be changed or rotated more frequently with ADHD than with normal children, given the perchant of the former for more rapid habituation or satiation to response consequences, apparently rewards in particular.
(vii) Anticipation is the key with ADHD children.

From Barkley (1990).

control. Patients are encouraged to become more independent from the situational factors and are taught to actively control their behaviour.

Self-observation

Initially, the patient needs to learn how to perceive his own behaviour and the current situation. Self-observation skills can be learnt and this may involve the patient being asked to record the frequency of interactional conflicts during the day. If the patient's age and intellectual ability permit, the results of the behaviour can also be recorded. The process of perfecting monitoring results in improved self-appraisal, which, in turn, helps the patient's self-reinforcement skills (Kanfer, 1975). The very structuring effect of systematic monitoring is frequently underestimated. It can, however, play an important role both in the assessment and treatment of hyperkinetic behaviour.

Self-instruction

Self-instruction is based on a modification of self-observation techniques. This type of training for hyperkinetic children is a well-established treatment for the disorder (Meichenbaum and Goodman, 1971; Meichenbaum, 1977; Kendall and

Table 26.4. The steps of self-instruction training

(i)	The child is asked to observe a model (usually the therapist, or a fellow-patient) who practises self-verbalization to do tasks successfully ('congnitive modelling').
(ii)	Then the child is asked to do the same task, following the model's verbal instructions ('overt external guidance').
(iii)	The the child is then asked to do the task while speaking the instructions out loud, thus imitating the model's self-instructions ('overt self-guidance').
(iv)	Then the child is asked to whisper the self-instructions to himself while doing the task ('faded overt self-guidance').
(v)	Finally the child is asked to do tasks while guiding himself by means of his 'inner voice' ('covert self-instruction').

From Meichenbaum (1977).

Braswell, 1985). It emphasizes the effect which 'self-talk' may have on an individual's actions, particularly in childhood. The training includes the following steps:

Problem definition
Initially the task itself should be considered ('Stop! What is this all about?').

Focusing of attention and planning
Solutions for the task should be sought ('What can I do? How should I proceed?').

Reaction control
Self-intruction (Table 26.4) should be undertaken ('First, I will do this, then I will do that . . .').

Correction of errors
Coping with frustration and failure should also be addressed ('I have made a mistake, now I will try a better way').

Self-appraisal
This should be undertaken as self-reinforcement ('I did the task well, it worked out very well').

This approach to treatment may appear very straightforward; however, it contains several difficulties. First, it is demanding in terms of time, several sessions may be needed every week, perhaps for as long as 2–3 months. This requires considerable motivation on the patient's behalf, which may be difficult with hyperkinetic children. In addition, self-instruction training needs to be adapted to the patient's individual needs, as an entirely standardized approach to treatment is unlikely to succeed.

Social competency training

Because most hyperkinetic patients have social and interactional difficulties, it will usually be helpful to use group setting for treatment. Being part of a group requires observing certain social rules. These tend to be difficult and complex, they make demands on the child and require him to acknowledge other individuals' rights. Hyperactive children usually have difficulties perceiving subtle rules in social situations. They tend to demonstrate little sympathy or empathy for the feelings and reactions of other individuals. It is therefore, essential to spell out precisely what is expected of them. Rules should be kept simple and the consequences of certain behaviour should be made clear. Rules may relate to personal interaction, e.g. not to hurt anybody's feelings, to verbalize needs and wishes, to ask when something is wanted, to take turns, etc. The aim of systematically practising such interactional skills in a small group setting is to improve the degree of social behaviour.

Systematic training programmes designed to encourage social competency have two main goals. First, to improve the understanding of social contexts, e.g. by better learning to perceive how their behaviour will affect the behaviour of others. Secondly, to attenuate those social skills which are lacking in the child's repertoire or which are only present to a rudimentary degree. It may nevertheless be difficult to generalize improvements to extend to behaviours in everyday life (Guevremont, 1990).

Functional training of specific deficits

Many hyperkinetic children have additional impairments, learning disorders or developmental deficits, involving language, perception or visual–motor skills (Minde, 1985). Such impairments usually require additional specific treatment. This may involve individual support or specific functional training. Several standardized treatment programmes are available (Lauth and Schlottke, 1993).

Table 26.5. lists guidelines which may be helpful for situations in which hyperkinetic children are confronted with demands or expectations (Wagner, 1989). They are fairly non-specific and may be used in a variety of different situations (Quaschner, 1990).

Occupational therapy may also be used as functional treatment and will often incorporate a number of the techniques described above. Working with

Table 26.5. Guidelines for hyperkinetic children when confronted with demands

(i)	Create a relaxed atmosphere
(ii)	Work with many short training phases
(iii)	Avoid distraction
(iv)	Gradually increase the difficulty of tasks
(v)	Provide attractive material to work with
(vi)	'Self-talk', i.e. self-instruction to facilitate actions
(vii)	Help the child to discover mistakes himself
(viii)	Praise and encourage the child instead of criticizing him and being impatient
(ix)	Begin with individual sessions only
(x)	Progress to include group settings

From Wagner (1989).

different materials involves the use of different senses and as well as helping fine motor skills, encourages patience and persistence. Constructing something and finishing the task properly may improve self-esteem. Working together with other individuals requires the children to accept social rules and keep them.

Play therapy

Non-directive play therapy alone is not the most suitable approach to treating hyperkinetic behaviour. It tends to make no difference or restrictions upon the child and is not very helpful in improving rule-abiding behaviour. However, due to the many emotional symptoms which many hyperkinetic children have, it is worth considering whether play therapy might be an appropriate adjuvant to treatment. When play therapy is integrated in a multidimensional treatment programme, it may be useful, and certain elements of play therapy have found their way into several treatment programmes (Döpfner and Sattel, 1991; Quaschner, 1990).

Medication

In many cases, medication is a great help as part of a comprehensive treatment programme. However, the exclusive use of medication is usually inadequate, and this approach must inevitably be combined with other steps. It is important to remember that many parents, teachers, and even nursing staff are prejudiced against the use of medication in the treatment of the disorder. Such prejudices tend to be tenacious and difficult to dispel. However, medication can be an important part of treatment, which does not preclude other approaches.

Good results have been achieved with psychostimulants, e.g. methylphenidate. However, other psychoactive substances may also be used, such as neuroleptics, e.g. chlorpromazine, thioradizine, antidepressants (particularly imipramine) and lithium (Remschmidt, 1992).

Environmental techniques

Therapeutic setting

Situational factors have a great influence on hyperkinetic behaviour. It is therefore helpful to select an 'appropriate' therapeutic setting which may involve outpatient treatment, partial hospitalization or inpatient treatment. Further institutions may also need to be be involved, e.g. schools, residential homes, therapeutic communities, etc.

Outpatient treatment

The success of outpatient treatment depends not only upon the patient's individual qualities, e.g. age, severity of the disorder, motivation, but also his parents' willingness and ability to cooperate with treatment. Frequently, the chances of outpatient treatment being successful are overestimated and precious time may be wasted. Problems may occur if treatment is not intensive enough, or if treatment techniques are not sufficiently well integrated, resulting in ineffective and uneconomical treatment. It may be more helpful to undertake outpatient treatment in the clinic of a facility which offers a wider spectrum of treatment techniques. An alternate way of supplementing outpatient treatment is to combine it with home treatment sessions. Thus, the outpatient setting is extended beyond the premises of the institution to cover the patient's home (Remschmidt and Schmidt, 1988).

Treatment in non-clinical settings

Non-clinical treatment settings include kindergartens, schools, nurseries, residential homes, etc. Several treatment programmes intended particularly for use in schools have been developed, with the aim of involving teachers and other educational professionals in treatment (Barkley, 1998). However, working together with such institutions may also be associated with considerable problems, and cooperation between therapeutic and non-clinical institutions may be better focused on prevention and recognition rather than on treatment.

As with parents, cooperation with teachers and educators is likely initially to focus on providing information about the symptoms of the disorder. It is not uncommon to be confronted with ideologically distorted or outdated ideas and misconceptions about the disorder, which should be addressed. This alone, however, will not solve the problem and recognition alone is unlikely to result in automatic improvement of the child's hyperkinetic behaviour. However, information may enable parents and teachers to view the child's behaviour from a new perspective, thus preparing the ground for specific measures which may have therapeutic effects.

It is of vital importance to coordinate the interdisciplinary efforts made to improve the child's behaviour. Due to the nature of the disorder, children require a broad approach to treatment, involving the coordinated action of many individuals (parents, teachers, therapists, etc.). This consistency and coordination of efforts also helps to prevent parents from feeling insecure about the treatment of their child.

Inpatient treatment

Inpatient treatment may be undertaken in institutions in which the patient is hospitalized or partially hospitalized for specific treatment. Children usually spend only a limited period of time in such an environment.

Partial hospitalization, e.g. day clinic has particular advantages, especially for younger children, as they can return home for the evening and night, remaining essentially in the family environment. This approach also enables the parents to become more involved in the treatment, particularly when they live close by. Some clinical institutions have developed specific treatment programmes for hyperkinetic children, and the execution in optimal environmental conditions allows these programmes to be followed exactly and thoroughly evaluated (Döpfner and Sattel, 1991; Quaschner, 1990).

Admission to hospital may be the last resort when outpatient treatment or partial hospitalization have failed to bring about any improvement. The severity of the disorder may require removing the child from his usual environment in order to provide respite to the individuals concerned: the patient, parents, other care-givers, etc. Admission is a good opportunity to commence a more intensive treatment programme. Because hyperkinetic disorders usually persist for years, admission to hospital may also provide an opportunity to plan future ways of dealing with the disorder, e.g. removing the child from the family environment and continuing treatment in a foster family or residential home.

Cooperation with parents

Cooperation with parents is important regardless of the setting in which the child is being treated. The treatment technique will determine the nature of this; however, the importance of working together with parents is of undisputed value in almost every case. Standardized parent training programs have been developed to influence the parent's style of upbringing, however, these tend to be discontinued by a large proportion of parents (Barkley, 1998). It is usually more helpful to adopt a more flexible approach which may be adapted to the particular needs of individuals. This approach usually involves three steps outlined below.

Step 1: Providing information and general advice

It is important to provide parents with the information they require about the nature of the hyperkinetic disorder. Possible causes, factors which may influence the course and prognostic considerations may need to be explained.

As treatment commences, the common guilty feelings which many parents have should be addressed. Frequently the parents' entire social network (relatives, friends, neighbours, teachers) blames the child's 'atrocious' behaviour on the parents' inablity to bring up their children properly, and the therapist should aim to unburden the family of these thoughts.

Step 2: Behavioural assessment

The parents of hyperkinetic children tend to perceive only the negative aspects of the child's behaviour. Therefore, parents need be helped to modify their perception of their child. Asking parents to record the child's behaviour and also their own reactions in detail may help them in this, which is the first step in defining treatment aims. Treatment aims should be derived from the child's positive behavioural characteristics.

Step 3: Undertaking treatment steps

The results of an assessment (step 2) suggest the points which should be addressed in the child's treatment. For instance, the following steps may be undertaken in pursuing treatment goals.

Structuring the patient's daily life

This is not only the basis for further therapeutic steps, but is a therapeutic step in itself.

Direct feedback on the patient's behaviour

Because hyperkinetic children have difficulties anticipating the sequelae of their behaviour, rules and expectations need to be made very clear and feedback should be given immediately.

Consistency in the style of upbringing
In dealing with hyperkinetic children, many different styles of upringing are practised, ranging from strictness and punishment to toleration of almost any behaviour. The parents should attempt to conform to a single style of upbringing in order to prevent the child from becoming disorientated. It is important to emphasize that both parents practise consistent styles of upbringing.

Interrupting escalating behaviour
This is an effective way of preventing excessive hyperkinetic behaviour. It may be helpful to use the 'time-out' technique, which can be adapted for effective use at home in the family context (Barkley, 1989).

Step-by-step approach to treatment, defining partial aims
In dealing with hyperkinetic children, adhering to the all-or-none law usually results in disappointment and deteriorating symptoms. Parents need to realize that hyperkinetic behaviour is a chronic condition and accept intermediate treatment goals and gradual improvements in symptoms.

Evaluation

As we have seen, there is no single approach to the treatment of hyperkinetic disorders. This is reflected in the findings of studies which have assessed the efficacy of different treatment techniques. A combination of several techniques, including behavioural therapy and medication, seems to achieve the best results. Intensive work with parents, e.g. parent training and psychoeducative measures are also helpful. Treatment steps focusing directly on the patient, such as self-control techniques, also appear to be effective. However, such techniques may have poor generalization qualities (Guevremont, 1990).

The treatment of hyperkinetic disorders not only requires a combination of several treatment techniques, but also continuous treatment over a considerable length of time. The frequent interventions are extremely demanding on the patient, his parents and the therapist. All individuals involved in such cases should be aware of the difficulties they will be confronted with in the course of treatment.

REFERENCES

Achenbach, T. M. and Edelbrock, C. S. (1983). *Manual for the child behavior checklist and revised child behavior profile*. Burlington, VT: University of Vermont, Department of Psychiatry.

Achenbach, T. M. and Edelbrock, C. S. (1987). *Manual for the youth self report and profile*. Burlington, VT: University of Vermont, Department of Psychiatry.

Barkley, R. A. (1989). Attention deficit-hyperactivity disorder. In *Treatment of childhood disorders*, ed. E. J. Mash, R. A. Barkley, pp. 39–72. The Guilford Press, New York.

Barkley, R. A. (1990). *Attention-deficit and hyperactivity disorder. A handbook for diagnosis and treatment*. New York: Guilford Press.

Barkley, R. A. (1998). *Attention-deficit and hyperactivity disorder. A handbook for diagnosis and treatment*, 2nd edn. New York: Guilford Press.

Conners, C. K. (1973). Rating scales for use in drug studies with children. *Psychopharmacological Bulletin*, **9**, 24–84.

Döpfner, M. and Sattel, H. (1991). Verhaltenstherapeutische Interventionen bei hyperkinetischen Störungen im Vorschulalter. *Zeitschrift für Kinder- und Jugendpsychiatrie*, **19**, 254–62.

Eisert, H. G. (1993). Hyperkinetische Störungen. In *Handbuch Verhaltenstherapie und Verhaltensmedizin bei Kindern und Jugendlichen*, ed., H-C. Steinhausen and M. von Aster, pp. 131–59. Weinheim: Psychologie Verlags Union.

Guevremont, D. (1990). Social skills and peer relationship training. In *Attention-deficit hyperactivity disorder*, ed. R. A. Barkley, pp. 540–72. New York: Guilford Press.

Hinshaw, S. P. and Erhardt, D. (1991). Attention-deficit hyperactivity disorder. In *Child and adolescent therapy*, ed. P. C. Kendall, pp. 98–128. New York: Guilford Press.

Kagan, J. (1966). Reflexion-impulsivity. The generality and dynamics of conceptual tempo. *Journal of Abnormal Psychology*, **71**, 17–24.

Kanfer, F. E. (1975). Self-management methods. In *Helping people change. A textbook of methods*, ed. F. H. Kanfer and A. P. Goldstein. New York: Pergamon.

Kendall, P. C. and Braswell, L. (1985). *Cognitive-behavioral therapy for impulsive children*. New York: Guilford Press.

Lauth, G. W. and Schlottke, P. F. (1993). *Training mit aufmerksamkeitsgestörten Kindern*. Weinheim: Psychologie Verlags Union.

Meichenbaum, D. H. (1977). *Cognitive-behaviour modification*. New York: Plenum.

Meichenbaum, D. H. and Goodman, J. (1971). Training impulsive children to talk to themselves. A means of developing self-control. *Journal of Abnormal Psychology*, **77**, 115–26.

Minde, K. (1985). Hyperaktives Syndrom. In *Kinder- und Jugendpsychiatrie in Klinik und Praxis*, vol. I, ed. H. Remschmidt and M. H. Schmidt, pp. 1–18. Stuttgart: Thieme.

Munden, A., and Arcelus, J. (1999). *The ADHD handbook. A guide for parents and professionals on attention deficit hyperactivity disorders*. London: Kingsley.

Quaschner, K. (1990). Die psychotherapeutische Behandlung und spezifische erzieherische Förderung von Vorschulkindern mit Hyperkinetischem Syndrom. *Frühförderung interdisziplinär*, **9**, 162–70.

Remschmidt, H. (1992). *Psychiatrie der Adoleszenz*. Stuttgart: Thieme.

Remschmidt, H. and Schmidt, M.H. (1988). Alternative Behandlungsformen in der Kinder- und Jugendpsychiatrie. Stuttgart: Enke.

Rosvold, H. E., Mirsky, A. F.; Sarason, J., Bransome, E. D. and Beck, L. H. (1956). A continuous performance test of brain damage. *Journal of Clinical and Consulting Psychology*, **20**, 343–50.

Schmidt, M. H., Esser, G. and Moll, G. H. (1991). Der Verlauf des hyperkinetischen Syndroms in klinischen und Feldstichproben. *Zeitschrift für Kinder- und Jugendpsychiatrie*, **19**, 240–7.

Taylor, E. (ed.) (1986). *The overactive child.* Oxford: MacKeith/Blackwell.

Wagner, I. (1989). *Aufmerksamkeitstraining mit impulsiven Kindern*, 3rd edn. Eschborn: Klotz.

World Health Organization (WHO) (1992). *The ICD-10 classification of mental and behavioural disorders. Clinical descriptions and diagnostic guidelines.* Geneva: WHO.

27 Autism

Doris Weber and Helmut Remschmidt

Characteristics of the disorder

Autistic disorders were first described independently by the Austrian/American child psychiatrist Leo Kanner (1943) and the Austrian pediatrician Hans Asperger (1944). The term autism had been previously introduced by Eugen Bleuler (1911), who used it to describe a symptom of schizophrenia. However, as autistic children do not actively withdraw into their own imaginary world, but rather are unable to develop normal social skills, the term 'autism' does not quite apply in Bleuler's sense. It has nevertheless become the most widespread term for describing the disorder described by Kanner and Asperger (Weber, 1985).

Classification and clinical characteristics

In ICD-10 (WHO, 1992), both autistic syndromes (childhood autism [= Kanner's syndrome] and Asperger's syndrome) are classified among the pervasive developmental disorders (F84). Both are defined according to behaviour, and must therefore be considered psychopathological syndromes. The diagnostic criteria for childhood autism are summarized in Table 27.1.

The manifestations of childhood autism (Kanner's syndrome) should be present before the child is 3 years old. The syndrome is characterized by impairment in three specific areas: reciprocal social interaction, patterns of communication and spectrum of interests. The child may also have stereotyped behaviours, phobic anxieties, sleeping and eating disorders, aggressive outbursts without apparent cause, and self-injury. These symptoms may change in the course of individual development. Other features which may be present include (Weber, 1970):

- a wide variation in intelligence (about 75% of patients have a marked intellectual impairment),
- sensory abnormalities,

Table 27.1. Diagnosic criteria of childhood autism (F84.0)

A. Before the age of 3 a pervasive developmental disorder occurs, characterized by at least one of the following symptoms:
   (i) disturbance of speech expression and reception, such as is required in social communication,
   (ii) development of highly selective social attention or abnormal reciprocal social interaction,
   (iii) functional or symbolic play patterns.

B. At least six symptoms from the following list are required to make the diagnosis. At least three symptoms from part (i), and at least one symptom each from parts (ii) and (iii) are required:
   (i) Qualitative impairment of mutual social interaction in at least three of the following points:
      (a) inability to use eye contact, facial expression, posture, or gestures to regulate social interaction;
      (b) inability to establish social contact with peers, engage in activites, establish mutual interests and express emotions appropriately;
      (c) impairment in reciprocal social interaction and inadequate appreciation of socioemotional cues (lack of response to other people's emotions and/or lack of modulation of behaviour to social context; poor use of social signals and a weak integration of social, emotional, and communicative behaviours);
      (d) inability spontaneously to express joy, interests or the wish to undertake activities with others.
   (ii) Qualitative impairment of communication skills in one or more of the following points:
      (a) developmental disorder of speech, without compensating for the deficit by gestures or facial expression;
      (b) poor synchrony and lack of reciprocity in conversational interchange;
      (c) poor flexibility in language expression;
      (d) impairment in make believe and social imitative play.
   (iii) Restricted, repetitive and stereotyped patterns of behaviour, interests and activities in at least one of the following points:
      (a) stereotyped preoccupations with particular limited interests, which may be abnormal or pursued with unusual intensity;
      (b) obsession with the performance of particular routines in rituals of a non-functional character;
      (c) stereotyped and repetitive motor mannerisms such as beating something with their hand or fingers, going through complicated motions, posturing, or motor stereotypies;
      (d) stereotyped preoccupations with parts of particular objects or a specific interest in non-functional elements of objects (such as their smell or feel).

From WHO (1992).

- specific speech abnormalities (retarded speech development, echolalia, pronoun reversal),
- motor abnormalities (psychomotor retardation, walking on tiptoes, stereotyped behaviour),
- marked fear of change, which can make the care of these children rather difficult to manage.

Some degree of autisitc behaviour is common in the development of healthy children, e.g. echolalia, fear of the unknown, stereotyped behaviour, rituals of non-functional character, symbiotic bonding, walking on tiptoes. However, in autistic children such behaviours occur at inappropriate developmental stages or are of increased severity or duration (Weber, 1985).

In addition to childhood autism, ICD-10 also classifies a syndrome known as atypical autism. Under this syndrome it is possible to classify autism, which has a different age of manifestation or lacks the full complement of diagnositic criteria required for the diagnosis of childhood autism.

Asperger's syndrome differs from the other two psychopathological syndromes by the absence of delayed speech and impaired intellectual development. However, patients are often unable to use their intellectual ability in a meaningful manner and tend to pursue highly specialized interests, e.g. learning timetables by rote, focusing all their interest on dinosaurs, etc.

Epidemiology

Studies with unselected samples showed a prevalence of about 4–5 per 10 000 children. The highest prevalence rate for autism has been reported by Gillberg (1989) with 10 autistic children per 10 000 children. There is a predominance of autism in boys, with a ratio of 3 to 1.

There are no prevalence studies of Asperger's syndrome. Whilst severe manifestations of the disorder are rare, mild cases are probably much more common. There is again a predominance of boys with a ratio of 8 to 1.

Assessment and differential diagnosis

Although examination is required for accurate diagnosis, which in turn will determine the most appropriate management, psychological tests such as the Childhood Autism Rating Scale (CARS) (Schopler et al., 1980) can also be helpful. A physical history, in particular neurological examination, should be undertaken including observation of the child at play and a mental state examination. Investigators may include EEG, visual and auditory activity, blood tests and chromosomal analysis.

Differential diagnosis

In differentiating Asperger's syndrome and Kanner's syndrome, the following points should be borne in mind. First, children with Asperger's syndrome lack the characteristic language delay which occurs in childhood autism (Kanner's syndrome). Nevertheless, the communicational function of language is also abnormal in these children.

Secondly, Asperger's syndrome is regarded by some as a personality disorder (Remschmidt, 1985), in which personality traits become fixed at a very early stage, changing only quantitatively. In contrast, Kanner's syndrome is an abnormal process which is very variable and subject to change.

The validity of the diagnosis of Asperger's syndrome or whether it simply represents Kanner's syndrome with normal intelligence remains unclear.

Autism must be distinguished from other disorders characterized by severe disturbances of interpersonal relations and other symptoms of childhood autism. These include childhood schizophrenia, symbiotic psychosis (Mahler), several types of mental retardation, disintegrative disorder (Heller's disease), Rett's syndrome, receptive–expressive language disorder, sensory deficits, elective mutism and psychosocial deprivation.

Aetiology and pathogenesis

Childhood autism (Kanner's syndrome)

Both organic factors and genetic factors are relevant in the aetiology and pathogenesis of childhood autism. The incidence of childhood autism is increased in a number of organic disorders, e.g. untreated phenylketonuria, rubella embryopathy, tuberous sclerosis as well as several chromosomal and metabolic abnormalities.

Studies with twins and families have demonstrated a significant role of genetic factors. Monozygotic twins have a much higher concordance rates than dizygotic twins, and childhood autism is 60–200 times more common among siblings of autistic children (Smalley, 1988).

Autistic personality disorder (Asperger's syndrome)

As Asperger (1968) suspected, and more recent family studies have shown, there is an important genetic influence on the aetiology of Asperger's syndrome. Asperger himself considered the autistic personality an 'extreme variant of male character' (Weber, 1988).

Psychotherapeutic techniques

Psychotherapy of autism needs to focus on the individual patient, while following certain principles (Cohen and Volkmar, 1997). Psychotherapy or any other type of treatment requires an accurate diagnosis. Delayed diagnosis, despite multiple consultations, is unfortunately still not uncommon, neither is misdiagnosis, e.g. 'developmental delay', which may have negative sequelae for both the child and his parents. There remains a need for better information to be made available to doctors, psychologists, parents, teachers, and kindergartens (Weber, 1985).

As soon as the diagnosis is made, the parents and other care-givers should be fully informed about the disorder (Remschmidt, 2000). It should be clearly stated that autism is a severe disorder, which can, however, be influenced positively by the appropriate treatment. The guilty feelings which many parents initially have should be addressed. Some parents attribute autism to genetic influences, others to the way they have treated their child in early childhood. Such feelings date back to earlier theories which see autism as a purely psychoreactive disorder. These psychoanalytic theories proposed that autism was caused by emotionally cool and intellectuallizing parents, who pass on these personality traits to their children, aggravating the traits by their style of upbringing. Today, this view is no longer tenable.

The considerable potential iatrogenic harm which families with autistic children may suffer has been emphasized by van Krevelen (1964).

General considerations

Although autism is a syndrome whose aetiology has major genetic and organic components, this does not preclude a psychotherapeutic approach to treatment. Psychotherapy can make a significant contribution to improving development, as well as to integration into an appropriate social environment. The aim is reciprocal adaption between the child and his environment.

There is no known psychological or physical cure for autism; however, novel treatments for autism are regularly developed claiming improvement or even cure. The majority of such approaches lack an empirical basis; however, parents are often seduced by these optimistic claims.

Several treatments have now, however, been found to be of benefit in controlled studies. These approaches are based on a number of basic principles and may be helpful in several different therapeutic contexts. They may be applied to all three categories of autistic behaviour.

(i) Behaviourally orientated approaches with an emphasis on structuring have been shown to be more effective than those which allow the child more freedom (Schopler et al., 1971; Schopler, 1989).

(ii) The child's environment should be structured and organized rather than being excessively permissive (Bartak, 1978; Schopler et al., 1971; Schopler, 1989).

(iii) Autistic children with marked developmental retardation respond better to a structuring approach to treatment than those with a more normal developmental level.

(iv) Treatment should always be structured to the child's developmental level. Treatment needs to focus on the patient's specific needs, and will usually aim to improve several different aspects of the disorder, e.g. facilitating steps towards more normal play, encouraging speech development, increasing autonomous action, reducing stereotyped and autoaggressive behaviour.

(v) Therapeutic techniques should be integrated into a larger treatment plan, which should serve to integrate individual techniques and focus therapetuic efforts on the ultimate goals of treatment.

(vi) The parents or other care-givers should always be involved in the treatment of autistic children. Treatment steps need to be continued at home and a structured environment will allow treatment gains to be built upon.

(vii) During adolescence a number of typical developmental problems commonly arise. These problems, such as lability of mood, aggressive behaviour, and sexual impulses may be later as compared to normal adolescents, but tend to occur eventually. In childhood autism (Kanner's syndrome), self-harm, epileptic seizures and occasional pychotic episodes also occur with increased frequency.

(viii) Psychotherapy of autistic children and adolescents should always be in keeping with the child's educational situation, i.e. the school or work place, residential home or other educational facility (Wing, 1966).

(ix) Autistic children and adolescents also require appropriate upbringing, supported by education. Programmes aimed at meeting these needs should include the following:
- a structured daily schedule with constructive psychological guidance,
- adequate time for recreational activities,
- activities which allow for the child's developmental status, language skills and communication capacity.

Early intervention

Early intervention is recommended in all autistic syndromes with the aim of achieving an accurate diagnosis as early as possible and optimizing environmental conditions to promote age-appropriate normal behaviour. Although many parents realize that there is a problem at an early stage, intervention commences only at the age of 3–4. This is often related to non-recognition by professionals or misdiagnosis.

The premise for the value of early intervention is based on the assumption that a child's development is influenced significantly by environmental factors. Autistic children require considerable support and external stimulation. Early intervention also aims to prevent or minimize disability and usually includes the following steps.

(i) The collection of all available information to enable an accurate diagnosis to be made.

(ii) The offering of information and support to parents regarding the nature of the disorder and the possible approaches to treatment. This often requires several sessions and will often be continued for several years.

(iii) A full assessment of the child's developmental status will include observation in several different situations (video recordings can be helpful), contact behaviour and social interaction with parents and other care-givers, as well as standardized psychological tests including an intelligence test, an assessment of sensory function, a neurological examination, EEG and further laboratory tests if indicated.

(iv) A treatment and developmental programme is set up in cooperation with the parents. Treatment should be adapted to the patient's abilities and take account of the parents' capabilities. It should be set up in conjunction with any other institutions involved in the care of the child, e.g. kindergarten, preschool.

(v) Time plays an important role in planning the programme. It is sensible to plan initially in shorter periods, e.g. up to a year as early on the prognosis will still be uncertain. Once the therapist gets to know the child better, a more reliable opinion on the prognosis may be given.

Behavioural therapy approaches

Establishing a behavioural therapy programme requires a functional behaviour analysis. The relevant behaviour must be defined and one must determine the frequency, severity and situational or predisposing factors of the behaviour. The behaviour should be interpreted with regard to its context. If, for instance, an autistic child expresses distress through self-harm, there is little point in addressing the self-injurious behaviour without addressing the distress (Howlin and Yates, 1989).

In behaviour therapy, as in early intervention, it is important to involve the parents and keep them informed about the rationale for treatment. Many experts consider home treatment with parents to be the ideal approach, as the child's needs can be determined in the context of the whole family (Howlin, 1989).

There are, however, risks with this family-orientated therapy. It is important to avoid excessive demands being placed on siblings, who play a co-therapeutic role. They should spend a limited amount of time 'caring' for the patient. The family's life should not revolve exclusively around the autistic child, and time needs to be be managed carefully. The therapist may help in pointing out ways of improving the effectiveness of care (Howlin, 1989). It is also important to remember that not all parents are ideally suited for the role of co-therapist.

The approach to behavioural therapy in autism is essentially the same as in other psychiatric disorders. The prinicples of behavioural therapy are explained in detail in Chapter 6 and need not be repeated here. However, the techniques may require modification and adaptation to the needs of autistic children and adolescents. Lovaas (1987) was one of the first to use behavioural techniques in the treatment of the disorder and offered the following guidelines (Janetzke, 1993).

(i) Autism is not primarily a disturbance of interpersonal relationships, but of perception and cognition (information processing). In Asperger's syndrome, however, the disturbance of interpersonal relationships is more marked, and may be considered a part of the autistic personality.

(ii) The aetiology of autism remains unknown, thus treatment cannot be focused directly on the cause of the disorder. However, behaviour modification is nevertheless possible. Behaviour modifications aim to enhance desired behaviours whilst reducing undesired behaviours.

(ii) In addition to professionals, parents and other care-givers can make a significant contribution to behavioural therapy once they have understood the principles on which it is based.

A wide spectrum of behavioural therapy techniques has subsequently been developed, including operant conditioning (using reinforcement and adverse stimuli), prompting, shaping and fading.

The small number of adolescents with childhood autism and average or above-average intelligence have behavioural abnormalities similar to those with Asperger's syndrome. They usually wish to have more social contact, particularly to the opposite sex, but are unable to show appropriate behaviour because of the disturbances in their social interaction and communication.

One adolescent with normal intelligence said: 'What should I do if I see a girl I like? Should I approach her and say: "Hello, would you like to go to the cinema with me?" And if she declines, how do I start a conversation? How do I discover whether she is interested in what I am saying?'

Other adolescents with autism unwittingly make socially inappropriate comments such as the 15-year-old autistic who interrupted his parents whilst they were entertaining in order to ask his mother about the facts of life.

A certain amount of improvement may be expected of behavioural training including role play and video feedback. However, many patients find it hard to generalize any role learnt and to know when to adapt behaviours in order to have appropriate interactions (Howlin and Yates, 1989).

It is important to distinguish between reinforcement and reduction of behaviours. Behaviours which should be reinforced include: language skills, communicational abilities and interactional competency. Inappropriate behaviours which should be reduced include self-stimulation, stereotyped behaviour, self-harm, tantrums or physical aggression.

Table 27.2 lists the general aims of treatment and the behavioural therapy techniques which are commonly used. All the techniques mentioned here have been shown to be effective. However, all also have limitations.

- The effectiveness of the methods is very variable, and to a large extent is dependent on general factors such as cooperation, intelligence, environmental factors, etc.
- The extent to which treatment success generalizes to cover other situations is very variable, but obviously crucial. The more similar therapeutic tasks are to everyday situations, the more likely is generalization to occur.
- Behavioural therapy can only form a part of an overall management plan (which may also include medication, counselling of parents or other caregivers, etc.).

Approaches other than behavioural therapy have also been developed and can often be a helpful addition in the treatment of autistic syndromes.

Physiotherapy

Impairment of motor function meriting specific treatment is common in all autistic syndromes. This may often be combined with music therapy.

Sports

Sports such as ball games, jumping games, horse-riding, swimming and activities on the climbing apparatus all help to improve motor skills in autistic children.

Music therapy

This is often helpful, especially when combined with movement exercises.

Table 27.2. Behavioural therapy techniqes for childhood autism

	Area of use	Aims of treatment	Behavioural technique
Reinforcing behaviours	Language development and encouragement of verbal communication	Non-verbal imitation, improving speech, using language for communication	Operant conditioning, discriminatory learning, prompting, fading
	Encouraging social interaction and communication	Perceiving and recognizing emotions, appropriate interactive behaviour in ordinary situations	Modelling, learning of rules, operant conditioning
Reducing behaviours	Reducing self-stimulation, stereotyped behaviours and self-harm	Influencing disturbed behaviour in individual sessions, groups and other social situations	Treatment with adversive stimuli, combination of adversive stimuli and reinforcing behavioural alternatives, e.g. in self-injurious behaviour, sensory extinction programmes, combination of behavioural therapy and medication
	Tantrums and aggressive outbursts	Attempting to identify the cause, directly influencing the disturbed behaviour and the context in which it is shown	Avoiding situations in which the behaviour is triggered

Play therapy

As well as offering these organized activities, it is important to encourage the child to use his imagination to initiate and engage in self-motivated activities.

Physically orientated approaches to psychotherapy (childhood autism and atypical autism)

These approaches use physical means to encourage the development of new, positive behaviours and reduce abnormal behaviours. Several different approaches have been proposed.

Sensory integration therapy is a functional technique which aims to try to compensate for the deficits caused by the child's impaired sensory abilities. The method emphasizes the coordination of the senses, and the child is taught to improve his perceptive capability of situations, thus facilitating his ability to react appropriately.

A developmental programme set up by Delacato (1974) is claimed to help the child to catch up in areas in which there is developmental delay through a physically based programme. This approach is, however, extremely demanding on all concerned and there is a danger of too many demands being made of the child.

Integrative physical therapy uses physical means in an attempt to broaden the child's personality. The importance of the child experiencing intense positive emotions such as warmth, security, protection and empathy is emphasized.

Many other therapeutic approaches have been suggested, and two of these are discussed in more detail below.

Holding therapy

This treatment was developed by the American child psychiatrist Maria Welch (1984) and is based on the assumption that the autistic child's resistance to closeness and physical contact can be overcome by holding the child until he gives up his resistance. After this resistance has been overcome, the child's anxiety of closeness will be reduced significantly.

'Holding' autistic children initially leads to intense aggression, defensiveness and resistance. However, when a state of exhaustion has been reached, the child may be able to interact with his parents in a different manner, often without signs of extreme autistic behaviour.

The technique of holding therapy has been summarized by Innerhofer and Klicpera (1988).

- The care-giver is instructed to hold the child tightly.
- The autistic child usually then begins to resist this.
- The care-giver should not give in to the child's resistance, but continue to hold the child tightly and attempt to establish eye contact with the child.
- The child will often put up a vehement struggle and become quite excited, resulting in screaming, spitting, scratching and other self-defensive actions.
- The care-giver must continue to hold the child tightly, releasing him only when a state of exhaustion is reached. The subsequent state of relaxation allows a different type of interaction between the child and the care-giver.
- Holding therapy is undertaken on a daily basis and one session usually lasts about 1 hour. Holding may also be used in-between sessions when the care-giver has the impression that the child is unhappy.

Tinbergen and Tinbergen (1984) have developed a theory which explains the mechanism by which holding therapy works. They suggest that childhood autism is an emotional disorder, which has its origin in a hostile social environment during early childhood. The disturbances of perception and all other abnormalities are considered secondary. The child thus lacks primal trust from the first weeks and months of his life. As a result of this, they are on hostile terms with others in their environment. Holding therapy, they propose, helps the child to develop a sense of trust by the clear demonstration, physically of love and attention.

The effect of tightly holding the child may be understood in terms of exposure by flooding. The muscular and nervous tension which builds up during the struggle, whilst holding the child, is followed by profound relaxation once exhaustion is achieved, thus overcoming anxiety as the two are incompatible with one another. The close proximity of the mother or care-giver whilst holding the child enables the child to associate positive feelings of security and trust with her.

A number of problems are associated with holding therapy. First, there is a dramatic, almost violent interaction between adult and child. Secondly, parents often feel a sense of guilt, partly as a result of feeling responsible, and partly because of the nature of the intervention required. The therapist needs to be prepared for dealing with these feelings.

The efficacy of the method has been demonstrated in several trials. Stereotyped behaviour, self-harm, and social withdrawal have all been reported to improve, resulting in children being quieter and more open to communication, with better social and interactional capabilities (Prekop, 1983).

Whilst its efficacy should not be overestimated (Innerhofer and Klicpera, 1988), holding therapy can be a helpful adjuvant to the therapeutic repertoire, reducing anxiety and optimizing the potential for other treatment techniques.

Table 27.3. Possible causes of crises in patients with autistic syndromes

(i)	Changes in the individual's environment
(ii)	Communicational misunderstandings
(iii)	Change occurring in the course of development
(iv)	Changes in the nature of the autistic disturbance

Crisis intervention (childhood autism and atypical autism)

A crisis may occur when an individual is challenged by problems which differ significantly from his or her previous experience for which there is no readily available coping strategy. The occurrence of such crises may cause considerable distress and hopelessness in those involved.

There are four major causes of crises in patients with autistic syndromes (Table 27.3).

(i) Sudden changes in the individual's environment may cause states of restlessness and severe excitation, particularly if the autistic child or adolescent has not been prepared to expect change.

(ii) Communication misunderstandings may cause a crisis with reciprocal misunderstanding of either verbal or non-verbal material. This is illustrated in the following vignette.

An autistic adolescent was brought to a day-care centre by taxi every day. On the way, a river had to be crossed on a small ferry. One day, the taxi was almost at the ferry when the traffic lights turned red; however, in order to reach the ferry on time it did not stop. This deviation from the normal course of events, including a breach of rules, so upset the boy that he became restless and excited. He shook the taxi driver's shoulder, which the driver misinterpreted as an assault. The patient, in turn, could not understand the commotion which resulted. Following this, the taxi driver and his colleagues refused to continue taxiing the autistic adolescent to the day-care centre any longer.

(iii) Change occurring in the course of normal development may also lead to crises in autistic individuals. For example, many autistic adolescents are unable to deal appropriately with sexual impulses or the changing demands placed on them as they mature.

(iv) Changes in the nature of the autistic disturbance may occur, thus affecting the individual's behaviour. Co-morbidity is common in autism and may take many forms, resulting in a broad spectrum of behavioural abnormalities culminating in crises.

Crisis intervention aims to terminate the crisis or at least prevent dangerous situations from occurring. Thus, it should not be seen as treatment, but rather the management of acute situations.

In autism, crisis intervention is frequently required and may be considered a psychotherapeutic technique. The approach differs from the normal approach to therapy and rehabilitation and all action taken in the course of crisis intervention needs to be undertaken swiftly and in a focused manner. It may be classified according to the type of approach.

Measures directed at the patient's environment

Such crises can, to some extent, be prevented by avoiding abrupt environmental changes which can cause restlessness and excitement when change is necessary. Crises can be managed by creating an environment in which the patient feels comfortable. Such steps are relatively easy if one knows the patient well. The presence of a well-known object, e.g. a favourite toy can contribute significantly to pacifying the autistic child as can the presence of familiar individuals.

Measures directed at the patient's behaviour

Behavioural techniques are usually directed at the patient. It is initially important to distinguish between behaviour which puts the patient and others at risk, e.g. states of anxiety or excitement, self-injurious behaviour, aggression towards others and the tendency to withdraw, which is less commonly encountered. The use of reinforcing techniques, diversion to less dangerous behaviour and the active replacement of one behaviour with another may all be valuable, although often when a crisis has developed, medication may be required before these techniques can be brought into play.

Measures directed at the family

These measures may be utilized to prevent further crises, using past experience to prevent escalation of conflicts. Many crises and emergencies occur after a conflict has escalated because of inconsistent reactions to the autistic child. The detailed analysis of a particular situation usually reveals specific behaviours of the parents or care-givers which may have contributed to the conflict and which should be modified or avoided in future conflicts.

The inclusion of parents and care-givers in treatment programmes can often significantly reduce the frequency of crises (DeMyer, 1979).

The coincidental or systematic observations parents or care-givers make should always be analysed and incorporated into any treatment programme. Those involved in crisis intervention should always ask parents and care-givers of their experience in terminating stressful situations or reducing the severity of the autistic child's disturbed behaviour. This is illustrated in the following vignette.

The mother of an autistic child who was often very aggressive at home, especially towards his mother, discovered that she was able to stop the child's aggressive behaviour by leaving the room and saying: 'I am going away now.' At this, the boy became sorrowful and looked somewhat dejected. The mother was reluctant to repeat this 'technique' because of feelings of guilt; however, such an approach (often called 'time out') is commonly used in a therapeutic context or as part of an educational programme. After discussing this with the mother, the therapist was able to help her overcome her guilty feelings and gave her support to incorporate this intervention into the upbringing of her son.

Medication

Medication can be a great help in crisis intervention and can be combined with psychotherapeutic and educational measures. Several points to remember when using medication for crisis intervention are summarized below (Moll and Schmidt, 1991; Warnke, 1995).

- Medication does not directly influence the underlying cause of autistic syndromes.
- The use of medication always requires careful analysis of the problem and the potential benefits of medication should be weighed against its likely side effects.
- Medication should be considered symptomatic and chosen according to the specific symptom, e.g. anxiety, depression, aggression, self-injury.
- It is important for doctors treating autistic children (usually child and adolescents psychiatrists) to keep fully informed and up to date about the drugs which can be useful and to disseminate this knowledge amongst other health care professionals and parents. There has been considerable prejudice against medication and thus this can only be countered by sensible use and continuing education.

Course and prognosis

Childhood autism (Kanner's syndrome)

Firm opinions on prognosis should not be given prior to the age of 5 years. By this time, a more clear prognosis can be given, although improvements may occur after this age in some children and cannot necessarily be attributed to a particular therapeutic intervention. The following points are useful for assessing the prognosis in autistic children:

Table 27.4. Results of a follow-up study of three large groups of adolescents and adults with childhood autism

1–2%	Almost normal psychopathological status
5–15%	'Normal' within limits
16–25%	Fairly encouraging status
60–70%	Poor to very poor status (constantly dependent on help)

From DeMyer et al. (1985); Eisenberg (1956); Rutter and Lockyer (1967).

- IQ, particularly the performance subscore of the WISC (Rutter, 1970, 1978);
- overall severity of the disturbance;
- developmental status of language skills, particularly the ability to communicate;
- duration of the echolalia phase;
- developmental status of play behaviour;
- achievement at school.

Unfortunately the overall prognosis in autism is not good (Table 27.4). About half of all patients with autism never learn to speak. The prognosis is worse in those with epileptic seizures, psychotic episodes, aggressive outbursts, self-injury or ritualistic behaviour occurring during adolescence. Adult autistic patients who have normal intelligence are usually abnormal in other respects, and disturbed social interaction is the most debilitating abnormality in these individuals (Weber, 1987). There are very few reports in the literature of autistic adults who marry or live together with a partner.

Autistic personality disorder (Asperger's syndrome)

The difficulties of this group of individuals closely resemble the problems of those with childhood autism of normal intelligence. They are unable to lead a normal life, usually because of problems with communication and social interaction. Some are integrated quite well in a work environment, particularly in vocations which do not require much social interaction, but many individuals with Asperger's syndrome remain reclusive and solitary all their life.

Case reports

Case 1: Bernard – diagnosis: childhood autism and mental retardation of unknown aetiology

The physical examination was normal and the intelligence was in the upper range of mental retardation The WISC showed a very heterogeneous profile. Bernard was able to communicate quite well, could write his name and a few single words in capital letters. However, he did not understand the value of money. Since the age of 6 years and 9 months he had lived in a residential home for mentally retarded children. A brother was also mentally retarded, but not autistic.

Bernard lacked initiative and drive, and usually required considerable encouragement. He had no close friends among the other children and adolescents, but had a good relationship with the care-givers of the residential group. He was neither aggressive towards others nor himself, but when he became upset he was either obstinate or screamed and shouted.

At the age of 10, Bernard was asked to bring two bottles of mineral water from the central kitchen. On the way back he smashed the two bottles, and would not assist with picking up the pieces. He could not express any reason for his behaviour. The following day after lunch he swept all the plates within reach off the table with his arms. He appeared disturbed and anxious. Over the following several days Bernard did not appear in the dining room for his meals and refused to eat the food and drink which was brought to him in his room. He did not, however, lose weight and was observed taking food secretly from the refrigerator and drinking from the tap.

It became apparent that this was a reaction to a difficult situation which had arisen for Bernard in the home. The care-giver he particularly liked was about to leave and he was to be moved into a more demanding group. In addition, two new children had recently joined the residential group. The boy's reaction to these changes in his environment was characterized by helplessness, frustration and aggression. He was fearful of being punished for his behaviour (social anxiety) and generalized his anxiety onto objects made of glass or china. As a result of these anxieties, Bernard developed phobias, avoiding meals with the other children and other social situations. This avoidant behaviour, which initially seemed like an obsessional symptom, appeared to reduce his anxiety.

The treatment technique used was systematic desensitization. Bernard was given plastic tableware and was asked to sit at a table in a room next to the dining room. The door between the two rooms initially was kept closed. Bernard began to attend meals again, and after 8 days he allowed the door to be opened. Another 8 days later the table was moved into the doorway and Bernard was served dessert in a glass bowl. Eventually, all the plastic cups and plates were changed to normal tableware. Several days later, Bernard's usual place was set together with the other children and he joined them eagerly.

Bernard's cooperation with the treatment helped to improve the social situation. More than 8 years have since passed, and Bernard has not had a recurrence of anxious or phobic symptoms.

Case 2: Axel – diagnosis: childhood autism, mental retardation and suspected cerebral trauma during birth; no physical disability
Axel's birth was complicated by compression of the umbilical cord, cardiac arrest, vacuum extraction and cyanosis. A physical and neurological examination at the age of 2 years and 9 months was normal.

Intelligence as determined by the WISC was in the upper range of mental retardation (IQ = 56), but was very heterogeneous in profile. Axel was able to communicate quite well verbally, but was unable to read or write. He lived at home, working in a workshop for the disabled, which he enjoyed.

His father taught at an art school and his mother had previously studied literature. Both parents attended, collaborated with behavioural therapy and contributed constructively to the programme. A brother 4 years younger than Axel was of normal intelligence and was very good at sports. The brother had a friendly but rather distant relationship, and family interaction was usually good.

Axel is now 23 years old, and although his behaviour is plainly abnormal, he does not bother other people. He avoids eye contact, is somewhat clumsy, speaks little and then usually speaks to himself. If he answers questions, the answers are short. He usually has a sock with him, to which a string is tied. He winds and unwinds the string by turning the sock around. When left alone, he is without orientation, and thus is entirely dependent on other people. He enjoys going to concerts and exhibitions, visiting friends and going to cafés and restaurants. Axel is one of a group of autistic individuals who can participate in normal life to some degree and enjoy themselves with others.

Between the ages of 3 and 8 Axel had tantrums every day, throwing objects around and screaming and shouting for extended periods of time. At the age of 4, he became terrified of bathtubs. This fear lasted several weeks. He was afraid of being sucked down into the drainpipe. He would only have a shower standing up in the tub, with the plug in the plughole, and he would continue to observe the plug carefully. At the age of 14 years, this same fear reccurred. At this time he drew several pictures of the house in which the family lived, including the bathroom, bathtub, toilet and drainpipe, at the bottom of which he drew a bucket which would catch him. This anxiety disappeared after 3 weeks, and he stopped drawing pictures on this theme. It is tempting to speculate that the drawing of the pictures had a self-therapeutic effect.

REFERENCES

Asperger, H. (1944). Die 'autistischen Psychopathen' im Kindesalter. *Archiv für Psychiatrie und Nervenkrankheiten*, 117, 76–137.

Asperger, H. (1968). Autistische Psychopathen. In *Heilpädagogik*, ed. H. Asperger, pp. 177–205. Wien: Springer.

Bartak, L. (1978). Educational approaches. In *Autism, reappraisal of concepts and treatment*, ed. M. Rutter and E. Schopler, pp. 423–38. New York: Plenum Press.

Bleuler, E. (1911). Dementia praecox oder Gruppe der Schizophrenen. In *Handbuch der Psychiatrie*, section 4, part 1, ed. G. Aschaffenburg. Leipzig: Deuticke.

Cohen, D. J. and Volkmar, F. R. (ed.) (1997). *Handbook of autism and pervasive developmental disorders*, 2nd edn. New York: Wiley.

Delacato, C. H. (1974). *The ultimate stranger. The autistic child.* New York: Doubleday.

DeMyer, M. K. (1979). *Parents and children in autism*. Washington, DC: Winston.

DeMyer, M. K., Barton, S., DeMyer, W. E., Norton, J. A., Allen, J. and Steele, R. (1985). Prognosis in autism. A follow-up study. *Journal of Autism and Childhood Schizophrenia*, **15**, 389–97.

Eisenberg, L. (1956). The autistic child in adolescence. *American Journal of Psychiatry*, **12**, 607–12.

Gillberg, C. (1989). The aetiology of autism. In *Diagnosis and treatment of autism*, ed. C. Gillberg, pp. 63–82. New York: Plenum Press.

Howlin, P. (1989). Help for the family. In *Diagnosis and treatment of autism*, ed. C. Gillberg, pp. 185–202. New York: Plenum Press.

Howlin, P. and Yates, P. (1989). Treating autistic children at home. In *Diagnosis and treatment of autism*, ed. C. Gillberg, pp. 307–22. New York: Plenum Press.

Innerhofer, P. and Klicpera, C. (1988). Die Welt des frühkindlichen Autismus. München: Reinhardt.

Janetzke, H. R. P. (1993). *Stichwort Autismus*. München: Heyne.

Kanner, L. (1943). Autistic disturbances of affective contact. *Nervous Child*, **2**, 217–50.

Lovaas, O. I. (1987). Behavioral treatment and normal education and intellectual functioning in young autistic children. *Journal of Consulting and Clinical Psychology*, **55**, 3–9.

Moll, G. H. and Schmidt, M. H. (1991). Entwicklungen in der Therapie des frühkindlichen Autismus. Ergebnisse der Therapieforschung. *Zeitschrift für Kinder- und Jugendpsychiatrie*, **19**, 182–203.

Prekop, I. (1983). Das Festhalten als Therapie bei Kindern mit Autismus-Syndrom. *Frühförderung interdisziplinär*, **2**, 54–64.

Remschmidt, H. (1985). Persönlichkeitsstörungen. In *Kinder- und Jugendpsychiatric in Klinik und Praxis*, vol. III, ed. H. Remschmidt and M. H. Schmidt, pp. 204–12. Stuttgart: Thieme.

Remschmidt, H. (2000). *Autismus. Erscheinungsformen, Ursachen, Hilfen*. München: C. H. Beck.

Rutter, M. (1970). Autistic children. Infancy to adulthood. *Seminars in Psychiatry*, **2**, 435–50.

Rutter, M. (1978). Developmental issues and prognosis. In *Autism. A reappraisal of concepts and treatment*, ed. M. Rutter and E. Schopler, pp. 497–505. New York: Plenum Press.

Rutter, M. and Lockyer, L. (1967). A five to fifteen year follow-up study of infantile psychosis. I: Description of sample. *British Journal of Psychiatry*, **113**, 1169–82.

Schopler, E. (1989). Principles for directing both educational treatment and research. In *Diagnosis and treatment of autism*, ed. C. Gillberg, pp. 167–83. New York: Plenum Press.

Schopler, E., Brehm, S. S., Kinsbourne, M. and Reichler, R. J. (1971). Effect of treatment structure of development in autistic children. *Archives of General Psychiatry*, **24**, 415–21.

Schopler, E., Reichler, R. J., DeVellis, R. F. and Daly, K. (1980). Toward objective classification of childhood autism: childhood autism rating scale (CARS). *Journal of Autism and Developmental Disorders*, **10**, 91–103.

Smalley, S. L. (1988). Autism and genetics. *Archives of General Psychiatry*, **45**, 953–61.

Tinbergen, N. and Tinbergen, E. A. (1984). *Autismus bei Kindern*. Berlin: Paul Parey.

van Krevelen, D. A. (1964). Autismus und Iatrogenie. *Acta Paedopsychiatrica*, **31**, 129–33.

Warnke, A. (1995). Medikamentöse Therapie bei Menschen mit frühkindlichem Autismus. In *Autismus und Familie*, ed. Bundesverband Hilfe für das autistische Kind, Hamburg, pp. 200–9. Bonn: Reha-Verlag.

Weber, D. (1970). *Der frühkindliche Autismus unter dem Aspekt der Entwicklung*. Bern: Huber.

Weber, D. (1985). Autistische Syndrome. In *Kinder- und Jugendpsychiatrie in Klinik und Praxis*, vol. II, ed. H. Remschmidt and M. H. Schmidt, pp. 269–98. Stuttgart: Thieme.

Weber, D. (1987). Zur Prognose frühkindlich-autistischer Kinder. In *Prognose psychischer Erkrankungen im Kindes- und Jugendalter*, ed. G. Nissen, pp. 122–35. Bern: Huber.

Weber, D. (1988). Autistische Syndrome. In *Psychiatrie der Gegenwart*, vol. 7, ed. K. P. Kisker, H. Lauter, J. E. Meyer, C. Müller and E. Strömgren, pp. 57–87. Berlin: Springer.

Welch, M. G. (1984). Heilung vom Autismus durch die Mutter-und-Kind-Haltetherapie. In *Autismus*, ed. N. Tinbergen and E. A. Tinbergen, pp. 297–308. Berlin: Paul Parey.

Wing, J. K. (ed.) (1966). *Early childhood autism. Clinical, educational and social aspects*. Oxford: Pergamon Press.

World Health Organization (WHO) (1992). *The ICD-10 classification of mental and behavioural disorders. Clinical descriptions and diagnostic guidelines*. Geneva: WHO.

28 Schizophrenia

Helmut Remschmidt, Matthias Martin and Eberhard Schulz

Definition and classification

Schizophrenia is typically associated with disorder of thinking, perception, and with inappropriate or blunted affect. As the disorder progresses, it often ultimately leads to a disintegration of personality. Intellectual capacity and conciousness are usually initially normal, however, intellectual impairments are common over the course of the illness (Remschmidt, 2001).

Little is known about the causes of schizophrenia. The classification systems ICD-10 and DSM-IV (WHO, 1992; APA, 1994) base the diagnosis on the symptoms of the disorder and define specific time criteria for the onset and course of schizophrenia.

In ICD-10, a diagnosis of schizophrenia requires the presence of at least one of the symptoms 1–4 listed below (two or more symptoms are required if they are not very clear), or at least two of the symptoms 5–8 (WHO, 1992):

1. thought echo, thought insertion or withdrawal, and thought broadcasting;
2. delusions of control, influence, or passivity, clearly referred to body or limb movements or specific thoughts, actions, or sensations; delusional perceptions;
3. hallucinatory voices giving a running commentary on the patient's behaviour, or discussing the patient among themselves, or other types of hallucinatory voices coming from some part of the body;
4. persistent delusions of other kinds that are culturally inappropriate and completely impossible, such as religious or political identity, or superhuman powers and abilities, e.g. being able to control the weather, or being in communication with aliens from another world;
5. persistent hallucinations in any modality, when accompanied either by fleeting or half-formed delusions without clear affective content, or by persistent over-valued ideas, or when occurring every day for weeks or months on end;
6. breaks of interpolations in the train of thought, resulting in incoherence or irrelevant speech, or neologisms;

7. catatonic behaviour, such as excitement, posturing, or waxy flexibility, negativism, mutism, and stupor;
8. 'negative' symptoms such as marked apathy, paucity of speech, and blunting or incongruity of emotional responses, usually resulting in social withdrawal and lowering of social performance; it must be clear that these are not due to depression or to neuroleptic medication.

Several additional symptoms apply specifically to the classification of 'simple schizophrenia' (F20.6): a significant and consistent change in the overall quality of some aspects of personal behaviour, manifest as loss of interest, aimlessness, idleness, a self-absorbed attitude, and social withdrawal.

The diagnostic guidelines of ICD-10 distinguish the following clinical subtypes of schizophrenia:

F20.0 paranoid schizophrenia
F20.1 hebephrenic schizophrenia
F20.2 undifferentiated schizophrenia
F20.3 catatonic schizophrenia
F20.5 residual schizophrenia
F20.6 simple schizophrenia

Independent of this classification, other classifications have been developed using psychopathological criteria and course of illness (Leonhard, 1986; Crow, 1980; Andreasen, 1982; Kay, 1991). The concept of positive (Type I) and negative (Type II) schizophrenia seems to be particularly relevant to treatment in childhood and adolescence (Bettes and Walker, 1987; Remschmidt et al., 1991; Schulz et al., 1994). The most important psychopathological findings which characterize Type I and Type II schizophrenia are summarized in Table 28.1.

However, positive or negative symptoms are not specific to schizophrenia. They may also be found in organic personality and behavioural disorders, depression, personality disorders and neuroses (Angst et al., 1989). Negative symptoms dominate in children (5–10 years) with schizophrenia and intellectually impaired children and adolescents.

Epidemiology

A number of studies have been published on the epidemiology of schizophrenia in children, and the following conclusions can be drawn.

(i) The prevalence of schizophrenia in children under 11 years old is less than 1 child in 10 000 children. Thus, schizophrenia is rarer than autism in this age group (Burg and Kerbeshian, 1987).

Table 28.1. Subgroups of schizophrenia

	Type I schizophrenia (positive symptoms, 'productive' symptoms, acute symptoms)	Type II schizophrenia (negative symptoms, withdrawal)
Clinical symptoms	Hallucinations, delusions, thought disorder, overactivity, excitability, threats or violence, bizarre behaviour, increased speech, neologisms	Flatness of affect, underactivity, social and emotional withdrawal, apathy, decreased speech, anhedonia, disorders of the stream of thought, thought blocking

(ii) Schizophrenia in children (excluding adolescents) is 50 times rarer than schizophrenia in adults (Karno and Norquist, 1989).
(iii) Whilst schizophrenia is rare in childhood, the prevalence increases significantly during adolescence. In a study based on complete patient samples from all child and adolescent child psychiatric treatment facilities in a defined region in Germany, the age of onset was between 4 and 13 in only 2.4% of the cases, but between 14 and 18 in 22.1% of cases (Remschmidt, 1988a).
(iv) The sex distribution of schizophrenia is uneven. Whilst in children more boys are affected, in adolescence, the sex distribution appears to be equal (Remschmidt et al., 1994).

Course and prognosis

Schizophrenia with negative symptoms has a much poorer prognosis than schizophrenia with positive symptoms, during both inpatient treatment and over the course of rehablitation (Remschmidt et al., 1991, 1992, 1994). This is due to the poor response of negative symptoms not only to neuroleptic medication, but also to rehabilitation and social reintegration.

Altogether, the prognosis of schizophrenia with onset in childhood or adolescence is poorer than schizophrenia with onset in adulthood (Weiner, 1982). In 23% of adolescent patients, remittance is achieved. Partial improvement is achieved by 50% of adult patients and 25% of adolescents. In 52% of adolescents the schizophrenia takes a chronic course, compared to 25% of adult patients. Krausz (1990) undertook a study of 59 adolescents with schizophrenia who were 13–17 years old at onset. During the course of 5–11 years, 50% of the cases became chronic (Krausz and Müller-Thomson, 1993). Only 22% of patients showed marked improvement. Schmidt and Blanz (1992) undertook a follow-up study of the course of schizophrenia in 40 adolescents. The observation period was 5 years following discharge from the initial inpatient treatment facility. The authors found that 60% of the patients had an occupational standing inferior to what might be expected considering their level of education. Gillberg et al. (1993) suggest that schizophrenia has a poor prognosis when the onset is during adolescence. The age of onset, the type of initial symptoms, and the patient's personality structure before onset of schizophrenia appear to be the most important prognostic factors (Remschmidt et al., 1994; Schulz et al., 1994). When the age of onset is under 13 years, the prognosis of schizophrenia must be considered very poor, particularly in young children. The early manifestation of emotional abnormalities, e.g. an extremely introverted attitude, associated with developmental delays and a gradual onset of the negative symptoms of schizophrenia increase the likelihood of a poor prognosis. In a prospective study, Martin (1991) showed that the persistence of cognitive impairment and the presence of affective symptoms predict a poor prognosis. However, the classification of schizophrenia in the well-known clinical subtypes, e.g. hebephrenic or paranoid schizophrenia, etc. does not predict the course or outcome of the disorder in adolescents (Martin, 1991; Remschmidt et al., 1991; Schmidt and Blanz, 1992; Schulz et al., 1994).

Developmental psychopathology

Schizophrenia in childhood and adolescence always needs to be regarded in a developmental context (Volkmar, 1996). An individual's symptomatology can usually be understood only when taking into account developmental status. The manifestation of schizophrenia in childhood must be distinguished from that in adolescence. Age and the developmental status are the two factors which determine, to the greatest extent, the clinical picture of schizophrenia in childhood and adolescence (Remschmidt, 1988b; Remschmidt et al., 1994). There are similarities between schizophrenia and the developmental psychopathology of specific childhood psychoses such as childhood catatonia (Leonhard, 1986), as well as between schizophrenia and the developmental psychopathology of psychoses in the transitional phase between late childhood and early adolescence. As proposed by Kanner (1943, 1957), classification of the childhood psychoses into childhood autism (no connection to schizophrenia), childhood disintegrative disorder (a result of encephalopathy) and childhood schizophrenia would seem appropriate.

Some knowledge of the cognitive and emotional developments taking place at any given age and the analysis of age-appropriate developmental steps is required in order to understand the psychosis and the likely specific symptoms, e.g. delusions, hallucinations. For example, hallucinations vary depending upon the child's age. In younger children, hallucinations tend to be unsystematic and largely determined by childlike fantasies. This may cause difficulties in distinguishing symptoms from normal experience.

During adolescence crises of personal development may occur, which can coincide with the onset of the schizophrenia and may initially obfuscate symptoms (Remschmidt and Martin, 1992). Such 'personality crises' are normal variants of behaviour during adolescence, during which many adolescents modify their attitude towards themselves (Remschmidt, 1992a). Such crises may be of such a degree that they result in self-injurious behaviour, suicide attempts, and oppositonal behaviour (Remschmidt, 1992b). The stress of the challenges of normal development may precipitate a psychotic episode, but this may be masked by the coincidental personal crisis. When symptoms develop, they are likely to be influenced by the adolescent's subjective situation. Individual vulnerability, personality traits prior to onset, current stressful life experiences, family influences and failure to cope with the challenges of normal development are generally regarded as contributing to the precipitation of schizophrenia in adolescents.

Increased vulnerability seems to occur in association with the following characteristics:

- impaired information processing skills (attention deficit, distractability, impaired selectivity);
- abnormal autonomic nervous response (under- or over-arousal, impaired habituation);
- impaired social competency;
- poorly developed coping mechanisms.

These characteristics can then interact with psychosocial stress factors, including emotional and cognitive factors in the family environment and important life events. Whilst sudden stressful experiences do not seem to play a major role, continual stress in the family environment seems to be much more important in precipitating psychosis (Dohrenwend et al., 1987). The treatment of schizophrenia is based on this vulnerability stress theory.

Treatment

Specific steps taken to treat schizophrenia should be considered as part of a larger treatment plan. In children and adolescents with schizophrenia, this normally comprises:

(i) treatment of the acute symptoms with medication,

(ii) psychopharmacological approach to prevent relapses,
(iii) psychotherapeutic work with the patient,
(iv) work with the parents and/or the wider family,
(v) specific rehabilitation programme (if necessary).

The psychopharmacological aspects of treatment are clearly important, but are beyond the scope of this book.

Individual treatment

During the acute phase, medication is the most important part of treatment; however, a psychotherapeutic approach to the patient is also recommended. Whilst extensive individual sessions with the patient aiming to uncover problems or interpret symptoms, e.g. delusions, hallucinations should not be undertaken, the establishment of a trusting and supportive relationship is helpful. Interaction with the patient should be frequent but brief, and should address the problems arising in everyday life. At this stage, psychoanalytically orientated approaches to treatment are contraindicated. Guiding the patient is not only the task of doctors or psychologists, but of the entire nursing staff. The following points are important.

Education

Once the acute symptoms have receded, psychotherapy should aim to educate the child or adolescent in what happened to him. Attempts should be made to help the patient to understand and cope with his psychotic symptoms to some degree. This should be undertaken in a stepwise manner which is not too emotionally stressful for the patient. Therapy should be supportive rather than attempt to reveal unconscious conflicts. Ideally, the patient should learn to cope with stressors in a way which does not precipitate a relapse. Stressors which commonly coincide with relapse include love affairs, fear of examinations, misjudgement of one's own abilities resulting in excessive self-imposed demands, and disagreements in the family involving autonomy or independence.

Cognitive restructuring and motivational therapy

Individual sessions with the patient may concentrate on coping facilities used to deal with specific residual sympotms, e.g. cognitive disturbance or medication-resistant hallucinations. They may also be used to promote better compliance with medication and other treatment or rehabilitation aims. It is also important to address issues relating to relapse prevention with the patient, such that new symptoms are recognized as being part of the disorder and brought to the attention of the therapist. Whilst insight is almost inevitably somewhat impaired in schizophrenia, a better understanding of the problem encountered, likely precipitants and sources of help can be encouraged.

Treating secondary psychosocial problems

Schizophrenia can result in a multitude of secondary problems, ranging from difficulties in social interaction, feelings of alienation, low self-esteem, and anxiety, to the practical problems of everyday life. It is an important task of the therapist to provide explanation and support the patient and allow him to the chance of experiencing success. These three aims should be kept in mind whilst choosing an appropriate therapeutic setting. The aims apply not only to sessions with the therapist, but to treatment as a whole. This should include occupational therapy and social skills training programmes for coping with everyday life, e.g. going shopping, organizing a party, attending school, vocational training, etc.

In the psychotherapy of adolescents with schizophrenia, the following aspects need to be considered (Werner and Mattejat, 1993).

- The relationship between the therapist and the patient should be characterized by personal presence and availability. The therapist should be caring, but able to state his views clearly and be assertive when necessary. At the same time, an appropriate distance must be maintained in the relationship. The patient should be approached politely and respectfully, and should experience the therapist as a caring individual. The therapist should present himself as someone with whom the adolescent can openly discuss his problems and anxieties, as well as a source of security and support.
- During therapy, the patient should have the opportunity to speak about his concerns. The therapist should discuss the issues brought up in a supportive manner. It is not advisable to reveal unconscious conflicts or offer psychoanalytic interpretations.
- The primary aim is to help the patient to cope with his most pressing symptoms. This will commonly revolve around issues such as cognitive disturbance, poor social competency, or obsessional symptoms. Behavioural techniques may also be utilized in the sessions.

Treatment approaches including the family

About 40% of adult patients with schizophrenia suffer a relapse during the first year after discharge from hospital, despite neuroleptic medication (Brown et al., 1972; Hogarty and Anderson, 1986). Relapse rates rise to 65% if psychopharmacological medication is not combined with psychotherapy and social

Table 28.2. Treatment approach and the risk of relapse in schizophrenia during the first year after discharge ($n = 103$; age: 17–55 years)

Type of treatment	Relapse rates (%)
Family therapy and long-term individual therapy	19
Social rehabilitation training and long-term medication	20
Family therapy, rehabilitation training and long-term medication	0
Long-term medication only	41

From Hogarty et al. (1986).

rehabilitation. Data from Hogarty et al. (1986) show the relationship between the treatment approach and the risk of relapse in schizophrenia (Table 28.2).

One concept developed to describe the family interactions and atmosphere is that of expressed emotions (EE). This concept comprises three essential parameters (Vaughn and Leff, 1976; Hahlweg et al., 1988).

Criticism

This includes any critical comment on the patient, either in terms of the words used, e.g. the expression of disagreement, dislike, or anger or the tone of voice used when speaking to the patient, e.g. debasing, undermining, or angry.

Hostility

This represents the degree to which the patient is made to feel rejected by family members.

Emotional over-involvement

This is the degree to which family members are emotionally involved with the patient and his life. Excessive worry or care in the sense of overprotection may contribute considerably to emotional overengagement.

Research on expressed emotions has revealed that the family atmosphere has an important influence on the course of schizophrenia, although it appears to have no relevance to the aetiology. The inclusion of the family in the treatment of schizophrenia results in a markedly reduced relapse rate. The importance of addressing these factors in order to reduce relapse is shown in Table 28.3.

The practical implication of this research is that the family of children and adolescents with schizophrenia should always be included in the treatment. Unfortunately, the use of family therapy in schizophrenia in the past, and the aetiological theories which arose from it, have resulted in family therapy being

Table 28.3. Relapse rates in studies focusing on expressed emotions (EE)

	Relapse rates %	
Type of therapy	9 or 12 months	24 months
Family therapy	8	20
Routine treatment	50	78
(Leff et al., 1982; 1985)		
Family therapy	6	17
Individual therapy	44	83
(Falloon et al., 1982, 1985)		
Patient group with high EE	33	
Control group with high EE	43	
Control group with low EE	20	
(Köttgen et al., 1984)		
Family therapy	19	32
Social competency training	20	42
Combined approach	0	25
Control group	41	66
(Hogarty et al., 1986; 1987)		
High EE		
family therapy		33
enactive	17	
symbolic	8	
educational programme only	43	
routine treatment	53	59
Low EE		
educational programme only	22	
routine treatment	20	33
(Tarrier et al., 1988; 1989)		

associated with negative connotations in relation to schizophrenia. Theories regarding 'double bind', i.e. a contradictory communication style, the 'schizophrenogenic mother' or 'psychotic families' have not been supported by recent research and it would also be an error to make the assumption that families with a schizophrenic child or adolescent in general are dysfunctional.

Collaboration with families should focus on improving the quality of communication within the family by 'psychoeducational' means. It is important to help the family with the emotionally stressful task of communicating and interacting with the patient in an appropriate manner. This has been shown conclusively to reduce the risk of relapse.

A further aim of family work is educational. The family should be advised how to deal with difficult situations and helped to develop strategies to deal with stress originating from within the family as well as external stressors. A structured treatment programme with the close family may prevent the patient from being exposed to excessive or adverse emotions from other family members. This approach is summarized in Table 28.4.

One can distinguish several different interventional levels. The emphasis and treatment aims are different in each of the three phases of therapy.

(i) The first step is to build up a trusting therapeutic relationship with the family. In the process, the family is educated and counselled about the disorder, aetiological factors, treatment options, medication and possible side effects.

(ii) The next step is supportive family therapy, aimed at preventing escalation of familial interaction, which is essential to minimize the risk of relapse. This involves interrupting the secondary interactional difficulties, conflicts, vicious circles, etc. which may have been precipitated by the psychosis, i.e. separation of symptoms from family interaction.

(iii) When the symptoms have improved and the family is no longer overly alarmed by them, additional problems may emerge. The final step involves family therapy, focusing on the patient's development and their increasing personal and emotional independence. This leads to attempts to reduce the patient's dependence on his parents, and facilitates his or her gradual detachment from the family. It is important, but often difficult for parents, to modify their view of the patient, releasing the adolescent from the patient role, and permit the adolescent to take more self-responsibility.

Rehabilitation

About 40% of children and/or adolescents with schizophrenia are unable to resume school or work and are prevented from returning home after discharge from hospital because of the severity of their symptoms or conflicts in the family. Such patients require a rehabilitation programme which aims to reintegrate patients over a period of 1–2 years. The programme should also include steps towards reintegration at school or at work. Programmes should be planned individually for each patient, taking into account their specific problems. One such rehabilitation programme has been established and evaluated (Martin and Remschmidt, 1983, 1984; Martin, 1991). Results showed that this type of rehabilitation programme is helpful and appropriate for the various

Table 28.4. Collaboration with the family of children and adolescents with schizophrenia

Interventional plane	Problems (focus)	Main aims of treatment	Typical techniques
(i) Family counselling (counselling of parents)	• Lack of information, uncertainty, hopelessness, guilty feelings	• Establishing a trusting therapeutic relationship	• Give support and orientation through information • Give positive connotations
(ii) Supportive and structuring family therapy	• Interaction between the symptoms and family communication (symptoms and malignant interactional patterns reinforce one another)	• Controlling symptoms (detaching the symptoms from family interaction) • Interrupting secondary interactional difficulties (secondary prevention)	• Clear agreements • Behavioural tasks • Behavioural 'contracts' ('directive' interventions)
(iii) Continued family therapy supporting the patient's development	• Relational patterns and family disagreements which impede development	• Expanding the available options of decision and action: supporting developmental potential	• Reframing • Paradoxical intervention and provocation techniques ('indirect techniques') • Conflict solving • Non-verbal and actional techniques

From Mattejat (1997).

Table 28.5. Treatment programme for children and adolescents with schizophrenia. The steps include inpatient treatment and rehabilitation

Acute phase (inpatient treatment)	Phase of remittance (inpatient treatment)	First rehabilitation phase (residential home)	Second rehabilitation phase (residential group)
Admission	Continued inpatient treatment	Depot medication Group therapy	Depot medication Increasing independence in the group
Neuroleptic medication Prompt activation Individual therapy and nursing care Occupational therapy Maintenance of contact with the family Group activities (if possible)	Neuroleptic medication Compulsory ward activities School attendance or individual instruction 'Reality training' Attention training, activities outside the hospital premises, increasing independence, home leave, family sessions	Individual therapy Practising daily routine School attendance 'Reality training'	Self-catering School attendance, semiskilled occupation or apprenticeship
Aim: Influence on acute symptoms, prevention of withdrawal and chronification	Aim: Reintegration within the hospital setting	Aim: Reintegration in a larger community, learning to adapt to reality, occupational orientation	Aim: Self-catering, occupational development

From Martin and Remschmidt (1983).

needs of adolescents with schizophrenia. Patients are helped through gradual steps to reattend school or work, and eventually return to the family environment or establish independent living.

A typical treatment programme for children and adolescents with schizophrenia is summarized in Table 28.5. It includes aspects of treatment, from the inital steps required in the acute phase through to the rehabilitation phase. The structure of our rehabilitation facility is shown in Fig. 28.1.

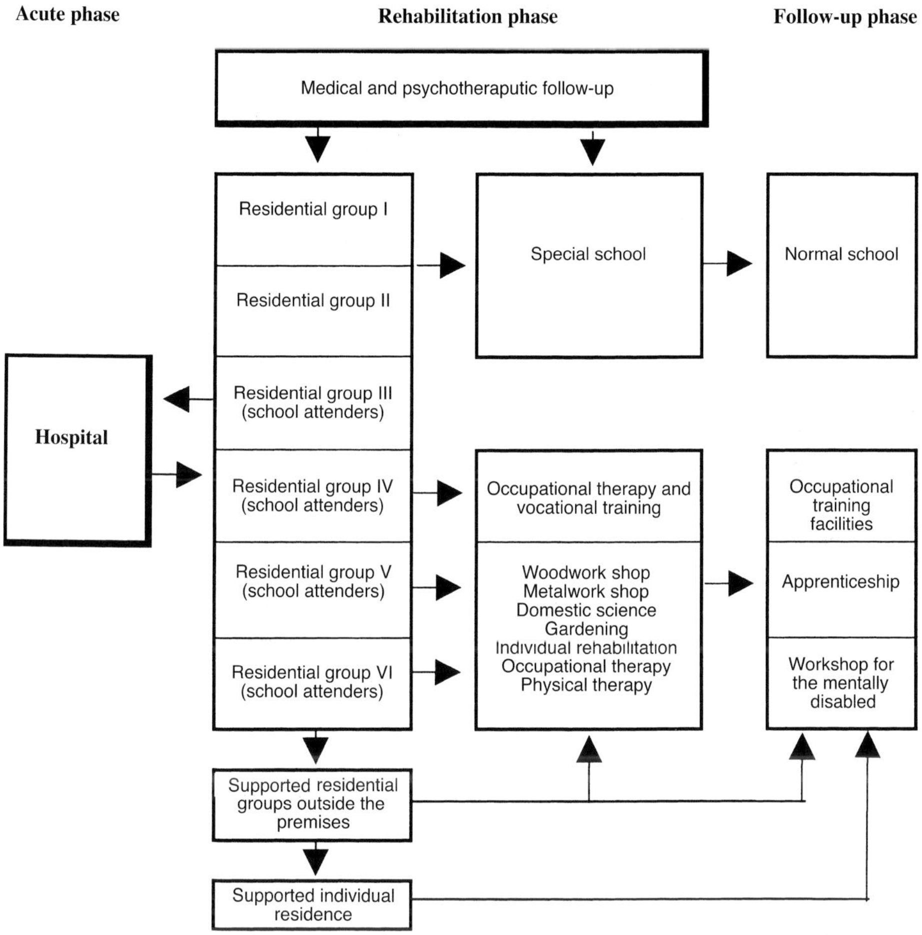

Fig. 28.1. Organization of a rehabilitation facility for children and adolescents with schizophrenia ('Leppermuhle', in Buseck, near Giessen, Germany).

It is important to consider a number of factors before initiating a rehabilitation programme.

- Negative symptoms often persist even after the initial symptoms have subsided, thus preventing discharge from hospital. Typical negative symptoms include: a loss of initiative, social withdrawal, blunting of emotional response, impaired social functioning, persistence of mild thought disorder, attention deficits, impaired concentration. The persistence of these symptoms are likely to prevent the patient from continuing school or work.
- An unstable course, with risk of relapse or residual symptoms is also an

indication for rehabilitation treatment. This applies to patients, in whom mild symptoms such as fragmentary delusional experiences, delusion of control, or hallucinations, persist despite extended inpatient treatment.

- Familial risk factors for relapse such as severe interpersonal problems within the family or psychiatric illness of close relatives, e.g. addiction, personality disorder, psychosis also contribute to an increased risk of relapse and can be considered an indication for rehabilitation.
- Other factors may also be indications for a rehabilitation programme, such as poor compliance with medication or follow-up appointments, co-morbidity (especially drug or alcohol dependency), or poor social integration.

Thus, rehabilitation treatment may be indicated either because of the patient, or his social environment and family. The aim of rehabilitation is to improve the remaining symptoms, and overcome the resulting social difficulties. Prior to rehabilitation, the following points should be considered (Wing, 1976).

- Assessment of the type and extent of the disability and social impairment.
- Definition of several limited treatment goals. The progress of specific treatment and the improvement of symptoms should be quantifiable by means of objective criteria.
- The treatment programme should be modified when necessary, depending on whether the goals have been attained or not. The goals may require modification over the course of treatment.

During the rehabilitation phase, children and adolescents need to be given the opportunity to cope not only with their disorder, but also to develop perspectives for the future. Psychotherapeutic help is therefore an essential part of rehabilitation treatment. After the acute psychotic symptoms have subsided, the patient needs to gradually develop a new view of himself, which incorporates experience of mental illness. In our experience, therapeutic sessions with children and adolescents with schizophrenia usually cover the following issues: the fear of losing one's identity, problems in the relationship with one's parents, particularly if symbiotic bonds are present, experiencing one's emotional deficits, coping with challenges in the future, the future in general, low self-esteem, particularly in connection with the mental illness, dealing with aggressive thoughts or impulses, and problems concerning partnership and sexuality. During this treatment phase, individual therapy sessions aim to determine to what extent the patient has recovered from the acute illness, continue to lead towards more reality, and support in coping with everyday situations.

During the long-term treatment of children and adolescents with schizophrenia, it is important to remember that excessive social stimulation may result in relapse, whilst insufficient social stimulation encourages secondary negative symptoms, which impede the progress of social reintegration. It is therefore advisable to commence psychoeducational steps, social skills training, communication training, problem coping training, and cognitive therapy at an early stage, but to pace this gradually so as not to overburden the patient. Such treatment is best undertaken by means of a multidimensional approach, which includes amongst others a psychotherapeutic technique and medication. The individual elements combined in this approach have been evaluated and are considered effective in the treatment of patients with schizophrenia (Alford and Correia, 1994; Harding and Zahniser, 1994; Hodel and Brenner, 1994; Kienzle and Martinius, 1992; Mari and Streiner, 1994; Resch, 1994; Rund, 1994; Rund et al., 1994).

The most important components of treatment have been outlined by Kienzle (1994).

(i) Optimizing cognitive differentiation: improving attention, concentration and the forming of ideas and concepts; improving abstract thought and differentiating language; influencing the ability to think and learn.
(ii) Improving social perception using visual therapy aids, e.g. pictures of situations in which a variety of effects plays a role.
(iii) Influencing verbal communication skills, e.g. by improving group interaction – active listening, appropriate interaction, communication techniques.
(iv) Improving social skills by means of a social competency training programme, e.g. role play.
(v) Conveying interpersonal problem-solving skills to enable the patient to cope with various difficult situations and to develop appropriate problem-solving techniques.

Case report

A 16-year-old female patient presented to our outpatient department for assessment. Her mother reported that her daughter had been increasingly 'confused' during the past few weeks, had given 'curious replies' to questions, suffered from sleep disturbance, and was unable to concentrate. Because of this behaviour, the patient had lost her work as an apprentice in a bakery. She had asked customers strange questions, was often late, and made errors when giving change. She had not slept the 2 nights before assessment, but had walked about the house talking to herself. She reported that she had seen the actress Grace Kelly in her parents' house.

Acute paranoid schizophrenia was suspected, and the patient was admitted to an inpatient unit for treatment.

There was no relevant family history for any relevant disorders. The patient's developmental history was normal, except that she had developed anxiety in connection with school and secondary night enuresis shortly after beginning the fourth year of primary school.

Findings

Physical examination including detailed neurological assessment, was normal. EEG and cranial CT were also normal. Two weeks after admission to hospital, whilst on neuroleptic medication, standardized psychological tests were performed. An assessment of intelligence and personality traits revealed several typical cognitive deficits and abnormalities: low stress tolerance, rapid exhaustibility, impaired concentration, thought disorder, and IQ test (WISC) results well below the average.

The preliminary diagnosis of acute paranoid schizophrenia was confirmed by observation of her behaviour in the inpatient setting and psychopathological assessments.

Course

The patient was initially treated with 30 mg of haloperidol and 120 mg of levomepromazine per day, commencing the day of admission. The delusional symptoms and hallucinations persisted under this regimen, the patient continued to be restless and overactive, with a persistent sleep disturbance. After the diagnosis was confirmed, sessions were undertaken with her parents. They were provided with information about the disorder, the possible course, treatment options and the prognosis. During the sessions, the patient's father expressed great shame and guilt about his daughter's disorder. These feelings were addressed on several occasions. The patient's mother considered the bond between herself and her daughter symbiotic and over-protective. Eventually, a trusting relationship was established between the therapist and both parents. Supportive family therapy was commenced, initially without the patient. As a result of their reduced distress, the parents were able to modify their interaction and behaviour towards the patient during the regular visits and periods of home leave. They complied fully with therapy and were able to discuss their thoughts and feelings freely, so that recurring anxieties could be addressed appropriately.

Unfortunately, the course of the illness caused problems. A relatively high medication dose was administered for several weeks, resulting in severe extrapyramidal side effects (tremor, acathisia), but despite this, the sleep disturbance persisted. Over the course of 4 months the neuroleptic medication was changed several times. The extrapyramidal side effects persisted, and the patient became increasingly depressed. This resulted in social withdrawal and severe negative symptoms. After 16 weeks, medication was changed to the atypical neuroleptic, clozapine. The dosage was gradually increased to 450 mg of clozapine per day.

During the first few weeks of treatment, short individual sessions were held with the patient, she attended occupational therapy for 45 minues four times per week, and individual activities were offered in order to motivate the patient to attend group activities and resume her previous hobbies. It proved very difficult to motivate the patient because of the persistent positive symptoms and negative symptoms such as social withdrawal and apathy.

Fortunately, the atypical neuroleptic medication resulted in the resolution of extrapyramidal side effects. The positive symptoms also improved rapidly. The patient was soon able to attend the hospital school, where she participated in group activities and attended occupational therapy for 1 hour every day. She also participated in a neuropsychological treatment technique aimed at training attention and concentration.

In the course of the following 10–12 weeks of treatment, the neuropsychological impairment, i.e. attention deficit, concentration difficulties, low stress tolerance persisted, despite improvements in the thought disorder and delusions. About 6 months after admission, rehabilitation treatment was recommended. The pros and cons of further treatment outside the family were discussed in family sessions, and the patient and her parents were asked to visit an appropriate rehabilitation facility. The whole family agreed, and she was soon transferred to the rehabilitation facility. Here, the atypical neuroleptic medication was continued, and she began rehabilitation in the facility's domestic science section. Her work tolerance increased gradually from 2 hours a day to a whole day. Family therapy sessions continued once every 2 weeks. The patient lived in a residential group together with eight other adolescents with schizophrenia. Regular group activities were undertaken to improve the patients' social and communicational deficits, and she also attended a special therapy programme aimed at improving the persistent cognitive deficits (Kienzle and Martinius, 1992).

Neuropsychological tests undertaken during hospital and rehabilitation treatment showed that the severe impairments present initially improved markedly over the course of rehabilitation. The patient eventually became independent enough to take up vocational training outside the rehabilitation facility, and 1 year after admission she was discharged back to her family environment. This step was carefully prepared, the parents had continued support through a parent group, and follow-up was arranged once a month for 2 years. The neuroleptic dosage was eventually reduced to 200 mg of clozapine per day. There has been no full-blown relapse during the 7-year follow-up, although an attempt to further reduce the dosage resulted in mood fluctuations, fleeting delusions of control and deterioration of cognitive abilities.

The patient has now become engaged to be married and is living together with her partner, an administrative employee. She successfully completed her vocational training and now works full-time. The couple wish to have children. Therefore, the risks of discontinuing the neuroleptic medication will need to be discussed with the couple.

REFERENCES

Alford, B. A. and Correia, C. J. (1994). Cognitive therapy of schizophrenia. Theory and empirical status. *Behavior Therapy*, **25**, 17–33.

American Psychiatric Association (APA) (1994). *DSM-IV. Diagnostic and statistical manual of mental disorders*, 4th edn. Washington, DC: APA.

Andreasen, N. C. (1982). Negative symptoms in schizophrenia: definition and reliability. *Archives of General Psychiatry*, **39**, 784–8.

Angst, J., Stassen, H. H. and Woggon, B. (1989). Effects of neuroleptics on positive and negative symptoms and the deficit state. *Psychopharmacology*, **99**, 41–6.

Bettes, B. A. and Walker, E. (1987). Positive and negative symptoms in psychotic and other psychiatrically disturbed children. *Journal of Child Psychology and Psychiatry*, **28**, 555–68.

Brown, G. W., Birley, J. L. T. and Wing, J. K. (1972). Influence of family life on the course of schizophrenic disorders. A replication. *British Journal of Psychiatry*, **121**, 241–58.

Burg, L. and Kerbeshian, J. (1987). A North Dakota prevalence study of schizophrenia presenting in childhood. *Journal of the American Academy of Child and Adolescent Psychiatry*, **26**, 347–50.

Crow, T. J. (1980). Molecular pathology of schizophrenia: more than one disease process? *British Medical Journal*, **280**, 66–8.

Dohrenwend, B. P., Shrout, P. E., Link, B. G. and Skodol, A. E. (1987). Social and psychological risk factors for episodes of schizophrenia. In *Search for the causes of schizophrenia*, ed. H. Häfner, W. F. Gattaz and W. Janzarik. Berlin: Springer.

Falloon, I. R. H., Boyd, J. L., McGill, C. W., Razani, J., Moss, H. B. and Gilderman, A. M. (1982). Family management in the prevention of exacerbations of schizophrenia. A controlled study. *New England Journal of Medicine*, **306**, 1437–40.

Falloon, I. R. H., Boyd, J. L., McGill, C. W. et al. (1985). Family management in the prevention of morbidity of schizophrenia. Clinical outcome of a two-year longitudinal study. *Archives of General Psychiatry*, **42**, 887–96.

Gillberg, I. C., Hellgren, L. and Gillberg, C. (1993). Psychotic disorders diagnosed in adolescence. Outcome at age 30 years. *Journal of Child Psychology and Psychiatry*, **34**, 1173–85.

Hahlweg, K., Feinstein, E., Müller, U. and Dose, M. (1988). Folgerungen aus der Expressed-Emotion-Forschung für die Rückfallprophylaxe Schizophrener. In *Die Schizophrenien. Biologische und familiendynamische Konzepte zur Pathogenese*, ed. W. P. Kaschka, P. Joraschky and E. Lungershausen, pp. 201–10. Berlin: Springer.

Harding, C. M. and Zahniser, J. H. (1994). Empirical correction of seven myths about schizophrenia with implications for treatment. *Acta Psychiatrica Scandinavica*, **90**, 140–6.

Hodel, B. and Brenner, H. D. (1994). Cognitive therapy with schizophrenic patients. Conceptual basis, present state, future directions. *Acta Psychiatrica Scandinavica*, **90**, 108–15.

Hogarty, G. E. and Anderson, C. M. (1986). Eine kontrollierte Studie über Familientherapie, Training sozialer Fertigkeiten und unterstützende Chemotherapie in der Nachbehandlung Schizophrener. Vorläufige Effekte auf Rezidive und Expressed Emotion nach einem Jahr. In *Bewältigung der Schizophrenie*, ed. W. Böker and H. D. Brenner (Hrsg.). Bern: Huber.

Hogarty, G. E., Anderson, C. M., Reiss, D. J. et al. and the EPICS research group (1986). Family psychoeducation, social skills training and maintenance chemotherapy in the aftercare treatment of schizophrenia. *Archives of General Psychiatry*, **43**, 633–42.

Hogarty, G. E., Anderson, C. M. and Reiss, D. J. (1987). Family psychoeducation, social skills training and medication in schizophrenia. *Psychopharmacological Bulletin*, **23**, 12–13.

Kanner, L. (1943). Autistic disturbances of affective contact. *Nervous Child*, **2**, 177–25.

Kanner, L. (1957). *Child psychiatry*, 3rd edn. Oxford: Blackwell.

Karno, M. and Norquist, G. S. (1989). Schizophrenia: epidemiology. In *Comprehensive textbook of psychiatry*, 5th edn, vol. 1, ed. H. I. Kaplan and B. J. Saddock, pp. 699–705. Baltimore: Williams & Wilkins.

Kay, S. R. (1991). *Positive and negative syndromes in schizophrenia. Assessment and research*. New York: Brunner-Mazel.

Kienzle, N. (1994). Kognitive Verhaltenstherapie mit schizophrenen Jugendlichen. In *Schizophrene Psychosen in der Adoleszenz*, ed. J. Martinius, pp. 109–23. Berlin: Quintessenz.

Kienzle, N. and Martinius, J.(1992). Modifikationen und Adaptationen des IPT für die Anwendung bei schizophrenen Jugendlichen. In *Integriertes psychologisches Therapieprogramm für schizophrene Patienten (IPT)*, ed. V. Roder, H. D. Brenner, N. Kienzle, B. Hodel, Weinheim: Psychologie Verlags Union.

Köttgen, C., Sonnichsen, I., Mollenhauer, K. and Jurth, R. (1984). Results of the Hamburg Camberwell family interview study I, II, III. *International Journal of Family Psychiatry* **5**, 61–94.

Krausz, M. (1990). Schizophrenie bei Jugendlichen. Eine Verlaufsuntersuchung. *Psychiatrische Praxis*, **17**, 107–14.

Krausz, M. and Müller-Thomson, T. (1993). Schizophrenia with onset in adolescence. An 11-year follow-up. *Schizophrenia Bulletin*, **19**, 831–41.

Leff, J. P., Kuipers, L., Berkowitz, R., Eberlein-Vries, R. and Sturgeon, D. (1982). A controlled study of social intervention in families of schizophrenic patients. *British Journal of Psychiatry*, **141**, 121–34.

Leff, J. P., Kuipers, L., Berkowitz, R. and Sturgeon, D. (1985). A controlled study of social intervention in families of schizophrenic patients. A two year follow-up. *British Journal of Psychiatry*, **146**, 594–600.

Leonhard, K. (1986). *Aufteilung der endogenen Psychosen und ihre differenzierte Ätiologie*. 2nd edn. Berlin: Akademie-Verlag.

Mari, J. D. and Streiner, D. L. (1994). An overview of family interventions and relapse on schizophrenia. Meta-analysis of research findings. *Psychological Medicine*, **24**, 565–78.

Martin, M. (1991). *Der Verlauf der Schizophrenie im Jugendalter unter Rehabilitationsbedingungen*. Stuttgart: Enke.

Martin, M. and Remschmidt, H. (1983). Ein Nachsorge- und Rehabilitationsprojekt für jugendliche Schizophrene. *Zeitschrift für Kinder- und Jugendpsychiatrie*, **11**, 234–42.

Martin, M. and Remschmidt, H. (1984). Rehabilitationsbehandlung jugendlicher Schizophrener. In *Psychotherapie mit Kindern, Jugendlichen und Familien*, ed. H. Remschmidt. Stuttgart: Enke.

Mattejat, F. (1997). Familien- und Systemtherapie. In *Kinder- und Jugendpsychiatrie Systematisch*, ed. U. Kñlker, F. Mattejat and M. Schulte-Markwort, pp. 167–74. Bremen: Uni Med.

Remschmidt, H. (1988a). Die Entwicklung und ihre Varianten in der Adoleszenz. In *Psychiatrie der Gegenwart*, 3rd edn, vol. 7, ed. K. P. Kisker, M. Lauter, I. E. Meyer and E. Strömgren, pp. 291–316. Berlin: Springer.

Remschmidt, H. (1988b). Schizophrene Psychosen im Kindesalter. In *Psychiatrie der Gegenwart*, 3rd edn, vol. 7, ed. K. P. Kisker, M. Lauter, I. E. Meyer and E. Strömgren, pp. 89–117. Berlin: Springer.

Remschmidt, H. (1992*a*). *Adoleszenz. Entwicklung und Entwicklungskrisen*. Stuttgart: Thieme.

Remschmidt, H. (1992*b*). *Psychiatrie der Adoleszenz*. Stuttgart: Thieme.

Remschmidt, H. (ed.) (2001). *Schizophrenia in children and adolescents*. Cambridge: Cambridge University Press.

Remschmidt, H. and Martin, M. (1992). Die Therapie der Schizophrenie im Jugendalter. *Deutsches Ärzteblatt*, **89**, A387–A396.

Remschmidt, H., Schulz, E. and Martin, M. (1992). Die Behandlung schizophrener Psychosen in der Adoleszenz mit Clozapin (Leponex). In *Clozapin. Pharmakologie und Klinik eines atypischen Neuroleptikums*, ed. D. Naber and F. Müller-Spahn, pp. 99–119. Stuttgart: Schattauer.

Remschmidt, H., Martin, M., Schulz, E., Gutenbrunner, C. and Fleischhaker, C. (1991). The concept of positive and negative schizophrenia in child and adolescent psychiatry. In *Negative versus positive schizophrenia*, ed. A. Marneros, N. C. Andreasen and M. T. Tsuang, pp. 219–42. Berlin: Springer.

Remschmidt, H., Schulz, E., Martin, M., Warnke, A. and Trott, G-E. (1994). Childhood onset schizophrenia. History of the concept and recent studies. *Schizophrenia Bulletin*, **20**, 727–45.

Resch, F. (1994). Psychotherapeutische und soziotherapeutische Aspekte bei schizophrenen Psychosen des Kindes- und Jugendalters. *Zeitschrift für Kinder- und Jugendpsychiatrie*, **22**, 275–84.

Rund, B. R. (1994). Cognitive dysfunctions and psychosocial treatment of schizophrenics. Research of the past and perspectives on the future. *Acta Psychiatrica Scandinavica*, **90**, 9–16.

Rund, B. R., Moe, L., Sollien, T. et al. (1994). The Psychosis Project. Outcome and cost-effectiveness of a psychoeducational treatment programme for schizophrenic adolescents. *Acta Psychiatrica Scandinavica*, **89**, 211–18.

Schmidt, M. H. and Blanz, B. (1992). Behandlungsverlauf und Katamnesen von 122 Psychosen in der Adoleszenz. In *Endogene Psychosyndrome und ihre Therapie im Kindes- und Jugendalter. Psychiatriehistorische, entwicklungspsychiatrische, psychopathologische, katamnestische, humangenetische, prognostische, psychotherapeutische und psychopharmakologische Aspekte*, ed. G. Nissen, pp. 163–77. Bern: Huber.

Schulz, E., Martin, M. and Remschmidt, H. (1994). Zur Verlaufsdynamik schizophrener Erkrankungen in der Adoleszenz. *Zeitschrift für Kinder- und Jugendpsychiatrie*, **22**, 262–74.

Tarrier, N., Barrowclough, C., Vaughn, C. E. et al. (1988). The community management of schizophrenia. A controlled trial of a behavioural intervention with families to reduce relapse. *British Journal of Psychiatry*, **153**, 532–42.

Tarrier, N., Barrowclough, C., Vaughn, C. et al. (1989). Community management of schizophrenia. A two-year follow-up of a behavioural intervention with families. *British Journal of Psychiatry*, **154**, 625–8.

Vaughn, C. E. and Leff, J. P. (1976). The influence of family social factors on the course of psychiatric illness. *British Journal of Psychiatry*, **129**, 125–37.

Volkmar, F. R. (ed.) (1996). *Psychoses and pervasive developmental disorders in childhood and adolescence*. Washington, DC: American Psychiatric Press.

Weiner, I. B. (1982). *Child and adolescent psychopathology*. New York: Wiley.

Werner, W. and Mattejat, E. (1993). *Psychotherapie in der Langzeitbehandlung schizophrener Jugendlicher*. In *Gefährdung der kindlichen Entwicklung*, ed. F. Poustka and U. Lehmkuhl, pp. 251–5. München: Quintessenz.

Wing, J. K. (1976). Eine praktische Grundlage für die Soziotherapie bei Schizophrenie. In *Therapie, Rehabilitation und Prävention schizophrener Erkrankungen*, ed. G. Huber. Stuttgart: Schattauer.

World Health Organization (WHO) (1992). *The ICD-10 classification of mental and behavioural disorders. Clinical descriptions and diagnostic guidelines*. Geneva: WHO.

29

Conduct disorders, antisocial behaviour, delinquency

Beate Herpertz-Dahlmann

Definition and classification

The terms conduct disorder and antisocial behaviour are used to describe behaviour which deviates from generally accepted social norms, whereas the term delinquency is used to describe breaches of law. These definitions cover a wide spectrum of behavioural disorders ranging from frequent arguing, lying, running away and playing truant, through to violent crime (Sholevar, 1995; Quay and Hogan, 1999).

ICD-10 (WHO, 1992) distinguishes six types of 'conduct disorder' (F91). These are: 'conduct disorder confined to the family context' (F91.0), 'socialized conduct disorder' (F91.1), 'unsocialized conduct disorder' (F91.2), 'oppositional defiant disorder' (F91.3) and two remaining categories for 'other' and 'unspecified' conduct disorders.

F91.0 and F91.3 most frequently occur in younger children and may have a better prognosis. F91.1 and F91.2 are determined by the nature of the child's or adolescent's bonding, rather than whether the antisocial behaviour occurs alone or in a group.

Conduct disorders may also be classified under other diagnostic categories, such as 'hyperkinetic conduct disorder' (F90.1) and 'mixed disorders of conduct and emotions' (F92). Because of their specific features, these disorders usually require a different approach to treatment.

Epidemiology

Conduct disorders are common in childhood and adolescence. Depending on the sample, the reported incidence of conduct disorder ranges from 5 to 25% (Malmquist, 1991). One study (Remschmidt and Walter, 1989) which included an entire clinical sample (all in- and outpatients from a rural area with a total population of 450 000) found conduct disorder to be the most common diagnosis (20%) among 12–17-year-old patients.

Aetiology

The aetiology of conduct disorders and antisocial behaviour is multifactorial and comprises biological, psychological and social factors (Stoff et al., 1997; Quay and Hogan, 1999). It is important to consider all aetiological factors, because they each suggest different treatment approaches, e.g. self-control programmes, family therapy, steps addressing the social environment.

The biological causes include genetic, sex-related, organic and neuropsychological factors. Adoption studies have demonstrated the role of genetic factors. A Swedish study followed-up 862 illegitimate boys who were adopted by non-relatives. Individuals with one delinquent but non-alcoholic, biological parent were at a 1.9 times greater risk of delinquency than individuals from the control group (Cloninger et al., 1982). The higher prevalence of antisocial behaviour in boys suggests additional sex-related causes of conduct disorder. Several studies have found that serum levels of androstendione and testosterone correlate with antisocial and aggressive behaviour (Susman et al., 1987; Olweus et al., 1988).

Neuropsychological impairment found in conduct disorder involves memory, attention, abstract thought, planning ability, concentration and logical thought. Dyslexia has been found to be more common among delinquents than among normal individuals (Weinschenk, 1985). In American studies, the prevalence of specific learning disorders in delinquent adolescents was 25–26% compared to 7–10% in the normal population (Keilitz et al., 1979).

The aetiologically relevant psychological factors include cognitive distortion and dysfunctional thoughts. In comparison to a control group of normal boys, Guerra and Slaby (1989) found that aggressive boys are more likely to view their social problems as a result of the adverse behaviour of others, to find fewer and less effective solutions when conflicts occur, and were unable to anticipate the sequelae of their aggressive behaviour.

Factors suggesting psychopathology in the family (alcoholism, delinquency, marital discord, absent father) are more common in families of children with conduct disorder. Also typical of these families is an excessively hard or inconsistent style of upbringing, inadequate control or supervision and the acceptance of selfish and aggressive behaviour.

Socioeconomic factors such as low family income and large families also play

Table 29.1. Types of inappropriate conduct occurring during childhood and adolescence

(i)	Inappropriate conduct due to inadequate or abnormal upbringing
(ii)	Inappropriate conduct as a result of a temporary disturbance of an already unstable mental state:
	(a) situational, social, educational
	(b) as a result of temporary neglect
(iii)	Primary inappropriate conduct during adolescence
(iv)	Inappropriate conduct as a result of low intelligence, learning disorder, brain disease or other types of brain damage
(v)	Inappropriate conduct as a symptom of physical disorder
(vi)	Inappropriate conduct as a result of psychosis
(vii)	Inappropriate conduct as a result of neurotic conflict ('neurotic conduct disorder')

From Hart de Ruyter (1967).

a role in the aetiology of conduct disorders and antisocial behaviour (West and Farrington, 1973).

Differential diagnosis

Antisocial or oppositional behaviour may occur in a number of other psychiatric disorders or may be related to other medical, social or familial factors (Table 29.1). Treatment should be guided by these factors.

When abnormal upbringing, neglect or serious developmental issues play a role (points (i) and (iv) in Table 29.1), the course tends to be chronic. Thus, unless the primary issue can be assessed, therapy is unlikely to cause significant improvement, whereas when symptoms arise as a result of adolescent conflicts or temporary issues (points (ii) and (iii) in Table 29.1), treatment tends to be more successful due to the important developmental aspects. When the conduct disorder is a symptom of physical disorder or psychosis, treatment naturally consists of addressing the primary physical disorder, e.g. epilepsy. Similarly, conduct disorder in dyslexic patients requires appropriate treatment of the dyslexia in addition to psychotherapy (see Chapter 24). Likewise, neurotic conflicts must be addressed according to the needs of the individual patient.

Treatment

Many approaches to treating antisocial or oppositional behaviour have been developed (Sholevar, 1995; Stoff et al., 1997; Quay and Hogan, 1999), although no single technique has conclusively been shown to be effective (Kazdin, 1987; Lewis, 1991). This is probably because children and adolescents with antisocial behaviour have individual vulnerability factors and usually have more than one abnormal behaviour, e.g. lying, stealing, running away. This results in a complex picture requiring a combination of several treatment techniqes (Remschmidt, 1989). The techniques commonly combined are summarized in Table 29.2.

Psychotherapeutic approaches to treatment are discussed in detail below. They may be classified as follows: (i) techniques directed at the patient, (ii) techniques directed at parents and the family, and (iii) techniques addressing the patient's environment.

Techniques directed at the patient

Techniques have been developed based on the theory that aggressive children have deficient social perception and information-processing abilities. The more ambiguous the situational conflicts are, the greater is the role which such deficits play (Dodge, 1985). Aggressive children tend to retaliate, whilst non-aggressive children tend to show some degree of understanding for the actions of peers. The cognitive deficits hypothesized to be present in antisocial children and adolescents include:

- inadequate empathy;
- narrow repertoire of options for resolving quarrels;
- poor understanding of the motives of other individuals;
- difficulty in anticipating situations in which conflicts may arise;
- poor degree of self-control;
- the tendency to focus more on their ultimate aims rather than thinking of useful intermediate steps.

Problem-solving training aims to modify social perception and the resulting behaviour in situations in which the child is provoked or frustrated. This technique is applied in the following way:

(i) The patient is helped to learn how to:
  - anticipate the interactional process (differentiated perception);
  - plan the individual steps of action (self-management);
  - develop rules and structure tasks (control of actions).

(ii) The therapist should actively encourage the process.

Table 29.2. Aims of treatment and the therapeutic techniques used to treat antisocial behaviour

	Technique	Focus	Main therapeutic processes
Techniques aimed at the patient	Individual psychotherapy	Intrapsychic bases of antisocial behaviour, particularly conflicts, and processes that were adversely affected during psychological development	A trusting therapeutic relationship is the mainstay of treatment; it should help the patient to gain some understanding of his disorder, attempt new behaviours and make corrective emotional experiences
	Group therapy	Similar to individual psychotherapy; reinforcement by peers, feedback, and empathy for the emotions of others contribute to improvement; therapy may also focus on group interaction, e.g. cohesion and leadership	Trusting relationship to the therapist and peers; group processes help the patients to develop an understanding for the experience of others and give them the opportunity to assess and correct their views and behaviours
	Behavioual therapy	Treatment is aimed at specific behavioural abnormalities; social behaviour may be trained	New behaviours are gradually developed using direct practice, role play, and behavioural modification techniques such as modelling and reinforcement; specific situational training at home and in the patient's environment, resulting in behaviour modification.
	Problem solution training	Cognitive processes and problem-solving skills are considered the basis of social interaction	Problem-solving skills are taught in steps using modelling, direct practice, repetition, role play, self-instruction training or 'internal dialogue' in order to identify prosocial problem solving strategies

	Medication	Biological factors which influence behaviour (based on empirical findings on neurotransmitters, biological cycles, and other physiological parameters which influence aggressive behaviour)	Administration of psychoactive medication to treat antisocial behaviour; use of lithium and neuroleptics because of the antiaggressive effects; more recently use of serotonin reuptake inhibitors, e.g. fluoxetine
	Inpatient treatment (residential home)	Use of several techniques during partial hospitalization or inpatient treatment	Several different therapeutic techniques; separation from the family or the usual environment in order to interrupt recurring interactional patterns
Techniques aimed at parents and the family	Family therapy	Treatment should focus on the family system as a whole rather than the patient alone: familial relationships, role functions, organization and dynamics of interaction	Communication, relationship and structure within the family; development of autonomy, problem-solving and interactional skills
	Parents' training	Interaction between the child and parents at home; particularly the child's behavioural abnomalities which are sustained or reinforced (involuntarily) by his parents' behaviour	Direct training of parents with the aim of modifying the child's abnormal behaviour; use of social learning techniques
Techniques aimed at the patient's social environment	Interventions aimed at the local environment	Local activities and treatment programs to improve social competency and encourage stable relationships	Activities encourage prosocial behaviour and the development of relationships with peers; such activities are incompatible with antisocial behaviour

Modified after Kazdin (1987).

Anticipating the actions of other individuals and recognizing one's reactions in certain situations may be practised by means of video recordings or picture stories. Role play and the practising of certain skills is more appropriately undertaken in group settings (Ross and Peterman, 1987). The therapist helps by verbalizing treatment steps, reminding the patient of self-instructions, and helping the patient to discover solutions to problems. In addition, the therapist should offer feedback by directly praising or criticizing the patient, and in certain circumstances also use mild punishments when necessary, e.g. withdrawing privileges.

This approach has been shown to be effective in clinical samples. However, it should not yet be considered a generally effective treatment for any type of antisocial behaviour. The approach is based on empirically proven theories of aggressive behaviour in children, and may eventually lead to a generally effective treatment approach.

Coie et al. (1991) used a cognitive behavioural treatment programme to treat three samples of boys from lower social classes with antisocial behaviour. The boys were treated for 1 year. The treatment programme was improved continuously, and the best results were achieved in the final sample. After the training, the boys received feedback both by peers and teachers.

Evaluation of the treatment programme undertaken by Peterman and Peterman (1993) with 5–13-year-old aggressive children showed good results which persisted for 6 months after discontinuing treatment.

Techniques directed at parents and the family

Behavioural training for parents of children with antisocial and aggressive behaviour is based on the theory that parents often involuntarily fail to emphasize the importance of appropriate social behaviour, on the one hand, whilst severely punishing antisocial behaviour, on the other (Patterson, 1982). This type of interaction between parents and children has been described as the 'reinforcement trap' (Kazdin, 1987). The child's antisocial behaviour may ultimately be reinforced by punishment: the parents are temporarily relieved when the child stops the behaviour; however, in the long run, the antisocial behaviour is even more likely to reccur.

Training programmes have been devised to help parents modify their behaviour during interactions with their child (Innerhofer and Warnke, 1980). This includes establishing rules, reinforcing adaptive behaviour (praise, rewards, token economy), making agreements, drawing up behavioural contracts, and the use of mild punishments ('time-out', withdrawal of privileges). Treatment is mainly undertaken by the parents and the therapist is not usually required to intervene with the child. The aim of treatment is to help parents to identify difficult behaviour in their children, define it, and recognize the behaviour which may be relevant for treatment. Parents are asked to use the technique at home and report results to the therapist.

Parent training has been used as a technique with children of different age groups and a variety of conduct disorders. The technique has been evaluated and shown to be effective during follow-up periods of up to 1 year. However, aggressive children seem to respond better to the treatment than children with non-aggressive conduct disorders, e.g. theft, fraud (Patterson, 1982).

Success depends on the duration of treatment (occasionally 50–60 sittings may be required), adequate comprehension and motivation in the parents, the severity of disturbed family interaction, the family's socioeconomic situation, and the social support of the child by individuals outside the family. Parent training requires a considerable amount of motivation of the parents and is not suitable for treating 'multiproblem families' (Lewis, 1991). The combination of problem solution training for the child and parent training has been shown to be effective (Kazdin et al., 1987).

In contrast to the assessment of behavioural training in parents, there is a paucity of studies on functional family therapy. The theoretical basis of this treatment approach is derived from systems theory, behavioural science and cognitive psychology. The approach is based on the assumption that the child's antisocial behaviour serves to sustain other functions in the family system, e.g. regulating closeness and distance among family members. As families with an antisocial adolescent tend to interact defensively and give one another less mutual support, treatment should focus on direct communication, positive mutual reinforcement, achieving constructive agreements and solution-seeking together. Functional family therapy requires a considerable degree of cooperation from all family members.

Techniques addressing the patient's social environment

Such techniques are intended to facilitate the transfer of the progress made during individual or group psychotherapy to the patient's usual social setting. They may also help to reinforce prosocial behaviour by giving the patient the opportunity to learn by imitating. As opposed to treatment in institutions, in this approach adolescents are not put together with other disturbed adolescents, but rather are integrated into a group of normal adolescents by way of group activities. In a study of 150 adolescents with conduct disorder undertaken by Feldman et al. (1983), the best results were obtained by experienced therapists using behavioural therapy methods in 'mixed' groups, i.e. adolescents with and without conduct disorders.

Techniques addressing the social environment have been used successfully to prevent antisocial behaviour in high-risk groups.

Case report

The treatment of a patient with antisocial behaviour using a combination of several of the techniques explained above is reported here.

Nine-year-old Thomas presented for assessment at the outpatient clinic. He had been adopted when he was 10 days old. As far as was known, pregnancy and birth had been without complications. As an infant, Thomas had been rather restless and was described as a difficult toddler. He had difficulties in settling into kindergarten, and this was even more marked when he started school. At the slightest irritation he would be abusive and aggressive, he was frequently oppositional, and his behaviour was often felt to be inappropriate and childish. After disagreements, he would withdraw for hours at a time. He was reported to have had no friends.

Psychological assessment revealed normal intelligence. Thomas drew a picture portraying himself and his family as animals. This proved to be revealing: Thomas saw his father as being weak and his mother as excessively aggressive and rejecting. He viewed his parents' relationship as tense. In the picture he portrayed himself as a turtle in its shell, standing between his parents. Thomas referred to himself as 'the worst of all monstrosities'. Personality testing revealed a tendency to overestimate his own capacity, and a tendency to avoid social contact. In the clinical interview he expressed the wish 'not to have a cruel heart, and to be able to love other people'. Because of the severity of symptoms, he was admitted to our day-hospital for treatment.

Thomas soon began to show the behaviour described by his parents. A behaviour schedule was drawn up for his time at the hospital school (Fig. 29.1). It was agreed that Thomas would earn one sticker for each morning he was not aggressive towards teachers or peers, e.g. quarreling with his neighbour, calling the teacher names. According to the contract drawn up between himself, the therapist, and his parents (Fig. 29.2), Thomas could exchange the points for specific rewards and privileges, e.g. going for a boat ride, buying a new toy car.

After school, Thomas was assigned to a small group where he could practise, for example: reacting to provocative behaviour, permitting others to finish with what they have to say, and agreeing on the rules of a game. Then, the therapist discussed the patient's behaviour using video recordings of the group situation. In individual sessions, problem-solving strategies were developed with the aid of video recordings, role play and discussions of day-to-day conflicts. Thomas was asked to think of solutions to a problem, go through the necessary steps, and consider the conse-

Behaviour schedule

	Monday	Tuesday	Wednesday	Thursday	Friday
Week 1	☺	☺			
Week 2		☺		☺	
Week 3		☺			☺
Week 4	☺	☺	☺		☺

I called my teacher by his/her proper name.
I spoke during lessons only after I was asked.
I got up from my chair only with permission.
I was kind to the other children.

Fig. 29.1. The patient's behavioural schedule for school.

quences and the effect they may have on other individuals. A short dialogue from an individual therapy session illustrates this approach (T. = Thomas; Ther. = therapist):
T.: 'Petra [a nurse] said that I messed up the play room and asked me to tidy it up. She was really annoyed. But I didn't use the room!'
Ther.: 'What are you going to do now?'
T.: 'I'm going to tell her that I didn't use the room, so I'm not going to tidy it up.'
Ther.: 'Well done! You didn't have a tantrum. I believe you when you say you didn't use the room, but perhaps Petra didn't believe you, because last week you did mess up the play room.'
T. [thoughtfully]: 'I could tell her that it wasn't me, but still help her to tidy it up.'
Ther.: 'What do you think Petra would say?'
T.: 'I think she would be glad. Perhaps next time she won't get annoyed with me.'
In addition to individual therapy, the parents were asked to participate in an intensive parent training programme. In particular, the patient's father learnt to be more assertive and react to Thomas' behaviour with praise or punishment, e.g. 'time-out' where appropriate. This relieved the patient's mother of a great amount of responsibility, enabling her to relinquish her exposed and dominant role within the family. This had a beneficial effect on her relationship with Thomas.

Eventually, Thomas was able to return to his usual school. Despite several relapses, his behaviour is sufficiently stable for him to continue there. He is still being treated regularly on an outpatient basis.

Delinquency

According to police reports, about 5% of all criminal suspects are children. The most common offence in children is theft, followed by burglary, damage to

Contract

I will try to keep the following rules:

Rules

1. I will call my teacher by his/her proper name.
2. I will speak during lessons only after I have been asked.
3. I will get up from my chair only with permission.
4. I will be kind to the other children.

If I manage to keep these rules for one whole lesson, my teacher Mr/Ms .... will give me a ☺. When I have collected 10 stickers, I can choose a reward.

Rewards include:

- going for a boat ride
- watching TV till 10 pm on Saturday
- buying a new toy car.

____

Child Mother/father

____

Teacher Therapist

Fig. 29.2. The contract which was drawn up together with the therapist, the patient and his parents.

property, assault, and arson. In adolescence, theft and burglary are the most common offences, followed by damage to property, assault, drug offences, public nuisance, and sexual offences (Remschmidt, 1992).

All the approaches mentioned above may also be used to treat delinquency. Because delinquency is frequently the result of conduct disorder gradually developing over the course of several years, the effect of therapy is usually limited. Therapeutic success depends on the individual, his family and the institutions involved in dealing with the delinquent adolescent.

Neurotic delinquency is an exception, the treatment of which is outlined in the following case report.

Case report

A 20-year-old man, Peter, presented for expert opinion in a court case. During the previous 6 months he had been apprehended for driving without a licence, grievous bodily harm, and interference with road traffic. Recently, he had been charged with theft and actual bodily harm to a witness. A youth welfare office report stated that he had expressed a generally pessimistic attitude and felt hopeless regarding his future. His delinquency could be understood in terms of his pessimistic attitude towards life in general.

Peter's history revealed that his father had committed suicide when he was 7 years old. Since that time his mother has suffered from alcoholism. Peter recalled that he had been his father's favourite child. He had been spoiled and given everything he wanted. His relationship with his mother had always been difficult.

When questioned about the theft, Peter was unable to explain his behaviour, although he realized that this did not improve his situation. He said that he had felt 'compelled to commit the theft and be caught in the very act'. He believed the offence was a result of the difficult relationship with his mother, and that he wanted to punish himself by being caught.

Psychological tests and mental state examination revealed that Peter had numerous mental and psychosomatic complaints. There was evidence of mental distress, low self-esteem, marked anxiety, and a tendency to depressive thoughts.

The conclusion of the assessment was that Peter had had a difficult early life, experiencing frequent conflicts and losses. This had led to a profound sense of insecurity, identity conflicts, the tendency to form inappropriate or insecure relationships and recurring feelings of worthlessness, hopelessness and depression.

This type of delinquency requires intensive psychotherapeutic input, ideally as client-centred counselling or individual psychodynamic-orientated psychotherapy.

Evaluation

It is beyond the scope of this book to discuss the outcome of individual techniques by which delinquency can be treated. Generally, however, the literature is not very encouraging. In a review (Lab and Whitehead, 1988) of studies undertaken between 1957 and 1984, about 50% reported no, or only a minor improvement of relapse rates with respect to delinquent behaviour. These results suggest that therapists and society will need to be content with modest improvements. Under these circumstances it would seem more appropriate to consider delinquency a chronic disorder requiring long-term treatment (Kazdin, 1987; Remschmidt, 1989).

Some studies have, however, demonstrated benefits of treatment. Gordon et al. (1988) studied 27 delinquents who received behavioural therapy together with their family in the home environment. Therapeutic success was determined by the number and severity of offences committed by the adolescents over the following $2\frac{1}{2}$ years. The group was compared with 27 delinquents who had received probationary sentences and were offered no treatment. Of those who received behavioural therapy, only 11% suffered relapse, compared to 67% of the group without treatment.

When assessing the therapeutic success of social training programmes in an outpatient setting, it is important to remember that the common observation period of 1 year is usually insufficient to detect any change in patients' problem-solving capacity (Busch et al., 1986). It is also open to discussion what measures should be used to assess the outcome of treatment methods. Over longer periods of follow-up, it may be more appropriate not only to look at relapse rates, but also at positive changes such as the commencement and completion of vocational training or employment.

REFERENCES

Busch, M., Hartmann, G., and Mehlich, N. (1986). *Soziale Trainingskurse im Rahmen des Jugendgerichtsgesetzes*, pp. 167–70. Bonn: Bundesministerium der Justiz.

Cloninger, C. R., Sigvardsson, S. and Bohman, M. (1982). Predisposition to petty criminality in Swedish adoptees II. Cross-fostering analysis of gene-environment interaction. *Archives of General Psychology*, **39**, 1242–7.

Coie, J. D., Underwood, M. and Lochman, J. E. (1991). Programmatic intervention with aggressive children in the school setting. In *Development and treatment of childhood aggression*, ed. D. J. Pepler and K. H. Rubin, pp. 389–410. Toronto: Erlbaum.

Dodge, K. A. (1985). Attributional bias in aggressive children. In *Advances in cognitive-behavioral research and therapy*, vol. 4, ed. P. C. Kendall, pp. 73–110. Orlando: Academic Press.

Feldman, R. A., Caplinger, T. E. and Wodarski, J. S. (1983). *The St. Louis conundrum. The effective treatment of antisocial youths*. Englewood Cliffs: Prentice Hall.

Gordon, D. A., Arbuthnot, J., Gustavson, K. E. and McGreen, P. (1988). Home-based behavioral-systems family therapy with disadvantaged juvenile delinquents. *American Journal of Family Therapy*, **16**, 243–55.

Guerra, N. G. and Slaby, R. G. (1989). Evaluative factors in social problems solving by aggressive boys. *Journal of Abnormal Child Psychology*, **17**, 209–19.

Hart de Ruyter, T. (1967). Zur Psychotherapie der Dissozialität im Jugendalter. *Jahrbuch für Jugendpsychiatrie*, **6**, 79–108.

Innerhofer, P. and Warnke, A. (1980). Elterntrainingsprogramm nach dem Münchner Trainings-

Modell. Ein Erfahrungsbericht. In *Familiäre Sozialisation und Intervention*, ed. H. Lukesch, M. Perez and K. Schneewind, pp. 417–39. Bern: Huber.

Kazdin, A. E. (1987). Treatment of antisocial behavior in children. Current status and future directions. *Psychological Bulletin*, **102**, 187–203.

Kazdin, A. E., Esveldt-Dawson, K., French, N. H. and Unis, A. S. (1987). Problem-solving skills training and relationship therapy in the treatment of antisocial child behavior. *Journal of Consulting and Clinical Psychology*, **55**, 416–24.

Keilitz, J., Zaremba, B. A. and Broder, P. K. (1979). The link between learning disabilities and juvenile delinquency. Some issues and answers. *Learning Disability Quarterly*, **2**(2), 2–11.

Lab, S. P. and Whitehead, J. T. (1988). An analysis of juvenile correctional treatment. *Crime and Delinquency*, **34**, 60–83.

Lewis, D. O. (1991). Adolescent conduct and antisocial disorders. In *Textbook of child and adolescent psychiatry*, ed. J. M. Wiener, pp. 298–308. Washington, DC: American Psychiatric Press.

Malmquist, C. P. (1991). Conduct disorder. Conceptual and diagnostic issues. In *Textbook of child and adolescent psychiatry*, ed. J. M. Wiener, pp. 279–87. Washington, DC: American Psychiatric Press.

Olweus, D., Mattsson, A. and Schalling, D. (1988). Circulating testosterone levels and aggression in adolescent males. A causal analysis. *Psychosomatic Medicine*, **50**, 261–72.

Patterson, G. R. (1982). *Coercive family process*. Castilia: Eugene.

Petermann, F. and Petermann, U. (1993). Training mit Jugendlichen. Förderung von Arbeits- und Sozialverhalten. Weinheim: Psychologie Verlags Union.

Quay, H. C. and Hogan, A. E. (ed.) (1999). *Handbook of disruptive behavior disorders*. New York: Kluwer Academic.

Remschmidt, H. (1989). Antisocial disorders, behaviour and delinquency. *Current Opinion in Psychiatry*, **2**, 490–6.

Remschmidt, H. (1992). *Psychiatrie der Adoleszenz*. Stuttgart: Thieme.

Remschmidt, H. and Walter, R. (1989). *Evaluation Kinder- und Jugendpsychiatrischer Versorgung*. Stuttgart: Enke.

Ross, A. O. and Petermann, F. (1987). *Verhaltenstherapie mit Kindern und Jugendlichen*. Stuttgart: Hippokrates.

Sholevar, G. P. (ed.) (1995). *Conduct disorders in children and adolescents*. Washington, DC: American Psychiatric Press.

Stoff, D. M., Breiling, J. and Maser, J. D. (ed.) (1997). *Handbook of antisocial behavior*. New York: Wiley.

Susman, E. J., Inoff-Germain, G. and Nottelmann, E. D. (1987). Hormones, emotional disposition, and aggressive attributes in young adolescents. *Child Deviations*, **58**, 1114–34.

Weinschenk, C. (1985). *Die erbliche Lese-Rechtschreibschwäche und ihre sozialpsychiatrischen Auswirkungen*. Bern: Huber.

West, D. J. and Farrington, D. P. (1973). *Who becomes delinquent?* London: Heineman Educational.

World Health Organization (WHO) (1992). *The ICD-10 classification of mental and behavioural disorders. Clinical descriptions and diagnostic guidelines*. Geneva: WHO.

30 Physical abuse and neglect

Helmut Remschmidt

Definition and epidemiology

The term physical abuse is used to describe non-accidental physical injury to a child or adolesent caused by a parent or other care-giver. The term child neglect describes inadequate care and attention given to a child.

In the literature, numerous related terms are used (Briere et al., 1996; Lutzker, 1998). The most common terms are: child abuse, child neglect, non-accidental trauma (NAT). The term battered child syndrome has also been used (Kempe and Helfer, 1972), emphasizing the phenomenon of child abuse in a broader social context than just the abusing individual. Recently, the term child abuse has focused on the family, because unfortunately this is the context in which child abuse occurs most commonly.

Emotional abuse by parents usually ensues from an adverse attitude towards the child who is rejected because of gender, physical appearance, or psychological abnormalities (Stutte, 1971). Forms of emotional child abuse comprise rejection (chronic denigration), social isolation, terrorizing by the threat of abandonment, chronic deprivation of attention, corruption by exposure to deviant child care practices and 'adultification', which involves making age-inappropriate demands upon the child (Finkelhor and Korbin, 1988). Emotional child abuse may reach sadistic proportions and can result in severe mental disturbance.

Child abuse is a criminal offence in most countries. About 4% of children under the age of 12 are brought to the attention of professionals or child protection agencies (Skuse and Bentovim, 1994). The number of unknown cases is presumed to be very high. About 10% of children who present for treatment of physical injury are thought to have suffered child abuse. A further 10% are thought to have been neglected (Friedman and Morse, 1974).

The prevalence of emotional child abuse is unknown. Cases of extreme abuse have been reported in the literature. In one case, a father punished his son by killing his favourite pet (a rabbit) in front of his eyes, and then forcing

Table 30.1. Types of violence and abuse which may occur in families

(i)	Violence between spouses (or partners)
	(a) violence against the spouse
	(b) rape in a marital relationship
	(c) retaliatory violence against the spouse
	(d) sequelae for children who witness marital violence
(ii)	Violence between parents and children
	(a) physical violence and neglect
	(b) emotional maltreatment
	(c) emotional abuse and incest
	(d) violence by children against their parents
(iii)	Violence between siblings
(iv)	Violence against elderly family members

From Remschmidt et al. (1990).

the child to keep the dead pet in his bed (Stutte, 1971). However, incidental reports do not allow conclusions to be drawn about the prevalence of emotional abuse in the general population.

Characteristics of the disorder and assessment

Physical child abuse and neglect, together with sexual abuse, are best understood in a context of 'violence in families', because child abuse is rarely the only manifestation of violence in the natural or reconstituted family.

The various types of violence and abuse which may occur in families are summarized in Table 30.1. These are all of considerable importance; however, here we will focus on violent behaviour of parents against children.

Abnormalities in the child

Child abuse or neglect should be suspected in the following circumstances:

- inexplicable physical complaints or signs of previous injury;
- the signs of physical or emotional neglect which cannot otherwise be explained, e.g. nutritional problems;
- abnormal anxiousness in a child;
- failure to seek protection from the parents or inappropriate attachment behaviour;
- defiant behaviour such as refusing to speak during disagreements or excessively compliant behaviour.

In some cases, the clinical picture may have the following characteristics: physical injury, delayed growth, intellectual impairment, emotional disturbance, behavioural abnormalities and impairment of personality development.

Abnormalities in the parents

As mentioned above, violence against the child is rarely the only abnormality in the family, and child abuse or neglect needs to be considered in the following instances (Kempe and Helfer, 1972):

- discrepancies between clinical findings and the history given by the child's parents;
- uncooperative or hostile behaviour of the parents;
- refusal or delayed parental consent to a physical examination of the child;
- inappropriate reaction to the child's injury;
- the suggestion of irritability or poor self-control in the parents;
- few or no visits by parents when children are in hospital;
- a history of abuse and neglect in one or both of the parents;
- inappropriately infantile marital relationship or partnership;
- a tendency towards social isolation of the family with avoidance of contact with the neighbours;
- unrealistic expectations of the child;
- frequent change of doctors or hospitals;
- alcohol abuse in the parents.

In many cases of child abuse or neglect, several of these factors are present. Parents frequently live in difficult social situations, often with concurrent unemployment, social discrimination or other social conflicts.

A detailed history can be decisive in revealing child abuse or neglect. However, for obvious reasons, histories tend to be unreliable, and in some cases may not be forthcoming at all.

Aetiology and pathogenesis

The causes of child abuse and neglect are generally considered multifactorial. In the individual case, these factors contribute to a varying degree. Empirical studies have shown that the factors summarized in Table 30.2 play a role in the aetiology of child abuse and neglect. These factors influence either the child, his parents or the family as a whole. The factors influencing the family are particularly important because they contribute to the cause of the disturbance, but also suggest an approach to treatment which is most likely to result in improvement.

Table 30.2. Factors which contribute to child abuse or put children at risk of maltreatment

Child	Parents	Family traits
Low birth weight and immaturity (30%)	History of having been abused themselves	Low income
Malformation, deformity	Physical punishment is accepted	Unemployed father
An unwanted child	Inappropriate child-rearing practice	Family with many children
Abnormal and unexpected behaviour	High rate of aggressive behaviour	Social isolation
Youngest sibling	Low rate of positive interaction, high rate of negative interaction	Disagreements and marital conflict
Stepchild	Relatively low educational level	Reconstituted family
	Psychiatric disturbance (alcoholism, psychosis, personality disorder)	
	Certain personality traits (impulsivity, irritability, tendency to withdraw, high anxiety level)	

From Remschmidt (1985).

The different theoretical approaches to understanding child abuse and neglect may be summarized in the following way:

- theories which focus on the individual patient; this approach assumes that the cause of the disturbance is with the patient's immediate care-givers (usually his parents);
- psychosocial theories, according to which the leading cause is the social environment;
- theories of interaction, which assume the interaction between several factors to be the leading cause of the disturbance.

The interactional approach is widely considered most appropriate, because it best explains the phenomenon of child abuse and neglect. Such an approach is based on the following assumptions.

Absence of an appropriate style of upbringing
Parents tend to have abnormal affective bonds. They have usually not learnt to deal with conflicts or stressful situations and have frequently themselves been abused.

Peculiarities of the abused child
Children may have characteristics, idiosyncracies or abnormalities which predispose them to being victimized (Table 30.2).

Style of social interaction which encourages abuse
Any tendency in the parents towards abuse may be attenuated by particular traits in the child. Thus, both factors may combine to reinforce one another, resulting in an escalation of violence against the child.

Tendency to violent interaction as a result of environmental factors
Such factors include emotional stress in the family, psychiatric disorders in one or both parents, low income, social isolation, etc.

Thus, child abuse and neglect tend to occur when these factors combine. Unexpected additional stress on parents or other care-givers may occur simultaneously, thus intensifying the problem. When additional problems occur, the resulting tension may cause an aggressive outbust towards the weakest member of the family, which is the child. When viewed in this way, child abuse is usually the result of parents or other care-givers being unable to react appropriately to the child's needs.

Treatment, rehabilitation and prevention

Acute intervention and indication for treatment

Those who care for abused and neglected children usually consider themselves advocates for the children. These individuals tend therefore, to take immediate legal action in cases of child abuse or neglect, such as withdrawing parents' care and custody. However, it is important to understand that such steps should be taken only as a last resort, rather than as the first step in dealing with child abuse.

In most countries, child abuse and neglect will have legal consequences. However, it is also an important role of health care professionals and child protection agencies to determine how the abuse was able to occur and identify treatment options.

For instance, it makes a great difference whether the child has been

Table 30.3. Proposals for the treatment and prevention of violence in families

(i) Legal steps
Zero tolerance of violence in general and veto of physical punishment in child-rearing
The right and obligation to report child abuse
Combination of the obligation to report child abuse and compulsory treatment
Criminalization of matrimonial rape
Improvement of extrajudicial strategies for solving conflicts
(ii) Administrative and institutional steps
Police action, e.g. crisis intervention in acute situations with professional support, 'crisis teams'
Establishing and improving specific support
child protection centres
centres for abused women
family crisis centres (primary prevention)
(iii) Steps aimed at the family and its environment
Modification of living conditions
Family support
family education programmes
social support services
(iv) Psychotherapeutic steps
Treatment of parents or couples
Psychotherapy focusing on the child, e.g. individual therapy, family therapy

From Remschmidt et al. (1990).

systematically abused in a sadistic way, or whether a mother of five children felt so overwhelmed with excessive demands, that a crisis resulted, during which she hit one of her children, injuring him seriously.

All individuals involved in reducing child abuse and neglect should consider carefully in each case not only appropriate redress, but also what can be done to improve the individual child's and his family's situation (Olbing et al., 1989; Briere et al., 1996; Lutzker, 1998). An independent commission of the German government has made proposals on how to prevent and combat violence in families. The proposals are summarized in Table 30.3.

When deciding which approach to treatment is appropriate, the following issues should be considered (Remschmidt, 1985).

(i) A risk assessment should be undertaken as to whether abuse and neglect are likely to continue. If this is the case, the child may need to be removed from the family.

(ii) It should be determined whether or not the parents have a psychiatric disorder. If this is the case, appropriate referrals should be made.

(iii) A careful appraisal of the individual case should contain the nature of any abuse or neglect, and determine whether the parents or other care-givers are likely to be able to cooperate with treatment. If they are, cooperative work should ideally begin during the child's hospitalization. The progress over the course of treatment will usually determine whether adequate cooperation is likely to continue on an outpatient basis.

Over recent years many institutions have increased their efforts to limit the acute risks to which abused children are exposed. Hospitals (paediatric hospitals, child and adolescent psychiatric departments) play a major role, as do child protection centres and centres for abused women. The latter are particularly important when the abused child's mother is herself a victim of abuse. In a large proportion of cases, alcohol consumption plays an important role, more usually involving the father, but sometimes the mother.

Psychotherapy with parents and families

The aim of such treatment is to modify the behaviour of parents and families, compensate for the abuse and neglect they may have experienced during childhood ('re-parenting'), and uncover reasons for the abuse and neglect of their children. This approach is usually accompanied by behavioural treatment programmes, which take effect more rapidly. Psychodynamic approaches aimed at uncovering early childhood conflicts and the causes for abusive behaviour are unlikely to be effective alone, because the technique does not address and bring about behavioural change, which is essential for a rapid improvement of the family situation. Individual psychotherapy is advisable when severe psychopathology is present, such as personality disorder or disturbed socialization.

The following treatment techniques have been used successfully (Remschmidt et al., 1990).

Individual treatment of the abusing parent

This technique should be combined with social skills training in the family setting, and include the spouse. Studies have shown that about three-quarters of affected families improve significantly. Individuals learn to deal appropriately with internal conflicts, resulting in a reduced risk of child abuse.

Marital therapy

This type of treatment aims to improve the marital relationship (or partnership), resulting in a reduced risk of abuse in the family.

Non-professional counsellors

Such individuals are given the task to establish a trusting relationship with parents, thus fulfilling their need for protection and care ('re-parenting'). Non-professional counsellors also have the role of helping parents deal with practical problems of everyday life. Parents usually experience them as less threatening than professionals. Non-professional counsellors usually manage to give intensive help and are less of a financial burden. This approach may be very helpful if the non-professional counsellors are selected carefully, prepared well for their task, and closely supervised (Engfer, 1986).

Self-help groups

Studies examining the effectivity of self-help groups have been encouraging. This approach is generally considered very helpful by the participants, because they are together with individuals who have to cope with similar problems as themselves and have frequently suffered the same fate.

Evaluation

The success rates of treatment by non-professionals, including self-help groups, are higher than other types of treatment. The benefits of parent therapy are not so clear. In one follow-up study looking at the success rates of treating abusing parents, the children were no longer seriously abused $4\frac{1}{2}$ years after the child abuse became known, but 68% of children were still suffering hostility, rejection, and/or physical punishment. It is an error to assume that parents will automatically discontinue the abuse once they become aware of the cause. Unfortunately, psychotherapy frequently fails to focus on the way behavioural change can be brought about after a problem has been discussed and understood. Thus, training programmes tend to be more successful than insight-orientated therapy with parents.

Individual psychotherapy with the child

Subsequent to experiencing abuse, many children show emotional disturbances, and persistent personality disorders may develop. Therefore, the abused child requires individual and specific psychotherapeutic help (Briere et al., 1996; Lutzker, 1998). Such assistance is important because it can help to interrupt the abusive cycle, which otherwise tends to result in the abused child eventually becoming an abusing parent. The psychotherapeutic techniques explained below have been used successfully (Remschmidt et al., 1990).

Individual treatment of the abused child

Individual psychotherapy needs to take into account the child's age. Younger children may benefit from play therapy, whereas verbal intervention is more appropriate with older children. The aim of treatment is to help the child to express his anxieties and conflicts, to learn to deal with them, to restore the lost trust in adults and to restore the child's self-esteem. Younger patients tend to respond better to such a therapeutic offer. The chances of therapeutic success improve if the parents manage to accept the change taking place in the child and are able to modify their own behaviour (Martin and Beezley, 1976). Thus, changes which occur in the child are intimately related to changes which occur in the parents.

Group psychotherapy

Group therapy is an appropriate treatment technique for children from the age of 8, who have particular difficulties in interacting with peers.

Psychotherapy with the whole family

Child abuse and neglect and other types of violence in families are usually the result of a persistent disturbance of family communication and interaction. In this situation, family therapy where possible, may be most appropriate. Family therapy needs to take into account the specific family structure, to challenge excessively rigid boundaries in the family system, support family members towards age-appropriate independence and assertiveness, help family members to understand the situation of the abused child, and support the family in developing new communicational and interactional strategies once the abuse has ceased. Several techniques may be used to achieve this goal. However, it is important to emphasize that this must be undertaken by experienced therapists, as there is a significant risk that intervention may contribute to an escalation of problems in the family (Larson, 1986).

Outpatient and inpatient family therapy may be combined with training programmes for the parents alone or for the whole family (Remschmidt et al., 1990).

(i) During inpatient family therapy the whole family spends several weeks or months living in a special family unit, where the family is cared for by specially trained nursing staff and therapists. Initially, treatment focuses on relieving the family of the ordinary duties of everyday life, enabling the parents to concentrate on improving the parent–child relationship ('re-parenting'). During the following phase, both individual family members and the family as a whole are helped to improve patterns of family interaction. Family interaction is analysed, for instance, by means of role play, which may include situations in which child abuse typically occurs. Alternative strategies to cope with such situations and new ways of behaviour are subsequently developed together with the family.

This approach requires considerable resources, but has the advantage that the family is kept together. Assessments can be made of the family's motivation for change, and difficult situations may be analysed in role play with the whole family. There is a danger, however, that families become dependent on the treatment facility, and the entire treatment is undertaken under rather artificial conditions. It is far from clear whether the success achieved during treatment will generalize and persist in ordinary family situations.

(ii) During outpatient family therapy, a similar approach is used. This approach is less demanding in terms of resources and is usually compatible with the parents' daily work. However, treatment will necessarily be of shorter duration and less intense compared to inpatient treatment. Not every family is suitable for family therapy. This type of treatment requires relatively well developed verbal skills, trust in the therapist and a high level of motivation.

Psychotherapy with parents

Psychotherapy with parents usually focuses on the conflicts and problems the parents have together, and the relationship between them and their children. The following problems usually need to be discussed.

(i) Abuse and neglect in the parents' own childhood:
  (a) marital problems or difficulties in partnership
  (b) the family's social situation
  (c) relationship between parents and the child
  (d) rejection of the child

(ii) Physical or mental impairment of the child

(iii) Analysis of situations in which the impulse to use violence arises.

The aim of this approach is to reconstruct the relationship between parents and child, whilst taking into account the parents' own biography, personality and child-raising behaviour. If this approach is impossible or likely to fail, legal consequences will ensue, resulting ultimately in the withdrawal of the parents' custody of the child. The child will then require alternative care on a permanent basis, e.g. foster family or residential home.

Preventing recurrence (secondary prevention)

At an early stage, the decision must be made as to whether the child is at risk for further abuse. Abuse is always damaging to the child and may frequently be life threatening. It is not easy to assess the risk of further abuse, and it may be helpful to consider the following points.

Personality of parents and the sequelae of abuse

The risk of the abuse continuing is increased when parents (or one parent) have a psychiatric disorder or an 'irritable' or impulsive personality structure. In such cases it is usually necessary to remove the child from his family initially because of the high risk of continued abuse, which may result in severe injury of the child. The feelings of guilt which many parents have after abusing their child play a major role, particularly if parents are unable to work through their guilt. The risk of recurrence is also high when a parent (or both parents) suffers from alcoholism. The severity of injury must also be considered when balancing the risks of recurrence. When there is disagreement between the parents as to how to manage the child, it is likely that, as the weakest member of the system, the child will suffer continued maltreatment.

Personality of the child and the sequelae of abuse

The child may show behaviour which tends to perpetuate the abusive cycle, such as anxiousness, failure at school, decreasing ability to meet parents' expectations or disturbance of psychosocial development, e.g. secondary encopresis or enuresis. Such behaviour is likely to contribute to parents' rejection of the child and continued maltreatment, particularly in situations in which parents feel frustrated with their child.

Type and extent of abuse

Some types of abuse are so extreme that removal of the child from the family is mandatory, at least initially. In such cases, the severity of the abuse influences the risk assessment. Such types of abuse include life-threatening practices such as strangling, inflicting severe cranial injury, beating the child with dangerous objects and extremely sadistic acts. However, it is important not to be dismissive of 'less severe' types of abuse, which are often likely to be chronic, and in these cases the risk of continued maltreatment may nevertheless be high.

Ability and willingness of parents and families to cooperate

In cases where family members do not appear to understand that child abuse is wrong, play it down, justify it or put forward poor excuses for the child's injuries, the risk of continued maltreatment is high. The same applies to families who refuse to cooperate or continue to demonstrate an emotionally cold and brusque manner of communication with the child who has been maltreated.

Administrational steps and cooperation

The success of most treatment steps depends upon the cooperation of the individuals involved. This applies to families and the abused child, health care professionals, youth welfare offices, child protection centres, social services, kindergartens, schools, and in some cases the legal authorities. It is important that the first person involved in a case of abuse passes on essential information to the appropriate authorities. This is usually the youth welfare office and the individual closest to the child. If serious injury has occurred, one must consider whether it is appropriate to involve the legal authorities. From a psychiatric perspective, it is essential to approach the problem in a way which is helpful to the child. However, in severe cases, e.g. sadistic acts, continued maltreatment immediate legal action may be required. Care of the child and the family is ideally placed in the hands of the institution with the most experience in dealing with child abuse and neglect, usually a child and psychiatric department or hospital, a child protection centre, or a similar child protection agency.

Prevention (primary prevention)

Recently, attempts have been made to improve primary prevention by identifying those children, parents and families at increased risk for child abuse. In order to identify these individuals, it has been helpful to determine those factors in the child, parent or family which indicate an increased risk (Table 30.2).

Standardized questionnaires have been developed, with which the risk of parents abusing their child can be determined objectively (Kempe and Kempe, 1978; Dodge et al., 1990). Attempts have also been made to identify factors at birth which indicate a high risk for child abuse (Altemeier et al., 1979, 1982, 1984; Olds and Henderson, 1989).

REFERENCES

Altemeier, W., Vietze, P. M., Sherrod, K. B., Sandler, H. M., Falsey, S. and O'Connor, S. (1979). Prediction of child maltreatment during pregnancy. *Journal of the American Academy of Child Psychiatry*, **18**, 205–18.

Altemeier, W., O'Connor, S., Vietze, P., Sandler, H. and Sherrod, K. (1982). Antecedents of child abuse. *Journal of Pediatrics*, **100**, 823–9.

Altemeier, W., O'Connor, S., Vietze, P., Sandler, H. and Sherrod, K. (1984). Antecedents of child abuse. A prospective study of feasibility. *Child Abuse and Neglect*, **8**, 939–400.

Briere, J., Berliner, L. Bulkley, J. A., Jenny, C. and Reid, T. (ed.) (1996). *The APSAC handbook on child maltreatment*. Thousand Oaks, CA: Sage.

Dodge, K. A., Bates, J. E. and Pettit, G. S. (1990). Mechanisms in the cycle of violence. *Science*, **250**, 1678–83.

Engfer, A. (1986). *Kindesmisshandlung. Ursachen, Auswirkungen, Hilfen*. Stuttgart: Enke.

Finkelhor, D. and Korbin, J. (1988). Child abuse as an international issue. *Child Abuse and Neglect*, **12**, 2–24.

Friedman, S. B. and Morse, C. B. (1974). Child abuse. A five-year follow-up of early case findings in the emergency department. *Pediatrics*, **54**, 404–10.

Kempe, C. H. and Helfer, E. R. (1972). *Helping the battered child and his family*. Philadelphia: Lippincott.

Kempe, R. and Kempe, C. H. (1978). *Child abuse*. London: Fontana / Open Books.

Larson, N. R. (1986). Familientherapie mit Inzestfamilien. In *Sexueller Missbrauch von Kindern in Familien*, ed. L. Backe, N. Leick, J. Merrick and N. Michelsen, pp. 104–17. Köln: Deutscher Ärzteverlag.

Lutzker, J. R. (ed.) (1998). *Handbook of child abuse research and treatment*. New York: Plenum Press.

Martin, H. P. and Beezley, P. (1976). Therapy for abusive parents: its effect on the child. In *The abused child. A multidisciplinary approach to developmental issues and treatment*, ed. H. P. Martin, pp. 251–63. Cambridge, MA: Ballinger.

Olbing, H., Bachmann, K-D. and Gross, R. (ed.) (1989). *Kindesmisshandlung. Eine Orientierung für Ärzte, Juristen, Sozial- und Erzieherberufe*. Köln: Deutscher Ärzteverlag.

Olds, D. L. and Henderson, C. R. (1989). The prevention of maltreatment. In *Child maltreatment. Theory and research on the causes and consequences of child abuse and neglect*, ed. D. Chiccetti and V. Carlson, pp. 722–63. New York: Cambridge University Press.

Remschmidt, H. (1985). Kindesmisshandlung und -vernachlässigung. In *Kinder- und Jugendpsychiatrie in Klinik und Praxis*, vol. III, ed. H. Remschmidt and M. H. Schmidt, pp. 366–73. Stuttgart: Thieme.

Remschmidt, H., Hacker, F., Müller-Luckmann, E., Schmidt, M. H. and Strunk, P. (1990). Ursachen, Prävention und Kontrolle von Gewalt aus psychiatrischer Sicht. In *Ursachen, Prävention und Kontrolle von Gewalt*, ed. H. D. Schwind, J. Baumann et al., pp. 157–292. Berlin: Duncker & Humblot.

Skuse, D. and Bentovim, A. (1994). Physical and emotional maltreatment. In *Child and adolescent psychiatry. Modern approaches*, ed. M. Rutter, E. Taylor, L. Hersov. Oxford: Blackwell Science.

Stutte, H. (1971). Probleme der körperlichen und seelischen Kindesmisshandlung. *Jahrbuch für Jugendpsychiatrie und Grenzgebiete*, **8**, 122–33.

31

Sexual abuse and sexual maltreatment

Helmut Remschmidt

Definition and epidemiology

The term child sexual abuse is used to describe the involvement of dependent and developmentally immature children and adolescents in sexual activities which they do not fully comprehend, and to which they are unable to give informed consent, and that violate the social taboos of family roles (Schechter and Roberge, 1976). Thus sexual abuse is present in such cases even if the child does not actively oppose the sexual advances and the offender does not use force.

The term sexual maltreatment is used when the use of force or violence is present and sexual activity is brought about against the child's will. One common type of sexual maltreatment is incest, a term used to describe sexual activity between family members. Sexual relationships between father and daughter and uncle and niece are the most common forms of incest. Child sexual abuse always results in a highly asymmetrical power distribution and a situation of dependency to the child's distinct disadvantage.

Every third or fourth adult is said to have experienced some type of sexual abuse as a child. According to statistics from USA, 5–10% of women report incestuous relationships. Such relationships cannot be considered single occurrences, as they are reported to have lasted an average of 2–3 years.

In Germany about 15 000 cases of child sexual abuse are reported to the police every year, involving more than that number of children, of which 77% are girls. These data clearly indicate that, in a considerable number of cases, an episode of sexual abuse involved more than one child. According to German police statistics, children are involved in 36% of all sexual offences. Of all sexual offences, 24% involve exhibitionism, 22% rape, and about 8% the sexual abuse of dependants, including incest.

The victims of sexual abuse and sexual maltreatment are frequently girls, 80% of whom are less than 14 years old. The offenders are most commonly men between 25 and 40 years (Remschmidt, 1989).

Characteristics of the disturbance

Child and adolescent sexual abuse occurs in a variety of forms and situations (Veltkamp and Miller, 1994). A useful breakdown distinguishes intrafamilial from extrafamilial child sexual abuse, both of which may occur with varying degrees of force.

The sexual abuse of minors most commonly occurs without the use of physical force. However, there is often a considerable amount of psychological pressure applied, which may result in equally severe emotional disturbance as the use of physical force may have done. When physical force is used, it may involve children being forced to perform or engage in sexual acts, and they may be raped, mutilated or even killed.

It is difficult to be accurate about the relative frequency of different types of sexual abuse. As sexual abuse is a taboo subject, there are great fluctuations in reporting, and many offences are kept a secret. Intrafamilial sexual abuse is particularly likely not to be reported, either because of fear, or concerns about the family being blamed or financially penalized (the perpetrator is often the family breadwinner).

Because of difficulties in obtaining accurate reports, epidemiological data on child sexual abuse relies to a great extent on retrospective reports of adults. These suggest that vaginal or anal intercourse is the most common type of abuse, followed by forced oral intercourse in boys and genital manipulation of female victims. Other sexual practices show no sex gradient.

Assessment

Sexual abuse is often not the presenting complaint, and the first step in assessment is recognition. The therapist needs to be open to cues and take seriously any suspicion that abuse has taken place. The following are the common means by which sexual abuse comes to the attention of professionals:

- the child's report,
- behavioural disturbance or inexplicable changes in behaviour,
- physical signs or symptoms,
- other types of maltreatment,
- accusations made by parents, relatives or other concerned adults.

Those criteria are often in themselves only pointers to the possibility of sexual abuse. Damon et al. (1992) have suggested using the following criteria to determine the likelihood of abuse having occurred. A careful assessment of these issues is required:

- age-inappropriate sexual behaviour or inappropriate knowledge in the child,

- the child's report of sexual abuse or incest,
- physical findings suggestive of sexual abuse,
- the report of a sibling or other informant that sexual abuse has occurred.

Assessment is often difficult and complicated. Only a small percentage of victims show physical signs of having been abused, and psychiatric assessment is therefore an important part of the validation of any accusations. Data need to be gathered from several different sources before forming an opinion. There are no pathognomonic features of sexual abuse in either child or offender, and there are no reliable diagnostic instruments. One-quarter to one-third of 'incestuous fathers' appear entirely normal in their behaviour, and psychopathology is not forthcoming on interview. Furthermore, the abused child is often confused and disturbed, complicated by ambivalent emotions toward the perpetrator.

In the course of assessment, the following general principles need to be taken into account.

(i) The way in which assessment is undertaken and its thoroughness needs to be in proportion to the degree of suspicion. A high degree of suspicion will justify a full pediatric and psychiatric assessment. If suspicion is low, asking the child and his parents a few screening questions may be sufficient. The necessity of probing further will depend on the nature and content of the answers given. This stepwise approach to assessment avoids unjustified zeal, and should prevent abuse being overlooked when it has actually occurred.

(ii) Additional traumatization of the patient during physical examination should be avoided. Examination should be postponed initially if the child does not cooperate, and physical contact should be kept to a minimum.

(iii) Multiple tests and examinations should be avoided. The child should be given the opportunity to choose an individual he trusts to accompany him to the tests and examinations (Fegert, 1993).

(iv) External sources of information should be used when available. The aim is to assess changes in the child's behaviour in an objective way, without prematurely raising the suspicion of sexual abuse.

(v) The credibility of the child's or adolescent's statements needs to be assessed. False testimony is rare in children, but more frequent in adolescents. False accusations must be borne in mind, particularly if the child or adolescent has a psychiatric disorder.

Sequelae of sexual abuse of children and adolescents

It is helpful to distinguish the short-term sequelae of sexual abuse from its intermediate and long-term sequelae, which are usually a result not of the offence itself, but of the circumstances surrounding the case, e.g. the use of force, the perpetrator being a family member, secrecy surrounding the offence, etc.

The short-term sequelae are well known: physical injury, pain, disappointment, distrust, resignation and depression, destruction of self-esteem, helplessness, failure at school, social withdrawal, suicidal thoughts or attempted suicide.

Sexual abuse within the family context regularly results in victims (usually girls) experiencing severe loyalty conflicts with their parents. If the offender is the child's father or stepfather, the child is usually put under pressure not to speak about the offence to her mother. This often results in a consequent disturbance of the relationship between mother and daughter. This secrecy imposed upon the child is a heavy burden. As the weakest individual involved, the child feels helpless and is unable to find ways of protecting herself either physically or psychologically. In many cases the child's mother is aware of the occurrence of the sexual abuse, but also feels helpless and powerless to intervene, sometimes out of the fear of financial ruin or of losing the partner.

The intermediate and long-term sequelae of child sexual abuse can be divided into three main areas.

Impairment of sexual gratification and disturbance of relationship

Sexual abuse may be the child's or adolescent's first sexual experience with a 'partner'. Perpetrators may be of either sex but are usually much older than the victims. Apart from the unpleasant circumstances and the use of physical force, the imbalance in power also contributes to the destruction of the victim's first sexual experience. The abusive acts are generally associated with feelings of vulnerability, helplessness and submission, with loss of any sense of self-determination or self-initiative. Such interactional patterns are frequently repeated in subsequent relationships and can only be modified in the presence of considerable support and empathic understanding.

Disturbance of the development of personal identity

The development of personal identity and the gender role may be severely disturbed through persistent sexual abuse. For instance, sexual abuse by the victim's father or stepfather will not only influence her perception of that individual, but will also distort her concept of a male partner in general, and influence her view of the relationship between her parents. As the marital relationship between parents serves as a model for heterosexual relationships and gender roles in general, victims of sexual abuse tend to become insecure and are often unable to cope with age-appropriate identification processes.

Emotional disturbance and mental disorder

Sexually abused and maltreated children suffer not only from short-term psychiatric sequelae following the abuse, but frequently develop chronic conflicts or severe psychiatric disorders in the long-term, especially when sexual abuse has continued for several years. Abuse may result in depression with appetite and sleep disturbances, suicidal thoughts or acts, school difficulties, attention deficits, antisocial behaviour, running away from home, oppositional behaviour, avoidance of close family relationships, hysterical reactions and conversion syndromes. In his early work, Freud considered incest as a leading cause of hysteria, which he later modified to 'incest fantasy'. In severe crises of self-esteem attempted suicide or self-injury may occur.

Victims often progress through several phases following sexual abuse. Summit (1981) describes these four phases as secrecy, helplessness, accomodation, and discovery.

Aetiology and pathogenesis

Many theoretical viewpoints have been proposed to explain the aetiology and pathogenesis of sexual abuse (Veltkamp and Miller, 1994). These tend to focus on the individual, or emphasize interactional and social factors.

Theories which focus on the individual

These theories propose that both offender and victim have specific traits which make them vulnerable as offenders or perpetrators. The perpetrators tend to be introverted, reluctant, passive and socially isolated men who form part of the victims' close social environment. They are likely to have been physically or sexually abused during their own childhood, suffer from low self-esteem, and tend to be narcissistic and autocratic in their interaction with other family members. Their social skills are often deficient and they are unable to establish age-appropriate sexual relationships as they perceive women as dominant. They usually support rigid moral opinions and values (Marquit, 1986). As in perpetrators of physical abuse and substance abuse, this narcissistic personality structure seems to be of central importance.

Interactional theories

According to interactional theories, sexual abuse in families is seen as a sign of disturbance in the whole family system. Thus incest is considered a result of severely disturbed family communication rather than the cause. Families in which incest occurs tend to have difficulties in accepting one another's individual boundaries ('overinvolved families'). Such families freqently draw rather rigid boundaries between the family and the social environment, so that typically all activities occur strictly within family limits, whilst others are excluded. This results in social isolation and excessive interdependence of family members. Intergenerational boundaries and specific roles tend to become blurred. Children may feel compelled to take over adult roles, whilst adults may have inappropriate expectations of their children, such that they are required to carry inappropriate responsibility, or expected to gratify their parents' emotional or sexual needs. Sexual abuse is facilitated by the overinvolvement of family members and the tendency towards the development of symbiotic bonds. At the same time, revelation of sexual abuse is threatening because of the degree to which the offending parent depends upon the abused child. Sexual abuse thus typically plays an important role in avoiding or regulating family conflicts.

Social theories

Beyond economic factors and poor socialization processes, Finkelhor (1982) has emphasized a variety of changes in society which may have contributed to the high prevalence of sexual abuse in today's society. Sexuality is no longer a taboo subject, and the boundaries between permitted and prohibited sexual practices have been blurred with increased opportunities for sexual gratification. In addition to this, emancipation of women has resulted in threats to the traditional dominant role of the male in the family, resulting in the consequent fear of female sexual demands. Divorce and reconstituted families are increasingly common. In these families opportunities for abuse is heightened by the co-habitation of a step-parent and a biologically unrelated young girl. Finally, the increasing social isolation of families, as a result of the trend towards small family units, limits the protective factors of extended family and the community.

All available studies suggest that sexual abuse occurs most frequently within the family setting or by acquaintances of the family. More than one-half of all cases of sexual abuse of girls occur within the victim's family, and an additional third are committed by acquaintances of the family. The data regarding male victims are similar, although the proportion of unknown offenders is slightly higher.

Treatment, rehabilitation, prevention

Treatment needs to address both the current situation and the potential long-term sequelae of sexual abuse (Veltkamp and Miller, 1994; Briere, 1996). Psychotherapy needs to be integrated into a larger treatment plan. This should be set up in conjunction with all individuals and institutions involved in the case, e.g. youth welfare authorities, law courts, hospitals, etc. Thus psychiatric intervention should consist not only of psychotherapy, but comprise a spectrum of wide-ranging steps directed as appropriate for the context in which the abuse has occurred.

Immediate intervention and indication for treatment

It is initially necessary to establish the nature and extent of sexual abuse, and assess the risk of continued abuse. In most cases, it will be necessary to separate the victim from the perpetrator in order to prevent further abuse. This will usually require legal action in order to protect the child. In deciding upon further action, the following options must be weighed up (Fürniss, 1989).

Penalizing the offender

This approach separates the victim from the perpetrator and holds the perpetrator responsible for his actions. Nevertheless, the whole family will be affected by his punishment, not only by the invariable consequent financial difficulties, but also as a result of the loss of a father figure in the family, which may have a potentially detrimental effect on individual family members.

Protection of the child

This approach aims to protect the child from the entire family, implying that both parents are responsible and must be assumed to have failed in appropriately caring for their child. The child may be removed not only from the offending parent, but also from the non-offending parent with whom he has ostensibly maintained a good relationship. A common outcome in such situations is that the parents are distracted from their own problems, and tend to develop new solidarity in the 'battle' for custody of the child. The child, in turn, may feel guilty, and will tend to consider the removal from the family to be her fault.

Therapeutic intervention

The aim of primary therapeutic intervention is to include the whole family in the treatment, whether or not the child is removed from the family. Treatment

Table 31.1. Therapeutic steps when treating child sexual abuse

(i)	Further sexual abuse must be prevented.
(ii)	The child's father (the offender) is expected to accept total responsibility for the abuse, thus assuming his responsibility as a parent.
(iii)	Both parents should accept equal responsibility for the child's general well-being. Appropriate boundaries between the generations are thus re-established.
(iv)	The relationship between the child and her mother is strengthened. The issue of alienation, rejection and rivalry with the mother must be addressed.
(v)	The parental emotional and sexual conflicts must be addressed. These may be interwoven with emotional immaturity and dependence.
(vi)	The relationship between the child and her father is addressed. Common themes are the child's emotions such as hatred, love, helplessness or power, and her father's envy and desire to dominate.

From Fürniss, 1989.

aims to normalize family relationships rather than penalizing the offender. The six basic therapeutic steps of this approach are shown in Table 31.1.

The first goal is to prevent further sexual abuse. This will often necessitate the perpetrator being removed from day-to-day contact the child.

The next important prerequisite is that the perpetrator (often the father) should accept responsibility for his wrong-doing. This is not only important in terms of the father's rehabilitation, but also permits the child to modify her concept of a father.

For the third step, the parents are encouraged to re-assume full responsibility for the upbringing of their child. It is important to ensure that both parents are involved at this stage, including the offending parent. The collaborative involvement of both parents allows the child to review and modify her image of the family and the role of parents and children within it. Nevertheless, this should be kept separate from the issue of protection of the child. Involvement in the child's upbringing does not necessitate living together.

The fourth step attempts to improve the relationship between child and mother. The child frequently feels disappointed and let down because of her mother's failure to protect her. A supportive and trusting relationship between mother and child is likely to be the most effective way of preventing further abuse. In any future situation where the risk of further abuse is present, the child will be able to turn to and seek protection from her mother, which may, in the past, not have been true.

The fifth goal is strengthening the parental relatonship, which involves addressing the inevitable sexual conflicts. When a case of abuse is revealed, both parents may decompensate. Partner roles and parent roles tend to become confused. The offending parent may react by attempting suicide, abusing alcohol or precipitously leaving the family. The other parent may contemplate divorce or flee the family home. These crises must be dealt with to enable the underlying marital problems, which may have contributed to the sexual abuse, to be addressed.

The final step addresses the relationship between the child and the abusing parent. This is extremely important for the victim's own psychosexual development. If this is not achieved, there is a high likelihood of problems being carried over into adulthood, e.g. ungratifying sexual relationships, prostitution. This issue is as relevant for boys as for girls.

If circumstances of the individual case render primary therapeutic intervention impossible, for example, because of a pending court case or the involvement of other agencies, the above model will have to be modified. Nevertheless, psychotherapeutic intervention can be useful at many stages of the process, and is advisable in every case encountered.

Psychotherapy with the sexually abused individual

Even when the whole family is available for treatment, individual or group psychotherapy for the child remains extremely important. It is advisable to begin with individual treatment, progressing to group work with other abused children. In the individual sessions, it is helpful to facilitate expression with the use of toys. Later, and in older children, verbal intervention is usually possible. The aims of both approaches are the following (Fürniss, 1989):

- helping the child speak about the sexual abuse;
- educating the child about sexual organs and development;
- building up the child's self-esteem;
- helping the child to develop more independence and decisiveness. This will help the child to overcome the feelings of helplessness so often present in children who have been abused.

Individual treatment of sexually abused children needs to take into account the type of abuse and the duration, as well as the accompanying circumstances. The following approaches are appropriate and have been used successfully (Engfer, 1986; Remschmidt, 1992):

Reduction of guilt

The child needs to understand and believe that she is responsible neither for the sexual abuse or incest, nor for any consequent break-up of the family.

Separation of victim and perpetrator

In most cases the perpetrator (usually the victim's father) will have to leave the family in order to prevent further abuse.

Development of an empathic therapeutic relationship

Trust is necessary not only to encourage the sharing of information, but is also the basis for psychotherapy.

Sex education

This can be a sensitive issue when a child has been sexually abused; however, despite their experience, many children remain either ignorant or misinformed and need accurate information in order to be able to form appropriate sexual relationships in the future.

Issue of autonomy

This focuses on themes such as self-control, locus of control, self-determination, coercion, and needs and preferences within relationships.

Psychotherapy with the perpetrator

In many cases, the perpetrator will also benefit from psychotherapy, particularly in cases where there is associated psychopathology such as personality disorder or poor social skills. Cognitive behavioural therapy programmes are the most effective approach for treating individuals who commit paedophilia, incest, and indulge in exhibitionism (Marshall et al., 1991). In some cases, antiandrogens are also administered as adjuvant treatment in combination with psychotherapy.

Family therapy

It is generally accepted that sexual abuse and maltreatment frequently arises as a result of a persistent disturbance in family communication. When family therapy is used, it should aim to bring about modifications in the style of family communication:

- dissolution of the rigid boundaries between the family and its environment;
- improvement of the independence and self-determination of individual family members;
- provision of an explanation of the sexually abused child's situation;
- discussion of the appropriateness of individual treatment for the child and/or perpetrator;

- assessing the likelihood of treatment being successful in reconstructing family relationships.

Achieving the open discussion of these issues is a difficult task in these families and therapists need to be not only flexible in terms of the techniques they use, but also experienced. In the hands of an unexperienced therapist, escalation of family conflicts and scapegoating is likely.

Legal steps

Experience in many countries has found that penalizing the perpetrator without offering treatment achieves little. Thus the principle of 'therapy rather than punishment' has become fashionable. This guiding principle cannot be applied in all cases, however, and it has been necessary recently to modify this guideline. When the sexual abuse is severe, chronic, or when the perpetrator refuses to cooperate with treatment, penalization is inevitable and therapy must be worked around this. It has been shown, especially in the USA, that the obligations to report sexual abuse and compulsory treatment are not incompatible. The advantage of such a system is that a larger proportion of cases of sexual abuse become known about, and compulsory treatment reduces the likelihood of subsequent family break-up.

REFERENCES

Briere, J. (1996). *Therapy for adults molested as children. Beyond survival.* New York: Springer.

Damon, L. L., Card, J. A. and Todd, J. (1992). Incest in young children. In *Assessment of family violence. A clinical and legal sourcebook*, ed. R. T. Ammerman and M. Hersen, pp. 148–72. New York: Wiley.

Engfer, A. (1986). *Kindesmisshandlung. Ursachen, Auswirkungen, Hilfen*. Stuttgart: Enke.

Fegert, J. M. (1993). *Sexuell missbrauchte Kinder und das Recht*, vol. 2, Ein Handbuch zu Fragen der kinder- und jugendpsychiatrischen und psychologischen Untersuchung und Begutachtung. Köln: Volksblatt.

Finkelhor, D. (1982). Sexual abuse. A sociological perspective. *Child Abuse and Neglect*, **6**, 95–102.

Fürniss, T. H. (1989). Krisenintervention und Therapie bei sexueller Kindesmisshandlung in der Familie. Erfahrungen aus Grossbritannien. In *Kindesmisshandlung. Eine Orientierung für Ärzte, Juristen, Sozial- und Erziehungsberufe*, ed. H. Olbing, K-D. Bachmann and R. Gross, pp. 77–89. Köln: Deutscher Ärzteverlag.

Marquit, C. (1986). Der Täter. Persönlichkeitsstruktur und Behandlung. In *Sexueller Missbrauch von Kindern in Familien*, ed. L. Backe, N. Leick, J. Merrick and N. Michelsen, pp. 118–36. Köln: Deutscher Ärzteverlag.

Marshall, W. L., Jones, R., Ward, T., Johnston, P. and Barbaree, H. E. (1991). Treatment outcome with sex offenders. *Clinical Psychology Review*, **11**, 465–85.

Remschmidt, H. (1989). Sexuelle Kindesmisshandlung. Epidemiologie, Erscheinungsformen und Begleitumstände sexueller Kindesmisshandlungen. In *Kindesmisshandlung. Eine Orientierung für Ärzte, Juristen, Sozial- und Erziehungsberufe*, ed. H. Olbing, K.-D. Bachmann and R. Gross, pp. 71–6. Köln: Deutscher Ärzteverlag.

Remschmidt, H. (1992). *Psychiatrie der Adoleszenz*. Stuttgart: Thieme.

Schechter, M. D. and Roberge, L. (1976). Sexual exploitation. In *Child abuse and neglect. The family and the community*, ed. R. E. Helfer and C. H. Kempe. Cambridge, MA: Ballinger.

Summit, R. (1981). Beyond belief. The reluctant discovery in incest. In *Women in context*, ed. M. Kirkpatrick. New York: Plenum Press.

Veltkamp, L. J. and Miller, T. W. (1994). *Clinical handbook of child abuse and neglect*. Madison, CT: International Universities Press.

Part IV

The practice of psychotherapy in various settings

32 Inpatient psychotherapy

Matthias Martin

Introduction

Inpatient psychotherapy is a common approach to treatment of psychogenic disorders in Germany, where more beds for inpatient psychotherapy are available in special hospitals for psychogenic and psychosomatic disorders than in all other countries together (Schepank, 1987; Schepank and Tress, 1988). In contrast, child and adolescent psychiatric hospitals have very few specific psychotherapy units for children and adolescents. Therefore, inpatient psychotherapy in childhood and adolescence is usually undertaken on general child and adolescent psychiatric wards.

Fig. 32.1 shows the age and sex distribution of inpatients treated at the Hospital for Child and Adolescent Psychiatry, University of Marburg (Germany). The majority (73%) of inpatients were 12 years old or older. A breakdown of patients by diagnosis (Fig. 32.2) shows that over half were admitted for the treatment of disorders which are overwhelmingly psychotherapeutically managed, e.g. anorexia nervosa, neuroses, specific emotional disorders, adjustment disorders. This serves to demonstrate the central role of psychotherapy in the management of children admitted to child and adolescent psychiatry departments.

Indications for inpatient psychotherapy

After the indication for inpatient treatment has been decided upon (see Chapter 2 for choice of treatment), the issue of selecting an appropriate treatment modality needs to be addressed. It is possible to distinguish four different treatment modalities:

- inpatient treatment,
- partial hospitalization (day-patient treatment),
- treatment in the usual environment (home-treatment), and
- outpatient treatment.

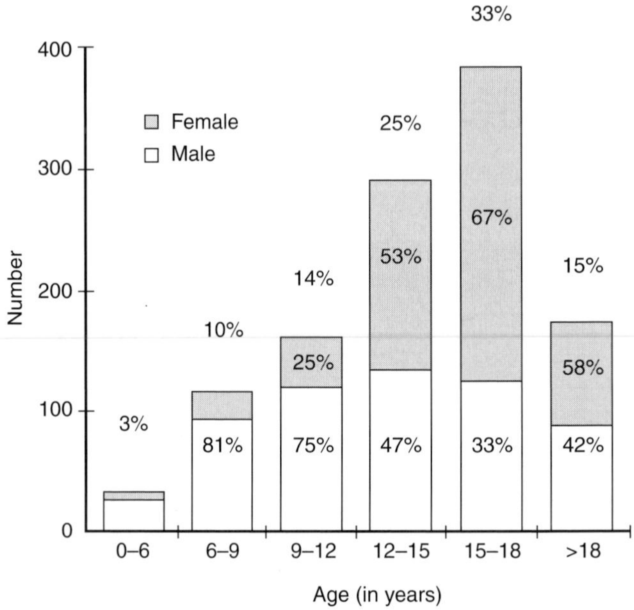

Fig. 32.1. Age distribution of inpatients at the Hospital for Child and Adolescent Psychiatry, University of Marburg (Germany), during a period of 5 years (1988–1992). The bars show a breakdown of the distribution by sex.

The duration of treatment will depend on the selected treatment modality and may vary from a few days to several years. Typically, both inpatient and outpatient psychotherapy require 3 to 6 months (Mattejat et al., 1994; Remschmidt et al., 1994).

The indications for the various approaches to treatment have been discussed in general by Remschmidt (1988) and by Hersov (1994) with emphasis on inpatient therapy.

Inpatient psychotherapy requires considerable resources in terms of mental effort, organization and finances. It is important to recognize that there are both positive and negative aspects of the patient's separation from his usual environment (friends, family, school). Inpatient treatment should therefore be reserved for severe and moderate mental disorders, and for when other approaches to treatment involve excessive risk, or are unlikely to succeed (little chance of success or previous failure), or cannot be undertaken for other reasons. Whilst considering the appropriateness of inpatient psychotherapy, both the patient's psychological symptoms and his environment, including risks he may be subjected to, need to be taken into account. In some cases the patient himself may be a risk to others. When the most important aim of treatment is to protect the patient from the detrimental influences of his

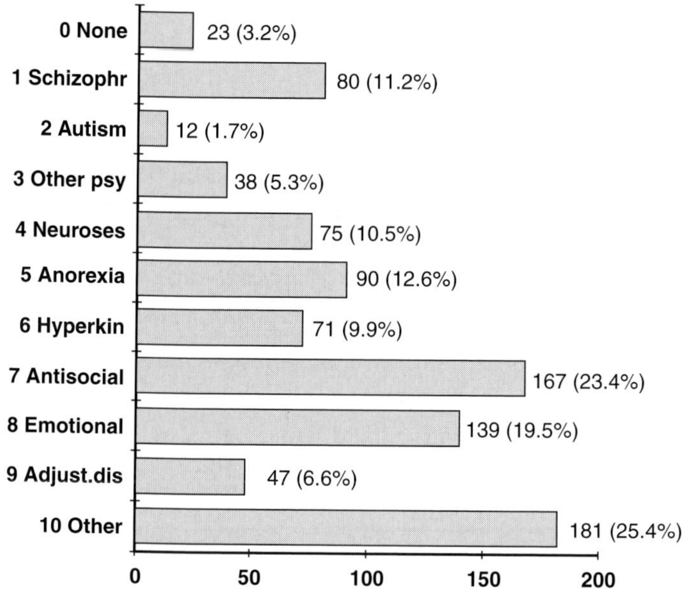

Note on abbreviations:

0: No disorder on first axis.
1: Schizophrenia.
2: Typical psychoses of childhood.
3: Other psychosis.
4: Neuroses.
5: Anorexia nervosa.
6: Hyperkinetic syndrome.
7: Antisocial behaviour disorder.
8: Specific emotional disorder.
9: Adjustment disorder and reaction to severe stress.
10: Other diagnoses.

Fig. 32.2. Disorders classified on the first axis of a multiaxial classification system (Rutter et al., 1975) according to ICD-9 during a period of 5 years (1988–1992). Total number of patients: 714.

environment, e.g. in cases of neglect, maltreatment or abuse, out-of-home placement in cooperation with youth welfare authorities may be appropriate, e.g. in a foster family or residential home. In such cases, inpatient treatment should never serve as a substitute for appropriate out-of-home placement.

Criteria for inpatient treatment

Inpatient treatment is essential in potentially life-threatening disorders, e.g. overdoses, severe anorexia nervosa and in disorders associated with the risk of self-harm or injury to others, e.g. acute psychosis, extreme excitement, severe self-injury. Inpatient treatment is also indicated when a period of observation, the close monitoring of treatment, or the efforts of a multidisciplinary team is required, e.g. in severe anorexia nervosa, psychosis, hyperkinetic syndrome. Inpatient treatment may also be necessary when previous outpatient treatment has failed and there is a risk of the disorder becoming chronic. Inpatient (psychotherapeutic) treatment is also advisable when outpatient treatment is unlikely to succeed as a result of poor or reluctant parental cooperation or a continuing detrimental family environment. In some cases, it will be necessary to separate the patient from his family temporarily in order to facilitate treatment, e.g. in separation anxiety, and in exceptional situations it may be necessary to undertake treatment on an inpatient basis when outpatient treatment is difficult or impossible to organize, e.g. when day-treatment is advisable but facilities are unavailable or when the distance between the patient's home and the outpatient treatment facility is too great. It has been shown that the duration of hospitalization of patients from areas with inadequate outpatient treatment facilites tends to be twice as long as when patients come from areas with good outpatient treatment facilities (Remschmidt and Walter, 1989).

Finally, hospitalization may be neccessary in order to undertake a thorough diagnostic appraisal, e.g. to assess the risk of self-harm or threat to others, in cases of suspected child abuse, or to assess whether out-of-home placement is required. In summary, the following factors may influence the decision to admit the patient:

- severity and/or chronicity of the disorder;
- risk of self-harm or injury to others;
- need to separate the patient from his family;
- lack of appropriate outpatient treatment facilities;
- inpatient treatment facility nearby.

The disorders most likely to require inpatient therapy include bulimia nervosa with frequent binges and subsequent vomiting, depression with risk of suicide, repeated self-injurious behaviour, severe obsessive-compulsive disorder, psychosis, conversion symptoms and separation anxiety. When symptoms are mild or moderate, outpatient treatment can be considered; however, if symptoms are severe or chronic, admission must be considered. The only realistic alternative for such disorders is a convenient day treatment facility.

Characteristics of inpatient psychotherapy

Inpatient psychotherapy can be more comprehensive and specific than outpatient psychotherapy and should not be considered merely as psychotherapy in a hospital setting (Schepank, 1987). The following definition of inpatient psychotherapy has been suggested (Schepank, 1987): 'The planned use of specific psychological treatment techniques for the intensive treatment of psychogenic disorders. Treatment should be undertaken in a specially adapted hospital setting with the cooperation of the patient himself, the institution, the agency financing treatment, the patient's family and his educational or occupational background. The aim of treatment is to improve symptoms and achieve prompt recovery. It is important that psychotherapy is undertaken continuously in a clearly predefined way. The various interventions (verbal and non-verbal) need to be coordinated and used to complement one another. The techniques used should be established theoretically and interventions individually dosed. Other steps, such as additional medical treatment, medication or custodial measures should be avoided where possible. Full cooperation of all involved working together towards the psychotherapeutic goals is essential. This requires clear allocation of tasks, exchange and sharing relevant information among those involved in treatment (and along appropriate hierarchial lines when neccessary), competency and the appropriate use of specifc and empirically proven treatment techniques, as well as clearly defined treatment goals.'

Inpatient psychotherapy in practice

A single psychotherapeutic method is usually inadequate in treating children and adolescents. Several treatment techniques combined to constitute a comprehensive treatment programme is likely to be more helpful in bringing about significant improvement in symptoms. Psychodynamic therapy (individually or in a group setting), behavioural therapy techniques, family therapy or more basic educational sessions for the family may all be part of a treatment plan and contribute to therapeutic success (Table 32.1). These approaches can be combined with relaxation training, projective techniques, psychodrama groups or role play. The treatment of anorexia nervosa is a good example of the coordination of different treatment techniques and gradual modification of the treatment plan (see Chapter 21).

One therapist alone will be unable to undertake all aspects of treatment, so that a multidisciplinary team should be available, who should work in close cooperation with one another, such that disparate aspects do not conflict with one another.

Initially, a detailed treatment plan should be drawn up in order to focus all measures on specific therapeutic goals. The treatment plan should clarify the patient's symptoms, define treatment goals and specify the treatment techniques to be used. Drawing up the treatment plan is also an important task for

Table 32.1. Outline for an inpatient treatment plan

Symptoms, patient's problems

(i) Parents' or care-givers' view

(ii) Patient's view (ranking of severity of problems, motivation for therapy with respect to the different symptoms or problems)

Patient's behaviour on the ward

Suspected diagnosis, assessment of problems

Treatment goals

(i) Goals for the patient
  Main symptoms
  Modification of behaviour towards adults
  Modification of behaviour towards other patients
  Modification of behaviour towards parents
  Modification of behaviour at school
  Modification of self-appraisal and self-esteem

(ii) Goals for cooperation with parents

Treatment planning

(i) Steps for the patient
  Psychotherapy with doctor/psychologist/therapist
  Behaviour of nursing staff
    in general
    towards specific symptoms or problems
  Activities and behaviour on the ward
  Physical therapy
  Occupational therapy and functional treatment
  Medication
  School
  Other, e.g. social steps

(ii) Steps for the family, other individuals important to the patient, institutions
  Family issues
  Institutional areas
  Legal requirements

Contact with the authorities, e.g. youth welfare office, school, etc.

Time schedule

(i) Presumed duration of diagnostic appraisal

(ii) Presumed duration of therapy
  Short-term treatment (inpatient therapy)
  Intermediate treatment (about 1 year)
  Long-term treatment (about 3 years)

From Remschmidt (1988).

the therapist who can use the process to help clarify and structure the approach to treatment. The plan should be drawn up following a period of initial diagnostic appraisal, usually no later than 2 weeks after admission. It should detail all individuals involved with the patient, define specific tasks and indicate and order all treatment steps precisely. Any difficulties which occur in drawing up such treatment plans need to be discussed within the ward team and any resulting modifications should be included in the plan. Optimal cooperation can be achieved only when the ward team is in agreement with the principles on which treatment is to be undertaken. It is important to consider the feasibility of any plan in addition to any desired goals (Remschmidt, 1988).

When planning and undertaking inpatient therapy, it is important to consider the therapeutic milieu. Hersov (1994) defined the therapeutic milieu as 'a structured environment that provides a variety of human relationships, satisfactory emotional interactions, opportunities for new learning and experiences, mastering of new situations and the development of personal and social competence'. Establishing and maintaining an appropriate therapeutic milieu will require ongoing support of all individuals involved in treating and caring for patients on the ward. Ideally, this will meet two requirements:

- first, training in specific professional skills with the aim of improving understanding of the patient's behaviour;
- secondly, improving the understanding of one's own behaviour and reactions, particularly on an emotional level.

The second of these areas, most often known as 'supervision' is important for the whole team. It should:

- focus on the patient and the therapeutic tasks;
- not come into conflict with the institution's organizational structure;
- be connected with the field of psychotherapy and meet professional needs;
- not replace therapy sessions nor resemble self-experience groups.

Supervision should be undertaken only by individuals with wide experience in child and adolescent psychotherapy. It may take the form of periodic individual sessions or team supervision, which focuses on the ward team encouraging their sense of autonomy.

Practical problems

Establishing a therapeutic milieu on a ward demands a considerable amount of flexibility from the staff and willingness to cooperate. They require a good working knowledge about psychiatric disturbances including psychogenic and psychosomatic disorders and approaches to treatment. Time needs to be made available for ward rounds, handovers, feedback, supervision, etc. Handovers need to be undertaken daily between shifts in order to pass on relevant information, which should be detailed and complete. It is essential to record all relevant information in written form. Ward rounds should involve all relevant members of the ward staff and should relate to both patients and treatment methods. Focusing on the patient involves therapists and nursing staff discussing any significant progress or problems, whilst focusing on the method involves reviewing the treatment techniques and defining the roles of the staff involved, e.g. Who will undertake behavioural training with the patient? How should the rewards for appropriate behaviour be awarded? What is the focus of play therapy in a particular patient? What problems does the family have to cope with? How is treatment affecting behaviour at school?. It is usually helpful to define one member of the nursing staff who will be primarily responsible for the patient ('primary nurse') who will establish a particularly trusting relationship with the patient.

It is important that suicidal behaviour is discussed openly when a patient is at risk. Ward rounds are good opportunities to discuss issues such as how to deal with suicidal, self-harming and aggressive patients.

It is equally important to address the issue of how to deal with parents of inpatients. The ward staff should always treat parents with compassion, respect and empathy.

Overemphasizing the role of disturbed family interaction in the aetiology of psychiatric disorders may result in parents being blamed and undermined, particularly by less experienced members of the ward staff. This may result in rivalry, emotional overinvolvement and inappropriate interaction between parents and ward staff.

Frequently, rivalry also occurs between the different professional groups working on a ward, e.g. the supposedly privileged role of therapists or teachers, whose opinion and theoretical background differs from that of the nursing staff. That such conflicts are common, and to some extent normal, needs to be remembered by therapists and supervisors.

Finally, it is important to recognize the limitations of psychotherapy and discuss this issue with the ward staff to avoid a sense of hopelessness and self-blame when dealing with these severe problems. This is a responsible task for the more senior therapists, particularly when supervising younger and less experienced members of the team.

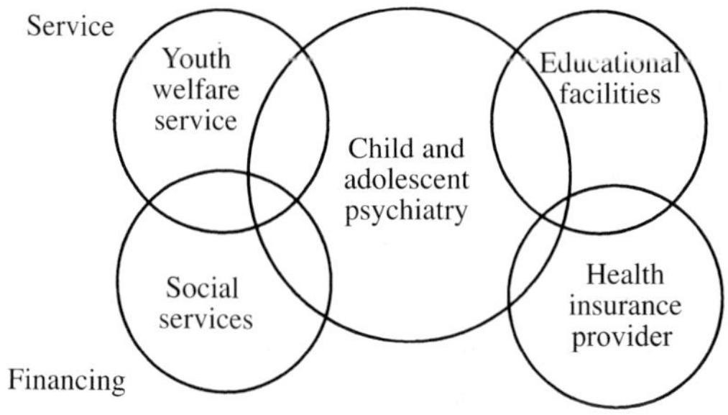

Fig. 32.3. The relationship between child and adolescent psychiatry and other related institutions.

Psychotherapy in complementary institutions

Not all psychiatric disorders which occur in childhood and adolescence can be successfully treated alone by means of short (3–6 month) inpatient psychotherapy such that the patient can be discharged back to his home environment. It is therefore necessary to establish a cooperative system of treatment facilities and complementary institutions to care for those children and adolescents unable to return home following inpatient treatment. Maintenance of training and ongoing education of staff in these institutions is difficult in most countries because of the insufficient number of places in residential homes or groups for children and adolescents with psychiatric disorders, yet this is of vital importance and may be facilitated by good links between institutions (see Fig. 32.3).

An example of a comprehensive treatment and rehabilitation programme for children and adolescents with psychiatric disorders has been established in association with the Hospital for Child and Adolescent Psychiatry, University of Marburg (Germany). A complementary rehabilitation facility has been established outside hospital premises, which offers care and rehabilitation for patients with chronic disorders requiring long-term treatment. The tasks of the facility include rehabilitation following discharge from hospital, e.g. for adolescents with autism, schizophrenia or mental retardation, ongoing psychotherapy in cases of chronic neurotic disorders, e.g. obssessive-compulsive disorder, anorexia nervosa, bulimia nervosa, continued educational or occupational support to children or adolescents who could not be reintegrated into their home environment, and helping patients to achieve gradually increasing autonomy following severe psychiatric illness in a series of successive steps towards rehabilitation, e.g. hospital, residential home, residential group, living alone.

There is an urgent need for long-term rehabilitation in a complementary institution following inpatient treatment. Whilst the primary aim of any child and adolescent psychiatric treatment is to treat and reintegrate the patient in his home environment as soon as possible, follow-up studies have shown that 20–35% of all child and adolescent psychiatric inpatients are unable to return home after discharge, so that out-of-home placement is neccessary. This out-of-home placement highlights the importance of child and adolescent psychiatric hospitals not only as places for treatment, but also as an institution in which important decisions for the patient's future are made following diagnostic appraisal, treatment and consideration of prognostic factors.

Treatment in a therapeutic home or residential group has the advantage that ongoing educational and psychiatric help can be offered to patients for an extended period of time, allowing treatment gains to be consolidated and built upon.

Collaboration between the child and adolescent psychiatric hospital and rehabilitation treatment facilities has the following advantages:

- the duration of psychiatric in-patient treatment can be reduced;
- therapeutic homes can cope with more severely disturbed patients if a hospital is available when crisis intervention is required;
- early discharge to the therapeutic home reduces the risks inherent in long-term hospitalization;
- treatment in therapeutic homes is less expensive than hospital inpatient treatment.

The involvement of social services is essential when planning rehabilitation treatment, because they usually play a major role both in selecting an appropriate institution as well as in financing rehabilitation. Planning requires close cooperation between the hospital, social services and the home or institution to which the patient is to be discharged. Patients placed out-of-home require not only a supportive and caring environment, but also ongoing treatment, requiring the close cooperation of doctors, psychologists, teachers and social workers. Such interdisciplinary collaboration requires members of the team to respect one another's professional competence. Breaching professional boundaries will lead to blurring of roles, resulting in substandard work. This issue has been addressed by Herzka (1980), who used the relationship between psychotherapy and education services as an example. A child with a psychological disorder requires psychotherapy because of the disorder and education because he is a child. Improving the collaboration of both fields is one of the principal tasks of child and adolescent psychiatry. Although good cooperation is the rule, controversy, misunderstandings and distrust between teachers and child and adolescent psychotherapists are still common. *A priori*, education and psychotherapy can be considered two equally important approaches to modifying children's behaviour. Both approaches have their own rules, which may at times be contradictory, but only together do they make up one whole. In treating children with psychiatric disorders, one approach is incomplete without the other. It is important that teachers and especially those with particular experience in teaching disturbed children, nevertheless remember that the child has a psychiatric disorder. Teachers should therefore be familiar with therapeutic considerations and take them into account when interacting with the child. In turn, therapists should not fail to appreciate the importance of the child's educational needs.

The average duration of stay in a rehabilitation facility is about 2–3 years. It is therefore of paramount importance that a stable relationship is built up between the children and adolescents and the educational staff who care for them. The staff's tasks include defining the rules for living together and making sure they are kept, providing appropriate role models, encouraging the development of normal social interaction and personal relationships, and conveying the impression that the children and adolescents are accepted as individuals despite the problems or difficulties they may have.

Although educational work with adolescents with social deficits or antisocial behaviour can be difficult, this is less the case in those with neurotic or psychosomatic disorders, who may require modification of overadaption and inhibitions. Thus, each patient will usually require an individual educational plan. Creating a therapeutic milieu also implies establishing an appropriate educational atmosphere which facilitates access to patients' emotional problems without losing contact with reality. The complex educational task which care-givers and teachers face makes considerable demands on those involved and requires careful planning and review processes.

Treating patients in a therapeutic home has considerable advantages. It can serve as a valuable intermediate step between inpatient and outpatient treatment. Treatment in the home can be much more intensive that outpatient treatment, and the home may be an important substitute for inadequate family support. Patients' families may view treatment in the home either with criticism, or consider it helpful. Competitive situations with professional care-givers may occur, and parents may gradually be discharged of the responsibility of participating in bringing up their child. It is therefore important to keep good levels of communication with the patient's family, addressing any family conflicts early in order to establish a stable basis for ongoing work with the patient (Arendt and Bosselman, 1981).

Psychotherapy in complementary treatment facilities generally makes the same demands on both therapist and patient as inpatient treatment. However, the role of educational influences and the interpersonal relationship between patients and care-givers is even more relevant than in a hospital setting. Psychotherapeutic measures should be undertaken by educationally qualified nursing and educational staff, and the rules for collaboration between therapists and educational staff must be clearly defined. Therapeutic and educational measures need to match and support one another in order to bring about improvement in the patient, especially in cases of chronic psychiatric disorder. The ultimate aim is to enable the child or adolescent to optimize his scholastic, professional, and personal competencies. Therapists who work in an institution should play a major role in establishing the therapeutic milieu, maintaining a relatively consistent therapeutic concept.

Specific subspecialization of rehabilitation facilities implies that they have special expertise in the types of disorder which they treat. This does not imply that therapeutic homes are required which, for example, exclusively treat eating disorders, sexually abused girls or patients with obsessive-compulsive disorder. However, the rehabilitation concept of an institution treating adolescents with schizophrenia will be quite different from the requirements for treating patients with psychosomatic disorders such as eating disorders, or neurotic disorders. In comparison, adolescents with antisocial behaviour require entirely different educational and therapeutic strategies. Thus it is probably appropriate to distinguish between different rehabilitation facilities according to their scope. Age is an additional problem which needs to be addressed when considering the most appropriate placement.

In the planning and undertaking of inpatient psychotherapy, it is important to select the most appropriate setting. The guiding principle should be that the interruption of the everyday activities of normal life due to hospitalization should be as brief as possible. Transfer to a less restrictive environment, such as a therapeutic residential group, should be undertaken as soon as possible. The better the collaboration regarding therapeutic approach of the relevant institutions, the better will be the chances of successful long-term outcome.

REFERENCES

Arendt, G. and Bosselmann, R. (1981). Familientherapie im Heim. *Unsere Jugend*, **5**, 208–16.

Hersov, L. (1994). Inpatient and day-hospital units. In *Child and adolescent psychiatry. Modern approaches*, 3rd edn, ed. M. Rutter, E. Taylor and L. Hersov, pp. 983–95. Oxford: Blackwell Science.

Herzka, H. S. (1980). Psychotherapie und Pädagogik. Eine Gegenüberstellung. *Acta Paedopsychiatrica*, **45**, 171–4.

Mattejat, F., Gutenbrunner, C. and Remschmidt, H. (1994). Therapeutische Leistungen einer kinder- und jugendpsychiatrischen Universitätsklinik mit regionalem Versorgungsauftrag und ihrer assoziierten Einrichtungen. Ein Beitrag zur Qualitätssicherung. *Zeitschrift für Kinder- und Jugendpsychiatrie*, **22**, 154–68.

Remschmidt, H. (1988). Gesichtspunkte zur Indikationsstellung therapeutischer Massnahmen. In *Kinder- und Jugendpsychiatrie in Klinik und Praxis*, vol. I, ed. H. Remschmidt and M. H. Schmidt, pp. 608–12. Stuttgart: Thieme.

Remschmidt, H. and Walter, R. (1989). *Evaluation kinder- und jugendpsychiatrischer Versorgung*. Stuttgart: Enke.

Remschmidt, H., Gutenbrunner, C. and Mattejat F. (1994). Zum Stellenwert verschiedener Therapieformen in einer kinder- und jugendpsychiatrischen Universitätsklinik und assoziierter Einrichtungen. Methodische und inhaltliche Aspekte der Therapiedokumentation im Rahmen der Qualitätssicherung. *Zeitschrift für Kinder- und Jugendpsychiatrie*, **22**, 169–82.

Rutter, M., Schaffer, D. and Shepherd, M. (1975). *A multiaxial classification system of child psychiatric disorders*. Geneva: World Health Organization (WHO).

Schepank, H. (1987). Die stationäre Psychotherapie in der Bundesrepublik Deutschland. Soziokulturelle Determinanten, Entwicklungsstufen und Ist Zustand, internationaler Vergleich. *Zeitschrift für Psychosomatische Medizin und Psychoanalyse*, **33**, 363–87.

Schepank, H. and Tress, W. (1988). *Die stationäre Psychotherapie und ihr Rahmen*. Springer: Berlin.

33 Day-patient psychotherapy

Andreas Warnke and Kurt Quaschner

The term 'partial hospitalization' is used to describe treatment of children and adolescents which is undertaken only during the day ('day-patient treatment') or night ('night-patient treatment'). Although night treatment is not particularly relevant in this age group, day-patient treatment has become increasingly important (Döpfner, 1993a). Day-patient treatment offers the many advantages of inpatient treatment, whilst allowing patients to spend the late afternoons, nights, and weekends in their usual home environment.

Indications and preconditions for day-patient treatment

Indications

The following indications for day-patient treatment have been suggested (Remschmidt, 1992; Remschmidt and Schmidt, 1988).

Avoidance of hospitalization

Day-patient treatment may be appropriate when outpatient treatment is impossible, has been only partially or unsuccessful, despite inpatient treatment being deemed unnecessary. This group may include children with emotional disturbance, hyperkinetic disorder, minimal brain dysfunction and severe specific learning disorders (such as dyslexia and dyscalculia). Day-patient treatment is particularly recommended when children are at risk of developmental disturbance or difficulties at school or work where the family is unable to provide sufficient support.

Curtailment of inpatient treatment

Day-patient treatment should be considered as a secondary treatment step in children who initially required inpatient treatment. Earlier discharge is often possible provided subsequent day-patient facilities are available, e.g. in psychosis, organic behavioural disorder due to brain dysfunction, anorexia nervosa.

Day-patient treatment may also be appropriate in the process of gradual reintegration into the family and school or work.

Refusal of inpatient treatment

In some cases, inpatient treatment may be considered advisable, but is refused by the patient or his parents. In such cases day-patient treatment may be an acceptable option. Even when the disorder is not life-threatening, outpatient treatment alone may prove inadequate. With some disorders, e.g. separation anxiety, symbiotic relationship between parents and child, and anorexia nervosa, there is a particular risk of the condition becoming chronic, and day-patient treatment may provide a useful 'way in' to treatment.

Preconditions for treatment and the spectrum of disorders

For day-patient treatment to be successful, several preconditions need to be met. The family needs to be available and willing to cooperate, so that family sessions can be undertaken at least every 2 weeks. The family is expected to be capable of bearing the responsibility for patient care during times of acute disturbance or conflict, and the child must be able to return home daily. The patient should also be in a position to tolerate group situations with peers in the open environment of the day-patient unit.

Contraindications for day-patient treatment include the treatment of disorders which are more appropriately treated in an inpatient facility, particularly if a secure unit is necessary, such as in severe depression, risk of suicide, acute psychosis, severe conduct disorder or delinquency with violence. Severe separation anxiety may result in unsurmountable difficulties every time the child is expected to leave home to attend day-hospital. Additionally, patients who are unable to keep rules in an open setting, e.g. those with acute addiction or severe anorexia and bulimia nervosa are also generally inappropriate for day-patient treatment.

The range of disorders which can be managed in a day-patient setting will depend, to a great extent, on available staff and financial resources, and the range is likely to vary according to the institution's conceptual emphasis. The following disorders are commonly treated in our unit: emotional disturbance, hyperkinetic conduct disorder, antisocial behaviour, and neurotic disorders. Emotional disturbances commonly occur together with difficulties in social interaction, and children often also have co-morbid conditions such as developmental or specific learning disorders (such as dyslexia and dyscalculia). Many of our children with hyperkinetic conduct disorder and antisocial behaviour, or specific learning disorder have a poor or inappropriate family environment and require day-patient treatment because they are at risk of being expelled from school. We also treat preschool children who frequently suffer from multiple developmental retardation.

In large cities, specific treatment facilities are usually available, e.g. day-patient treatment facilities for specific learning disabilities such as dyslexia or developmental speech disorders. Such facilities may be required for patients with normal general intelligence, who are unable to attend normal school and require psychotherapeutic help.

The age of patients in our day-hospital ranges from 5–18 years, the majority being between 7 and 12. The average duration of treatment is 5–6 months. Day-hospitals specializing in the treatment of adolescents, e.g. with schizophrenia or anorexia nervosa will obviously have a different age distribution.

Transport to our day-patient unit is varied. Some children use public transport, a few parents bring their child, and some children are brought by taxi, particularly preschoolers and children from places with poor public transport. The issue of covering these expenses needs to be discussed with health insurance providers beforehand (Eisert and Eisert, 1988; Schmidt, 1993).

Multimodal approach to partial hospitalization

A multimodal approach to treatment can address symptoms with different methods. The term 'multimodal' does not imply that treatment methods are used indiscriminately, but emphasizes the need to plan individually the approach to therapy, depending on the type of disorder ('differentiated treatment').

This approach is particularly appropriate for partial hospitalization because therapy can be much more intensive than outpatient treatment. In addition to the ('quantitative') issue of treatment intensity ('qualitative') considerations of the appropriate treatment also play an important role in planning treatment. Disorders are often complex and associated with a broad spectrum of symptoms, which requires a range of approaches to optimize outcome.

The multimodal approach takes into account not only the variety of symptoms, but also the fact that no single treatment technique is effective in all types of disorders.

Structure and distribution of tasks

General setting

The general setting, i.e. the day-patient unit's external and internal structure, including the daily schedule influences treatment to a considerable extent, regardless of the theoretical concept or therapeutic school on which treatment is based. This type of general setting (with appropriate 'spatial' and 'temporal' structures) is an important precondition for individually focused psychotherapy. The general setting may also be regarded as a 'therapeutic factor' in itself, contributing to operant conditioning techniques such as stimulus control, which may be part of a behavioural therapy programme.

Stimulus control aims to modify behaviour by influencing and minimizing problematic behaviour which is related to specific situations or stimuli. Stimulus control is the most common technique individuals use to bring about or prevent specific reactions in normal life. This technique is very relevant to day-patient treatment. It is possible to distinguish the following common types of stimuli, i.e. situational conditions (Hautzinger, 1993).

Discriminatory stimuli

Such stimuli have become associated with specific behaviours in the course of previous experience. For example, in a day-patient context, such stimuli might include the following sequence: mealtime → washing hands → praise. A great variety of such sequences can be introduced into daily routines. Behaviour gradually becomes 'automatic' as patients adopt the sequence and consider the resulting behaviour natural.

Verbal stimuli, rules and regulations

These include verbally agreed rules, e.g. to 'stop' when aggression is about to break out. Patients are rewarded when rules are kept and privileges are withdrawn when rules are broken.

Stimuli which encourage behaviours

These include helping patients with tasks and bringing about situational conditions which encourage specific behaviour, e.g. modifying the size or composition of a group in order to improve group interaction and the therapeutic effect of group activities.

Motivational conditions

The role of a specific behaviour is enhanced and reinforcement improved by modifying a situation in advance, e.g. temporarily withdrawing social contact and prohibiting play.

External structure

The external structure of day-patient treatment includes the unit's premises and greatly determines the general atmosphere. The rooms need to meet functional, educational and therapeutic requirements. A day-patient unit for about 12 children should resemble the following structure:

- a large central entrance hall which may be used as a multipurpose room: it also functions as an entrance hall, giving access to the other rooms, and can be used as a waiting room or modified for festivities. It contains the cloakroom, tables and seats, and a small play corner. The hall is also used to exhibit patients' art work or work produced in occupational therapy;
- a kitchen with dining room used for breakfast, lunch and afternoon snack. The kitchen is fitted with a sink, two cookers, two ovens, a dishwasher, a refrigerator and several cupboards. Thus facilities are also available to cook meals with a group;
- a group room with a cupboard containing games, a small library, and a play corner either for use during free time, or for individual or group psychotherapy sessions;
- a play therapy room;
- a gym which can be used for games or gymnastics, with an attached room for equipment;
- an occupational therapy room with work benches and appropriate tools;
- a large group therapy room equipped with a video system, suitable for role play, family therapy, parent training, team conferences, professional training, etc.;
- individual offices for one doctor and one psychologist;
- a school room, also suitable for:
  - (i) group sessions,
  - (ii) individual sessions,
  - (iii) play and relaxation;
- an office for the staff and secretary;
- outdoor activities such as sports may be undertaken on the large lawn outside the building, and gardening is possible on a small plot nearby.

Internal structure (interventions and daily schedule)

An example of a daily schedule is shown in Fig. 33.1. It reflects the approach to treatment in our day-patient unit. The schedule comprises an internal structure, which incorporates the therapeutic concept and the relevant patient interventions.

8.00 - 8.30	Children arrive, received by staff, hanging up coats, changing clothes when necessary
8.30 - 8.50	Breakfast
8.50 - 9.00	Cleaning teeth, washing hands, preparation for school; patients are accompanied to the school room
9.00 - 12.00	(a) Lessons for school-aged children, individual sessions, work with parents (b) Preschoolers are involved in play sessions or treatment sessions individually or in small groups. Preschoolers may attend school for some lessons
12.00 - 12.45	Lunch
12.45 - 13.30	Play
13.30 - 14.00	Homework for school-aged children
14.00 - 16.00	Group activities, group psychotherapy (usually in a small group), work with parents
16.00 - 16.15	Afternoon snack
16.15 - 16.30	Departure for home

Fig. 33.1. The day-patient unit's schedule.

Daily life activities

General measures are intended to improve the patient's ability to cope with everyday life. The neccessary practical skills include appropriate eating behaviour, tidy clothes and general hygiene. All meals are usually taken together. Each child is expected to sit in his own place, e.g. three children and one supervisor at each table, and the children are expected to keep certain rules:

- behaviour during the meal, e.g. Who will serve the food? Are the children allowed to speak, sing, play or get up during meals?;
- rules on beginning and ending meals, e.g. Which group is allowed to get up first and go to wash their hands?;
- table manners, e.g. Is it compulsory to eat with knife and fork? What are the consequences of refusal to eat, playing with food, spilling drinks?;
- clearing the table, e.g. Who is expected to help? What needs to be done?;
- rules related to hygiene, e.g. When is the appropriate time for washing hands, cleaning teeth etc.?

Meals are generally commenced together. We favour serving the food in serving dishes so that children can help themselves, as at home. Some patients may require individual assistance while eating.

A further area which is given particular weight is dressing skills, e.g. buttoning garments, tying shoelaces and hygiene skills, e.g. washing hands, appropriate toilet behaviour, cleaning teeth, etc. This may be particularly difficult for patients with mental retardation or antisocial behaviour. Toilet training is an important part of specific treatment programmes for patients with enuresis and encopresis.

Educational measures

School attendance is compulsory, and children are also provided with supervised homework sessions, with associated treatment when neccessary, e.g. for specific learning disorders such as dyslexia or dyscalculia. Some children may also take part in individual remedial sessions, e.g. for spelling or speech, whilst the others continue in the classroom. If a patient is unable to take part in a whole morning's lessons, he may be permitted to return to the day-patient unit early. This may occur in the case of school refusal or misbehaviour which disturbs other children in the class. Educational goals need to be discussed with teachers and care-givers in order to make homework supervision relevant and effective.

Recreational facilities

Recreational activity is an important part of treatment. Therapy cannot be undertaken all day long – no child would tolerate this, and it would also contradict the idea of improving patients' autonomy and independence. Recreational activity is therefore scheduled throughout the day. Many patients have difficulties playing alone or persistently quarrel with others, therefore, daily recreational activities are also organized to create a 'flexible recreational programme'. Such activities include birthday celebrations or goodbye parties prior to discharge, swimming in summer or tobogganing in winter, season's celebrations such as Easter or Christmas, out of doors or indoor games, etc. This type of flexible recreational programme requires special planning efforts and good supervision by nursing staff.

Recreational activities are coordinated with treatment sessions, both in terms of time and the interventions used. Periods of recreational activity may conveniently interlock with individual therapy sessions.

More specific therapeutic intervention

Ideally, the daily schedule should include both individual and group psychotherapy sessions.

Individual psychotherapy

Individual psychotherapy is offered to most patients and undertaken by the doctor or psychologist on the unit. It may include general techniques such as play therapy, and/or more symptom orientated approaches such as cognitive or behavioural therapy. Counselling is also offered by the unit staff.

Functional treatment

Functional treatment for specific learning disorders such as dyslexia or dyscalculia is an important part of the multimodal therapy approach. Functional treatment is important because many patients suffer from a specific learning disorder, even though it may be a secondary disorder rather than the primary reason for treatment. Scholastic difficulties are frequently due to specific difficulties such as dyslexia, dyscalculia, attention deficit, or sensory impairment. Functional treatment of these deficits is important, because if they remain untreated the risk of secondary symptoms such as emotional and behavioural disturbances is high.

Physiotherapy is not usually emphasized in day-patient treatment, although in some cases psychomotor function may need attention.

Occupational therapy is useful for improving manual skills and may contribute to improving self-esteem.

Speech therapy should also be offered in a day-patient setting for patients with speech disorders.

Group psychotherapy

Much day-patient treatment takes place in group settings. The group setting can be considered in itself a therapeutic factor, which may have an effect in a variety of situations. Specific group psychotherapy has two main applications. First, improving social competency and interpersonal skills, which may be undertaken using role play or very small groups. Secondly, 'creative' groups can be formed, in which creative or occupational techniques are used to improve specific skills.

Informal groups are also important, despite not having strictly 'therapeutic' aims. Informal groups offer a degree of freedom and enable children to engage in a wider range of activity. These groups are not so disrupted if patients have to leave the group for individual therapy sessions.

In addition to individual and group psychotherapy in the unit, the patient's experiences and world outside the day hospital premises should also be included in treatment. Thus, cooperation with parents is particularly important, and collaboration with other institutions is also required in most cases.

Cooperation with parents

An important task of those involved in day-patient treatment is to coordinate the various educational milieus and direct personal influences to which the patient is subjected. Obviously, this task will have to include the patient's parents. Thus, cooperation with parents is one of the most important aspects of day-patient treatment. Prior to admission, the issue of cooperation needs to be addressed and discussed with parents. Parents are required to participate in weekly sessions, although even then good cooperation is not guaranteed, and unforeseen difficulties may arise in the course of treatment.

The neutral term 'cooperation with parents' is intended to indicate that the aim of cooperation is not the realization of a particular theoretical concept. The term reflects the fact that cooperation can include many different aspects, be more or less intense, have various goals, and be a two-way process.

On a basic level, 'cooperation' simply means exchanging information. How does the patient behave at home? How does he behave in the day-hospital? What difficulties and problems occur? Which treatment steps are being undertaken and which steps are planned?

A secondary level is, however, the issue of parental education, although the boundary between the levels is very blurred. The main focus is to offer full explanation about the disorder and support the parents. Both therapist and parents need to agree on strategies of dealing with the patient in order to facilitate the transfer of behaviour modifications from day-hospital to the home environment.

When the disorder is not only an individual problem but involves the whole family, more intense cooperation is necessary. In some cases, formal parent training or family therapy may be advisable (see Chapters 12 and 13). Issues which need to be addressed and modified usually include family relationships, interaction, attitudes and communicational styles.

The broad range of ways to cooperate with parents is reflected in the general therapeutic setting. The frequency of sessions ranges from weekly family therapy including all members of the family to offering advice to one or both parents briefly every 2–3 weeks.

Cooperation with other institutions

Both prior to admission and following discharge, day-patient units usually need to cooperate with various other institutions such as schools, residential homes or other hospital departments, e.g. the speech therapy department of an ENT hospital.

When follow-up treatment is to be undertaken by a different facility, the day-patient needs to prepare for discharge and future treatment with that facility.

In some cases, cooperation with youth welfare agencies may be necessary, particularly when the patient is a foster child or comes from a residential home. Sometimes, out-of-home placement is required following day-patient treatment, in which case the youth welfare office usually needs to be involved.

The staff and its tasks (teamwork)

The make up of the staff team in day-patient units is generally interdisciplinary and multiprofessional. The range of therapy and educational help which can be offered takes into account the staff's qualifications and professional experience, although material considerations (facilities and funds) are also important for any day-patient unit's work. In our experience, the following staff mix has been useful:

- one doctor or psychologist, supervised by a senior therapist, to undertake psychotherapy and parental work. They are usually also primarily responsible for cooperation with complementary institutions, e.g. schools, youth welfare agencies. With a major responsibility for new referrals, they must also be clear about the indications for day-patient treatment, and will be involved in the assessment, drawing up treatment plans and documenting all steps;
- one occupational therapist to assist patients in developing practical skills, e.g. eating behaviour, dressing, sensory training;
- one nurse to take on tasks such as distributing any necessary medication, accompanying children to hospital for investigations, weighing patients, drawing blood, assistance with EEG, etc. The nurse also has a particular involvement in patients with 'physical' symptoms, e.g. enuresis, encopresis;
- one remedial teacher who provides additional help for children with specific learning disorders such as dyslexia, dyscalculia, motor impairment, attention deficit, perceptional disorders, etc.;
- one therapist for extra therapeutic work such as horse riding or music therapy;
- one physiotherapist for psychomotor training groups;
- one secretary for secretarial and specific organizational tasks;
- several teachers from the hospital special school for school lessons in the morning.

All staff members contribute to individual patient care, either for one or several patients. This involves participation in sessions with parents and specific therapeutic tasks such as work with a particularly aggressive patient or a child with mutism. It is important that all staff members contribute in the non-specific tasks such as supervising meals, play, or supervising home work.

Agreements on tasks and responsibilities must be made with all individuals involved when drawing up a treatment plan. This degree of cooperation is essential for the smooth running and therapeutic value of the unit. A number of weekly meetings are held:

- organizational conference ($1\frac{1}{2}$ hours) during which the daily and weekly schedules are discussed and the tasks for each staff member outlined;
- therapeutic conference and grand rounds with the supervising therapist (2 hours), during which a patient's history, clinical findings, diagnosis, behavioural observations, etc. are reviewed and discussed. Treatment goals are defined and incorporated in the treatment plan;
- staff meetings, at which any organizational issues, e.g. ordering material needed in the unit, coordinating work and holidays, etc. are discussed.
- teachers' conference (1 hour) during the term time only. Teachers and therapeutic staff have the opportunity to share observations made during lessons or in the day-patient unit. Issues concerning individual patients are discussed in detail, and strategies to help the child are developed. Organizational issues concerning school attendance after discharge are also addressed.

These meetings take up a considerable amount of time, but are essential for successful interdisciplinary cooperation and therefore of unquestionable value. The conferences must be well organized in order to be effective. The following suggestions may be helpful towards achieving this aim.

- An agenda and timetable should be prepared beforehand, perhaps by the individual responsible for keeping the minutes.
- The conference should begin and end on time, the agenda and timetable should be adhered to.
- One individual should be responsible for chairing the conference and focusing discussions.

It may be helpful to hold the conference in the following order: discussion of topics of general interest (time limited); introduction of new staff members or visitors; approval of the minutes from the last conference; modification of measures previously agreed upon; discussion of treatment progress, diagnostic appraisal, specific therapeutic issues, patient care, planning work with parents and organizational issues concerning the patient and other institutions.

The course of day-patient treatment

The steps involved in day-patient treatment are shown in Fig. 33.2. Individual steps are discussed below.

Indication for treatment and subsequent preparation of admission

↓

Admission, diagnostic appraisal, observation phase

↓

Therapeutic goals and treatment plan

↓

Treatment

↓

Discharge and follow-up

Fig. 33.2. The steps involved in day-patient treatment.

Indication for treatment and subsequent preparation of admission

Patients are usually admitted for day-patient treatment following diagnostic appraisal in the outpatient clinic or on the ward. Patients and their parents are generally permitted to visit the facility beforehand, and usually the therapist will undertake an interview prior to admission. The family should be asked about their expectations, hopes, treatment aims, etc. In some cases, other individuals who are familiar with the child, such as care-givers, teachers, previous therapists or grandparents may be asked to provide relevant additional information. The indication for day-patient treatment should be reassessed and the family's motivation to cooperate confirmed. The therapist should give an estimate as to the probable duration of treatment. If the family is willing, an admission date is agreed upon. The issue of who is to cover the cost of day-patient treatment must be addressed beforehand, including the issue of travel costs. Parents must understand the need to take their child home for the night, on weekends and public holidays. However, children do not remain at home during school holidays. Day-hospital runs continuously, not only during term-time. As the decision for day-patient treatment is made after an initial interview, the family has enough time to reconsider the decision if they wish.

Admission, diagnostic appraisal, observation phase

An initial assessment and observation phase lasting 2–4 weeks usually precedes treatment and includes the following steps:

- taking a child and adolescent psychiatric history on the day of admission;
- physical examination and additional investigations, e.g. EEG, laboratory studies;
- psychological assessment including standardized tests;
- behavioural observation in various situations.

The findings and test results are discussed among the staff, possibly with the aid of standardized behavioural observation scales and treatment goal questionnaires. They are the basis for further treatment plans.

Naturally, diagnostic appraisal continues throughout the course of treatment. As treatment proceeds, the therapist is likely to encounter additional information about the patient, his family and developmental capacity. The family's ability to cooperate, in particular, often only becomes clear after treatment has commenced.

Therapeutic goals and treatment plan

Problem behaviours are then defined and therapeutic goals discussed and defined in cooperation with the family. A treatment plan is then drawn up in order to coordinate the specific treatment steps considered appropriate for the individual patient.

Treatment

Treatment is regularly discussed in the team meeting, and individually supervised by a senior therapist. Individual, group and family therapy techniques are used and modified when necessary. There are special considerations to be borne in mind when working in a day-patient setting.

- Psychotherapy can be stressful to both child and family and should therefore be administered carefully and in the right 'dose' in order to prevent both 'overtreatment' and boredom. No child will tolerate therapy all day long. In addition to school and daily routine activity, psychotherapy should not exceed two individual psychotherapy sessions per day.
- Both time and activities should be organized carefully in order to avoid clashing timetables, delays, unavailable staff, inadequate supervision of patients, and general wasted time.
- Therapeutic techniques may be transferred from the day-patient setting to the school or home environment ('co-therapy'). For example, a nurse or educator may help a patient with dyslexia to read street names while taking a walk outdoors using the phonetic sign language which the patient was taught in therapy, thus facilitating treatment.
- Cooperation with parents contributes significantly to treatment success, particularly as the patient has to cope with two different environments (day-hospital and home).
- Treatment needs to address particularly those deficits and developmental delays which are amenable to therapy, i.e. compensating deficits, catching up

<table>
<tr><th>TIME</th><th>MONDAY</th><th>TUESDAY</th><th>WEDNESDAY</th><th>THURSDAY</th><th>FRIDAY</th></tr>
<tr><td>8.00</td><td colspan="5">Arrival</td></tr>
<tr><td>8.30</td><td colspan="5">Breakfast</td></tr>
<tr><td>9.00</td><td>School</td><td rowspan="2">School</td><td>School</td><td>School</td><td rowspan="2">School</td></tr>
<tr><td>11.30</td><td>Individual functional treatment</td><td>Individual functional treatment</td><td>Individual functional treatment</td></tr>
<tr><td>12.00</td><td colspan="5">Lunch</td></tr>
<tr><td>12.45</td><td colspan="5">Informal group</td></tr>
<tr><td>1.30</td><td colspan="4">Homework</td><td></td></tr>
<tr><td rowspan="2">2.00</td><td rowspan="2">Informal group</td><td rowspan="2">Individual psychotherapy</td><td>Weekly group discussion</td><td rowspan="2">Individual psychotherapy</td><td rowspan="2">Session with individual care-giver</td></tr>
<tr><td>'Tidying up'</td></tr>
<tr><td>3.00</td><td>Psychomotor training group</td><td>Role play in group</td><td>Occupational therapy group</td><td>Family session</td><td></td></tr>
<tr><td>4.00</td><td colspan="4">Afternoon snack</td><td></td></tr>
<tr><td>4.15–4.30</td><td colspan="4">Departure</td><td></td></tr>
</table>

Fig. 33.3. Example for a week's schedule (see case report).

on delays. This will assist the child to develop his natural potential, with its strengths and weaknesses.

Case report

10-year old Tony was admitted for treatment of hyperkinetic conduct disorder (classified as F90.1 in ICD-10) to our day-patient unit. In addition to the typical symptoms (attention deficit, hyperactivity) the patient showed abnormal social behaviour in that he breached normal social boundaries and demonstrated impulsive breaking of social rules. This resulted in severe disturbance of behaviour in groups, so that the patient was excluded from group situations several times. His parents described him as very restless, with an unstable temper and poor concentration. Home work was frequently associated with problems such as avoidance, constant misbehaviour, or refusal.

Diagnostic appraisal showed that the boy had normal intelligence but marked dyslexia (specific developmental reading and spelling disorder).

Subsequent treatment took a multimodal approach, which can be considered typical for day-patient settings. Individual treatment steps are shown in Fig. 33.3. In addition to the usual components of therapy, the treatment plan included interventions aimed at the individual patient. These interventions were tailored to meet the patient's specific needs.

Behavioural therapy techniques were the cornerstones of treatment. Operant reinforcement plans were used ('contingency management') and social competency training was undertaken in individual and group sessions ('role play group').

In Tony's case functional training of reading and spelling skills was particularly important in order to help his dyslexia. He was helped in reading and spelling skills in individual sessions at school.

In addition to the role play group, Tony was included in a very small occupational therapy group (three patients). He also attended a psychomotor training group aiming both to improve the ability to relax and activate patients.

Family therapy sessions were undertaken every two weeks during the entire course of day-patient treatment. They were not only part of the usual cooperation during treatment, but an essential component of therapy. The family conflicts which arose during treatment, including disagreements between parents and their children, required several additional sessions. However, collaboration with the family was excellent in spite of conflicts, the patient's parents were reliable and cooperative, and the accompanying difficulties were overcome to a large degree.

Over the course of treatment, Tony's symptoms improved gradually and slowly. Tony eventually gained some understanding of his behaviour in the context of other's behaviour. He understood why he should act more appropriately, which resulted in behavioural improvement, i.e. the number of conflicts he provoked in group situations and during social interaction was significantly reduced over his stay.

Discharge was planned at a relatively early stage. The designated school cooperated readily. The patient and his new class teacher had the opportunity to meet prior to discharge. Thus the patient was carefully prepared for the challenges of the new school.

Discharge and outpatient follow-up

The duration of treatment depends on the course, the patient's and his family's wishes, as well as organizational factors, e.g. start of school. The planning of follow-up treatment and the process of discharge are discussed with parents well beforehand. Out-of-home placement, should a child be unable to return home, is a serious step which requires careful consideration. Day-patient units usually do not offer follow-up treatment, but exceptions are permissible when there is no alternative.

Evaluation

Day-hospitals are fairly new among psychiatric health care facilities, particularly in child and adolescent psychiatry. Hence there is a paucity of empirical studies on the efficacy of day-patient treatment. However, those results which are available are encouraging (Döpfner, 1993b). One of the few studies in which different treatment techniques were compared (Remschmidt et al., 1988) comes to the conclusion that day-patient treatment can replace inpatient therapy in some cases. Some follow-up studies have suggested that treatment effects are relatively stable over time.

REFERENCES

Döpfner, M. (1993a). Konzeption einer teilstationären Behandlung. In *Kinderpsychiatrie: Vorschulalter*, ed. M. Döpfner and M. H. Schmidt, pp. 140–55. München: Quintessenz.

Döpfner, M. (1993b). Wirksamkeit teilstationärer Behandlung. In *Kinderpsychiatrie: Vorschulalter*, ed. M. Döpfner and M. H. Schmidt, pp. 156–74. München: Quintessenz.

Eisert, H. G. and Eisert, M. (1988). Stationäre Behandlung, teilstationäre Behandlung und home treatment. Möglichkeiten und konkrete Durchführung verschiedener Behandlungsmodalitäten. In *Alternative Behandlungsformen in der Kinder- und Jugendpsychiatrie*, ed. H. Remschmidt and M. H. Schmidt, pp. 14–28. Stuttgart: Enke.

Hautzinger, M. (1993). Stimuluskontrolle. In *Verhaltenstherapie*, 2nd edn, ed. M. Linden and M. Hautzinger, pp. 289–93. Berlin: Springer.

Remschmidt, H. (1992). *Psychiatrie der Adoleszenz*. Stuttgart: Thieme.

Remschmidt, H. and Schmidt, M. H. (1988). *Alternative Behandlungsformen in der Kinder- und Jugendpsychiatrie*. Stuttgart: Enke.

Remschmidt, H., Schmidt, M. H., Mattejat, F., Eisert, H. G. and Eisert, M. (1988). Therapieevaluation in der Kinder- und Jugendpsychiatrie. Stationäre Behandlung, tagesklinische Behandlung und home-treatment im Vergleich. *Zeitschrift für Kinder- und Jugendpsychiatrie*, **16**, 124–34.

Schmidt, M. H. (1993). Möglichkeiten und Grenzen teilstationärer Arbeit. In *Kinderpsychiatrie: Vorschulalter*, ed. M. Döpfner and M. H. Schmidt, pp. 134–9. München: Quintessenz.

34

Home treatment

Helmut Remschmidt and Andreas Warnke

Definition and concept

Home treatment involves therapeutic work with children, adolescents and families in their own familiar environment. Treatment may be undertaken in a natural, foster or adoptive family, residential home or group, or other institution which cares for children and adolescents. The term 'home treatment' does not imply any specific therapeutic approach, but may include a variety of techniques combined in a treatment plan. In practice, behavioural therapy and parent training are the most frequently used methods in home treatment. It is possible, however, to utilize other treatment methods in certain circumstances, if there is a more appropriate method for the disorder, symptoms are not severe, and there is sufficient motivation and support present.

Home treatment is based on the following general principles.

(i) The place in which treatment is undertaken is the patient's usual environment. Both diagnostic assessment and therapy are undertaken in the patient's home.

(ii) Sessions are undertaken by one or more therapists who visit the patient regularly. These include specific interventions involving the patient and his parents.

(iii) The patient's parents or care-givers often act as co-therapists. It is therefore essential that they are well informed and receive appropriate support from the therapist.

(iv) The course and improvement of symptoms in the patient and his family will usually be empirically evaluated. Standardized tests, questionnaires and specific problem-orientated notes can be very helpful.

(v) The therapist should be available by telephone in his practice or institution at defined times in case of unexpected difficulties or crises.

The relationship between individuals involved in home treatment are shown in Fig. 34.1. The relationship is triangular, involving the professional therapist (psychiatrist, psychologist), the 'immediate therapist' or co-therapist (usually the patient's mother and/or father), and the patient himself. There is usually

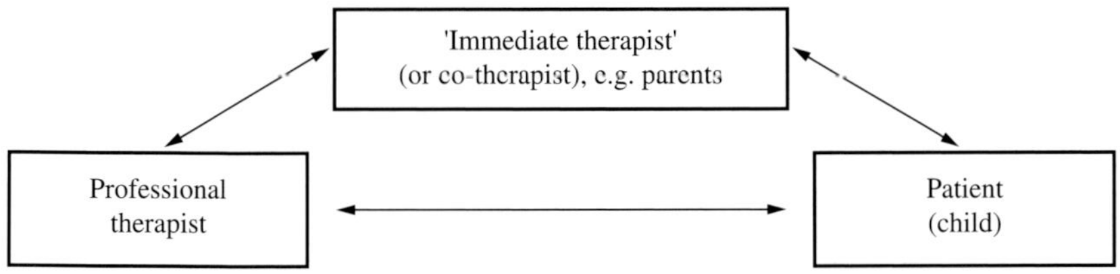

Fig. 34.1. The relationships between the individuals involved in home treatment.

first a discussion and agreement upon behavioural roles, followed by sessions of therapy and parent education. Feedback between the patient, therapist and co-therapists is essential because of the many steps involved in treatment, which range from understanding instructions to feeding back on the consequences for therapeutic interventions.

Home treatment has several *advantages* over other types of treatment if the technique is carefully targeted and appropriately applied. On the basis of these premises, it offers a realistic alternative to hospitalization or outpatient treatment (Reimer, 1983; Remschmidt and Schmidt, 1988).

(i) As treatment is undertaken in the patient's home, the therapist has the opportunity to observe the child's and family's situation much more closely. The therapist is able to gain a better understanding of the child's role in the family, the day-to-day workings of the family, and the degree to which the family is integrated within its social setting. This information can be difficult to obtain in outpatient or inpatient settings. The information often contributes significantly to the diagnostic process, and aids the therapist in selecting material to use in therapy.

(ii) Treatment is undertaken in the same setting in which the disorder arose. Thus the therapist has the opportunity of adapting treatment to the conditions at home. Parents are prevented from playing down issues, which often occurs with outpatient treatment or hospitalization. Thus, interventions are more likely to be realistic and appropriate.

(iii) Therapy is undertaken by two different types of therapists. First, the visiting professional psychotherapist, and secondly, the patient's parents or other care givers in their role as co-therapists. This approach has, of course, both advantages and disadvantages. The advantage is that those individuals most familiar with the child, who are affected most by the disorder and who have parental responsibility, are directly involved in treatment. Depending on their capability, however, they may be unable to maintain an appropriate 'therapeutic' distance to the patient, resulting in neglect of the child's own capabilities. This issue needs to be addressed when educating parents.

(iv) It has been suggested that involving parents in treatment of their own child allows them to take up responsibility for the improvements which occur, which encourages parents, improves their motivation as well as the relationship with the child (Gambrill, 1977). It is often easier to motivate parents for home-treatment than for hospitalization.

(v) Home treatment may contribute to prevention if it is commenced at an early stage. Thus the disorder is prevented from becoming severe or even chronic.

(vi) Finally, economical considerations may favour home treatment, being less expensive than hospitalization or day-hospital treatment, even having taken into account transport costs and the occasional need for additional personnel. Whilst the efficacy of home treatment has been demonstrated by studies (Reimer, 1983; Remschmidt and Schmidt, 1988), it is not covered by health insurance in many countries, including Germany. The home treatment programme reported here was undertaken as a research study (Remschmidt and Schmidt, 1988).

Indications and contraindications

Home treatment may be able to replace hospitalization or day-hospital treatment in certain cases, but is only likely to succeed if several specific external conditions are met (Eisert et al., 1985):

- at least one care-giver needs to be at home during certain predefined hours;
- a minimum family structure is required;
- sufficient space must be available for the therapist, such that he does not intrude too much in the family;
- the distance from the institution to the patient's home should not be too great (the therapist should not have to drive for longer than 30–40 minutes).

Treatment can only be undertaken with the parents' full cooperation. If the relationship between parents and child is too seriously impaired or if parents are unreliable, therapeutic interventions may not be possible in the therapist's absence.

Home treatment needs to be backed up by a larger institution with outpatient, day-hospital and inpatient facilities in order to make a switch from one treatment modality to another easier.

Home treatment is a realistic alternative to hospitalization or outpatient treatment if those requirements are met (Remschmidt and Schmidt, 1988; Remschmidt et al., 1988); however, only about 10–15% of patients typically presenting to a child and psychiatric university hospital meet these requirements.

Table 34.1. Approaches to home treatment

Method	Disorder or target behaviour
Behaviour therapy	Conduct disorders (aggressive outbursts, tantrums)
Parent training	Antisocial behaviour and delinquency
Informal support and family therapy	Hyperactive behaviour
Special educational support	Attention deficit
Support at school	Disorder of speech development
Parent education	Separation anxiety
Offering advice to parents	School anxiety
Drawing up contracts	Sibling rivalry
Role play	Enuresis
Programmed texts	Encopresis
Video feedback	Autistic behaviour

Table 34.1 shows several examples of therapeutic approaches useful in home treatment. In a study of 109 patients with a range of diagnoses, patients were randomly assigned to inpatient, day-patient or home treatment (Remschmidt and Schmidt, 1988; Remschmidt et al., 1988). The ICD-9 (WHO, 1978) diagnoses included: neuroses (300), anorexia nervosa (307.1), enuresis (307.6), encopresis (307.7), eating disorder (307.5), conduct disorder (312), conduct disorder with emotional disturbance (312.3), disturbance of emotions (313), emotional disorder with relationship problems (313.3), and hyperkinetic syndrome (314). The sample was highly selected and constituted 10–15% of patients who present to a child and psychiatric university hospital. Outcome was found to be generally good with conduct disorder, but also with more complex problems such as neurotic disorders or anorexia nervosa.

In this sample, home treatment was used to treat a much broader spectrum of disorders compared to reports in the literature (Remschmidt and Schmidt, 1988). Based on our experience, those patients suitable for home treatment may be characterized thus:

- symptoms too severe for outpatient treatment;
- admission for inpatient treatment regarded as in the absence of other facilities;
- partial hospitalization (day-hospital) or home treatment considered a realistic possibility;
- parents' cooperation is essential;
- manageable distance between the institution and the patient's home (not further than 20–30 km);
- absence of serious symptoms such as suicidality or threatening behaviour;

- younger children tend to cooperate better than adolescents and are therefore somewhat easier to manage;
- about 10–15% of patients who typically present to a child and psychiatric university hospital can be considered for home treatment.

Home treatment is contraindicated when hospitalization is required to treat a disorder appropriately or when other approaches to treatment are expected to show better outcome.

Approach to treatment

Although in theory almost any approach to treatment can be used for home treatment, only a few have been shown to be practicable, including behavioural therapy, parent training, family support and education, and in some cases family therapy (see Table 34.1).

Treatment steps

The following steps have been suggested when planning home treatment (Reimer, 1983).

Initial interview

This is undertaken by the therapist and may take two to three sessions. The aim is to obtain a comprehensive picture of the presenting problem, family situation and the relationship between the patient and other family members. It is usually necessary to speak with the child and his parents separately, especially to obtain a detailed history. It is often useful to ask both parents, and the child to describe and comment on the frequency of the symptoms.

A video recording of a session with the child and parents can be made, which can subsequently be reviewed and rated with standardized family diagnostic scales. This enables the therapist to obtain a better idea of the family dynamics and the role which the child's symptoms may be playing.

Physical examination and standardized psychological tests

Careful physical examination is just as important as performing standardized psychological tests, which should generally include assessment of general intelligence and personality traits. Additional assessment techniques may be used when appropriate, e.g. specific techniques to assess disturbance of body image and depression in anorexia nervosa, Matching-Familiar-Figures, Conners Scale in attention deficit hyperactivity disorder.

Behavioural observation in the family setting

A session of behavioural observation in the family context should be undertaken prior to initiating treatment. Informal observation in everyday situations, as well as observations of the child and parents in more structured situations, e.g. whilst playing a game or during the family Rorschach Test, may be valuable. These can also be video taped to enable informal and structured observation later.

Drawing up a treatment schedule

Before initiating therapy, a treatment schedule must be drawn up, if neccessary with the assisstance of a supervisor. This should be based on the information gathered and should contain the most important therapeutic goals as well as the steps required to reach this goal. The plan should be discussed with parents and the patient in an appropriate way, given the child's age and developmental stage. Therapeutic steps and the individual tasks should be discussed. The treatment schedule should also include the duration and structure of treatment, e.g. number of home visits, type and contingency of reinforcements.

Undertaking therapy

After the treatment schedule has been discussed, it is executed at home under the therapist's supervision. Parents should receive continued reinforcement about their role in therapy. They should also be asked to record the course of the symptoms appropriate to the nature of the disorder being treated. A minimum of at least one home visit per week should be undertaken by the therapist. He also needs to be available for telephone advice at predetermined times should problems arise.

Evaluation and follow-up

Treatment methods need to be evaluated, especially if they are relatively new, and therefore patients should be followed up. Ideally, evaluation should address outcome and the difficulties encountered during treatment (Table 34.2). Evaluation should be undertaken with appropriate standardized psychological tests and questionnaires in order to determine outcome and the course of the disorder objectively. General tests should be administered for all patients (regardless of the disorder), with additional specific diagnostic tests for the assessment of specific disorders. Tests may be completed by the therapist, patient, parents, care-givers or teachers, depending on the nature of the

Table 34.2. Psychological measures including standardized tests for evaluating the outcome of psychotherapy. The measures applied prior to treatment (pre), after treatment (post) and at follow-up

	Time	Rater
(a) General measures (suitable for all types of evaluation)		
(i) Personal data	Pre	Therapist
(ii) Symptom list	Pre / post / follow-up	Therapist
(iii) Checklist of psychosocial risks	Pre / post / follow-up	Therapist
(iv) Psychosocial competency	Goals pre / post	Therapist
(v) Clinical records	Pre / post	Therapist
(vi) Parent questionnaires, e.g. CBCL	Pre / post	Parents
(vii) Self-assessment scales	Post	Patient
(viii) Assessment of outcome	Post	Therapist
(ix) Parent satisfaction	Post	Parents
(x) Overall appraisal		Parents and teachers
(b) Specific measures (suitable for specific disorders)		
[in this example specific techniques for evaluating the hyperkinetic syndrome are listed]:		
(i) Matching Familiar Figures Test (pre / post)		
(ii) Attention assessment test (pre / post)		
(iii) Behaviour assessment scales for neurotic, emotional and conduct disorders (rated by care-givers pre / post)		
(iv) Conners-Scale (rated by teachers and parents pre / post)		
(v) Behaviour questionnaires (rated by teachers pre / post)		

problem, e.g. Matching Familiar Figures Test, Child Behaviour Check List, Conners Scale.

Principles of treatment and educational methods

Outcome depends largely on the extent to which parents and care-givers can grasp and cooperate with treatment techniques. The initial educative measures are of paramount importance. Several educational methods are shown in Table 34.1. Two basic principles are important:

(i) techniques and principles of treatment known to be effective, and
(ii) methods by which parents can be educated in these techniques.

Techniques and principles of treatment

Parents or other co-therapists should be fully informed of the principles by which treatment is undertaken and should be given the opportunity to practise these methods. Reimer (1983) has suggested the following behavioural methods for home treatment:

- positive reinforcement, e.g. material rewards, points on a behavioural schedule, social recognition or activities;
- appropriate punishment, usually by withdrawing privileges or recognition;
- differential reinforcement;
- making clear rules and expectations;
- communication training;
- role play;
- training exercises, e.g. attention or perception training.

Educational methods

The following educational methods have been used successfully to prepare parents for their role in treatment:

- modelling by the therapist in order to demonstrate the technique, after which parents are asked to practice the technique;
- video recordings of individuals who have participated in treatment in a similar case;
- feedback on parents' own video recordings made for their interaction with the child. This method helps to reinforce parental appropriate behaviour and correct any inappropriate behaviour without causing any unnecessary embarrassment to the parents.

Ways of organizing home treatment

The most important aspects of organizing home treatment have been explained above. Home treatment can generally be undertaken both by child and adolescent psychiatrists or psychotherapists in private practice and institutions. Until now, most has been undertaken as research by institutions. Therapists undertaking home treatment usually require the support of an institution, and competent colleagues and supervisors who can help with the complex issues which often arise during therapy. In many cases, diagnostic appraisal is neccessary in an institution with additional facilities, which is easier when the therapist is associated with such an institution.

Mobile home treatment services exist in some countries. One example is the mobile home treatment service which the Hospital for Child and Adolescent Psychiatry, University of Marburg (Germany) maintained for 10 years. The responsibilities of this unit included follow-up treatment of former inpatients, outpatient clinics in rural areas as well as home treatment (Remschmidt et al., 1986).

REFERENCES

Eisert, M., Eisert, H. G. and Schmidt, M. H. (1985). Hinweise zur Behandlung im häuslichen Milieu ('home-treatment'). *Zeitschrift für Kinder- und Jugendpsychiatrie*, **13**, 268–79.

Gambrill, E. D. (1977). *Behavior modification. Handbook of assessment, intervention and evaluation*. San Francisco: Jossey Bass.

Reimer, M. (1983). *Verhaltensänderung in der Familie. Home-treatment in der Kinderpsychiatrie*. Enke: Stuttgart.

Remschmidt, H. and Schmidt, M. H. (ed.) (1988). *Alternative Behandlungsformen in der Kinder- und Jugendpsychiatrie. Stationäre Behandlung, tagesklinische Behandlung und home-treatment im Vergleich*. Stuttgart: Enke.

Remschmidt, H., Walter, R. and Kampert, K. (1986). Der mobile kinder- und jugendpsychiatrische Dienst. Ein wirksames Versorgungsmodell für ländliche Regionen. *Zeitschrift für Kinder- und Jugendpsychiatrie*, **14**, 63–80.

Remschmidt, H., Schmidt, M. H., Mattejat, F., Eisert, H. G. and Eisert, M. (1988). Therapieevaluation in der Kinder- und Jugendpsychiatrie. Stationäre Behandlung, tagesklinische Behandlung und home-treatment im Vergleich. *Zeitschrift für Kinder- und Jugendpsychiatrie*, **16**, 124–34.

World Health Organization (WHO) (1978). *Mental disorders. Glossary and guide to their classification in accordance with the ninth revision of the classification of diseases*. Geneva: WHO.

Index

Numbers in italics indicate *tables* or *figures*